Breathing Disorders
Disorders
IN SLEEP

WALTER T MCNICHOLAS, MD, FRCPI, FRCPC
NEWMAN CLINICAL RESEARCH PROFESSOR,
CONWAY INSTITUTE FOR BIOMOLECULAR AND BIOMEDICAL RESEARCH,
UNIVERSITY COLLEGE DUBLIN AND
DIRECTOR, RESPIRATORY SLEEP DISORDERS UNIT,
ST. VINCENT'S UNIVERSITY HOSPITAL,
DUBLIN, IRELAND

ELIOT A PHILLIPSON, MD
CHAIR
DEPARTMENT OF MEDICINE, UNIVERSITY OF TORONTO,
TORONTO, ONTARIO, CANADA

SAUNDERS

LONDON EDINBURGH NEW YORK OXFORD PHILADELPHIA ST LOUIS SYDNEY TORONTO 2002

SAUNDERS
An imprint of Elsevier Science Limited

First published 2002
Reprinted 2003

ISBN 0 7020 2510 0

British Library Cataloguing in Publication Data
A catalogue record for this book is available from the British Library

Library of Congress Cataloging in Publication Data
A catalog record for this book is available from the Library of
Congress

Note
Medical knowledge is constantly changing. As new information
becomes available, changes in treatment, procedures, equipment and
the use of drugs become necessary. The editors/authors/contributors
and the publishers have taken care to ensure that the information
given in this text is accurate and up to date. However, readers are
strongly advised to confirm that the information, especially with
regard to drug usage, complies with the latest legislation and
standards of practice.

 ELSEVIER SCIENCE your source for books,
journals and multimedia
in the health sciences

www.elsevierhealth.com

The
publisher's
policy is to use
**paper manufactured
from sustainable forests**

Printed in China

TABLE OF CONTENTS

CONTENTS

PREFACE

Breathing disorders in sleep represent something of a paradox in clinical medicine. On the one hand, these disorders have been recognized only in recent decades and are still regarded as a niche interest by many clinicians, particularly those from clinical disciplines other than respiratory medicine, psychiatry, and otolaryngology. On the other hand, sleep-related breathing disorders such as the sleep apnea syndrome are now recognized as being very common. Indeed, current epidemiological data indicate that the sleep apnea syndrome is second only to asthma in the prevalence league table of chronic respiratory disorders. Furthermore, respiratory disorders such as chronic obstructive pulmonary disease can result in abnormalities of gas exchange during sleep that are even greater than those occurring during exercise or other forms of physiological stress.

These considerations clearly indicate that there is an ongoing need to educate physicians about breathing disorders during sleep, particularly since the prevalence of disorders such as sleep apnea is so high that the investigation and management of many patients involve clinicians outside specialized sleep centers.

The purpose of this book is to provide a broad overview of all aspects of breathing disorders during sleep, with each chapter written by a recognized expert in the field. The volume is intended to provide a comprehensive review of the topic but presented in such a fashion as to be of interest and value to the practicing clinician.

We are very grateful to the many experts who have contributed their time and expertise to producing the various chapters in this book. Most chapters include a number of boxes containing key points of information, which provide the core information contained within the chapter concerned. This feature is intended to allow the reader to gain quick access to the core information contained within the book.

Walter T McNicholas
Eliot A Phillipson
2001

CONTRIBUTORS

Sonia Ancoli-Israel, PhD
Professor of Psychiatry
Department of Psychiatry
University of California
San Diego
California
USA

T Douglas Bradley, MD
Toronto General Hospital
University Health Network
Toronto
Ontario
Canada

Dina Brooks, PhD, MSc, BSc (PT)
Research Associate
Department of Respiratory Medicine
West Park Healthcare Centre
Toronto
Ontario
Canada

Peter M A Calverley, FRCP, FRCPE
Professor of Medicine
Pulmonary and Rehabilitation Research Group
University Department of Medicine
University Hospital
Aintree
Liverpool
UK

Robert J O Davies, DM, FRCP
Senior Lecturer in Respiratory Medicine
Oxford Centre for Respiratory Medicine
Churchill Hospital
Oxford
UK

Lori Davis, BSc, RCPT (P), RPSGT
Manager
Sleep and Cardio-Pulmonary Diagnostic Laboratories
West Park Healthcare Centre
Toronto
Ontario
Canada

Jerome A Dempsey, PhD
Professor of Preventive Medicine, Physiology and
Kinesiology
Department of Preventive Medicine
University of Wisconsin-Madison
Madison
Wisconsin
USA

Neil J Douglas, MD, FRCP, FRCPE
Professor of Respiratory and Sleep Medicine
University of Edinburgh
Respiratory Medicine Unit, Department of Medicine
Royal Infirmary NHS Trust
Edinburgh
Scotland
UK

John A Fleetham, MB, BS, FRSP(C)
Professor of Medicine
Respiratory Division
Vancouver Hospital
Vancouver
British Columbia
Canada

W Ward Flemons, MD, FRCPC, FACP
Clinical Associate Professor of Medicine
University of Calgary
Foothills Hospital
Calgary
Alberta
Canada

Claude Gaultier, MD, PhD
Department of Physiology
Hôpital Robert Debré
Paris
France

Roger S Goldstein, MB, ChB, FRCP (UK), FRCP (C)
Professor of Medicine and Physical Therapy
University of Toronto
Sleep Laboratory and Cardio-Pulmonary Diagnostics
West Park Healthcare Centre
Toronto
Ontario
Canada

Ludger Grote, MD, PhD
Associate Professor of Medicine
Sleep Laboratory
Department of Pulmonary Medicine
Sahlgrenska University Hospital
Goteborg
Sweden

Ronald R Grunstein, MB, BS, MD, PhD, FRACP
Centre for Respiratory Failure and Sleep
Disorders
Royal Prince Alfred Hospital
Camperdown
Sydney
Australia

Christian Guilleminault, MD, Biol. D
Professor of Neurology
Stanford University Sleep Disorders Clinic
Palo Alto
California
USA

Jan Hedner, MD, PhD
Professor of Medicine
Sleep Laboratory
Department of Pulmonary Medicine
Sahlgrenska University Hospital
Goteborg
Sweden

Victor Hoffstein, MD, PhD, FRCPC
Professor of Medicine
University of Toronto
St Michael's Hospital
Toronto
Ontario
Canada

Jean Krieger, MD, PhD
Professor of Neurology
Clinique Neurologique
Hopitaux Universitaires de Strasbourg
Strasbourg
France

Patrick Lévy, MD, PhD, EFCR
Professor of Medicine
Sleep Laboratory
Grenoble University Hospital
Grenoble
France

Daniel I Loube, MD
Clinical Director
Sleep Medicine Institute
Swedish Medical Centre
Seattle
Washington
USA

Atul Malhotra, MD, FRCPC
Instructor in Medicine
Harvard Medical School
Department of Pulmonary and Critical Care
Medicine
Brigham and Women's Hospital and Massachusetts
General Hospital
Boston
Massachusetts
USA

Jennifer Martin
Joint Doctoral Program in Clinical Psychology
San Diego State University and University of
California, San Diego
San Diego
California
USA

Walter T McNicholas, MD, FRCPI, FRCPC
Newman Clinical Research Professor
Conway Institute for Biomolecular and Biomedical
Research
University College Dublin and
Director
Respiratory Sleep Disorders Unit
St. Vincent's University Hospital
Dublin
Ireland

Mary J Morrell, RGN, PhD
Lecturer in Sleep Physiology
Wellcome Trust Career Development Fellow
National Heart and Lung Institute
Imperial College of Science, Technology & Medicine
Royal Brompton Hospital
London
UK

Luciana Palombini, MD
Fellow
Stanford University Sleep Disorders Clinic
Palo Alto
California
USA

Jean-Louis Pépin
Assistant Professor
Sleep Laboratory
Grenoble University Hospital
Grenoble
France

Paul Peppard, PhD
Senior Scientist
Department of Preventive Medicine
University of Wisconsin-Madison
Madison
Wisconsin
USA

Eliot A Phillipson, MD
Chair
Department of Medicine
University of Toronto
Toronto, Ontario
Canada

Susan Redline, MD, MPH
Professor of Pediatrics
Cuse Western Reserve University
Rainbow Babies and Children's Hospital
Cleveland, Ohio
USA

Aaron E Sher, MD
Albany
New York
USA

Carl J Stepanowsky
Joint Doctoral Program in Clinical Psychology
San Diego State University and University of
California, San Diego
San Diego
California
USA

John R Stradling, MD, FRCP
Professor of Respiratory Medicine
Oxford Centre for Respiratory Medicine
Churchill Hospital
Oxford
UK

Kingman P Strohl, MD
Professor of Medicine
Case Western Reserve University
Director, Centre for Sleep Disorders Research
Louis Stokes VA Medical Center
Cleveland
Ohio
USA

William A WhiteLaw, MD, PhD, FRCPC
Professor of Medicine
University of Calgary
Foothills Hospital
Calgary
Alberta
Canada

David P White, MD, PhD
Associate Professor
Harvard Medical School
Sleep Disorders Program
Brigham and Women's Hospital
Boston
Massachusetts
USA

Terry B Young, PhD
Professor of Preventive Medicine
Department of Preventive Medicine
University of Wisconsin-Madison
Madison
Wisconsin
USA

GLOSSARY

(Plus chapter where first mentioned)
Apnea index (AI) (6)
Apnea-hypopnea index (AHI) (3)
Body mass index (BMI) (3)
Calgary Sleep Apnea Quality of Life Index (SAQLI) (5)
Central sleep apnea (CSA) (10)
Clinical prediction rules (5)
Critical pressure (6)
Epworth Sleepiness Scale (ESS) (2)
Esophageal pressure manometry (6)
Genioglossal advancement (GA) (9)
Hyoid myotomy and suspension (HM-1, HM-2) (9)
Hypocapnic apneic threshold (1)
Karolinska Sleepiness Scale (KSS) (2)
Laser assisted uvulopalatoplasty (LAUP) (9)
Laser midline glossectomy (LMG) (9)
Likelihood ratio (LR) (5)
Maintenance of Wakefulness test (MWT) (2)
Mallampati score (6)
Mandibular advancement (MA) (9)
Maxillofacial advancement osteotomy (MMO) (7)
Maxillomandibular advancement (MMA) (9)
Mean sleep latency (MSL) (2)
Multiple sleep latency test (MSLT) (2)
Nasal pressure transduction (or transducers) (6)
Negative intermittent positive pressure ventilation (NIPPV) (17)
Negative predictive value (5)
Non–rapid eye movement sleep (NREM) (1)
Obstructive sleep apnea syndrome (OSAS) (2)
Oral Appliance (OA)(11)
OSLER test (2)
Performance Vigilance Test (6)
Polysomnography (PSG) (6)
Positive predictive value (5)
Quality of life index (5)
Radiofrequency tongue base ablation (RFTBA) (9)
Rapid eye movement sleep (REM) (1)
Respiratory disturbance index (RDI) (5)
Respiratory effort related arousal (RERA) (6)
Respiratory inductance plethysmography (6)
Sensitivity (5)
SF-36 (5)

Sickness Impact Profile (5)
Slow wave sleep (10)
Specificity (5)
Stanford Sleepiness Scale (SSS) (2)
Tongue base reduction with hyoepiglottoplasty (TBRHE) (9)
Tongue-retaining devices (TRD) (11)
Transpalatal advancement pharyngoplasty (TPAP) (9)
Upper airway resistance syndrome (UARS) (2)
Uvulopalatopharyngoglossoplasty (UPPGP) (9)
Uvulopalatopharyngoplasty (UPPP) (7)
Velopharyngeal insufficiency (VPI) (9)

PART ONE
INTRODUCTION

1 IMPACT OF SLEEP ON VENTILATION

Mary J Morrell and Jerome A Dempsey

INTRODUCTION

The design of the central and peripheral elements of the nervous system is near ideal for purposes of controlling breathing. In an awake human at rest or during exercise this nearly perfectly engineered system ensures that each breath is produced with a minimum energy cost to the respiratory muscles and with a precise regulation of CO_2 and O_2 levels in arterial blood. If this precision is disrupted, for example by a sigh, changes in posture, prolonged expiration (as occurs with vocalization), swallowing, changes in airway caliber, or exercise, departure from normal or adequate ventilation is only momentary. In the vast majority of cases the control system is able to adjust within a matter of seconds and homeostasis and efficiency are restored.

Vigilance and high gain of chemical and mechanical sensory feedback are absolutely essential characteristics to ensure the fast, efficient regulation of breathing. Another key mechanism is the uniformity of distribution of efferent motor output (tonic and phasic) to the 'respiratory' musculature of the upper airway and to the thoracic pump. This uniformity means that during each breath the upper airway is stiffened, thus preventing narrowing in response to the generation of subatmospheric intrapleural pressure. Similarly, the activation of the intercostal musculature serves to stiffen the ribcage and thereby prevent any inefficient, inward motion of the ribcage while the diaphragm descends during inspiration.

During sleep many of the characteristics of the ventilatory control system are lost or greatly compromised. Thus, in an otherwise healthy human, sleep may unmask serious problems in both the efficiency and precision of ventilatory control. For example, 1) significant hypoventilation and a sustained respiratory acidosis are a normal response to sleep in health, whereas CO_2 retention of any magnitude is rarely tolerated during wakefulness; 2) airway resistance can be increased 3 to 4 times in sleep; 3) reflex effects, which normally protect airway patency or augment ventilatory drive to maintain ventilation in the face of increased mechanical loads, are lost or greatly suppressed in sleep; and 4) during sleep, cessation of breathing (apnea) occurs in response to small reductions in arterial P_{CO_2} ($PaCO_2$), leading to instabilities in ventilation. These fundamental effects of sleep on ventilatory control are manifested, in part, in the significant levels of sleep-disordered breathing (i.e., > 5 apneas or hypopneas per hour of sleep) in 4 to 9% of a normal (nonclinical) population between the ages of 30 to 60 years (1). These effects are also evident in the periodic breathing patterns that persist during sleep in the presence of environmental hypoxia in the healthy person (2) or in the patient with chronic heart failure (3). This chapter characterizes and attempts to explain some of these fundamental effects of sleep on ventilatory control in the human.

FUNDAMENTAL EFFECTS OF SLEEP ON THE VENTILATORY CONTROL SYSTEM

There are few unanesthetized animal models currently available in which chronic recordings can be made from medullary neurons in (and out of) phase with respiration, during both wakefulness and sleep (4). These valuable data, along with the relatively impure electromyogram (EMG) data in humans, have shown us that 'wakefulness' does indeed make a significant input to the total respiratory motor output; both pump and upper airway muscles. Medullary inspiratory cells show a reduction in their phasic electrical activity at the onset of non–rapid eye movement (NREM) sleep (4). These basic central neural effects of sleep on phrenic and hypoglossal nerve activity, along with secondary mechanical influences on the extrathoracic airway and chest wall, explain many of the sleep-related ventilatory changes outlined below.

SLEEP-RELATED CHANGES IN RESPONSES TO CHEMORECEPTOR FEEDBACK
NREM Sleep Decreases the Response to Chemical Stimuli

The slopes of the ventilatory responses to exogenous hypercapnia and hypoxia are reduced by 10–50% in NREM sleep. There are multiple causes of this reduced chemoresponsiveness, namely: 1) the loss of the 'wakefulness' input from suprapontine regions to the medullary respiratory controller diminishes the increase in respiratory motor output in response to chemoreceptor input, i.e., chemoreceptor resetting; 2) sleep-induced increases in upper airway resistance (R_{UA}) mean that the ventilatory response is diminished for any given increase in phrenic nerve activity or central respiratory motor output; and 3) the increase in cerebral blood flow in sleep means that the cerebrofluid partial pressure of carbon dioxide (P_{CO_2}) and concentration of hydrogen ions in the vicinity of the medullary chemoreceptors is reduced relative to $PaCO_2$. Therefore, the magnitude of the central CO_2 stimulus (in the true stimulus versus response curve) is actually less than that represented in the measured alveolar CO_2 ($PACO_2$) versus ventilatory response slope (5). The implication of these three factors during normal (air breathing) conditions is that, in sleep, CO_2 retention would occur in proportion to the change in chemoreceptor set point and to increasing airway resistance. In addition, the ventilatory responses to any degree of endogenous CO_2 retention or hypoxia (such as those after an apnea or hypopnea) would be reduced. Of course, many of these secondary ventilatory responses also promote transient arousals from sleep that enhance the ventilatory responsiveness, possibly to a level in excess of that in steady state wakefulness. Therefore, the ability to respond to and correct the chemical stimuli associated with transient underventilations in sleep also depends to a significant extent on how 'arousable' we are in response to chemoreceptor stimuli.

Hypocapnic Apneic Threshold

Ventilation can be increased via chemostimulation (e.g., with brief hypoxic exposure). When this occurs, withdrawal of the hypoxic stimulus results in ventilation remaining high and only slowly (> 1 min) returning to pre-stimulus control levels. This centrally mediated memory-like excitatory mechanism has been labeled short-term potentiation (6). This mechanism is obviously very important in maintaining stable breathing patterns (i.e., in preventing apnea after transient ventilatory overshoots, such as those associated with arousals). However, when a brief hypoxic stimulus is applied during NREM sleep and $PaCO_2$ is allowed to fall normally as ventilation increases, hypopnea or apnea occurs upon withdrawal of the excitatory stimulus. These findings suggest that hypocapnia, especially when it occurs during sleep, opposes this 'protective' stabilizing short-term potentiation mechanism.

Another experimental approach used to perturb breathing and CO_2 is mechanical ventilation. Using this technique to gradually reduce $PaCO_2$ during NREM sleep, it has been shown that apnea occurs when the $PaCO_2$ is decreased about 2–4 mm Hg below eupneic values, or roughly to the waking $PaCO_2$ level. In contrast, during wakefulness mechanical ventilator–induced hypocapnia may promote increases or decreases in respiratory motor output, reflecting behavioral inputs to ventilatory control associated with wakefulness. Thus, NREM sleep (or removal of the vigilance attending the waking state) unmasks a highly sensitive hypocapnea-dependent apneic threshold. In turn, this means that the reduced $PaCO_2$ accompanying any ventilatory overshoot overrides the excitatory short-term potentiation mechanism. Therefore apnea and instability in breathing pattern are promoted in sleep (Fig. 1.1A).

The importance of hypocapnia as a cause of breathing instability in sleep is further shown in periodic breathing during sleep in the hypoxic environment of high altitudes (2) or in idiopathic central sleep apnea syndrome (7), during which supplementing inspired CO_2 completely removes all central apneas and periodicities.

To recap, reductions in P_{CO_2} during sleep, secondary to transient ventilatory stimuli such as hypoxemia, cortical arousal, or changes in R_{UA} are probably a major cause of central hypopneas and apneas in sleep. Furthermore, not only does hypocapnia cause a reduction in phrenic nerve activity, it also reduces hypoglossal motor output to the muscles of the upper airway and, in persons with an already highly collapsible upper airway (e.g., snorers), will cause airway closure (8). Therefore, in many people, transient hypocapnia is likely to be a major cause of central

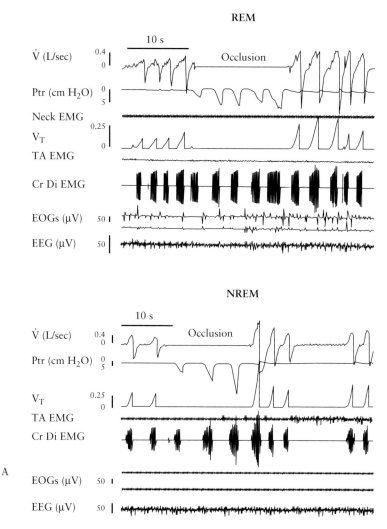

Fig 1.1 A, *Effects of REM and NREM sleep on respiratory motor output during and following an obstructive airway event. In REM, crural diaphragm (CrDi EMG) and inspiratory tracheal pressure (Ptr) are augmented during the occlusion but not in a systematic, progressive manner, in that the ventilatory overshoot (V) is smaller and no central apnea ensues compared to NREM. Note in NREM sleep the progressive increase in CrDi EMG and reduction in Ptr during occlusion, the ventilatory overshoot upon termination of the occlusion and the subsequent central apnea. V*T*, tidal volume; TA, transversus abdominis; EOG, electro-oculogram; EEG, electroencephalogram. Recordings were obtained during tracheal occlusion in a tracheostomized, sleeping dog. (From Xi L, Chin Moi Chow, Smith CA, Dempsey JA. Effects of REM sleep on the ventilatory response to airway occlusion in the dog. Sleep 1994; 17:674–687.) **B,** Disruption or 'fractionation' of diaphragm EMG (Di EMG) and its mechanical consequences on pressure generation and tidal volume during phasic REM sleep in the dog. Note disruptive effects of eye movements (EOG) on the ramp of diaphragm EMG activity, tracheal pressure, air flow and V*T* during eupneic breathing (left panel) and similar fractionation effects during airway occlusion (right panel). Contrast these effects in REM with the smooth ramp of Di EMG and tracheal pressure generation during inspiration in NREM sleep. (From Smith CA, Henderson KS, Xi L, et al. Neural-mechanical coupling of breathing in REM sleep. J Appl Physiol 1997; 83:1923–1932.)*

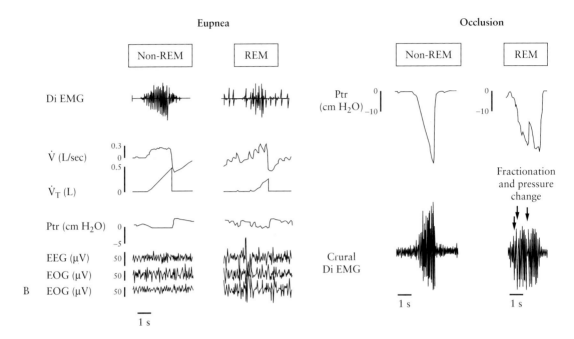

Fig 1.1B

apnea and may also contribute to the occurrence of obstructive apneas and hypopneas during sleep.

SLEEP-RELATED CHANGES IN COMPENSATION FOR MECHANICAL LOADS AND UPPER AIRWAY REFLEXES

Applying a mechanical load in wakefulness results in a highly variable ventilatory response within and between subjects (9). In the majority of cases, tidal volume and minute ventilation are maintained by an immediate prolongation of inspiratory time and an increase in the amount of inspiratory muscle activity (9–13). During sleep, any strategy adopted by the ventilatory control system must take into account the hypotonic state of the pharyngeal muscles, which makes the airway more compliant (15). Typically, application of a ventilatory load during sleep results in a significant fall in tidal volume and minute ventilation (9–13, 15). The sleep-related loss of immediate load compensation suggests that this compensatory mechanism is dependent upon consciousness, loss of which may act directly on the respiratory control system or via an influence on mechanoreceptors and reflex mechanisms (see below).

Application of mechanical loads for prolonged periods of time (41–50 breaths) during NREM sleep results in a progressive increase of respiratory effort plus a prolongation of inspiratory time, causing a return in ventilation toward pre-loaded levels (9, 11, 13, 14). The compensation to a sustained load is likely to be mediated by a rise in $PaCO_2$ coupled with a small fall in PaO_2 (16). The fact that a number of studies have found no increase in expired CO_2 with loading (13, 14) is not surprising since only minimal levels of hypercapnia (1–2 mm Hg) are required to produce a significant augmentation of respiratory drive, and changes of this magnitude are usually within the margin of error of most measurement systems.

The importance of chemostimulation on ventilatory load compensation during NREM sleep is illustrated by the study of Wilson and colleagues (9). These investigators applied a ventilatory load to people breathing a hyperoxic gas mixture. Under these conditions the return of ventilation toward pre-load levels was delayed for several breaths. Furthermore, removal of the load caused ventilation to fall to pre-load levels, whereas removal during normoxia resulted in hyperpnea (9).

An important 'dual' reflex effect for maintenance of upper airway patency occurs in response to imposition of a collapsing pressure to the upper airway (17). The deformation of the upper airway via negative pressure (1) augments hypoglossal nerve activity and EMG activity of genioglossus muscles, so that the airway is stiffened and resists collapse and (2) reduces central respiratory motor output, possibly causing apnea, which means that negative intrathoracic pressure or collapsing pressure is diminished and the airway is less likely to narrow or close. This important protective reflex has been demonstrated by exposing the isolated upper airway to square waves of negative pressure sufficient to initiate airway collapse. It has also been shown by application of a ramp of negative pressure, as would normally be experienced during inspiration (18), and by oscillating pressures of very low magnitude at high frequency (> 30 Hz; (19)), as might be experienced by a snorer. It is likely that these reflex mechanisms are critical to preventing airway collapse in many snorers during sleep; and they may also explain many prolongations of inspiratory or expiratory times in sleep.

A special case which may involve the reflex effects explained above is central apnea. During these events intrathoracic pressure does not become more negative; however, narrowing and even collapse of the upper airway have been shown to occur (20). Presumably the collapse and deformation of the upper airway would reflexively inhibit phrenic nerve activity and prolong the central apnea.

Protective reflex mechanisms have been shown to be present, although reduced in gain during NREM sleep (21, 22). However, in REM sleep it is not possible to activate the muscles of the upper airway in response to negative pressure, even when the airway is narrowed to the point of collapse (22). Certainly the underlying postural muscle atonia of REM sleep, together with this failure of reflex activated mechanisms in the upper airway, could explain the increased prevalence of airway obstruction and sleep-disordered breathing in REM sleep (see below).

ADDITIONAL INFLUENCES OF SLEEP AFFECTING VENTILATORY CONTROL

In addition to the sleep-related changes in neurophysiology, which in turn influence central respiratory motor output, there are other factors that could also perturb breathing during sleep. For example, sympathetic efferent vasoconstrictor activity is reduced with the onset of NREM sleep, and this change coincides with a reduction in systemic blood pressure. This reduced efferent sympathetic output may cause vasodilatation and vascular engorgement in the upper airway, leading to airway narrowing and increased R_{UA}. Thus, significant reductions in R_{UA} have been observed with local topical application of vasoconstrictor substances to the upper airway during sleep in snorers (23).

Assuming a horizontal position in sleep also means that functional residual capacity (FRC) will be reduced, which has two implications. First, the reduction in FRC will produce a lower oxygen 'reservoir' and thus, for any given apneic length, greater O_2 desaturation would be expected. In addition, the lower FRC will also mean less caudal traction on the trachea and a greater probability of increased and unstable R_{UA} (24, 25).

☞ Key points box 1.1

During sleep the normal regulatory mechanisms adopted by the ventilatory control system to maintain blood gas homeostasis in wakefulness are compromised.

- The loss of wakefulness reduces neural input from suprapontine areas to medullary respiratory neurons, thereby producing a fall in phrenic and hypoglossal activity.
- The responses to hypercapnia and hypoxia are reduced and a sensitive hypocapnic apneic threshold is unmasked.
- Immediately ventilatory compensation to mechanical respiratory loads is lost and there are sleep-related reductions in some upper airway protective reflexes; accordingly, upper airway patency and maintenance of normal waking $PaCO_2$ are jeopardized.

SLEEP-RELATED CHANGES IN VENTILATION

HOW DO CHANGES IN VENTILATORY CONTROL INFLUENCE THE LEVEL OF BREATHING DURING SLEEP?

In healthy humans, the shift from wakefulness to NREM sleep is associated with predictable changes in ventilation and blood gases, although the magnitude may vary.

Ventilation is Decreased

By the beginning of the twentieth century, it had already been noted that ventilation decreases during sleep (26). In 1963, Bulow published his comprehensive work characterizing spontaneous ventilation and respiratory responses to hypercapnia and hypoxia during different sleep states. Bulow's work, plus that of others, demonstrated that minute ventilation ($\dot{V}_I$) is reduced by between 0.4 and 0.9 L/min (6–11%) during NREM stage II sleep, and by 0.61 L/min (8%) during stage IV sleep, compared to wakefulness (27–30). REM sleep is also associated with a reduction in $\dot{V}_I$ from between 0.3 and 1.6 L/min (5–15%), compared to wakefulness (29, 31, 32). It has been argued the actual sleep-related decrement in ventilation has been overestimated. The contention is that accurately measuring breathing in relaxed awake subjects is difficult because ventilation may be stimulated, either by the emotional stress associated with the experimental protocol or by efferent feedback in response to the facemasks or nose clips. Nevertheless, when breathing was measured during wakefulness and sleep, in a carefully controlled environment using noninvasive techniques $\dot{V}_I$ still fell significantly during stage IV sleep (0.6 L/min; 10%) and REM sleep (0.9 L/min; 14%) compared to wakefulness (33).

PaCO$_2$ is Increased and PaO$_2$ is Decreased

The sleep-related reduction in $\dot{V}_I$ is associated with increases in alvelolar and arterial CO_2 of between 2 and 6.5 mm Hg (for review see Phillipson and Bowes [34]). To produce an increase in $PaCO_2$, alveolar ventilation must be reduced more than CO_2 production ($\dot{V}co_2$). During NREM sleep, both oxygen consumption ($\dot{V}o_2$) and $\dot{V}co_2$ are decreased compared to wakefulness ($\dot{V}o_2$: decrease 19.4 ml/min, 8.5%; $\dot{V}co_2$: decrease 23.9 ml/min, 12.3% [30]). The decrease in metabolism occurs in the first hour of sleep, and the magnitude of the decrease is similar during all stages of NREM and REM sleep (30, 35). A small but significant sleep-related reduction in arterial oxygen saturation also occurs during both NREM (stage IV sleep: SaO_2 96.5%) and REM sleep (SaO_2 96.2%), compared to wakefulness (SaO_2 97.3%) (33).

Breathing is Exceedingly Regular

In the deepest stages of sleep, breathing is exceedingly regular; tidal volume is reduced by approximately 12% compared to wakefulness, and respiratory frequency is either increased slightly or unchanged (26, 28, 29, 33,). In contrast, breathing during light sleep (stage I–II) is irregular (26). This variability, which occurs in both $\dot{V}_I$ and tidal volume, has been shown to be significantly correlated with electroencephalogram (EEG) frequency in elderly (36) and younger people (37). In situations in which sleep stage is fragmented with frequent transient arousals, such as in people with sleep-related periodic limb movements, ventilation becomes unstable. Thus, there is a positive feedback system with sleep fragmentation affecting ventilation and, in turn, changes in ventilation causing sleep state instability.

SLEEP-RELATED CHANGES IN UPPER AIRWAY RESISTANCE AND CALIBER

HOW DOES MODULATION OF EFFERENT ACTIVITY TO RESPIRATORY MUSCLES AFFECT THE UPPER AIRWAY?

R_{UA} increases during sleep, in part due to a reduction in neuronal drive to the upper airway muscles which is greater than that to the respiratory pump muscles (for review see Horner [38]). The size of the increase in R_{UA} varies depending on the individual subject and the sleep stage. In early studies, inspiratory R_{UA} increases of between 49 and 64% were recorded during stable NREM sleep (32, 39). However, subsequent work has revealed that the increases are not uniform among subjects; young non-obese persons who do not snore experience a relatively small sleep-related increase in total pulmonary resistance of 2.6 cm H_2O/L/s (40), whereas in people who snore the increase can be 20 times greater (increase in total pulmonary resistance, 9.3–70 cm H_2O/L/s; (39, 41). However, it is worth noting that at high resistances, when the pressure versus flow relationship is nonlinear (i.e., under conditions of flow limitation), relating theoretical measurements of resistance to the airway caliber can be problematic, owing to nonlaminar flow. In addition, resistance values vary depending on the point on the pressure-flow curve at which the values are calculated (e.g., fixed flow, peak pressure) (Fig 1.2) (42).

Upper airway caliber has been measured during sleep using direct imaging. These techniques have shown that the size of the pharyngeal airway lumen is reduced during sleep (43). Furthermore, dynamic imaging techniques have revealed a typical pattern of inspiratory and expiratory narrowing during NREM sleep in normal subjects,

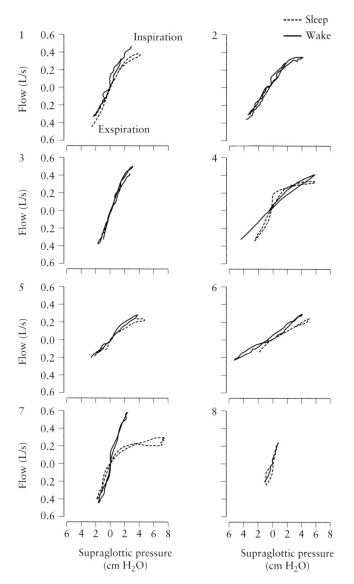

Fig 1.2 *Flow versus supraglottic pressure plots during wakefulness and sleep in six subjects with variable sleep-related changes in pharyngeal resistance. Note that in some subjects (7, 4) a single point estimate of upper airway resistance will vary according to the position of the measurement on the resistance curve. (From Badr MS, Kawak A, Skatrud JB, et al. Effect of induced hypercapnic hypopnea on upper airway patency in humans during NREM sleep. Respir Physiol 1997; 110:33–45).*

which is exacerbated in people who snore or who have a mild degree of sleep-disordered breathing (Fig 1.3A–D). During inspiration the airway lumen narrows substantial-

ly. At the transition between inspiration and expiration it then 'pops' open again, followed by a progressive narrowing during the middle to late expiratory period (44).

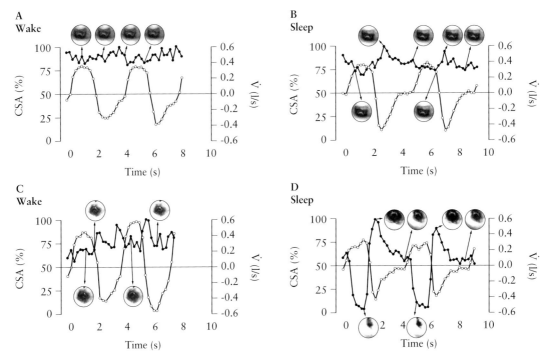

Fig 1.3 *Fiberoptic images of the retropalatal cross-sectional area (CSA) during different phases of the breathing cycle. Data show CSA (filled circles) and respiratory airflow ($\dot{V}$; open circles) in a normal healthy subject (A and B) and in a subject with mild sleep-disordered breathing (C and D) during wakefulness (A and C) and sleep (B and D). CSA is expressed as a percentage of the maximum CSA that occurred during the two breaths shown. (From Morrell MJ, Badr MS. Effects of NREM sleep on dynamic within-breath changes in upper airway patency in humans. J Appl Physiol 1998; 84:190–199).*

⊶ Key points box 1.2

Sleep-related changes in ventilatory control produce predictable alterations in ventilation and respiratory mechanics.

- Minute ventilation falls, $PaCO_2$ increases, and PaO_2 decreases.
- Breathing is very regular during stable sleep and irregular during light or fragmented sleep.
- Upper airway caliber is reduced, leading to an increase in upper airway resistance to airflow.
- Arousal from sleep stimulates ventilation and can lead to perpetuation of unstable breathing and sleep patterns.

WHAT CAUSES THE NORMAL SLEEP-INDUCED ALVEOLAR HYPOVENTILATION?

The dominant influence accounting for the normal hypoventilation accompanying sleep in normal subjects is the loss of significant neural input from supramedullary neurons to the medullary respiratory controller. In turn, this neural loss reduces respiratory motor output to 1) the thoracic pump muscles and 2) the muscles regulating the caliber of the upper airway, thereby leading to an increase in R_{UA}.

ROLE OF A SLEEP-RELATED REDUCTION IN THORACIC PUMP MUSCLE ACTIVITY

NREM sleep has a significant effect on respiratory motor output to the pump muscles, which contributes to the hypoventilation in all normal human subjects. Experimental evidence for this effect by itself (i.e., independent of changes in R_{UA}) is shown by 1) the hypoventilation that accompanies sleep in tracheostomized humans (45); 2) the very small sleep-related changes in R_{UA} in many healthy people; and 3) the lack of effect of nasal continuous positive airway pressure (CPAP) on ventilation in these healthy people with small increases in R_{UA} (40).

Another experimental approach to this question in humans has been the use of positive pressure mechanical ventilation. This intervention allows the investigator to hold constant any sleep-induced mechanical influences that may be secondary to increases in R_{UA} or chest wall compliance. Studies using this technique have shown that at any given PaCO$_2$ the inspiratory neural output is significantly reduced (below wakefulness) in NREM sleep (46). In other words, the set point of chemoresponsiveness is increased in NREM sleep, presumably because of reduced input from suprapontine areas to the medullary controller. A caveat to this interpretation is that sleep-induced increases in cerebral blood flow may also account for some of this reduced inspiratory motor output by reducing brain PCO$_2$ (relative to PaCO$_2$) and therefore central chemoreceptor input ((47); see above).

ROLE OF A SLEEP-RELATED INCREASE IN UPPER AIRWAY RESISTANCE

There is also evidence in support of the sleep-induced increase in R_{UA} as a cause of alveolar hypoventilation, at least in subjects who experience a doubling of R_{UA} in sleep. First, in NREM sleep, alveolar ventilation decreases in the face of increases in EMG activities of the diaphragm, intercostal muscles, and even accessory inspiratory muscles (scalenus) and abdominal expiratory muscles (16, 31, 48). Second, in people with large sleep-related increases in R_{UA}, when resistance was reduced using CPAP (41) or helium (49), within a few breaths ventilation increased, PCO$_2$ fell, and accessory plus diaphragm EMGs were markedly reduced.

The above experimental evidence has largely been collected during steady state conditions. However, an increased R_{UA} has also been shown to occur at sleep onset (i.e., during alpha to theta transitions) (50) (Fig. 1.4AB). These dynamic changes in R_{UA} occur coincident with the sleep-related sudden drop in ventilation but interestingly account

for only about 30–40% of the associated variation in ventilation within and across subjects (51, 52).

An overall view

Given the available evidence in humans, together with that in chronically instrumented animals, it can be concluded that sleep-induced alveolar hypoventilation in all humans is influenced to a significant extent by a loss of respiratory motor output to the thoracic pump muscles. In addition, many subjects experience at least a doubling of R_{UA} in sleep, and this added mechanical load also contributes to the alveolar hypoventilation, despite augmented respiratory muscle activity observed in NREM sleep.

☞ Key points box 1.3

Sleep-related alveolar hypoventilation can be produced by a number of factors; the relative importance of each factor may vary across individuals.

- In people who have only a small sleep-related increase in upper airway resistance, hypoventilation is due to a fall in thoracic pump muscle activity.
- In snorers sleep-related increases in upper airway resistance contribute to the hypoventilation.

WHAT ARE THE SPECIAL EFFECTS OF REM SLEEP ON VENTILATION?

Two major phenomena occur in REM sleep, presumably due in part to activation of the pontine reticular activation system, namely 1) posture muscle atonia, including muscles of the upper airway and ribcage, via active inhibition of motor neurons and 2) widespread flurries of activity (or 'phasic' events), which occur throughout the cortex and brainstem and are reflected in rapid eye movements (53). The effect on ventilatory control is profound. In all people, breathing frequencing generally increase and tidal volume falls, especially when REM events occur (i.e., so-called 'phasic REM'). Breath-to-breath variability is marked in both frequen-

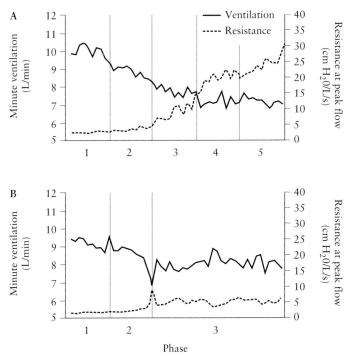

Fig 1.4 *Resistance calculated at peak inspiratory airflow (dashed lines) and ventilation (solid line) during the progression though sleep (x-axis, 5 'standardized' phases). A shows subjects who achieved slow wave sleep (n = 8); B shows subjects who did not (n = 5). (From Kay A, Trinder J, Kim Y. Progressive changes in airway resistances during sleep. J Appl Physiol 1996; 81:282 289.)*

cy and tidal volume; abdominal motion exceeds that of the ribcage because of the dominance of diaphragm over intercostal muscle activity; and upper airway compliance increases and the airway becomes more susceptible to closure via negative pressure. The ventilatory response to CO_2 or hypoxia becomes generally blunted, but the major change in these responses is the marked disorganization and the unpredictable ventilation from breath to breath.

CONSEQUENCES OF REM SLEEP ON VENTILATION

The enhanced variability of ventilatory control in REM can be observed during obstructive apneas (Fig. 1.1A,B). In NREM sleep, the rising chemical stimuli cause a progressive cycle-by-cycle increase in diaphragmatic EMG and decrease in pleural pressure during the obstruction, with a substantial ventilatory overshoot upon termination of the apnea and opening of the airway. However,

in phasic REM sleep there is evidence that the respiratory motor output does respond to increased chemical stimuli but that this occurs only when the chemical stimuli are very high (toward the end of the apnea); the increasing respiratory motor output is not systematic and progressive over the length of the apnea, as it is in NREM sleep. Note also in Figure 1.1A that the ventilatory overshoot upon termination of the obstruction is reduced in REM (versus NREM), and no central apnea occurs.

There are at least three reasons for the blunted and erratic response to chemical stimuli in REM. First, the postural muscle atonia of REM might increase chest wall compliance and cause its distortion during inspiratory efforts, thereby compromising neural-mechanical coupling in REM, so that a given inspiratory neural output produces less mechanical change in terms of pressure and flow rate. Certainly this chest wall distortion must play some role in diminishing ventilatory chemoresponsiveness in REM. However, the second and principal reason for this reduced ventilatory (and pressure) output is that REM phasic events interfere with the magnitude of medullary neural respiratory motor output in response to a rising chemoreceptor sensory input. Thus, the erratic and mostly reduced inspiratory pressure or tidal volume responses during and after airway obstruction in REM (versus NREM) coincide with erratic and generally diminished responses of the diaphragm EMG signal (54) (Fig 1.1A). In turn, the reduced amplitude of the diaphragm EMG occurs because inspiration is terminated early, coincident with the occurrence of REM activity. This 'interference' of REM events probably originates in the pons and has its impact at the level of the medullary and respiratory neuronal network.

A third influence of phasic REM events on neural respiratory motor output is the interruption or 'fractionation' of the ramp of diaphragmatic EMG activity during inspiration. Examples of this fractionation effect on the EMG of the diaphragm are shown during eupnea and during airway occlusion in REM in Figure 1.1B. Note the smooth ramp of diaphragmatic EMG and tracheal pressure during NREM as opposed to the interrupted diaphragmatic EMG with increased frequency of eye movements during REM. These fractionations have marked effects on mechanical output in the form of tracheal pressure and flow rate and the resulting tidal volume. In addition to reducing the magnitude of the diaphragmatic EMG and pressure responses during airway occlusion in REM sleep, the fractionations may mean that sensory input from the chest wall leading to cortical arousal is also reduced in REM. Perhaps this explains in part why occlusive apneas are much longer in REM than in NREM sleep, before a lightening of sleep state or arousal occurs to end the apneic period (55).

The above discussion emphasizes the inhibitory effects of REM events on the magnitude of respiratory motor and therefore ventilatory output. However, the phasic events of REM may also be excitatory and thereby prevent hypocapnia-induced central apnea. Firstly, the reduced chemoresponsiveness to the asphyxia of airway occlusion (see Fig 1.1A) means that the subsequent post apnea overshoot of ventilation is blunted in REM. The blunting of the overshoot lessens the probability of sufficient hypocapnia being produced in the postocclusion period in REM to cause a subsequent apnea or hypopnea. In addition, even for a given

level of hypocapnia in REM, inspiratory efforts occur coincident with eye movements and prolongation of expiratory time is prevented. Thus hypocapnia-induced apnea, which occurs even with very small reductions in $PaCO_2$ in NREM, is much harder to elicit in REM sleep (56). This apparent 'excitatory' effect of REM on respiratory rhythm explains why periodic breathing and central apneas occur so very rarely in REM sleep in such conditions as chronic heart failure (3); sleep in hypoxic environments (2), or idiopathic central sleep apnea (7).

⊙—⛏ Key points box 1.4

- REM sleep causes (1) postural muscle atonia (including upper airway); (2) widespread cortical and medually neuronal activity; and (3) intermittent disruption of diaphragm EMG activity.

- The ventilatory consequences are (1) an increased breathing frequency and greater dependence on diaphragmatic contraction; (2) a highly variable and usually depressed response of respiratory motor output to chemical stimuli; (3) a more collapsible upper airway; (4) longer duration of obstructive apneas; and (5) reduced susceptibility to central apneas.

SLEEP DISORDERED BREATHING IN THE UNDIAGNOSED, HEALTHY POPULATION

THE OCCURRENCE OF APNEA AND HYPOPNEAS

In addition to the sleep-induced alveolar hypoventilation and increased R_{UA} in sleep, many healthy subjects aged 30 to 60 years also experience disordered breathing events in the form of apneas and hypopneas at rates of more than 5–10 per hour of sleep (for details, see chapter by Young on Epidemiology in this book). These events (see Fig. 1.5) are caused by one or more of the fundamental effects of sleep on the regulation of motor output to the pump muscles and/or the upper airway, as detailed above. Skeletal and soft tissue dimensions of the upper airway, together with body mass, age and gender all are risk factors in the

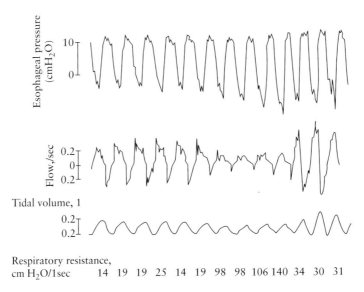

Fig 1.5 *Transient increase in upper airway resistance during sleep as a cause of hyponea. Note the sudden reduction in the flow rate and the more negative esophageal pressure as resistance increases transiently (possibly due to changes in sleep state) and V_T is reduced during NREM sleep. Resistance values listed are measured at the pressure nadir reached at peak inspiration. (From Dempsey JA, Smith CA, Harms CA, Chow C, Saupe KW. Sleep-induced breathing instability – state of the art review. Sleep 1996; 19(3):236–247.)*

prevalence and severity of these sleep-disordered breathing events in the undiagnosed population.

Each respiratory event causes arterial oxyhemoglobin desaturation and CO_2 retention. They are also often self-perpetuating because of the ventilatory overshoot which often follows the apnea. The hyperventilation, in turn, will lead to hypocapnia and yet another ventilatory depression (see Fig 1.1A).

Terminations of many of these sleep-disordered breathing events give rise to transient arousals from sleep and to significant increases in sympathetic efferent vasoconstrictor activity, cardioacceleration and increased systemic blood pressure. Indeed, these nocturnal events may even lead to chronic (daytime) elevation in blood pressure – although it remains undetermined whether the occurrence of sleep-disordered breathing events at a rate of < 20/hour actually cause significant hypertension in otherwise healthy humans.

Upper Airway Resistance Syndrome

Even in the absence of multiple discreet sleep-disordered breathing events in the form of apneas or hypopneas, it has been suggested that increased airway resistance, *per se*, may have significant effects on daytime sleepiness (57). The rationale here is that increased R_{UA} will lead to increased inspiratory muscle effort, thereby increasing sensory input to the medulla and cortex causing arousals and disrupting sleep. This so-called 'upper airway resistance syndrome' seems to be clinically important, producing significant daytime sleepiness. However, given the lack of immediate load compensation in sleep (see above) we think it more likely that the source of the augmented inspiratory effort is chemoreceptor stimulation, i.e., analogous to that produced experimentally by sustained external loading of the airway (see above). Therefore, in these people the primary event is a hypopnea or sustained hypoventilation with accompanying levels of O_2 desaturation and CO_2 retention that are undetectable or do not reach conventional criteria for 'events' detection. Thus the increased inspiratory effort and sensory input leading to arousals in the presence of high R_{UA} are likely to be secondary phenomena, attributable to increased chemoreceptor stimuli.

In terms of how one views homeostatic control, these sleep-disordered breathing events are evidence of a marked failure of our apparently normal regulatory system. Notably, these 'failures' occur night after night, even in healthy individuals who have adequate structural capacities of their lung, airways and nervous system to permit function at a highly efficient and precise level in the waking state, even under conditions of heavy exercise. The significant prevalence of this sleep-disordered breathing among normal subjects underscores the profound effects of the state of consciousness on homeostatic regulation.

⊶ Key points box 1.5

- In a non-clinical population aged 30–60 years, during sleep 9% of males and 4% of females experience a significant number of apneas and hypopneas. These events occur in addition to the usual hypoventilation present in all subjects and the increase in upper airway resistance that is present in many.

- This sleep-disordered breathing is accompanied by arousals and increases in blood pressure and commonly has effects on daytime sleepiness.

- These important consequences of sleep-disordered breathing underscore the profound effects of sleep state on ventilatory control, a system which functions near-perfectly during wakefulness.

ACKNOWLEDGMENTS

M.J. Morrell is supported by a Wellcome Trust Research Career Development Fellowship; J.A. Dempsey's research is funded by NHLBI.

REFERENCES

1. Young T, Palta M, Dempsey J, et al. The occurrence of sleep-disordered breathing among middle-aged adults. N Engl J Med 1993; 328:1230–1235.

2. Berssenbrugge A, Dempsey J, Iber C, et al. Mechanisms of hypoxia-induced periodic breathing during sleep in humans. J Physiol (Lond) 1983; 343:507–524.

3. Hanly PJ, Millar TW, Stejes DC, et al. Respiration and abnormal sleep in patients with congestive heart failure. Chest 1989; 96:480–488.

4. Orem J, Osorio I, Brooks E, et al. Activity of respiratory neurons during NREM sleep. J Neurophysiol 1985; 54:1144–1156.

5. Parisi RA, Neubauer JA, Santiago TV, et al. Brain blood flow and control of respiratory muscles during sleep. Acta Biol Med Exp 1986; 11:115–126.

6. Eldridge FL, Millhorn DE. Oscillation, gating, and memory in the respiratory control system. In: The handbook of physiology the respiratory system. Control of breathing, vol 2. Bethesda, MD: American Physiological Society, 1986; 93:114.

7. Xie A, Wong B, Phillipson EA, et al. Interaction of hyperventilation and arousal in the pathogenesis of idiopathic central sleep apnea. Am J Respir Crit Care Med 1994; 150:489–495.

8. Warner G, Skatrud JB, Dempsey JA. Effect of hypoxia-induced periodic breathing on upper airway obstruction during sleep. J Appl Physiol 1987; 62:2201–2211.

9. Wilson PA, Skatrud JB, Dempsey JA. Effects of slow wave sleep on ventilatory compensation to inspiratory elastic loading. Resp Physiol 1984; 55:103–120.

10. Iber C, Berssenbrugge A, Skatrud JB. Ventilatory adaptations of resistive loading during wakefulness and non-REM sleep. J Appl Physiol 1982; 52:607–614.

11. Wiegand L, Zwillich C, White D. Sleep and the ventilatory response to resistive loading in normal man. J Appl Physiol 1988; 64:1186–1195.

12. Hudgel DW, Hulholland M, Hendricks C. Neuromuscular and mechanical responses to inspiratory resistive loading during sleep. J Appl Physiol 1987; 63:603–608.

13. Badr MS, Skatrud JB, Dempsey JA, et al. Effect of mechanical loading on inspiratory and expiratory muscle activity during NREM sleep. J Appl Physiol 1990; 68:1195–1201.

14. Remmers JE, DeGroot WJ, Sauerland EK, et al. Pathogenesis of upper airway occlusion during sleep. J Appl Physiol 1978; 44:931–938.

15. Gugger M, Molly J, Gould GA, et al. Ventilatory and arousal responses to added inspiratory resistance during sleep. Am Rev Respir Dis 1989; 140:1301–1307.

16. Henke KG, Badr MS, Skatrud JB, et al. Load compensation and respiratory muscle function during sleep. J Appl Physiol 1992; 72:1221–1234.

17. Mathew OP. Control of upper airway muscle activity. In: Regulation of breathing. Dempsey JA, Pack AI, eds. New York: Marcel Dekker; 1994:1064–1134.

18. Eastwood PR, Curran AK, Smith CA, et al. Effect of upper airway negative pressure on inspiratory drive during sleep. J Appl Physiol 1998; 84:1063–1075.

19. Eastwood PR, Satoh M, Curran AK, et al. Inhibition of inspiratory motor output by high-frequency low-pressure

oscillations in the upper airway of sleeping dogs. J Physiol 1999; 517:259–271.

20. Badr MS, Toiber F, Skatrud JB, et al. Pharyngeal narrowing/occlusion during central sleep apnea. J Appl Physiol 1995; 78:1806–1815.

21. Horner RL, Innes JA, Morrell MJ, et al. The effect of sleep on reflex genioglossus muscle activation by stimuli of negative pressure in humans. J Physiol (Lond) 1994; 476:141–151.

22. Harms CA, Zeng YJ, Smith CA, et al. Negative pressure-induced deformation of the upper airway causes central apnea in awake and sleeping dogs. J Appl Physiol 1996; 80:1528–1539.

23. Wasicko MJ, Leiter JC, Erlichman JS, et al. Nasal and pharyngeal resistance after topical mucosal vasoconstriction in normal humans. Am Rev Respir Dis 1991; 144:1048–1052.

24. Van deGraaff WB. Thoracic influence on upper airway patency. J Appl Physiol 1988; 65:2124–2131.

25. Begle RL, Badr S, Skatrud JB, et al. Effect of lung inflation on pulmonary resistance during NREM sleep. Am Rev Respir Dis 1990; 141:854–860.

26. Smith E. (1860). Cited by Bulow K. Respiration and wakefulness in man. Acta Physio Scand 1963; 59:7–9.

27. Bulow K. Respiration and wakefulness in man. Acta Physiol Scand 1963; 59:7–9.

28. Gothe B, Altose MD, Goldman MD, et al. Effect of quiet sleep on resting and CO_2 stimulated breathing in humans. J Appl Physiol 1981; 50:724–730.

29. Douglas NJ, White DP, Pickett CK, et al. Respiration during sleep in normal man. Thorax 1982; 37:840–844.

30. White DP, Weil JV, Zwillich CW. Metabolic rate and breathing during sleep. J Appl Physiol 1985; 59:384–391.

31. Tabachnik E, Muller NL, Bryan AC, et al. Changes in ventilation and chest wall mechanics during sleep in normal adolescents. J Appl Physiol 1981; 51:557–564.

32. Hudgel DW, Martin RJ, Johnson B, et al. Mechanics of the respiratory system and breathing pattern during sleep in normal humans. J Appl Physiol 1984; 56:133–137.

33. Stradling JR, Chadwick GA, Frew AJ. Changes in ventilation and its components in normal subjects during sleep. Thorax 1985; 40:364–370.

34. Phillipson EA, Bowes G. Control of breathing during sleep. In: The handbook of physiology: the respiratory system. Control of Breathing, vol 2, part 2. Bethesda, MD: American Physiological Society, 1986: 62–648.

35. Brebbia DR, Altshuler KZ. Oxygen consumption rate and electroencephalographic stage of sleep. Science 1965; 150:1621–1623.

36. Pack AI, Cola MF, Goldszmidt A, et al. Correlation between oscillations in ventilation and frequency content of the electroencephalogram. J Appl Physiol 1992; 72:985–992.

37. Trinder J, VanBeveren JA, Smith P, et al. Correlation between ventilation and EEG-defined arousal during sleep onset in young subjects. J Appl Physiol 1997; 83:2005–2011.

38. Horner RL. Motor control of the pharyngeal musculature and implications for the pathogenesis of obstructive sleep apnea. Sleep 1996; 19:827–853.

39. Skatrud JB, Dempsey JA. Airway resistance and respiratory muscle function in snorers during NREM sleep. J Appl Physiol 1985; 59:328–335.

40. Morrell MJ, Harty HR, Adams L, et al. Changes in total pulmonary resistance and PCO_2 between wakefulness and sleep in normal human subjects. J Appl Physiol 1995; 78:1339–1349.

41. Henke KG, Dempsey JA, Kowitz JM, et al. Effects of sleep-induced increases in upper airway resistance on ventilation. J Appl Physiol 1990; 62:617–624.

42. Badr MS, Kawak A, Skatrud JB, et al. Effect of induced hypocapnic hypopnea on upper airway patency in humans during NREM sleep. Respir Physiol 1997; 110:33–45.

43. Horner RL, Shea SA, McIvor J, et al. Pharyngeal size and shape during wakefulness and sleep in patients with obstructive sleep apnea. Q J Med 1989; 72:719–735.

44. Morrell MJ, Badr MS. Effects of NREM sleep on dynamic within-breath changes in upper airway patency in humans. J Appl Physiol 1998; 84:190–199.

45. Morrell MJ, Harty HR, Adams L, et al. Breathing during wakefulness and NREM sleep in humans without and upper airway. J Appl Physiol 1996; 81:274–281.

46. Simon PM, Dempsey JA, Landry DM, et al. Effect of sleep on respiratory muscle activity during mechanical ventilation. Am Rev Respir Dis 1993; 147:32–37.

47. Parisi RA, Edelman NH, Santiago TV. Central respiratory carbon dioxide chemosensitivity does not decrease during sleep. Am Rev Respir Dis 1992; 145:832–836.

48. Lopas JM, Tabachnik E, Muller NL, et al. Total airway resistance and respiratory muscle activity during sleep. J Appl Physiol 1983; 54:773–777.

49. Skatrud JB, Dempsey JA, Badr S, et al. Effect of airway impedance on CO_2 retention and respiratory muscle activity during NREM sleep. J Appl Physiol 1988; 65:1676–1685.

50. Kay A, Trinder J, Bowes G, et al. Changes in airway resistance during sleep onset. J Appl Physiol 1994; 76:1600–1607.

51. Kay A, Trinder J, Kim Y. Individual differences in relationship between upper airway resistance and ventilation during sleep. J Appl Physiol 1995; 79:411–419.

52. Hudgel DW, Hamilton HB. Respiratory muscle activity during sleep-induced periodic breathing in the elderly. J Appl Physiol 1994; 77:2285–2290.

53. Pack A. Changes in respiratory motor activity during REM sleep. In: Dempsey JA, Pack AI, eds. Regulation of Breathing New York: Marcel Dekker; 1995; 983–1010.

54. Smith CA, Henderson KS, Xi L, et al. Neural-mechanical coupling of breathing in REM sleep. J Appl Physiol 1997; 83:1923–1932.

55. Glesson K, Zwillich CW, White DP. The influence of increasing ventilatory effort on arousal from sleep. Am Rev Respir Dis 1990; 142:295–300.

56. Xi L, Smith CA, Saupe KW, et al. Effects of rapid-eye movement sleep on the apneic threshold in dogs. J Appl Physiol 1993; 75:1129–1139.

57. Guilleminault C, Stoohs A, Clerk M, et al. A cause of excess daytime sleepiness. The upper airway resistance syndrome. Chest 1993; 104:781–787.

2 ASSESSMENT OF THE SLEEPY PATIENT

Jean Krieger

INTRODUCTION

With the increasing awareness of the frequency of sleep disorders, sleepiness has become a concern because of its potential risks for the individual person and for society (1, 2). It is therefore important that the clinician dealing with problems of respiratory related sleep disorders keep in mind that these are not the only cause of excessive daytime sleepiness and be able to identify other possible disorders.

For the Oxford Advanced Dictionary, 'sleepy' means 'needing, ready for, sleep.' Being sleepy is a physiological condition, which occurs in a normal subject at least once a day. Actually, the normal sleep propensity is maximum during the usual sleep period when the body temperature and plasma cortisol level are minimal. There is a secondary trough in vigilance during the midafternoon hours. One of the difficulties in studying sleep disorders is identifying when this condition is pathological (or excessive). Decisions can be based on self-evaluation or instrumental evaluations, none of which is ideal, and probably the gold standard for the identification of excessive daytime sleepiness remains to be described. The second problem is identifying the cause of excessive sleepiness. The cause may be related to a dysfunction of the sleep generating system itself (narcolepsy, idiopathic hypersomnia) or be the consequence of a disturbance of sleep structure caused by a factor internal to the body (sleep apneas or possibly periodic limb movements in sleep) or external to the body (environmental).

This chapter addresses the following problems: 1) how to identify the sleepy patient, and 2) the possible causes of abnormal sleepiness.

DEFINITION AND TOOLS FOR THE INVESTIGATION OF EXCESSIVE DAYTIME SLEEPINESS

SUBJECTIVE (INTROSPECTIVE) SLEEPINESS

The first proposed definition described sleepiness as an 'elemental feeling state' (3), meaning that only the subject is able to know, by introspection, whether he or she is sleepy or not. The Stanford Sleepiness Scale (4) or the Karolinska Sleepiness Scale (5) and many visual analog scales are based on such an approach. This provides an instantaneous picture of the subject's feeling. It has proved useful in experimental designs, when the question is whether the experimental situation has an impact on the subject's feeling. The approach is much less useful in clinical situations, in which an evaluation of a more chronic condition is sought and in which the question is whether the subject's feeling is normal or pathological. In addition, it may be difficult for the subject to differentiate actual sleepiness (i.e., readiness to fall asleep) from feelings of fatigue. A good example of this dissociation is given by most insomniac subjects, who rate themselves as sleepy (not feeling refreshed) but prove unable to fall asleep when they are given the opportunity to do so (6).

OBJECTIVE SLEEPINESS

For these reasons, the definition of sleepiness most commonly used in clinical situations is based on a more objective concept of sleepiness, relying on the actual occurrence of a sleep episode. This definition is based on the postulate that the more sleepy a person is, the more likely he or she is to fall asleep; thus sleepiness is defined by a behavior, which can be objectively assessed by various approaches. One set of approaches consists of instrumental ones; examples are the Multiple Sleep Latency Test (MSLT) or the Maintenance of Wakefulness Test (MWT), in which the likelihood of falling asleep is measured by the speed with which the subject falls asleep under standardized, presumably sleep-inducing conditions, with sleep being detected with electrophysiological variables; a variant of this type of approach is the OSLER test (7), in which sleep is identified by a change in behavior. Another approach is to measure the likelihood of falling asleep by the frequency of the occurrence of sleep episodes under the more naturalistic conditions of usual life; this can be done by the subject himself or herself as is the case with the Epworth Sleepiness Scale and can be termed self-evaluation of objective sleepiness. Although this is often called subjective sleepiness, it would be better called a subjective evaluation of objective sleepiness, as the concept is basically different from what was defined as subjective sleepiness earlier.

Multiple Sleep Latency Test

The MSLT is based on the postulate that the sleepier a person is, the faster he falls asleep. This postulate has been questioned, and some authorities have suggested that it was possible to fall asleep quickly under the conditions of the test without other signs of sleepiness (8). The test was first described for the investigation of the effects of various manipulations of sleep (mainly sleep deprivation and pharmacological interventions), and there are numerous publications showing that the test is sensitive to such manipulations (9–11; see 12 for a minireview). However, its validation as a tool for measuring absolute sleepiness is much less well established; no normative data have been published. It is often accepted that a mean sleep latency longer than 10 min is normal, between 5 and 10 min is the gray zone and shorter than 5 min is pathological. However, this statement was initially based on a study that investigated only 14 control subjects (compared with 27 narcoleptic patients [13]), and the presently accepted normal cut-off of 10 min is consensus-based rather than data-based.

Several studies investigated the MSLT in normal samples, selected for the absence of sleep disorders complaints: in a study of over 100 young adults screened for normal sleep habits and absence of sleep pathology, 32% had a mean sleep latency (MSL) ≤ 5 min, and only 40% had MSL > 10 min (14). Another study of normal subjects found an overall MSL of 11 min in younger subjects

(18–29 years) and 12.5 min in older subjects (30–80 years), with more than 10% in both groups having MSL < 5 min (15). These results could throw doubt on the rule that an MSL ≤ 5 min (10 min) is abnormal, but they were considered to be indicative of chronic sleep deprivation in those subjects with short latencies, even though there were no other signs of sleepiness on performance tests (16) and the MSL did not reach the normal range of > 10 min when subjects with latencies shorter than 6 min were given the opportunity to lengthen sleep duration to 10 hours for 6 nights (17). Clearly, the debate on whether our society is sleep deprived (18, 19) is still open, and the meaning of short sleep onset latencies remains ambiguous.

In practice, the subject is given the instruction to 'Please lie quietly, keep eyes closed, and try to fall asleep' four to five times a day, every 2 hours starting at 0930 or 1000. To maintain the sleep-inducing conditions, the room should be quiet and dark, with all sources of noise removed, at constant comfortable temperature, without alcohol or caffeine on the day of the test; the patient lies in a comfortable bed, in his or her preferred sleep position. The electroencephalogram (EEG) is recorded under the standard Rechtschaffen and Kales (20) conditions. Between the trials, the patient stays out of bed and is prevented from sleeping. As it is important that the guidelines are strictly followed (see Table 2.1), the reader is referred to the detailed description of the conditions of the test in the published guidelines (21) and their review by the American Sleep Disorders Association (ASDA) (22).

There are two versions of the protocol, an experimental one and a clinical one; some confusion has occurred between the two, and it might be useful to specify that the clinical test is designed as follows (12): the test is terminated 15 min after sleep onset (or after 20 min if no sleep has occurred), sleep onset being defined as the first epoch scored as sleep (whatever the sleep stage, including stage 1). The sleep latency is the elapsed time from lights-out to the first epoch of sleep. The prolongation of the test for 15 min is designed to assess the occurrence of a rapid eye movement (REM) sleep episode, which is important for the diagnosis of narcolepsy (23). The REM latency is the time from sleep onset (as defined above) to the first epoch of REM sleep. All definitions of sleep epochs are based on the strict application of Rechtschaffen and Kales' criteria (20).

One of the problems that have been emphasized (24) is that the MSLT, although the test is repeated four to five

Table 2.1 Specific procedures for the MSLT (clinical version)*

Measure	Time	Procedure
	Prior to testing	
	30 min	Suspend tobacco smoking
	15 min	Suspend vigorous physical activity
	10 min	Prepare for bed
		Remove shoes
		Loosen constricting clothing
	5 min	In bed hooked up
		Calibration series
	45 s	Introspective sleepiness measure
	30 s	Assume comfortable position for falling asleep
	5 s	'Please lie quietly, keep your eyes closed, and try to fall asleep'
	Following lights out	
	0 min	Lights out
Sleep latency	x_1 min	First epoch of sleep (including stage 1)
REM latency	x_2 min	First epoch of REM sleep
	x_1 + 15 min	End the test if sleep has occurred
	20 min	End the test if no sleep has occurred

* Modified after Carskadon MA. Measuring day time sleepiness. In: Kryger MH, Roth T, Dement WC, eds. Principles and practice in sleep medicine, 2nd edn. Philadelphia. WB Saunders 1994: 961–966.

times throughout a day, provides a picture only on that specific day, which does not necessarily reflect overall sleepiness, which should be evaluated over weeks or months for clinical purposes. In addition, the guidelines require that the subject spend the previous night in the hospital with a polysomnographic recording in order to evaluate his or her sleep duration and quality. This requirement certainly makes sense for experimental situations. However, it is also possible that the sleep disturbance induced by the night in the sleep laboratory alters the results of the test, although no study has systematically investigated this point.

Another problem that has been emphasized is that the identification of a sleep episode is based on Rechtschaffen and Kales' criteria (20), which require that the EEG changes indicative of a change in vigilance test last for at least half an epoch (i.e., 15 s in most United States sleep laboratories or 10 s in most European laboratories). It is likely that a lapse in vigilance shorter than 15 s may cause serious accidents and be perceived by the subject.

This may be one of the reasons for the poor correlations between MSLT data and other evaluations of sleepiness. A more disturbing paradox is that MSLT is poorly correlated with factors expected to influence sleepiness in clinical populations such as age, total sleeptime, percentage of delta sleep, wake after sleep onset (25, 26). Also, it is difficult to understand why a measure of sleepiness is not correlated with the number of sleep-disturbing events or the number of sleep disruptions—for instance, in the obstructive sleep apnea syndrome (27)—whereas it is universally recognized that the elimination of these events improves somnolence.

Even though the MSLT is probably not the gold standard for the evaluation of absolute sleepiness in clinical situations, it has been shown to be useful for the evaluation of treatment efficacy (28–30).

Maintenance of Wakefulness test

Because ability to stay awake may be more relevant clinically and conceptually than ability to fall asleep, an alternative multiple nap approach was proposed (31), with the major difference that the patient was instructed to stay awake, to sit comfortably throughout the test; this procedure addresses the criticism on sleepability discussed above. This MWT is less standardized than the MSLT: the duration of each trial was 20 min (or after 10 min of sleep) in early reports (31–33), then prolonged to 40 min in later studies (34, 35). The criterion for sleep onset was either sustained sleep (i.e., three consecutive epochs of stage 1 or one epoch of any other stage [31–34]) or one epoch of any stage (35).

The MWT in its 40 min version was on average ± standard deviations (SD) 25.9 min ± 11.8 in a group of 322 obstructive sleep apnea syndrome (OSAS) patients; in a subgroup of 24 patients treated with continuous positive airway pressure (CPAP) it increased from 18 ± 12 min to 32 ± 10 min (34); in its 20 min version it was 11.0 ± 4.8 min in 12 OSAS patients (32) and 10.7 ± 5.3 min (33), 11.0 ± 5.6 min 51), and 9.9 ± 6.1 min (31) in 11, 12, and 10 narcoleptic patients, respectively.

Correlations between MSLT and MWT, although statistically significant, are weak (r = 0.41; i.e., 17% of the variance [35]), leading to the conclusion that the two tests measure different abilities. An alternative explanation could be that the measures have intrinsic variability, unrelated to what they are supposed to measure. Correlation of MWT with apnea-hypopnea index (AHI) is no better than with MSLT (r = − 0.35) (34).

The MWT has the advantage of having normative data, albeit on only 64 subjects in a multicenter study involving six centers (36). In its 40 min version, the mean sleep latency to the first epoch of sustained sleep (i.e., three consecutive 30 s epochs of sleep) was 35.2 ± 7.9 min, with a lower normal limit (= mean −2 SD) of 19.4 min. Calculation of the data on the basis of a 20 min trial duration yielded very similar MSL whether sleep onset was defined as brief sleep (10 s or one epoch of any sleep stage, 18.1 ± 3.6 min, lower normal limit: 10.9 min) or sustained sleep (18.7 ± 2.6 min, lower limit: 13.5 min), in agreement with mean values between 18 and 19 min reported previously in smaller groups in normal controls (31–33) using 20 min trials. These values were significantly higher than those reported in patient groups. The authors (36) concluded that the MWT separates normal controls from patients and recommended the use of the MWT with 20 min trials with sleep onset defined as the first occurrence of one epoch of any stage. Other recommendations were for a dark room with a light source behind the subject's head delivering 0.10–0.13 lux at the corneal level, with the

patient sitting in bed, back and neck supported by a bedrest, at a room temperature of 22°C, trial termination at sleep onset or after 20 min, and an instruction to the patient to 'Please sit still and remain awake as long as possible; look directly ahead of you, do not look directly at the light.' Under these conditions, impairment of wake ability exists if the MSL is less than 11 min.

The MWT is probably closer to what the clinician is interested in, but still the conditions of the test, although they are supposed to mimic the boring situation in which patients are most likely to doze off, are far from being realistic.

In addition, the MWT also suffers from the above-mentioned difficulties related to the definition of a sleep episode according to Rechtschaffen and Kales (20), which does not take into account micro – sleep episodes shorter than 15 s.

Osler test

The principle of the Oxford Sleepiness Resistance (OSLER) (7) test is very similar to that of the MWT: the subject is requested to stay awake in the dark for four times 40 min. However, sleep onset is identified on behavioral criteria (rather than electrophysiological criteria): the subject is asked to press a switch in response to a light emitting diode (LED); the absence of response to 7 LED illuminations defines 'sleep onset' and ends the test. There have been so far very few validation studies, but the test has been shown to discriminate persons with sleep apnea from normal subjects, and is simpler to administer than the MWT. It has the advantage that sleep onset is defined automatically and bypasses the discussions on the electrophysiogical criteria for the definition of sleep onset.

Epworth Sleepiness Scale

The Epworth Sleepiness Scale (ESS) is based on principles very similar to those of the MSLT or the MWT. The actual occurrence of a sleep episode is used as a marker of sleepiness. However, there are several differences, some of which constitute an advantage, others a drawback over the instrumental tests.

The first difference is that the frequency of occurrence (rather than the speed of onset) of a sleep episode is taken as a measure of sleepiness. The second difference is that the conditions of normal daily life (rather than artificial laboratory situations) are used: eight different situations, which are supposed to be experienced by anyone, are proposed; the subject rates on scale of 0–3 how likely he or she is to fall asleep in any of these conditions. This is certainly an advantage in that the test is more naturalistic; but it also has the drawback of introducing more variability related to subject's personal interest in the proposed activity. Sleepiness can be evaluated over a prolonged period of time (in contrast to a single day with the instrumental tests). It poses a problem when a subject does not experience some of the proposed situations. The protocol in this case proposes that the patient make a guess of what it would be, which is probably one of the weak points of the test. Another, and probably the main weak point, is that it is a self-evaluation, which means that the test is sensitive to misperception of sleep episodes; yet it should be noted that there is a high correlation between the patients' and their partners' independent reports (37). The test is also sensitive to cheating, which may become a problem when losing a job or a driving license is at stake.

The test has a high test-retest reliability (38). It also has the advantage of being inexpensive, as it requires only pen and paper.

In practice, the individual scores are totaled, ending up in a minimum total score of 0 and a maximum score of 24 (Table 2.2).

Normal subjects have scores lower than or equal to 10. Scores higher than 12 are considered to be pathological (6).

ESS scores do correlate significantly with instrumental measures of sleepiness, but again the correlations are

---

⟳ Key points box 2.1

Identification of exessive daytime sleepiness

- The identification of the sleepy patient relies on clinical complaints.
- Various tools designed to quantify sleepiness may help objectify the complaint, but there is presently no gold standard to measure 'absolute' sleepiness.
- The Epworth Sleepiness Scale (ESS) and the maintenance of wakefulness test (MWT) are the most adequate tests, but clearly there is a need for rethinking the assessment of sleepiness.

Table 2.2 Procedure for the Epworth Sleepiness Scale*

How likely are you to doze off or fall asleep in the following situations, in contrast to feeling just tired? This refers to your usual way of life in recent times. Even if you have not done some of these things recently try to work out how they would have affected you. Use the following scale to choose the *most appropriate number* for each situation:

0 = would never doze   1 = *slight* chance of dozing

2 = *moderate* chance of dozing   3 = *high* chance of dozing

Situation	*Chance of dozing*
Sitting and reading	—
Watching TV	—
Sitting inactive in a public place (e.g. a theater or a meeting)	—
As a passenger in a car for an hour without a break	—
Lying down in the afternoon when circumstances permit	—
Sitting and talking to someone	—
Sitting quietly after a lunch without alcohol	—
In a car, while stopped for a few minutes in the traffic	—

Thank you for your cooperation

* After Johns MW. A new method for measuring daytime sleepiness – the Epworth Sleepiness Scale Sleep 1991; 14:540–545.

not very strong, with a range of 15 to 25% of the variance of one test 'explained' by the other one (39–41). Correlations between ESS scores and AHI or indices of sleep fragmentation are no better than with the MSLT (ranging from 0.21 to 0.36), (42).

CLINICAL DIAGNOSIS OF EXCESSIVE DAYTIME SLEEPINESS

Despite the difficulties in defining a gold standard able to provide an absolute measure of sleepiness that would be valid in any situation, clinically the diagnosis is often obvious: the patient complains of being unable to stay awake under soporific conditions, and his or her inability to stay awake has caused awkward situations, such as falling asleep at meetings, during social intercourse, or even while driving or under other hazardous circumstances. More often, sleepiness is not the primary complaint of the patient; and, in patients investigated for another reason (often heavy snoring or witnessed apneas), the clinician is led to seek the presence of excessive daytime sleepiness. Sleepiness is often denied or minimized by the patient. The report of the spouse then proves useful.

Defined as the inadequate occurrence of a sleep episode, excessive daytime sleepiness is in principle easy to differentiate from other conditions characterized by a feeling of not being refreshed, not feeling energetic, or having lost interest in doing things. These feelings typically characterize fatigue and depression. However, in some instances, fatigue and loss of energy are symptoms of conditions that also cause excessive sleepiness.

Therefore, it may not be easy to differentiate symptoms related to chronic fatigue or depression from symptoms related to a cause of excessive daytime sleepiness. Under those circumstances, a gold standard for the absolute measure of sleepiness would be useful.

The choice of the best suited test depends on the clinical situation: if the patient is not likely to exaggerate (consciously or not) his sleepiness, an ESS is certainly the least expensive next step. Otherwise, or if the ESS is in contradiction with the conclusions of the clinical data, an instrumental test is required. The MWT is probably better suited to the clinical question, especially if the conclusions may have medicolegal implications. There is no simple interpretation of a discordance between MWT and ESS.

CAUSES OF EXCESSIVE DAYTIME SLEEPINESS

In the general population, the prevalence of excessive daytime sleepiness is poorly investigated: in a review of the literature (43) it was observed that the prevalence ranged from 0.3 to 13.3%, depending on definition and on the age and sex of the population studied. The effect of age, however, was not uniform, as some studies found a maximum in the 18–30 year (44) or 10–19 year (45) age group, whereas others found an increasing prevalence with age (46, 47). The main conclusion of the review was that methodological problems precluded any firm conclusion. More recent studies of excessive daytime sleepiness indicate prevalence rates of 11% in women and 6.7% in men of daytime sleepiness every day or almost every day in a Finnish population sample of 11354 adults (33–60 years [48]). It is more frequently reported in an elderly population over 65 years (20% 'usually sleepy in the daytime' [49]). Both studies found sleepiness to be associated with depression, insomnia, and sleep-disordered breathing.

According to a national United States cooperative study involving 11 sleep-wake disorders clinics and nearly 5000 patients, excessive daytime sleepiness was the largest overall diagnostic category, accounting for 51% of all the 3090 diagnoses made (50). The most prevalent diagnoses in this category were sleep apnea syndromes (43%), narcolepsy (25%), idiopathic hypersomnia (i.e., unexplained hypersomnia [9%]), no hypersomnia abnormality (5%), other hypersomnia (5%), psychiatric disorders (essentially depression [4%]), periodic limb movements in sleep (4%), and other causes, including medical, toxic, environmental, and psychophysiological (5%). These data are probably biased, as it seems obvious that in the general population the ratio of OSAS to narcolepsy is not 2 to 1. The following section broadly outlines the main diagnostic criteria for the major causes of sleepiness (Fig. 2.1).

SLEEP RESTRICTION

Sleep restriction is certainly by far the most frequent cause of occasional sleepiness, and certainly it is a frequent cause of chronic sleepiness. As it is not considered a 'medical' condition, it is likely that most sleep-deprived people do not seek medical advice for their sleepiness. Because of its nonmedical status, the patients often omit to mention it. Usual bedtimes and rising times should be systemati-

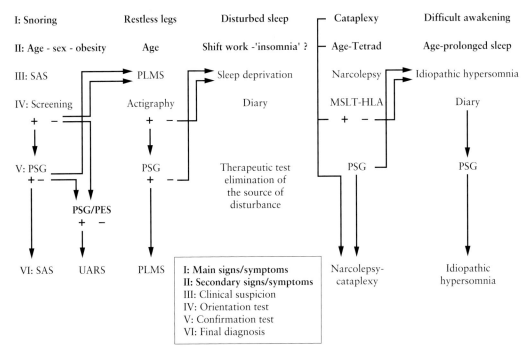

Fig 2.1 *Decision tree for the diagnostic of excessive daytime sleepiness. SAS= sleep apnea syndrome; PSG = polysomnography; PES= oesophagel pressure; PLMS = periodic leg movement syndrome; MSLT = multiple sleep latency test.*

cally recorded, and a sleep diary should be obtained from any sleepy patient.

OBSTRUCTIVE SLEEP APNEA SYNDROME

OSAS and the related upper airway resistance syndrome (UARS) constitute the topics of this book and will not be detailed here.

NARCOLEPSY

Typically narcolepsy symptoms begin during the second decade and rarely start after the age of 40 years. However, the disorder can go undiagnosed until later ages. It is often considered a rare disorder; however, its prevalence (about 0.05%) is twice that of multiple sclerosis or half that of parkinsonism, neither of which is taken as a rare disorder.

The narcoleptic episodes (narcolepsy means 'sleep attack') last several tens of minutes during which the patient has increasing difficulty remaining awake; if he or she tries to oppose the sleepiness, his or her behavior may become maladapted (illegible writing, blurred speech,

automatic behavior). When the patient has an opportunity to take a nap, it has a refreshing value, and the patient again feels alert for a couple of hours. The clinical profile of sleepiness is thus different from that observed in sleepiness from other causes.

The cataplectic episodes constitute the clinical signature of the disorder. They are episodes of decreased muscular tone, typically elicited by situations that involve both surprise and an emotional load, the most typical of which is laughter. The loss of tone can involve the lower limbs, causing the patient to collapse, or to feel a need to sit down, or it can be restricted to the upper limbs or to the facial muscles. These episodes last about 1 min but may be much shorter. It is important to note that there is no loss of consciousness, but sometimes a cataplectic episode continues into a sleep episode in very sleepy patients.

Sleep paralysis and hypnagogic hallucinations, the other two elements of the narcoleptic tetrad, are less frequent but are of great clinical value if cataplexy is missing (which is the case in about 10% of cases).

Night sleep is often of poor quality and interrupted by frequent awakenings. In extreme cases the severely disrupted night sleep can be hardly distinguished from the sleepy 'wake' period.

Sleep-onset REM periods (SOREMPs) are the electrophysiological signature of the disorder. The MSLT provides several opportunities for detecting SOREMPs throughout the day. It is generally considered that at least two naps should include a REM sleep onset, but it should be kept in mind that these are not absolutely specific and can be observed in other sleepy patients, including those with OSAS (32). Therefore, the diagnosis of associated narcolepsy and sleep apnea should be accepted only if REM sleep onset episodes persist after sleep apneas have been eliminated with an adequate treatment.

The diagnosis is typically based on the clinical features. It may be difficult to make a diagnosis, especially when cataplexy is missing, or atypical. In this case, an MSLT proves useful when it demonstrates sleep-onset REM episodes. HLA typing has no positive predictive value, but a patient whose HLA phenotype would not be DRB1*1501 – DQB1* 0602 would have little chance to be narcoleptic.

IDIOPATHIC HYPERSOMNIA

The nosologic situation of idiopathic hypersomnia (IH) is far from clear or consensual. The concept was derived from the initial description by Roth (51), who subdivided non-narcoleptic functional hypersomnia into three categories: (1) monosymptomatic IH, characterized by prolonged nocturnal sleep and daytime hypersomnia; (2) polysymptomatic IH with the same symptoms plus prolonged confusion and disorientation upon awakening; and (3) neurotic hypersomnias. The concept was then extended to all sorts of conditions, including sleepiness or hypersomnia, when no specific cause could be identified. This resulted in a heterogeneous group, from which the upper airway resistance syndrome has been extracted recently. There are at present two tendencies: one is to include under this term all conditions of excessive sleepiness, prolonged sleep episodes, or excessively deep sleep, without an obvious cause and normal polysomnography, which is the option of the International Classification of Sleep Disorders (52) and of some researchers (53). Other researchers (54, 55) instead favor a more restrictive definition, closer to Roth's initial description. In this case, IH appears as a relatively well defined clinical entity characterized by the early onset (usually before the age of 20 years) of prolonged sleep need, typically longer than 10 hours, with difficulty awakening, especially when sleep is shortened for social reasons, and non-refreshing daytime naps. With this definition, there is often a family history of prolonged sleep or sleepiness.

The diagnosis relies on the clinical history; a sleep diary may prove useful, although it is often obscured by social constraints. Polysomnography is mandatory to exclude other possible causes and ideally should include a quantitative evaluation of respiratory effort to exclude upper airway resistance syndrome. It shows a normal sleep macrostructure and microstructure, with a prolonged sleep duration.

⊶ Key points box 2.2

Causes of excessive daytime sleepiness
- There are many possible causes of excessive daytime sleepiness, which require systematic investigation, based on clinical interview, sleep diary, and polysomnography: sleep-disordered breathing, periodic limb movements in sleep, chronic sleep deprivation, narcolepsy, and idiopathic hypersomnia are among the most frequent ones.

PERIODIC LIMB MOVEMENTS IN SLEEP

Periodic limb movements in sleep is classically considered a possible cause of excessive daytime sleepiness. The syndrome has a polygraphic definition (56, 57): a periodic activation of flexor muscles in the lower limbs (the most often recorded muscle is the muscular tibialis); by definition, the activation should last for more than 0.5 s and less than 5 s and be repeated in series of at least five activations, separated by more than 5 s and less than 90 s. The diagnosis is considered positive if at least five activations are present per hour of sleep. The muscles most often involved are the dorsal flexors of the toes and the flexors of the ankle; the flexors of the knee or even the flexors of the hip may be involved, as well as upper limb flexor muscles. The periodic movements aZre related to micro-arousals, but there is disagreement as to whether arousal precedes and causes the movement or the converse.

It has been shown that periodic limb movements in sleep can be highly prevalent in subjects without complaints about sleep, especially in older subjects (58, 59), which opened the debate over whether periodic limb movements should always be considered pathological. More recently, on the basis of the absence of a correlation between the number of periodic limb movements in sleep and the severity of sleepiness, it was suggested (60) that the presence of periodic limb movements in sleep did not preclude the diagnosis of idiopathic hypersomnia. This debate is strangely reminiscent of the debate concerning sleepiness and sleep apnea: some OSA patients do not complain of excessive daytime sleepiness and realize that they were sleepy only once they are treated. There is only a poor correlation between the number of respiratory events and the severity of excessive daytime sleepiness.

In conclusion, although it may be difficult to separate physiological from pathological sleepiness, excessive daytime sleepiness is a frequent symptom with many possible causes, some of which may not be obvious. Only a systematic stepwise evaluation makes it possible not to miss a treatable cause.

REFERENCES

1. Dement WC. The perils of drowsy driving. N Engl J Med 1997; 337:783–784.

2. Mitler MM, Crarskadon MA, Czeisler CA, et al. Catastrophes, sleep, and public policy: consensus report. Sleep 1988; 11:100–109.

3. Dement WC, Carskadon MA, Richardson G. Excessive daytime sleepiness in the sleep apnea syndrome. In: Guilleminault C, Dement WC eds. Sleep apnea syndromes. New York: Alan R Liss; 1978: 23–46.

4. Hoddes E, Zarcone V, Smythe H, et al. Quantification of sleepiness: a new approach. Psychophysiology 1973; 10:431–436.

5. Akerstedt T. Subjective and objective sleepiness in the active individual. Int J Neurosci 1990; 52:29–37.

6. Johns M. Rethinking the assessment of sleepiness. Sleep Med Rev 1998; 2:3–15.

7. Bennett LS, Stradling JR, Davies RJO. A behavioural test to assess daytime sleepiness in obstructive sleep apnoea. J Sleep Res 1997; 6:142–145.

8. Harrison Y, Horne JA. 'High sleepability without sleepiness.' The ability to fall asleep rapidly without other signs of sleepiness. Neurophysiol Clin/Clin Neurophysiol 1996; 26:15–20.

9. Carskadon MA, Dement WC. Effects of total sleep loss on sleep tendency. Percept Mot Skills 1979; 48:495–506.

10. Carskadon MA, Dement WC. Cumulative effects of sleep restriction on daytime sleepiness. Psychophysiology 1981; 18(2):107–113.

11. Dement WC, Seidel W, Carskadon M. Daytime alertness, insomnia, and benzodiazepines. Sleep 1985; 5:528–545.

12. Carskadon MA. Measuring daytime sleepiness. In: Kryger MH, Roth T, Dement WC eds. Principles and practice in sleep medicine, 2nd Ed. Philadelphia: WB Saunders; 1994: 961–966.

13. Richardson GS, Carskadon MA, Flagg W, et al. Excessive daytime sleepiness in man: multiple sleep latency measurement in narcoleptics and in control subjects. Electroencephalogr Clin Neurophysiol 1978; 45:621–627.

14. Bonnet MH. The effect of varying prophylactic naps on performance, alertness and mood throughout a 52-hour continuous operation. Sleep 1991; 14:307–315.

15. Levine B, Roehrs T, Zorick F, et al. Daytime sleepiness in young adults. Sleep 1988; 11:39–46.

16. Manni R, Ratti MT, Barzahi, et al. Daytime sleepiness in healthy, university students: a multiparametric study. Ital J Neurol Sci 1991; 12:203–209.

17. Roehrs T, Timms V, Zwyghuizendoorenbos A, et al. Sleep extension in sleepy and alert normals. Sleep 1989; 12:449–457.

18. Bonnet MH, Arand DL. We are chronically sleep deprived. Sleep 1995; 18:908–911.

19. Harrison Y, Horne JA. Should we be taking more sleep? Sleep 1995; 18:901–907.

20. Rechtschaffen A, Kales A. A manual of standardized terminology, techniques and scoring system for sleep stages of human subjects. Los Angeles: Brain Information Service, Brain Research Institute, 1968.

21. Carskadon MA, Dement WC, Mitler MM, et al. Guidelines for the multiple sleep latency test (MSLT): a standard measure of sleepiness. Sleep 1986; 9:519–524.

22. American Sleep Disorders Association. The clinical use of the multiple sleep latency test. Sleep 1992; 15:268–276.

23. Aldrich MS, Chervin RD, Malow BA. Value of the multiple sleep latency test (MSLT) for the diagnosis of narcolepsy. Sleep 1997; 20:620–629.

24. Johns MW. A new method for measuring daytime sleepiness—the Epworth Sleepiness Scale. Sleep 1991; 14:540–545.

25. Chervin RD, Kraemer HC, Guilleminault C. Correlates of sleep latency on the multiple sleep latency test in a clinical population. Electroencephalogr Clin Neurophysiol 1995; 95:147–153.

26. Kronholm E, Hyyppa MT, Alanen E, et al. What does the multiple sleep latency test measure in a community sample? Sleep 1995; 18:827–835.

27. Chervin RD, Aldrich MS. Characteristics of apneas and hypopneas during sleep and relation to excessive daytime sleepiness. Sleep 1998; 21:799–806.

28. Engleman HM, Cheshire KE, Deary IJ, et al. Daytime sleepiness, cognitive performance and mood after continuous positive airway pressure for the sleep apnoea hypopnoea syndrome. Thorax 1993; 48:911–914.

29. Kribbs NB, Pack AI, Kline LR, et al. Effects of one night without nasal CPAP treatment on sleep and sleepiness in patients with obstructive sleep apnea. Am Rev Respir Dis 1993; 147:1162–1168.

30. Rajagopal KR, Bennett LL, Dillard TA, et al. Overnight nasal CPAP improves hypersomnolence in sleep apnea. Chest 1986; 90:172–176.

31. Mitler MM, Gujavarty KS, Sampson MG, et al. Multiple day-time nap approaches to evaluating the sleepy patient. Sleep 1982; 5:S119–S127.

32. Browman CP, Krishnareddy KS, Sampson MG, et al. REM sleep episodes during the maintenance of wakefulness test in patients with sleep apnea syndrome and patients with narcolepsy. Sleep 1983; 6:23–28.

33. Browman CP. Evaluation of daytime somnolence: objective measures of sleep-wake tendency. J Electrophysiol Techn 1986; 13:233–239.

34. Poceta JS, Timms RM, Jeong DU, et al. Maintenance of wakefulness test in obstructive sleep apnea syndrome. Chest 1992; 101:893–897.

35. Sangal RB, Thomas L, Mitler MM. Maintenance of wakefulness test and multiple sleep latency test – measurement of different abilities in patients with sleep disorders. Chest 1992; 101:898–902.

36. Doghramji K, Mitler MM, Sangal RB, et al. A normative study of the maintenance of wakefulness test (MWT). Electroenceph Clin Neurophysiol 1997; 103:554–562.

37. Johns MW. Sleepiness in different situations measured by the Epworth sleepiness scale. Sleep 1994; 17:703–710.

38. Johns MW. Reliability and factor analysis of the Epworth sleepiness scale. Sleep 1992; 15:376–381.

39. Hardinge FM, Pitson DJ, Stradling JR. Use of the Epworth Sleepiness Scale to demonstrate response to treatment with nasal continuous positive airways pressure in patients with obstructive sleep apnoea. Respir Med 1995; 89:617–620.

40. Johns MW. Daytime sleepiness, snoring, and obstructive sleep apnea—The Epworth sleepiness scale. Chest 1993; 103:30–36.

41. Olson LG, Cole MF, Ambrogetti A. Correlations among Epworth Sleepiness Scale scores, multiple sleep latency tests and psychological symptoms. J Sleep Res 1998; 7:248–253.

42. Pitson DJ, Stradling JR. Autonomic markers of arousal during sleep in patients undergoing investigation for obstructive sleep apnoea, their relationship to EEG arousals, respiratory events and subjective sleepiness. J Sleep Res 1998; 7:53–59.

43. D'Alessandro R, Rinaldi R, Cristina E, et al. Prevalence of excessive daytime sleepiness—an open epidemiological problem. Sleep 1995; 18:389–391.

44. Bixler EO, Kales A, Soldatos CR, et al. Prevalence of sleep disorders: a survey of the Los Angeles metropolitan area. Am J Psychiatry 1979; 136:1257–1262.

45. Lugaresi E, Cirignotta F, Zucconi M, et al. Good and poor sleepers: an epidemiological survey of the San Marino population. In: Guilleminault C, Lugaresi F, eds. Sleep/wake disorders: natural history, epidemiology, and long-term evolution. New York: Raven Press, 1983; 1–12.

46. Partinen M, Rimpela M. Sleeping habits and sleep disorders in a population of 2016 Finnish adults. Yearbook Health Ed Res 1982. Helsinki: The national Board of Health, 1982; 26:253–260.

47. Klink M, Quan SF. Prevalence of reported sleep disturbances in a general population and their relationship to obstructive airways diseases. Chest 1987; 91:540–546.

48. Hublin C, Kaprio J, Partinen M, et al. Daytime sleepiness in an adult, Finnish population. J Intern Med 1996; 239:417–423.

49. Whitney CW, Enright PL, Newman AB, et al. Correlates of daytime sleepiness in 4578 elderly persons: the cardiovascular health study. Sleep 1998; 21:27–36.

50. Coleman RM, Roffwarg HP, Kennedy SJ, et al. Sleep-wake disorders based on a polysomnographic diagnosis: a national cooperative study. JAMA 1982; 247:997–1003.

51. Roth B. Functional hypersomnia. In: Guilleminault C, Dement WC, Passouant P, eds. Narcolepsy. New York: Spectrum, 1976; 333–349.

52. Diagnostic Classification Steering Committee. International classification of sleep disorders: diagnostic and coding manual. Rochester, Minnesota: American Sleep Disorders Association, 1990.

53. Aldrich MS. The clinical spectrum of narcolepsy and idiopathic hypersomnia. Neurology 1996; 46:393–401.

54. Billiard M. Idiopathic hypersomnia. In: Aldrich MS, ed. Neurobase sleep disorders. La Jolla, CA: Arbor Publishing, 1994.

55. Bruck D, Parkes JD. A comparison of idiopathic hypersomnia and narcolepsy-cataplexy using self report measures and sleep diary data. J Neurol Neurosurg Psychiatry 1996; 60:576–578.

56. Coleman RM. Periodic movement in sleep (nocturnal myoclonus) and restless legs syndrome. In: Guilleminault C, ed. Sleeping and waking disorders, indications and techniques. Boston: Addison-Wesley Publishing Company; 1982; 265–295.

57. Coleman RM, Pollak C, Weitzman ED. Periodic movements in sleep (nocturnal myoclonus): relation to sleep-wake disorders. Ann Neurol 1980; 8:416–421.

58. Ancoli-Israel S, Kripke DF, Mason WJ, et al. Sleep apnea and PMS in a randomly selected elderly population final prevalence results. Sleep Res 1986; 15:101.

59. Coleman RM, Bliwise DL, Sajben W, et al. Epidemiology of periodic movements during sleep. In: Guilleminault C, Lugaresi E eds. Sleep-wake disorders: natural history, epidemiology and long-term evolution. New York: Raven Press; 1983; 217–229.

60. Nicolas A, Lesperance P, Montplaisir J. Is excessive daytime sleepiness with periodic leg movements during sleep a specific diagnostic category? Eur Neurol 1998; 40:22–26.

PART TWO

OBSTRUCTIVE
SLEEP APNEA

3 Epidemiology of Obstructive Sleep Apnea

Terry B Young and Paul Peppard

Introduction

The high prevalence of undiagnosed obstructive sleep apnea (OSA) in the general adult population is now well established. Of particular importance, the range of severity, commonly measured by the frequency of apnea and hypopnea episodes per hour of sleep (apnea-hypopnea index, AHI), is wide. Figure 3.1 shows how a typical adult population is distributed on AHI status. The figure, based on data from a population sample of 1299 middle-aged adults, none of whom had been diagnosed as having sleep apnea, shows AHI values range from 0–84, with the distribution greatest for lower AHI values (1). The clinical importance of this is twofold: a significant number of cases of severe OSA warrant identification and treatment, and there is a large number of people with mild

OSA for whom the benefits and costs of diagnosis and treatment are not yet clear (2–7). Furthermore, there is evidence that the lowest end of the OSA spectrum should include the very common condition of heavy snoring without apneic and hypopneic events and episodic upper airway resistance (8–10). If these conditions are added to the population prevalence of OSA, the burden is staggering.

Recent media coverage of the high prevalence of sleep apnea and educational campaigns on sleep disorders are bringing a great deal of public attention to disrupted breathing during sleep and heavy snoring, often with the message that these conditions should be discussed with the person's health care provider. One consequence of this rather sudden uncovering of OSA in the general population is that clinicians, particularly in primary care, are

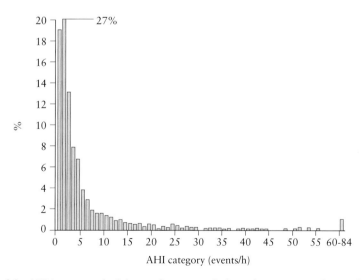

Fig 3.1 Distribution of the AHI in a general adult population sample from the Wisconsin Sleep Cohort Study (N=1299).

being faced with growing numbers of patients seeking help who have OSA at the milder end of the spectrum (5, 11). With increased public awareness and clinical recognition, this trend is likely to escalate. To address the potential public health and clinical burden of OSA, epidemiological studies are needed to describe its patterns of occurrence, risk factors, and natural history (i.e., the course of untreated OSA over time).

This chapter focuses on OSA prevalence, progression, and risk factors, using findings primarily from population-based studies. Subsequent chapters cover epidemiological findings on morbidity and mortality outcomes. The term 'OSA' in this chapter reflects its typical usage in population studies as a condition of recurrent episodes of obstructive apnea and hypopnea, with or without symptoms. It has been suggested that episodes of upper airway resistance be considered the same as apnea and hypopnea events in calculating an event index (e.g., AHI), but no population studies to date have done so (12). Consequently, the measures of OSA are based on apneic and hypopneic events unless stated otherwise. The acronym for obstructive sleep apnea syndrome (OSAS) will indicate clinically diagnosed OSA (presumed symptomatic).

PREVALENCE

The earliest studies, prior to 1990, showed that the occurrence of apnea and hypopnea episodes in nonclinic samples was not as rare as previously believed; OSA was estimated to occur in 1 to 5% of middle-aged men (13). Some of these studies sought to estimate the 'lower limit' of prevalence by conducting polysomnography on small subsets comprising only people with self-reported OSA symptoms selected from survey samples and then assuming that all the cases of OSA had been identified (14). Although these studies were undermined by the low sensitivity of screening questions, even these lower limits of prevalence established the importance of studying OSA further. Since then, studies on much larger samples have shown even higher prevalences.

Age- and sex-specific prevalences over a range of OSA severity were first estimated for middle-aged men and women by the ongoing population-based Wisconsin Sleep Cohort Study (1). The study found that, based on a sample of 625 employed adults, 9% of women and 24% of men had at least mild OSA as evidenced by an average of five or more apnea and hypopnea events per hour of sleep. OSA accompanied by extreme daytime sleepiness that impaired daily functions was estimated to be 2% in women and 4% in men. The results from this study are particularly helpful in estimating the potential clinical burden of OSA because the study used in-laboratory polysomnography conducted according to clinical standard guidelines.

Studies of OSA prevalence in many countries have been completed, but due to variation in methodology, direct comparisons are limited. Different measurement techniques, definitions of abnormal events, and cut-off points on the continuum of the summary measure (e.g., AHI ≥ 5 events/hr) will obviously affect the magnitude of the prevalence estimates. The equivalence of AHI measured by standard in-laboratory polysomnography, unattended polysomnography in the home, and monitors restricted to a few parameters, such as oxygen desaturation and oral-nasal airflow, has not been established (15). Furthermore, studies vary in the definitions used, particularly for hypopneic events (16). Work has been under way to begin standardizing the measurement and definitions, including severity guidelines, for OSAS. A report recently released by an international task force has recommended that OSAS diagnosis be based on overnight monitoring demonstrating five or more obstructed breathing events (apnea, hypopnea, or respiratory effort related arousals) per hour of sleep in combination with symptoms of excessive daytime sleepiness or other sleep and daytime problems. Recommendations for ranking severity of OSAHS are based on both AHI cut-off and impairment of social or occupational functioning (Table 3.1) (12).

Some prevalence studies have used roughly similar definitions and cut-off points to indicate mild or worse OSA (AHI ≥ 5) and to approximate OSAS (AHI ≥ 5 and complaints of daytime sleepiness). As seen in Table 3.2, it appears that OSA of at least mild severity occurs in 5% or more of many adult populations, and OSA that would meet minimal clinical criteria occurs in at least 1%, leaving little doubt that regardless of the population studied, a significant proportion of adults have OSA over a wide range of severity (1, 14, 44, 86, 92, 93).

In contrast to the high prevalence of screen-detected OSA in the general population, the prevalence of clinically diagnosed OSAS is low. Chart surveys and other clinic-based studies have shown that recognition is particularly low in primary care settings (11). In a

Table 3.1 Proposed severity criteria for OSAHS (12)

A. Sleepiness
  1. Mild: Unwanted sleepiness or involuntary sleep episodes occur during activities that require little attention (such as watching TV or reading). Symptoms produce only minor impairment of social or occupational function.
  2. Moderate: Unwanted sleepiness or involuntary sleep episodes occur during activities that require some attention (such as attending concerts or meetings). Symptoms produce moderate impairment of social or occupational function.
  3. Severe: Unwanted sleepiness or involuntary sleep episodes occur during activities that require active attention (such as eating, driving). Symptoms produce marked impairment in social or occupational function.
B. Sleep-related obstructive breathing events
  (apnea, hypopnea, and respiratory effort–related arousals)
  1. Mild: 5–15 events/hour of sleep
  2. Moderate: 15–30 events/hour of sleep
  3. Severe: greater than 30 events/hour of sleep

Adapted from American Academy of Sleep Medicine Task Force (W. Flemons, Chair), Sleep-related breathing disorder in adults; recommendations for syndrome definition and measurement techniques in clinical research. Sleep 1999; 22:667–689.

Table 3.2 Prevalence estimates for any OSA (mild to severe, AHI ≥ 5) and OSAS (any OSA and excessive daytime sleepiness)

Reference	Population	N	Monitoring method	Prevalence estimate for: AHI ≥ 5	AHI ≥ 5 + excessive sleepiness
Lavie (92)	Israel, men	78	Polysomnography	5.3%	0.9%
Gislason et al. (14)	Sweden, men	61	Polysomnography		1.4%
Marin et al. (93)	Spain, men	597	Home oximetry*	15%	2.2%
	Spain, women	625	Home oximetry*	6%	0.8%
Stradling and Crosty (44)	UK, men	1001	Home oximetry	5.1%	1.3%
Bearpark et al. (86)	Australia, men	311	Respiratory monitor	26%	3%
Young et al. (1)	US, men	352	Polysomnography	24%	4%
	US, women	250	Polysomnography	9%	2%

* Estimates based on ≥ 10 desaturation events/hour.

study comparing clinically diagnosed and screen-detected cases of OSA in the general population sample of the Wisconsin Sleep Cohort Study, 82% of men and 93% of women meeting the recommended criteria for moderate or worse OSAS (AHI ≥ 15, often or almost always extremely sleepy in daytime) remained undetected (17).

In addition to highlighting the large burden of unrecognized disease, the disparity in screen-detected and clinic-diagnosed prevalence illustrates the importance of population-based studies to determine the causes and consequences of OSA. When only a very small portion of a condition is manifested in clinic patient populations, it is likely that many selection factors are operating. In addition to the obvious selection factor of symptom severity, many factors such as comorbidity, referral patterns, public and provider awareness, and socioeconomic status can influence whether a person who truly has OSAS will actually be evaluated and diagnosed. Consequently, risk factors and outcomes found from studies on patient samples can easily be due to biases and may fail to reflect true associations.

○┐ Key points box 3.1

- Obstructive sleep apnea is prevalent in the general adult population
- The severity spectrum of undiagnosed OSA ranges from mild to very severe
- 80–90 % of OSAS is undiagnosed
- An estimated 9% of women and 24% of men have sleep-disordered breathing of at least mild severity
- 1–4% of middle-aged adults have OSA that meets the criteria for OSAS
- OSA is very common in older adults; symptoms and outcomes may differ from those in middle-age

---

INCIDENCE AND PROGRESSION

Incidence and progression estimates require baseline and follow-up data from which changes in OSA status over time can be determined. While prevalence is the proportion of people in a population with the condition of interest, incidence refers only to the development of new disease per unit time in a given population at risk for that disease. Incidence has not yet been estimated, and only preliminary data on progression are available thus far. Four year and eight year follow-up data from the Wisconsin Sleep Cohort Study show an average increase from baseline AHI for women of 1.0 event/hour after 4

years, and 2.2 events/hour after 8 years, and for men of 1.7 events/hour at 4 years, and 5.0 events/hour at 8 years. After eight years, the prevalence of AHI ≥ 15 increased by 10% for men and by 16% for women; the prevalence of at least mild OSA at AHI ≥ 5 increased by 23% for men and 30% for women (T. Young, unpublished data). These preliminary data indicate that there is a tendency for OSA to worsen over time. The net increase in severity may be a result of additional risk factor exposure, such as weight gain, as well as natural progression of the pathophysiology present at baseline.

Individual change is reflected in Figure 3.2, in which 8 year follow-up AHI is plotted against baseline AHI for a sample of 200 Sleep Cohort Study participants. Participants treated for OSAHS (n = 2) were eliminated. Note that most change was toward greater AHI after 8 years (points lie above the line of identity); very few people showed a significant decrease in OSA severity. These data do suggest that considerable worsening can occur in 8 years, and that there is little chance that the OSA will simply 'go away.' However, there was some regression, indicating that exogenous factors may act to decrease severity. Nevertheless, some portion of the observed individual AHI changes in either direction is likely to be the result of measurement error, including intrasubject night-to-night variability. Further follow-up of this cohort will allow more precise measurement of AHI change over time.

A progressive trend in OSA severity was also reported from a 10 year follow-up of a subgroup (n = 38) of a population sample. Lindberg et al. found that in the men who had not been treated for sleep apnea during the 10 year period, the mean AHI rose from 2.1 to 6.8 events/hour (p < .01), and the percentage with AHI ≥ 5 events/hour increased from 14% to 45% (18). Although sleepiness was reported to be worse than at baseline, the authors caution that these data were based solely on recall of baseline sleepiness. Of the few clinic-based studies in which patients who had refused treatment were restudied after a period of time, two studies, based on patients with mild to moderate OSAS, found significant progression (19, 20), but in a study of patients with relatively severe OSAS (mean AHI = 52), no net progression, and some individual regression, was seen after 5 years (21). Interpretation is limited due to methodological weaknesses in the clinic-based studies, including the lack of adequate prospective design features, such as assessment of

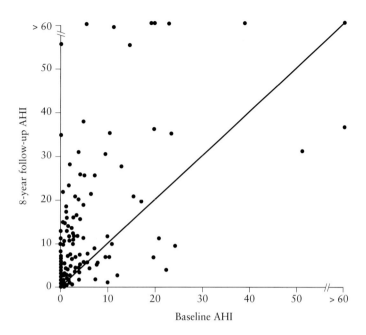

Fig 3.2 *Eight year follow-up data versus baseline AHI in the Wisconsin Sleep Cohort Study (N=192). The diagonal line is a line of equality: follow-up, indicating where points would lie if AHI did not change.*

bias due to incomplete follow-up and low study power. However, the available data from both population and clinic studies suggest that change in severity, mostly toward progression, does occur in individuals with mild or moderate OSA.

Significant change in OSA severity over relatively short time periods is particularly important as it indicates that identification of the determinants of change may lead to effective intervention to reduce or halt OSA progression. In addition, information on progression, particularly the degree to which OSA in asymptomatic people with lower levels of AHI (e.g., 5–15) worsens over time, would be of great help in deciding if treatment should be initiated or could be postponed.

○┅ Key points box 3.2

- Most untreated mild to moderate OSA progresses in severity over time
- Some OSA regresses in severity, but rarely disappears

DEMOGRAPHIC PATTERNS OF OCCURRENCE

Knowledge of the occurrence of OSA by sex, age, geographic region, and race may be helpful clinically in targeted case-finding and in providing clues to causation. There is, however, danger in locking into stereotypes so that a significant number of OSA cases is ignored. An example of this is the previous lack of attention paid to women with OSA symptoms, discussed below.

SEX

In the past, OSAHS was thought to be a disease predominantly of men (22), and the basis for evaluation and treatment was developed almost entirely from clinical observations of, and research on, male patients. The ratio of men to women OSAS patients seen in sleep clinics was typically 8:1 or greater. More recently, population studies that have included women revealed that OSA was not rare in women; the population ratio of OSA, even at higher severity levels, was approximately 2:1 (1, 23). This indicated that a bias favoring men for evaluation and diagnosis of OSAS had been operating. To correct this problem, it is necessary to identify the reasons that have led to underdiagnosis of OSAS in women relative to men. There are several possible explanations.

First, women may have different symptoms. Since clinical guidelines were based on observations of men, the adequacy of this symptom profile for women was unknown. In a population-based study to investigate this (24), the clinical indications for OSAS evaluation were found to be as appropriate for women as they were for men. Habitual snoring, reported breathing pauses, and daytime sleepiness were the best predictors of both mild and moderate OSA for women and men; there were no OSA symptoms unique to women.

A second explanation is that women are unaware of their snoring or are reluctant to acknowledge it. This would result in less help-seeking for OSA and reduced likelihood of a referral for sleep evaluation from primary or other care settings. Two studies of community samples have indicated that the sensitivity of habitual snoring as the sole predictor of OSA at a severity level of AHI $\geq$ 15 is less for women than for men. Redline et al. found that among study participants with an AHI of 15 or greater, 76% of the men and only 41% of the women reported snoring (23). Similarly, Young et al. found that 83% of the men and 62% of the women with AHI $\geq$ 15 reported snoring (24). On the other hand, the specificity of snoring appears to be lower for men. In the Young et al. study, 30% of men and only 11% of women with AHI $<$ 2 reported habitual snoring.

Raising the awareness in women of their own snoring and encouraging their acknowledgment of it would indeed be a step forward in better detection of OSAS in women, but underreporting by women does not account for the bulk of the gender inequity in the clinical detection of OSAS. A remaining explanation is that health care providers in primary care are failing to refer women who report snoring for OSAS evaluation or are failing to ask the appropriate follow-up questions for sleep apnea screening when women complain of daytime problems that may be due to OSA. The former may particularly hold true if women coincidentally have psychological problems in addition to the classic OSAS features and these problems become the focus for further evaluation, rather than the sleep apnea.

Although the excess occurrence of OSAS in men has always been clinically noted, few studies to investigate the underlying role of sex in OSAS have been conducted. Past research has mostly focused on hypotheses of sex hormones as risk factors. The role of estrogen and proges-

terone on breathing during sleep has been investigated, but these studies have been inconclusive (25, 26).

Another line of research took advantage of menopause-related hormonal differences. A number of studies have compared pre-and postmenopausal OSAS patients to investigate possible risk factor differences (27). These studies concurred that premenopausal women were more likely to be morbidly obese (28–30) and found that the premenopausal women tended to have structural abnormalities of the upper airway (28). These studies were limited, however, by small sample sizes; age was not adequately accounted for; and selection bias affecting the findings may have been present. Furthermore, since the onset of OSAS was unknown, it is possible that OSA had been present in the postmenopausal women while they were still premenopausal.

Although menopause is often listed as an established risk factor for OSA, there is no evidence as yet from studies designed specifically to test this hypothesis (31). Previously, comparison of OSA by menopausal status in the ongoing Wisconsin Sleep Cohort Study had suggested that menopause is a risk factor for OSA, but after adjustment for age and body mass index (BMI), the association was not statistically significant. We have now accrued a larger sample size and have found that even after adjustment for age and BMI, women of peri- and postmenopausal status, compared to premenopausal status, are four times as likely to have OSA (odds ratio for having AHI $\geq$ 15 versus AHI $\geq$ 2 = 4.2 (95% confidence interval = 1.3 to 13.9) (T. Young, unpublished data). This finding, although preliminary, is statistically significant (p = .01) and provides the first strong evidence that menopause is an independent risk factor for OSA. Further cross-sectional analyses investigating number of years postmenopausal and use of hormone replacement, as well as longitudinal analyses of data from intensive follow-up evaluation at 6 month intervals, should more definitively characterize the role of menopause in sleep apnea.

Although research on menopausal status is vital to understanding the role of hormones in OSA for women, it does not directly address the reasons why men are at greater risk of sleep apnea. In addition to those hypotheses based on the protective effect of female hormones, others focus on morphological factors (27). Gender differences in body fat distribution, especially in the waist and neck region, and in craniofacial dimensions (9), are well established. These differences have been proposed as the underlying causes of the increased male risk, but evidence is not conclusive.

⊶ Key points box 3.3

- The male:female ratio for OSA prevalence is 2:1
- Snoring and sleepiness are the strongest predictors of OSA for both men and women
- Women probably underreport their snoring
- Menopause is a risk factor for OSA, independent of age and weight for height

---

AGE

Based on clinic observations, OSAS prevalence was thought previously to increase in middle age to a peak around 60 years of age. However, some of the earliest community studies showed a very high prevalence of OSA in older people. Using home monitoring techniques, Ancoli-Israel et al. found 62% of 427 community-dwelling adults over age 65 years old had an AHI of 10 or greater(32). This degree of high prevalence was unsuspected, since most patients evaluated for OSAS were middle-aged, and it necessitated a new look at conditions concomitant with aging. Epidemiology studies continue to point to an increasing prevalence with age. There are several possible explanations. The higher prevalence may simply reflect the accumulation of cases from a constant incidence rate acting on the additional years of life experienced by older populations. OSA is thought to be a lifelong condition, so unless people with OSA die at a much higher rate, prevalence would have to increase with increasing time at risk. Or, prevalence may increase because the incidence rate truly increases, perhaps due to a dramatic increase in exposure to risk factors directly or indirectly related to aging (e.g., losing tone of critical tissue or lack of exercise). Finally, it is possible that increased OSA in older adults is the result of a new form of OSA distinct from OSA in younger people, with onset at a much older age. Several diseases, such as breast cancer, have a bimodal distribution with respect to age, in which incidence plateaus in young or middle age, and then peaks again at a much older age. Often the etiology and natural history for such disorders are different for the young- and old-age onset diseases. If a 'new' form of OSA with a high incidence rate appears at older ages, the important question is whether this OSA is of clinical significance in older people (e.g., should older people be evaluated or treated differently from younger people?) (33–35). Differences in symptoms and outcomes have been noted. Snoring, a concomitant feature of OSA, has been shown in many studies to decrease after the age of 65 years (36). This may indicate that OSA events are predominantly central rather than obstructive, but it is also possible that older people do not report snoring accurately. Of particular importance, some studies of older people have failed to find the associations of OSA with health outcomes found in studies of younger people (36, 37). This has raised one point of view that if OSA in older people carries less health risk, diagnosis and treatment may not be warranted. Nevertheless, the high prevalence of OSA in older people, virtually none of whom have typically been seen in sleep clinics, indicates that older people with OSAS are being missed to a serious extent. Further work is needed to understand OSA in older people and to determine how this should be clinically addressed.

GEOGRAPHIC LOCATION AND RACE

OSA differences by country of origin or race may be due to exogenous risk factor exposure as well as to genetics. Thus far, the only risk factor that has been considered with regard to international differences in OSA prevalence is obesity. Variation in weight has been considered a potential explanation for the lower OSA prevalence in Sweden, Israel, and United Kingdom, where obesity is less common, compared to the United States and Australia (38, 39).

A great deal of interest has been expressed in whether African-Americans are at high risk for OSA, generated in part by suggestive evidence from two studies, and also because, if there is an elevated risk, it could potentially explain some of the higher rate of hypertension and mortality in African-Americans. Few studies have had the racial heterogeneity needed to investigate OSA risk in African-Americans. In the two exceptions, a higher prevalence was found in younger and in older age groups, but not in middle-aged groups. In a study of older community-dwelling adults, Ancoli-Israel et al. found that compared to Caucasians, African-Americans were 2.5 times more likely to have OSA at a severity level of AHI ≥ 30 (40). The number of people with AHI ≥ 30 was small, but the increased risk for African-Americans was statistically significant (p = .04). However, when comparisons were made using a lower AHI cut-off point, which included a larger number of people in the OSA positive category, a difference was not seen. Redline et al., using a family study sample, found that the youngest group (ages 3–25 years) were twice as likely as Caucasians to have AHI ≥ 5 (41). A comparison of the association of OSA and craniofacial measures on a subsample indicated that while many hard and soft tissue parameters were significant risk factors for OSA in Caucasians, tongue area and soft palate length were the only risk factors for OSA in African-Americans. The authors note that these findings may indicate a potential racial difference in effectiveness of surgical therapy. A large multicenter epidemiology study of OSA and cardiovascular risk, the Sleep Heart Health Study, includes a multiracial sample (42). Results are not yet available, but this study will be able to determine risk differences for African-Americans, Hispanics, and Native Americans.

RISK FACTORS

BODY HABITUS AND OBESITY

Few epidemiological studies of correlates of OSA fail to find a relationship with obesity. Obesity has been hypothesized to alter breathing during sleep via multiple mechanisms including alteration of upper airway structure and function, disturbance of the relationship between respiratory drive and load compensation, and obesity-related hypoxemia (43). A variety of body habitus measures including neck morphology (44–49), general obesity (50–52), and central obesity (50, 52–54) have been cross-sectionally associated with OSA in convenience samples of patients from sleep-disorders clinics or population-based studies. Although some of these studies seem to conflict with regard to what measure of obesity or body habitus is the 'best' predictor of OSA, it should be noted that all measures of body habitus are correlated, some highly so. Thus, any degree of ponderosity should be viewed as a risk factor or harbinger of OSA, whatever the measure used to assess body habitus.

A few prospective observational and weight loss studies have sought to examine relationships between weight change and OSA. Pendlebury et al. (20) followed 55 patients over a mean time of 17 months. They found no statistically significant correlations between change in polysomnographically measured AHI and change in BMI. Similarly, Sforza et al. (21) also report no correlation

between change in AHI and change in BMI in 32 OSA patients followed over a 5-year period. However, Peppard (55), in an analysis of Wisconsin Sleep Cohort data (n = 694), found highly statistically significant associations between change in BMI over a 4 year period and incidence and progression of OSA. Each 1 kg/m² increase in BMI yielded an estimated 30% increase (95% confidence interval 13 to 50%) in the odds of developing OSA (AHI ≥ 5 events/hour) over a 4-year interval. Among persons with OSA, a 1 kg/m² increase in BMI predicted a 9% (7–12%) increase in the AHI. Additionally, weight loss yielded analogous predictions of percentage AHI reduction among participants who lost weight.

Several studies have examined the effect of weight loss on measures of OSA. These studies were generally small (n < 30) and involved patients with severe obesity and OSA. Only a few had control groups. The studies either involved surgical (typically gastric bypass or gastroplasty) or dietary weight loss. Five uncontrolled studies of surgical weight loss (56–60) found that an average 25–50% weight loss yielded 70–98% average reductions in indices of OSA. Eight uncontrolled studies of dietary weight loss (59, 61–67) in obese patients found that mean 10–20% weight loss yielded mean 30–75% reductions in indices of OSA. Two controlled dietary weight loss studies (68, 69) found that mean weight losses of 9 and 17% yielded mean AHI decreases of 47 and 61%, respectively. These weight loss studies, as well as the analysis of weight change in the Wisconsin Sleep Cohort, all suggest that weight loss may, on average, yield clinically meaningful reductions in OSA. However, individual responses among studies were variable, with complete elimination of OSA in some participants and very little OSA response to weight change in others.

There is no question that excess body weight and OSA are associated. Based on biological plausibility, clinical observations, and epidemiological associations, the assumption is usually made that the association is causal. Since obesity is a growing world-wide health problem, it follows that OSA will continue to grow in prominence and that clinical and public health strategies utilizing weight control will be attractive approaches to the management of OSA. These findings have important clinical implications for overweight patients with mild to moderate OSA who are poor candidates for nasal continuous positive airway pressure (CPAP) therapy. Weight loss may be appropriate as an alternative strategy for improvement in daytime symptoms of OSA and to prevent the progression of OSA.

⊶ Key points box 3.4

- Obesity is a very strong risk factor for OSA
- All measures of obesity—neck and waist girths, weight, skin folds—predict OSA
- An increase of 1 kg/m^2 in BMI (e.g., a 7 lb. gain in a 5′ 10″ person) yields an estimated 30% increase in the odds of developing OSA
- An increase (decrease) of 1 kg/m^2 in BMI yields an estimated 9% increase (decrease) in the AHI

GENETICS

There is a paucity of research linking specific genetic syndromes and polymorphisms with OSA. A Japanese study (70) found a statistically significantly ($p < 0.05$) higher prevalence (81%) of HLA-A2 antigen in 32 obstructive sleep apnea syndrome patients relative to a normal control group (n = 32) and to the Japanese population (prevalence in the control group and Japanese population both 41%), suggesting a genetic basis for sleep apnea. A few genetic syndromes that exhibit abnormal craniofacial or upper airway anatomy and function (e.g., Marfan syndrome, Down syndrome) have been linked to disturbed nocturnal respiration (11).

Familial clustering of OSA or symptoms of OSA (e.g., habitual snoring) has been reported (71–76). Redline et al. (77), using polysomnographically determined OSA, estimated odds ratios for sleep apnea syndrome (SAS, 15 or more OSA events/hour with daytime sleepiness) as a function of the number of first degree relatives with OSA. Compared with subjects having no relatives with OSA, subjects having one relative with OSA had 1.6 times the odds of having SAS (95% confidence interval: 1.0 to 2.5), subjects with two relatives with OSA had 2.5 (1.1 to 6.0) times the odds, and subjects having three relatives with OSA had 4.0 (1.1 to 14.7) times the odds. All odds ratios were adjusted for age, sex, race, and BMI, removing, in part, heritable effects associated with race or obesity from the estimates. In addition, the authors estimated that roughly 40% of OSA variability could be explained by familial factors.

CRANIOFACIAL MORPHOLOGY

Various abnormalities of the bony and soft tissue structures of the head and neck may predispose to OSAS. Dysmorphisms related to mandibular size and position and to palatal height have been observed in OSAS patients, particularly those of normal body weight. Several predictive models of OSAS have included morphometric data (78, 79). Craniofacial risk factors may be endogenous or exogenous. Presence of enlarged tonsils and adenoids during childhood has been suggested as a cause of abnormal growth patterns of the lower face and jaw (e.g., 'adenoidal facies') that may predispose to OSA in later life (13). Although craniofacial abnormalities may be strong risk factors for OSA (e.g., over 50% of people with acromegaly are reported to have OSAS [26]), they probably account for a small fraction of the total prevalence of OSA.

SMOKING

Smoking is often mentioned as a risk factor for OSA, but few studies have been conducted to investigate this association. There are several mechanisms for a role of smoking in OSA. The upper airway inflammation and airway disease associated with smoking may increase vulnerability to OSA. The decline in nicotine blood levels during sleep may cause sleep instability, which in turn has been linked to OSA (80). In addition, nicotine has been shown to stimulate upper airway tone and decrease airway resistance; withdrawal of nicotine over the night may then result in changes in airway tone and resistance that favor OSA. Two epidemiological studies have found positive associations between self-reported cigarette smoking and OSA, and other studies have found a higher prevalence of snoring among smokers (81–83). If smoking does contribute to increased OSA, the effect seems likely to be reversible after cessation of smoking. In the Wetter et al. study (82), former smokers were not statistically significantly more likely to have OSA (AHI ≥ 5 events/hour) than those who had never smoked, whereas current smokers were three times (95% confidence interval: 1.4 to 6.4) more likely to have OSA than those who had never smoked. Furthermore, a dose-response relationship was evident, with heavier smokers more likely to have worse OSA than lighter smokers. If smoking is a cause of OSA, smoking cessation could be an important means of preventing OSA or decreasing its severity.

ALCOHOL

Adverse effects of alcohol on nocturnal respiration and OSA are typically seen in studies in which defined quantities of alcohol are administered to healthy subjects or to patients with OSA prior to bedtime. In these instances, OSA events could be initiated in healthy subjects or exacerbated in patients with OSA (31, 84). However, in a controlled cross-over experiment, moderate alcohol consumption near bedtime was not demonstrated to be important in determining the level of nasal CPAP pressure necessary to prevent apneas and hypopneas in 14 men with moderate to severe OSA (85). That is, roughly the same level of pressure was required to eliminate OSA on nights when the men consumed alcohol as on nights when they did not.

Observational epidemiological studies have not consistently demonstrated statistically significant associations between self-reported typical alcohol consumption and OSA, with some investigation finding associations (36, 81) but others failing to demonstrate any (48, 86, 87). Although the studies that involve administration of alcohol near bedtime strongly suggest the potential of alcohol to have an acute adverse impact nocturnal respiration, the effect of long-term alcohol use patterns on the development or progression of OSA is unknown.

NASAL CONGESTION

Nasal congestion at night, whether due to allergic rhinitis, acute upper respiratory infection, or anatomy, has been linked to OSA in both experimental and epidemiological studies (88). A comparison of OSA in seasonal allergic rhinitis patients during and after a symptomatic period of allergen exposure indicated that AHI was higher and the apneic events were of longer duration during the period with rhinitis (89). Two epidemiological studies have found history of chronic nasal congestion to be strongly related to snoring. Survey data on a sample of 4927 men and women from the Wisconsin Sleep Cohort Study showed that people with chronic nighttime nasal congestion versus those without were twice as likely to be habitual snorers (p < .0001) (88). In addition, among the subsample studied by laboratory polysomnography (n = 911), people with nasal congestion attributed to allergies versus those without allergies were 1.8 (p = .04) times more likely to have AHI ≥ 15. However, no link with OSA was found for nasal resistance at bedtime measured by rhinometry. Stradling and Crosby, in their study of

Oxford men (n = 1001), also found nasal congestion to be linked to habitual snoring, but they did not find a link with OSA measured by home oximetry (44). If it is causal, the role of nasal congestion due to rhinitis in OSA is particularly important: congestion could be alleviated pharmacologically and, if congestion were indeed a primary cause of OSA, a significant portion of OSA could be reduced.

O━ Key points box 3.5

Evidence for risk factors

Risk factors: strong evidence

- Obesity
- Male sex
- Middle age and older
- Craniofacial abnormalities

Risk factors: some evidence

- Menopause
- Family member with OSAHS
- Smoking
- Nasal congestion at night

CONCLUSIONS

It is clear that the high prevalence of undiagnosed OSA, particularly mild OSA, poses difficult clinical and public health questions. The resources needed for screening, case finding, clinical evaluation, and treatment of the known burden of OSA, including snoring, would be daunting (13, 90, 91, 92, 93). Yet, investigations into the medical care and social costs of untreated OSA indicate that perhaps early detection and treatment of OSA would result in less cost overall (6, 7). A pressing question that clinicians will continue to face is, what should be done for the asymptomatic patient with mild OSA? Epidemiological population-based studies, particularly those with longitudinal design, have begun to provide some of the information needed to address this question. Of particular importance, from a public health standpoint, is identifying cost-effective prevention and intervention strategies. Crucial to this is the identification of modifiable risk factors and then quantifying the degree to which reduction in exposure could limit the occurrence of OSA. At present, there is preliminary evidence from longitudinal data that weight reduction may decrease OSA severity and progression, and it may perhaps prevent its occurrence. Nasal congestion, hormonal change with menopause, and smoking are all promising as modifiable risk factors, but more investigation is needed. With the documented ongoing trend for obesity and overweight to increase, it is vital to begin to think about risk factor reduction strategies to stem what could only be an increase in the already high prevalence of OSA.

REFERENCES

1. Young T, Palta M, Dempsey J, et al. The occurrence of sleep-disordered breathing among middle-aged adults. N Engl J Med 1993; 328:1230–1235.

2. Olson LG, King MT, Saunders NA, et al. Emerging issues in sleep-disordered breathing. Med J Aust 1996; 165:107–110.

3. Pack A, Gottschalk A. Mechanisms of ventilatory periodicities. Ann Biomed Engineering 1993; 21.

4. Baumel M, Maislin G, Pack A. Population and occupational screening for obstructive sleep apnea: are we there yet? Am J Respir Crit Med 1997; 155:9–14.

5. Pack A, Gurubhagavatula I. Economic implications of the diagnosis of obstructive sleep apnea. Ann Intern Med 1999; 130:533–534.

6. Kapur V, Blough D, Sandblom R, et al. The medical cost of undiagnosed sleep apnea. Sleep 1999; 22:749–755.

7. Bahammam A, Delaive K, Ronald J, et al. Health care utilization in males with obstructive sleep apnea syndrome two years after diagnosis and treatment. Sleep 1999; 22:740–747.

8. Lugaresi E, Cirignotta F, Geraldi R, et al. Snoring and sleep apnea: natural history of heavy snorers disease. In: Guilleminault C, Partinen M, eds. Obstructive sleep apnea sydrome: clinical research and treatment. New York: Raven Press, 1990: 25–36.

9. Guilleminault C, Stoohs R, Kim Y, et al. Upper airway sleep-disordered breathing in women. Ann Intern Med 1995; 122:493–501.

10. Young T, Finn L, Hla KM, et al. Hypertension in sleep-disordered breathing. Snoring as part of a dose-response relationship between sleep-disordered breathing and blood pressure. Sleep 1996; 19:S202–S205.

11. Strohl KP, Redline S. Recognition of obstructive sleep apnea. Am J Respir Crit Care Med 1996; 154:279–289.

12. American Academy of Sleep Medicine Task Force (W. Flemons, Chair). Sleep-related breathing disorders in adults: recommendations for syndrome definition and measurement techniques in clinical research. Sleep 1999; 22:667–689.

13. Stradling JR. Sleep-related breathing disorders. 1. Obstructive sleep apnoea: definitions, epidemiology, and natural history. Thorax 1995; 50:683–689.

14. Gislason T, Almqvist M, Eriksson G. Prevalence of sleep apnea syndrome among Swedish men. J Clin Epidemiol 1983; 41:571–576.

15. Martin RJ, Block AJ, Cohn MA, et al. Indications and standards for cardiopulmonary sleep studies. Sleep 1985; 8:371–379.

16. Redline S, Sander M. Hypopnea, a floating metric: implications for prevalence, morbidity estimates and case finding. Sleep 1997; 20:1209–1217.

17. Young T, Evans L, Finn L, et al. Estimation of the clinically diagnosed proportion of sleep apnea syndrome in middle-aged men and women. Sleep 1997; 20:705–706.

18. Lindberg E, Elmsry A, Gislason T, et al. Evolution of sleep apnea syndrome in sleepy snorers: a population-based prospective study. Am J Respir Crit Care Med 1999; 159:2024–2027.

19. Svanborg E, Larsson H. Development of nocturnal respiratory disturbance in untreated patients with obstructive sleep apnea syndrome. Chest 1993; 104:340–343.

20. Pendlebury ST, Pepin JL, Veale D, et al. Natural evolution of moderate sleep apnoea syndrome: significant progression over a mean of 17 months. Thorax 1997; 52:872–878.

21. Sforza E, Addati G, Cirignotta F, et al. Natural evolution of sleep apnoea syndrome: a five year longitudinal study. Eur Respir J 1994; 7:1765–1770.

22. Guilleminault C, Tilkian A, Dement WC. The sleep apnea syndromes. Annu Rev Med 1976; 27:4645–4849.

23. Redline S, Kump K, Tishler PV, et al. Gender differences in sleep-disordered breathing in a community-based sample. Am J Respir Crit Care Med 1994; 149:722–726.

24. Young T, Hutton R, Finn L, et al. The gender bias in sleep apnea diagnosis. Are women missed because they have different symptoms? Arch Intern Med 1996; 156:2445–2451.

25. Manber R, Armitage R. Sex, steroids and sleep: a review. Sleep 1999; 22:540–554.

26. McNamara S, Grunstein R, Sullivan CE. Obstructive sleep apnea. Thorax 1993; 48:754–764.

27. Schwab R. Sex differences and sleep apnoea. Thorax 1999; 54:284–285.

28. Leech JA, Onal E, Dulberg C, et al. A comparison of men and women with occlusive sleep apnea syndrome. Chest 1988; 94:983–988.

29. Wilhoit S, Suratt P. Obstructive sleep apnea in premenopausal women: a comparison with men and with postmenopausal women. Chest 1987; 91:654–658.

30. Guilleminault C, Quera-Salva M, Partinen M, et al. Women and the sleep apnea syndrome. Chest 1988; 93:104–109.

31. Bresnitz EA, Goldberg R, Kosinski RM. Epidemiology of obstructive sleep apnea. Epidemiol Rev 1994; 16:210–227.

32. Ancoli-Israel S, Kripke D, Klauber M, et al. Sleep-disordered breathing in community-dwelling elderly. Sleep 1991; 14:486–495.

33. Bliwise DL. Chronologic age, physiologic age and mortality in sleep apnea. Sleep 1996; 19:275–276.

34. Ancoli-Israel S. Are breathing disturbances in the elderly equivalent to sleep apnea syndrome? Sleep 1994; 17:77–83.

35. Young T. Sleep-disordered breathing in older adults: is it a condition distinct from that in middle-aged adults? Sleep 1996; 19:529–530.

36. Enright PL, Newman AB, Wahl PW, et al. Prevalence and correlates of snoring and observed apneas in 5,201 older adults. Sleep 1996; 19:531–538.

37. Philip P, Dealberto MJ, Dartigues JF, et al. Prevalence and correlates of nocturnal desaturations in a sample of elderly people. J Sleep Res 1997; 6:264–271.

38. Kripke DF, Ancoli-Israel S, Klauber MR, et al. Prevalence of sleep-disordered breathing in ages 40–64 years: a population-based survey. Sleep 1997; 20:65–76.

39. Davies RJ, Stradling JR. The epidemiology of sleep apnoea. Thorax 1996; 51:S65–S70.

40. Ancoli-Israel S, Klauber M, Stepnowsky C, et al. Sleep-disordered breathing in African-American elderly. Am J Respir Crit Care Med 1995; 152:1946–1949.

41. Redline S, Tichler P, Hans M, et al. Racial differences in sleep-disordered breathing in African-Americans and Caucasians. Am J Respir Crit Care Med 1997; 155:186–192.

42. Quan SF, Howard BV, Iber C, et al. The Sleep Heart Health Study: design, rationale, and methods. Sleep 1997; 20:1077–1085.

43. Strobel RJ, Rosen RC. Obesity and weight loss in obstructive sleep apnea: a critical review. Sleep 1996; 19:104–15.

44. Stradling JR, Crosby JH. Predictors and prevalence of obstructive sleep apnoea and snoring in 1001 middle aged men. Thorax 1991; 46:85–90.

45. Davies RJ, Ali NJ, Stradling JR. Neck circumference and other clinical features in the diagnosis of the obstructive sleep apnoea syndrome. Thorax 1992; 47:101–105.

46. Shelton KE, Woodson H, Gay S, et al. Pharyngeal fat in obstructive sleep apnea. Am Rev Respir Dis 1993; 148:462–466.

47. Ferini-Strambi L, Zucconi M, Palazzi S, et al. Snoring and nocturnal oxygen desaturations in an Italian middle-aged male population. Epidemiologic study with an ambulatory device. Chest 1994; 105:1759–1764.

48. Olson LG, King MT, Hensley MJ, et al. A community study of snoring and sleep-disordered breathing. Prevalence. Am J Respir Crit Care Med 1995; 152:711–716.

49. Mortimore IL, Marshall I, Wraith PK, et al. Neck and total body fat deposition in nonobese and obese patients with sleep apnea compared with that in control subjects. Am J Respir Crit Care Med 1998; 157:280–283.

50. Bearpark H, Elliot L, Grunstein R, et al. Occurrence and correlates of sleep-disordered breathing in the Australian town of Busselton: a preliminary analysis. Sleep 1993; 16:S3–S5.

51. Levinson PD, McGarvey ST, Carlisle CC, et al. Adiposity and cardiovascular risk factors in men with obstructive sleep apnea. Chest 1993; 103:1336–1342.

52. Millman RP, Carlisle CC, McGarvey ST, et al. Body fat distribution and sleep apnea severity in women. Chest 1995; 107:362–366.

53. Grunstein R, Wilcox I, Yang TS, et al. Snoring and sleep apnoea in men: association with central obesity and hypertension. Int J Obesity Related Metab Disord 1993; 17:533–540.

54. Shinohara E, Kihara S, Yamashita S, et al. Visceral fat accumulation as an important risk factor for obstructive sleep apnoea syndrome in obese subjects. J Intern Med 1997; 241:11–18.

55. Peppard P. A population-based longitudinal epidemiologic study of the association of sleep-disordered breathing with body habitus and elevated blood pressure. Doctoral Dissertation, Department of Preventive Medicine, University of Wisconsin-Madison, Madison, WI; 1999:219.

56. Harman EM, Wynne JW, Block AJ. The effect of weight loss on sleep-disordered breathing and oxygen desaturation in morbidly obese men. Chest 1982; 82:291–294.

57. Peiser J, Peretz L, Ovnat A, et al. Sleep apnea syndrome in the morbidly obese as an indication for weight reduction surgery. Ann Surg 1984; 199:125–129.

58. Charuzi I, Ovnat A, Peiser J, et al. The effect of surgical weight reduction on sleep quality in obesity-related sleep apnea syndrome. Surgery 1985; 97.535 538.

59. Rajala R, Partinen M, Sane T, et al. Obstructive sleep apnoea syndrome in morbidly obese patients. J Intern Med 1991; 230:125–129.

60. Pillar G, Peled R, Lavie P. Recurrence of sleep apnea without concomitant weight increase 7.5 years after weight reduction surgery. Chest 1994; 106:1702–1704.

61. Rubinstein I, Colapinto N, Rotstein LE, et al. Improvement in upper airway function after weight loss in patients with obstructive sleep apnea. Am Rev Respir Dis 1988; 138:1192–1195.

62. Pasquali R, Colella P, Cirignotta F, et al. Treatment of obese patients with obstructive sleep apnea syndrome (OSAS): effect of weight loss and interference of otorhinolaryngoiatric pathology. Int J Obesity 1990; 14:207–217.

63. Suratt PM, McTier RF, Findley LJ, et al. Effect of very-low-calorie diets with weight loss on obstructive sleep apnea. Am J Clin Nutr 1992; 56:182S–184S.

64. Suratt PM, McTier RF, Findley LJ, et al. Changes in breathing and the pharynx after weight loss in obstructive sleep apnea. Chest 1987; 92:631–637.

65. Kiselak J, Clark M, Pera V, et al. The association between hypertension and sleep apnea in obese patients. Chest 1993; 104:775–780.

66. Nahmias JS, Karetzky MS. Ventricular dysfunction and pulmonary function in OSA syndrome. N J Med 1993; 90:538–544.

67. Noseda A, Kempenaers C, Kerkhofs M, et al. Sleep apnea after 1 year domiciliary nasal-continuous positive airway pressure and attempted weight reduction. Potential for weaning from continuous positive airway pressure. Chest 1996; 109:138–143.

68. Smith PL, Gold AR, Meyers DA, et al. Weight loss in mildly to moderately obese patients with obstructive sleep apnea. Ann Intern Med 1985; 103:850–855.

69. Schwartz AR, Gold AR, Schubert N, et al. Effect of weight loss on upper airway collapsibility in obstructive sleep apnea. Am Rev Respir Dis 1991; 144:494–498.

70. Yoshizawa T, Akashiba T, Kurashina K, et al. Genetics and obstructive sleep apnea syndrome: a study of human leukocyte antigen (HLA) typing. Intern Med 1993; 32:94–97.

71. Strohl KP, Saunders NA, Feldman NT, et al. Obstructive sleep apnea in family members. N Engl J Med 1978; 299:969–973.

72. El Bayadi S, Millman RP, Tishler PV, et al. A family study of sleep apnea: physiological and anatomic interactions. Chest 1990; 98:554–559.

73. Redline S, Tosteson T, Tishler PV, et al. Familial aggregation of symptoms associated with sleep-related breathing disorders. Am Rev Respir Dis 1992; 145:440–444.

74. Pillar G, Lavie P. Assessment of the role of inheritance in sleep apnea syndrome. Am J Respir Crit Care Med 1995; 151:688–691.

75. Mathur R, Douglas NJ. Family studies in patients with the sleep apnea-hypopnea syndrome. Ann Intern Med 1995; 122:174–178.

76. Guilleminault C, Partinen M, Hollman K, et al. Familial aggregates in obstructive sleep apnea syndrome. Chest 1995; 107:1545–1551.

77. Redline S, Tishler PV, Tosteson TD, et al. The familial aggregation of obstructive sleep apnea. Am J Respir Crit Care Med 1995; 151:682–687.

78. Jamieson A, Guilleminault C, Partinen M, et al. Obstructive sleep apneic patients have craniomandibular abnormalities. Sleep 1986; 9:469–477.

79. Kushida CA, Efron B, Guilleminault C. A predictive morphometric model for the obstructive sleep apnea syndrome. Ann Intern Med 1997; 127:581–587.

80. Pack AI, Cola MF, Goldszmidt A, et al. Correlation between oscillations in ventilation and frequency content of the electroencephalogram. J Appl Physiol 1992; 72:985–992.

81. Jennum P, Sjol A. Snoring, sleep apnoea and cardiovascular risk factors: the MONICA II Study. Int J Epidemiol 1993; 22:439–444.

82. Wetter DW, Young TB, Bidwell TR, et al. Smoking as a risk factor for sleep-disordered breathing. Arch Intern Med 1994; 154:2219–2224.

83. Bloom JW, Kaltenborn WT, Quan SF. Risk factors in a general population for snoring. Importance of cigarette smoking and obesity. Chest 1988; 93:678–683.

84. Partinen M. Epidemiology of sleep disorders. In: Kryger MH, Roth T, Dement WC, eds. Principles and practice of sleep medicine, 2nd edn. Philadelphia: W.B. Saunders Cy; 1994: 437–452.

85. Teschler H, Berthon-Jones M, Wessendorf T, et al. Influence of moderate alcohol consumption on obstructive sleep apnoea with and without AutoSet nasal CPAP therapy. Eur Respir J 1996; 9:2371–2377.

86. Bearpark H, Elliott L, Grunstein R, et al. Snoring and sleep apnea: a population study in Australian men. Am J Respir Crit Care Med 1995; 151:1459–1465.

87. Worsnop CJ, Naughton MT, Barter CE, et al. The prevalence of obstructive sleep apnea in hypertensives. Am J Respir Crit Care Med 1998; 157:111–115.

88. Young T, Finn L, Kim H. Nasal obstruction as a risk factor for sleep-disordered breathing. J Allergy Clin Immunol 1997; 99:S757–S762.

89. McNichols WT, Tarlo S, Cole P. Obstructive apneas during sleep in patients with seasonal allergic rhinitis. Am Rev Respir Dis 1982; 126:625–628.

90. Phillipson EA. Sleep apnea—a major public health problem. N Engl J Med 1993; 328:1271–1273.

91. Grunstein RR. Sleep apnoea—evolution and doubt. Eur Respir J 1994; 7:1741–1743.

92. Lavie P. Incidence of sleep apnea in a presumably healthy working population. Sleep 1983; 6:312–318.

93. Marin J, Gascon J, Gispert J. Prevalence of sleep apnea syndrome in the Spanish adult population. Int J Epidemiol 1997; 26:381–386.

4 PATHOGENESIS OF OBSTRUCTIVE SLEEP APNEA SYNDROME

Atul Malhotra and David P White

INTRODUCTION

Obstructive sleep apnea syndrome (OSAS) is a common disorder, affecting at least 4% of men, and 2% of women in North America (1). It is characterized by repetitive collapse of the pharyngeal airway during sleep, with each episode generally being terminated by arousal. The cessation (or substantial reduction) in airflow is associated with hypoxia and hypercarbia, while the respiratory arousal leads to sleep fragmentation and the consequences of sleep deprivation (2–4). Although the exact mechanisms for these events remain somewhat unclear, considerable work has been done addressing this pathophysiology. On the basis largely of imaging studies, patients with OSAS appear to have diminished pharyngeal anatomy, as evidenced by reduced luminal cross-sectional area and increased soft tissue mass around the airway (5–9). During wakefulness, airway patency can be maintained by increased neural activation of pharyngeal dilator muscles (10). However, at sleep onset, muscle activity falls, allowing upper airway collapse, most commonly at the level of the soft palate. Epidemiological factors that increase the risk of OSAS include obesity, aging, male sex, and alcohol consumption (11–23). In this chapter, we discuss the current state of knowledge regarding the pathogenesis of OSAS, including some discussion of the potential influence of these epidemiological variables on these mechanisms.

PHARYNGEAL ANATOMY

Some investigators speculate that the evolution of speech in humans, which demanded substantial laryngeal motility, led to the loss of rigid support of the hyoid bone, which is anchored to the styloid processes in most mammals. This rendered the pharyngeal airway of humans largely dependent on soft tissue and dilator muscle activation to maintain patency (24). The portion of the upper airway most vulnerable to collapse lies between the choanae and the epiglottis (Fig 4.1A,B).

During wakefulness, pharyngeal dilator muscles are generally able to maintain patency in this portion of the airway regardless of anatomy. However, the extent to which the airway is dependent on muscle activation is quite variable. A person with an anatomically large airway may have minimal requirement for pharyngeal muscle activity, whereas a patient with a small one may be critically dependent on dilator function to maintain patency. Thus, pharyngeal airway patency requires an interaction between anatomy and muscle physiology.

The majority of the evidence supporting an anatomic abnormality in OSAS patients is derived from imaging and endoscopic studies. Haponik et al. originally reported a substantially smaller minimal pharyngeal cross-sectional airway area in apnea patients than in controls when imaged during wakefulness, although the groups were not controlled for weight (5). Since this original report, numerous authors, using a variety of imaging techniques (computed tomography, magnetic resonance imaging, acoustic reflection, cephalometrics), have demonstrated a small pharyngeal airway in apnea patients, with the smallest airway luminal size generally occurring at the level of the velopharynx (behind the soft palate) in both patients and controls (6–9, 25–32). However, these studies suffer from two important limitations. First, they have focused, for the most part, on airway luminal size with little attention to airway soft tissue structures. Second, during wakefulness, airway lumen reflects not pure anatomy but the interaction between anatomy and muscle activation as stated above. Therefore, the available information on the determinants of upper airway anatomy is somewhat limited.

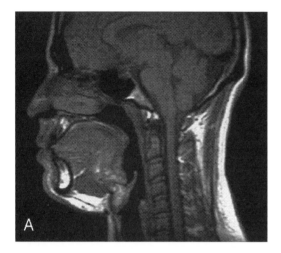

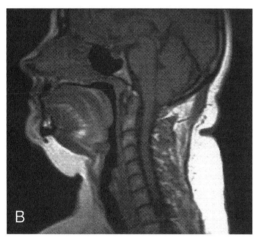

Fig 4.1 *Midsagittal MR image shows differences between normal subject (A) and patient with OSA (B). Note the limited airway lumen behind the soft palate of the apnea patient as compared to the normal subject. (From Schwab RJ. Upper airway imaging. Clin Chest Med 1998; 19[1]:33–54, 1998.)*

Variables affecting upper airway luminal size are likely numerous and include obesity, craniofacial deformity (e.g. retrognathia), jaw position, tongue size, tonsillar enlargement (especially in children) (33) and other, yet to be defined influences. As obesity is a strong determinant of sleep apnea prevalence, its influence on airway anatomy has been studied, with controversial results. Some authors have demonstrated preferential deposition of fat in the upper airway of apneics persons as compared to weight-matched controls, whereas others have found fat distribution to be nonspecific with no real upper airway propensity (34–37). As a result, the precise explanation for the rise in prevalence of OSAS with increasing weight remains to be elucidated, but almost certainly it relates to changing pharyngeal anatomy, as is discussed below (38).

The most definitive evidence supporting an anatomical abnormality in OSAS patients comes from Isono et al. (39). In this study, the authors measured the critical pressure (Pcrit) required to close (completely collapse) the upper airway of humans undergoing general anesthesia with complete neuromuscular paralysis. Under the condition of absent neuromuscular activity, the authors observed a positive Pcrit in OSAS patients, meaning that the airway was collapsed at atmospheric pressure and required positive pressure to reopen (39). Normal controls, on the other hand, had patent airways at atmospheric pressure and required suction (negative pressure) to collapse the pharynx (Fig 4.2). This observation strongly supports the existence of a biomechanical abnormality of the upper airway in apnea patients. In addition, the authors showed a strong correlation between Pcrit and the oxygen desaturation index, indicating a clear relationship between airway anatomy and apnea severity. Endoscopic evaluation also demonstrated a larger cross-sectional area of the velopharynx in controls compared to apneic patients, again suggesting deficient anatomy in the latter (39). One possible limitation of this otherwise unique and persuasive study is the potential development of atelectasis and reduced lung volume under conditions of anesthesia and hyperoxia (40–43). As is discussed below, lung volume can have a substantial influence on upper airway size, especially in apneic persons (28). In the Isono et al. study, the extent to which atelectasis and hyperoxia influenced lung volume and therefore upper airway size is potentially an important issue. However, based on multiple imaging and endoscopic studies, airway lumen size is clearly compromised in most apneic subjects.

The measurement of an upper airway Pcrit during sleep (not anesthesia) is increasingly appreciated as a useful measure of an individual person's propensity or vulnerability to pharyngeal collapse (44–47). The concept that apneic persons have an upper airway more prone to collapse during sleep is supported by the observation that OSAS patients often require positive pressure to maintain

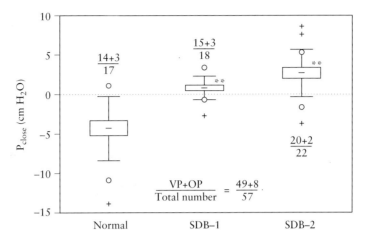

Fig 4.2 *Box plots illustrate observed closing pressure. Distribution of sites of primary closure was provided for each of the 3 groups: normals, SDB1 (patients with mild apnea), and SDB2 (patients with severe apnea). Mean values are indicated by horizontal bar within each box; bars above and below each box represent standard error. End of vertical line denotes standard deviation. ° or + symbols, outliers. VP, velopharynx; OP, oropharynx. **p < 0.01 versus normal group. (From Isono S, Remmers JE, Tanaka A, et al. Anatomy of pharynx in patients with obstructive sleep apnea and in normal subjects. J Appl Physiol 1997; 82[4]:1319–1326).*

airway patency during sleep (i.e., positive Pcrit, need for continuous positive airway pressure [CPAP] therapy during sleep). Patients with mild disease or simple snoring tend to have a slightly negative Pcrit, whereas normal controls have a substantially negative Pcrit (–10 to –15 cm H_2O). These Pcrit measurements, which reflect both anatomy and neuromuscular activity, also support an upper airway anatomic abnormality among patients with OSAS (48–52).

In addition to airway size, airway shape may also be an important determinant of upper airway collapsibility. Several studies have reported an oval shape of the pharyngeal airway in persons with OSAS when compared to controls (i.e., a relatively high anteroposterior–lateral luminal airway dimension) (25, 53). Leiter has also suggested a reduced ability of muscles to dilate the pharynx when it is oval in shape (54). Whether this shape represents an important component of apnea pathogenesis or is simply a marker of fat deposition in the fat pads lateral to the airway remains to be elucidated.

Finally, only recently have the soft tissues surrounding the upper airway been evaluated with the best studies utilizing magnetic resonance (MR) imaging techniques (6–9, 26, 55–57). Using sophisticated analyses of soft tissue variables, Schwab et al. (26) reported a significantly and

substantially increased thickness of the lateral pharyngeal walls, independent of fat pad thickness (at the level of the minimum axial airway lumen). This finding is helpful in explaining the reduced lateral diameter of the airway lumen in apneic patients as compared to non–weight-matched controls. No important skeletal differences were observed, implicating soft tissues as the major anatomical difference between apneic persons and controls. Schwab et al. (8, 9) have argued therefore that lateral wall thickening and ultimately collapse are important components in the pathogenesis of OSAS. Whether this will ultimately prove to be the case is unclear at this time. However, all evidence to date suggests that inadequate pharyngeal anatomy is an important component in the pathogenesis of OSAS.

CONTROL OF UPPER AIRWAY PATENCY

The crucial determinant of patency of the upper airway is the transmural pressure (Ptm). This pressure represents the difference between the luminal pressure and the surrounding tissue pressure (Pti). Although Pti is not often measured, it is useful conceptually to consider the pressures both inside and outside the pharyngeal lumen. In the absence of flow, the luminal pressure is atmospheric (i.e., zero).

curto respiratorio - mm inspiratorios

With the onset of inspiration, luminal pressure becomes subatmospheric (i.e., negative), favoring upper airway collapse. Pharyngeal dilator muscle activity therefore must increase to maintain patency. During expiration the luminal pressure becomes positive, thereby supporting the airway even in the absence of phasic muscle activity. In this section, we review the factors involved in the maintenance of upper airway patency, including muscles, lung volume, vascular effects, and timing of neuromuscular activation.

PHARYNGEAL DILATOR MUSCLES

Although the muscles responsible for maintaining upper airway patency and the mechanisms controlling their activity are at best understood only incompletely, certain generalizations can be made. The muscles of prime importance fall into three groups: (1) the muscle of the tongue (genioglossus), (2) the muscles influencing hyoid position (geniohyoid, sternohyoid, etc.), and (3) the muscles of the palate (tensor palatini, levator palatini, etc.) (58). The activity of many of these muscles resembles that of the diaphragm with increased activation during inspiration, thus stiffening or dilating the upper airway and counteracting the collapsing influence of intraluminal negative pressure (59). These are referred to as inspiratory phasic upper airway muscles, the best studied of which is the genioglossus. Inspiratory phasic muscle activation is likely influenced or produced by central respiratory neurons with an inspiratory phasic pattern of activation. Other upper airway muscles, such as the tensor palatini, do not generally demonstrate inspiratory phasic activity but remain at a relatively constant level of activation throughout the respiratory cycle (60). These muscles are called tonic, or postural muscles, and are also thought to play an important role in maintaining patency of the airway. Such pharyngeal muscles are likely influenced not by central respiratory neurons with primarily inspiratory firing but by neurons with a more continuous activation pattern.

The activity of pharyngeal dilator muscles is influenced by a variety of stimuli, the best studied being the negative pressure reflex (NPR). The application of negative pressure to the pharynx leads to a substantial increase in pharyngeal dilator muscle activity, thereby reducing the tendency for collapse. Local anesthesia studies in humans have determined that the major afferents for this negative pressure reflex are nasal and laryngeal (61–65). Although the NPR clearly can be induced with supraphysiological

pressures, the role this reflex plays in regulating upper airway muscle activity during normal tidal breathing in apnea patients and nonapneic controls is unclear. However, recent studies have demonstrated that pharyngeal anesthesia in normal subjects can diminish not only the NPR but basal genioglossal activation as well, suggesting an important role for local reflex control of dilator muscle activation during tidal breathing (66).

Arterial chemistry (PO_2 and PCO_2) may also influence upper airway muscle function. It has been known for years that progressive hypoxia leads to increased activity of pharyngeal muscles with a similar pattern to that of the diaphragm (67). More recently, McEvoy et al. (68) studied normal subjects under conditions of sustained and repetitive isocapnic hypoxia and found that repetitive intermittent hypoxia (RIH, similar to what apneic patients would experience) led to suppression of genioglossal electromyographic (EMG) activity, whereas no such suppression was observed with sustained hypoxia. This suppression of genioglossus activity with RIH may be one mechanism for the ongoing loss of upper airway patency experienced by untreated OSAS patients (68). This may also at least in part explain the improvement in apnea hypopnea index (AHI) experienced by some OSA patients with oxygen therapy alone (69).

Similarly, hypercapnia has been studied in both animal and human models and has been shown to substantially increase genioglossus muscle activity. Onal et al. (70) have demonstrated increased genioglossal activity with CO_2 rebreathing in humans with a fairly linear relationship between the genioglossal and diaphragmatic EMG (70). These authors suggested that both the diaphragm and genioglossus muscle share similar control mechanisms and that pharyngeal dilator activity was intimately related to the control of ventilation. More recently, Schwartz et al. (71) investigated the effects of hypercapnia on the isolated upper airway of a hyperoxic dog and found important increases in both inspiratory flow rate and inspiratory phasic muscle activity, although no change in tonic activity was observed. Therefore, carbon dioxide can importantly influence pharyngeal muscle dilator activity and airway patency. .

Although less well studied, several other physiological influences on pharyngeal muscle activity have been reported. As is discussed below, female hormones, particularly progesterone, seems to augment genioglossal activation and may protect women, to some extent, from the development of apnea (72, 73). In addition, lung inflation, probably through working through vagal mechanisms, inhibits dilator muscle activity (74, 75). Phasic volume feedback inhibits genioglossal activation whereas reducing inflation augments the activity of this muscle. As a result, upper airway muscles are under the control of numerous physiological control systems.

NEUROMUSCULAR COMPENSATION

Evidence that some combination of the mechanisms described above can lead to neuromuscular compensation for deficient pharyngeal anatomy in apnea patients comes from Mezzanotte et al. (76). These authors reported OSAS patients to have substantially greater genioglossal and tensor palatini activation than normal controls (Fig 4.3). These findings support the concept of inadequate anatomy in OSAS patients, who require increased dilator muscle activity during wakefulness to preserve luminal patency. Hendricks et al. (77) have subsequently also shown upper airway dilator muscle hyperactivity in English bulldogs, an animal model of obstructive sleep apnea (77). In addition, Series et al. (78) reported the musculus uvulae of human apnea patients both to be hypertrophic and to exhibit increased anaerobic enzyme capacity when compared to nonapneic snorers. Both findings suggest a highly trained muscle, presumably from the increased activation required by deficient anatomy.

The stimulus to this neuromuscular compensation in the apnea patient remains unclear at this time, although the negative pressure reflex has been proposed as a likely candidate. In favor of this is the observation that positive airway pressure can substantially reduce muscle activation in apnea patients during wakefulness (79, 80). In addition, as is discussed below, both the negative pressure reflex and neuromuscular compensation are substantially attenuated during sleep (63–65). On the other hand, apnea patients have minimally increased negative pressure in the upper airway during normal awake tidal breathing, with considerably greater negative pressure generally being required to activate the reflex. As a result, the relationship between the reflex and the augmented muscle activity of the apnea patient remains unclear.

It has even been suggested that the increased propensity for collapse of the upper airway in apneic persons could be a product of an abnormality in this negative pressure reflex. Mortimore and Douglas (81) reported that the response of

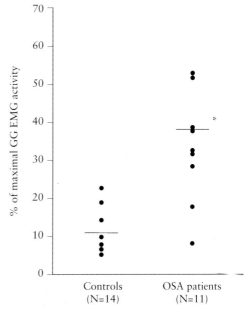

Fig 4.3 *Peak phasic genioglossus EMG activity. Under basal conditions, the genioglossus functions at a higher percentage of maximum in OSA patients than controls, *p < 0.05 versus controls. (From Mazzanote WS, Tangel DJ, White DP. Waking genioglossal electromyogram in sleep apnea patients versus normal controls [a neuromuscular compensatory mechanism]. J Clin Invest 1992; 89:1571–1579.)*

the levator palatini and palatoglossus muscles to negative pressure is compromised in apneic persons as compared to control subjects. After treatment of these patients with nightly CPAP, they were able to demonstrate a significant increase in the NPR of these two muscles (81). The mechanism of improvement with CPAP therapy (e.g., reduced upper airway edema, decreased sleep deprivation, etc.) is unclear. Despite these observations, apnea patients obviously have some mechanism driving neuromuscular compensation during wakefulness, yielding greater muscle activation. Whether this is the negative pressure reflex or some other mechanism awaits further study.

INFLUENCE OF SLEEP ON PHARYNGEAL MUSCLE ACTIVATION AND CONTROL

The influence of sleep on the mechanisms described above has not been thoroughly studied, yet, it is of obvious importance in the pathogenesis of obstructive sleep apnea. The best studied pharyngeal muscle control mechanism is the negative pressure reflex (NPR). This reflex has been demonstrated by several laboratories to be substantially attenuated if not lost during stable non-rapid eye movement (NREM) sleep (63–65, 82) (Fig 4.4). A more recent study has observed negative pressure to actually inhibit upper airway muscle activity during REM sleep, a reversal of the waking response. These same authors examined the NPR during the wake-sleep transition (first five breaths after the alpha-theta electroencephalogram [EEG] transition) and reported a decrement in muscle responsiveness, although this change did not reach statistical significance (83). Therefore, we might conclude that this

reflex is brisk awake, mildly diminished in the wake-sleep transition, substantially reduced during stable NREM sleep, and actually inhibitory during REM sleep. To the extent that this reflex drives neuromuscular compensation in the apnea patient, these changes during sleep could be quite important (Fig 4.5).

The chemical (PO_2, PCO_2) influence on upper airway muscle activity during sleep has not been extensively studied. However, the observations that genioglossal muscle activity rises during sleep in normal subjects after the placement of an inspiratory resistive load and over the course of an apnea in OSAS patients suggests an intact CO_2 response. In both instances, muscle activity increases over a time course, consistent with hypoventilation with

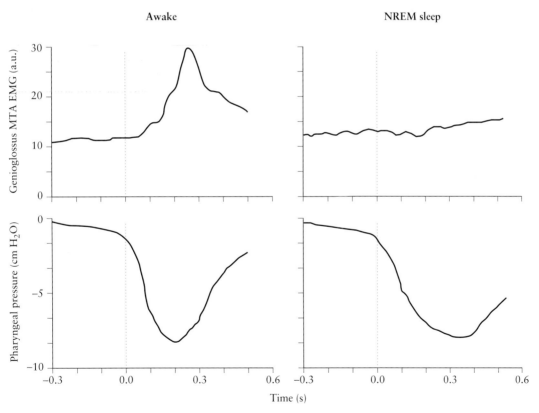

Fig 4.4 *Group signal averaged genioglossus muscle response. Mean group signal averaged response for the genioglossus moving time average (MTA) EMG and pharyngeal pressure for n = 5 both awake and during NREM sleep. Vertical dashed lines denote onset of the negative pressure pulse. Note large genioglossus EMG response during wakefulness which is markedly reduced during sleep. (From Wheatley JR, Mezzanotte WS, Tangel DJ, et al. Influence of sleep on genioglossus muscle activation by negative pressure in normal men. Am Rev Respir Dis 1993; 148[3]:597–605.)*

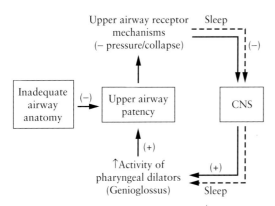

Fig 4.5 The Pathogenesis of Pharyngeal Obstruction in OSA. Inadequate upper airway anatomy negatively influences patency. During wakefulness this may trigger upper airway reflexes through the central nervous system (CNS) to increase the activity of pharyngeal dilator muscles, leading to increases upper airway patency. During sleep (dashed line), however, these reflex mechanisms are attenuated ultimately leading to the loss of pharyngeal dilator activity, which has a negative impact on pharyngeal patency.

subsequently rising PCO_2 (60, 84–86). The hypoxic response, on the other hand, has been minimally studied, but may be interactive with hypercapnia in both of the situations described (87–92).

The observations described above may also help explain the reported changes in genioglossal muscle activity during sleep reported in normal subjects. In a normal person a transient decrement in ventilation and genioglossal muscle activity occurs at sleep onset, which may represent a loss of wakefulness stimuli on muscle activity (93). However, over time, genioglossal activity recovers and is generally reported to be greater during stable NREM sleep than during wakefulness (84). This likely represents a response to the rising CO_2 level, which occurs during sleep even in normal subjects, primarily owing to increased upper airway resistance and a reduced ability to respond to such increments in resistance during sleep. Therefore, in a normal subject during stable NREM sleep ventilation is reduced, upper airway resistance is increased, PCO_2 is above awake levels, and genioglossal muscle activity is elevated (94, 95). Therefore, we cannot implicate falling genioglossal activity as the cause of increased airflow resistance in

normal controls during NREM sleep. During REM sleep, the genioglossal EMG level is quite similar to that seen during NREM sleep, other than during actual eye movements, during which there is transient inhibition of muscle activity (88, 96).

The cause of the increased upper airway resistance in normal subjects during sleep is unclear, but it has been associated with changes in the activity of other dilator muscles such as the tensor palatini. This nonphasic muscle loses activity at sleep onset, with further decrements as NREM sleep progresses, and has been correlated with increments in resistance (97). It would seem, therefore, that pharyngeal dilator muscles may behave quite differently during sleep, with some losing activity (tensor palatini), leading to increased resistance and hypoventilation, whereas others (genioglossus) respond to the resultant rise in PCO_2 (84).

In the apnea patient, the upper airway muscles behave quite differently. In general, a substantial loss of muscle activity (both genioglossus and tensor palatini) occurs at sleep onset associated with the development of an apnea or hypopnea (98) (Fig. 4.6). Over the course of the apnea, as hypoxia and hypercapnia develop, muscle activity rises until the patient ultimately awakens, which is associated with a huge burst of dilator muscle activity, thereby reestablishing airway patency. This process is then repeated again and again over the course of the night. It has been argued that this loss of muscle activity at sleep onset in the apnea patient represents a loss of the neuromuscular compensation present during wakefulness and is largely responsible for pharyngeal collapse. It has also been suggested, as addressed above, that these events occur due to a sleep-induced loss of the NPR, which may drive such neuromuscular compensation during wakefulness. However, to date it has not been convincingly demonstrated that neuromuscular compensation is a direct product of this reflex or that the reflex is immediately lost at sleep onset. Therefore, further investigation will be required to firmly document the relationship between sleep, the NPR, and muscle activation in the apnea patient. However, some association seems likely.

Finally, to complete a discussion of pharyngeal muscle function, some comment on the pharyngeal constrictors seems appropriate, as these constrictor muscles extend from the nasopharynx to the epiglottis. When activated these muscles tend to reduce pharyngeal luminal size,

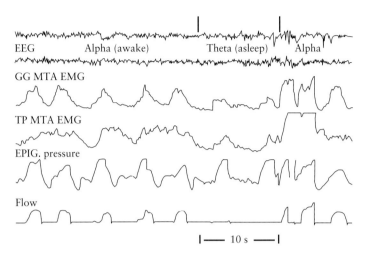

Fig 4.6 *Raw data demonstrating the effect of the alpha-theta transition on genioglossus (GG) and tensor palatini (TP) EMG in a representative OSA patient. At sleep onset there is a substantial decrement in both GG and TP EMG associate with an obstructive event. EEG, Electroencephalogram; MTA, moving time average; Epig. Press., epiglottal pressure. (From Mezzanote WS, Tangel DJ, White DP. Influence of sleep onset on upper-airway muscle activity in apnea patients versus normal controls. Am J Respir Crit Care Med 1996; 153[6 Pt 1]: 1880–1887.)*

although this may not always be the case. Kuna et al. (99, 100) have studied these muscles in normal controls and apneic persons and observed pharyngeal constrictors to activate in a similar fashion to pharyngeal dilator muscles during spontaneous and induced apneas (i.e., their activity does not increase during apnea, thereby contributing to pharyngeal closure). As a result, constrictor activity was not necessary to induce airway closure during NREM sleep (99, 100). This and other studies are convincing that constrictors likely do not play an important role in the pathogenesis of apnea.

OTHER FACTORS INFLUENCING UPPER AIRWAY PATENCY BOTH AWAKE AND ASLEEP

Although muscular factors are clearly important in the pathogenesis of OSAS, nonmuscular influences are also of interest and several are discussed here. First, the tissue pressure that surrounds the airway can compromise pharyngeal patency when it exceeds intraluminal pressure. In obese persons, the effect of gravity in the supine posture may lead to an increase in this tissue pressure, thus favoring luminal collapse (101). Studies in rabbit models using lard-filled bags placed on the neck demonstrated airway

compromise mediated by an increase in tissue pressure (102). This concept is supported by the frequent observation that apneas are more common in the supine posture (103–107). Tissue pressure can be reduced by sleeping in the lateral decubitus posture and minimized further in the upright position (107, 108). Thus tissue pressure, which can be influenced by position, may importantly affect apnea frequency.

Second, upper airway patency may be influenced by blood flow or vascular volume. Vascular perfusion is a dynamic process that can change quickly, leading to anatomical changes. Several studies have assessed the importance of blood flow in determining airway size, with differing results depending on the experimental model and the duration of perfusion changes. Chronic overperfusion or high central venous pressures may contribute to edema within the upper airway and potentially to luminal compromise (109). More acute changes may increase the stiffness of the upper airway, potentially making it less collapsible (e.g., during hypercarbia (110–112)). Finally, thigh strapping, which reduces preload, has been shown to increase the size of the upper airway (113). However, although blood flow may influence pharyngeal airway size and collapsibility, its importance in the pathogenesis of obstructive sleep apnea is currently speculative.

Finally, lung volume may importantly influence airway size and collapsibility. It has been clearly demonstrated in humans that the upper airway lumen is larger at high lung volumes and relatively smaller at low ones (28). This influence of lung volume on upper airway size is particularly pronounced in persons with OSAS. This may be quite important in obese subjects, who, especially in the supine posture, have a tendency for end expiratory volume to approach the residual volume of the lung owing to basilar atelectasis as well as abdominal weight limiting diaphragmatic excursion (114–117). This could have a substantial impact on upper airway dimensions. Most investigators believe that this effect of lung volume on pharyngeal patency is a product of tracheal traction or tug on the airway (118, 119). With minimal traction (low lung volume), the airway becomes quite compliant and collapsible while increasing traction stiffens the airway, making collapse less likely. This concept has been convincingly demonstrated in animals with a recent study suggesting that pharyngeal dilator muscles are ineffective at low lung volumes and increasingly effective as lung volume or tracheal traction increases (120). In addition, Begle et al. (74) have investigated the relationship between pulmonary resistance and lung volume during NREM sleep in normal subjects. Using a tank respirator, these authors demonstrated that increased lung volume leads to a decreased pulmonary resistance, independent of the activity of pharyngeal muscle dilators (74). They concluded that the change in resistance was mediated by traction on tissues of the neck caused by descent of mediastinal structures. Therefore, sleep-induced decrements in lung volume may importantly influence pharyngeal size and the ability of dilator muscles to maintain patency. One mechanism by which CPAP may work is by increased lung volume.

CENTRAL NEUROMUSCULAR MECHANISMS OF APNEA GENERATION

Although local factors are clearly important in the pathogenesis of upper airway collapse, changes in muscle activation and probably lung volume are obviously a product of changes in the central neural modulation. As a result, a number of investigators have focused on central neural mechanisms to explain the pathogenesis of OSAS. In this section, we review two neurotransmitter systems (sero-

tonin and adrenaline) as they relate to sleep apnea. In addition, we review the available evidence for differences in basic ventilatory control between normal subjects and apneic patients.

Serotonin (or 5-HT) has been proposed as both an important mediator of upper airway muscle activation and as a cause of falling dilator muscle activity during sleep. This interest in serotonin has evolved from a number of observations. First, serotonin is a known modulator of skeletal muscle activation in other (not upper airway) system (121, 122). Second, the raphe serotonergic neurons project to the hypoglossal motor nucleus (which controls genioglossal activity) and to other motor nuclei controlling pharyngeal dilator muscles (123). Third, both in vivo and in vitro studies indicate that 5-HT is excitatory to hypoglossal motor neurons (Fig 4.7). Fourth, the firing frequency of these raphe serotonergic neurons is highly dependent on state, with reduced firing during drowsiness, further reductions during slow wave sleep, and minimal firing during REM sleep. Therefore, 5-HT is a model neurotransmitter to downregulate to an important extent pharyngeal dilator muscle activity during sleep (124–130).

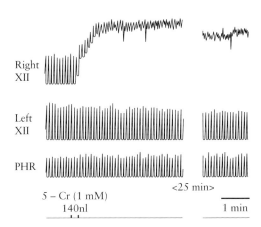

Fig 4.7 The stimulatory effect of 5-CT (serotonin agonist) on output by the hypoglossal motor nucleus via the hypoglossal nerve (Right XII, Left XII). This cranial nerve innervates important pharyngeal dilators such as the genioglossus muscle. (From Kubin L, Tojima H, Davies RO, et al. Serotonergic excitatory drive to hypoglossal motoneuron in the decerebrate cat. Neurosci Lett 1992; 139:243–248.)

Despite these observations, the importance of serotonin in this process must be questioned for a number of reasons (131, 132). First, genioglossal activity in normal subjects and hypoglossal motor neuron firing frequency in chronically instrumented cats is minimally, if at all, reduced during NREM sleep despite substantial decrements in raphe neuronal firing. Second, the decrement in dilator muscle activity in apnea patients occurring at sleep onset takes place very quickly (seconds) whereas the reductions in raphe neuron activity are quite slow (minutes). Finally, attempts to increase muscle activity during wakefulness and sleep with serotonin enhancing agents (mainly selective serotonin re-uptake inhibitors) have had minimal impact on apnea frequency in patients or on muscle EMG in normal controls (133–135). On the other hand, Veasey et al. (136) have demonstrated decreased dilator muscle activity and decreased airway size in English bulldogs after the administration of serotonin antagonists. As a result, serotonin remains the focus of considerable attention and research in this area.

Similarly, noradrenergic neurons in the locus ceruleus (LC) and pons show state dependence with progressive reductions in firing frequency from wakefulness to NREM sleep to REM sleep. These LC neurons project throughout the brain, including the hypoglossal nucleus, where they are thought to increase the excitability of the hypoglossal neurons. The withdrawal of this excitatory stimulus at the onset of sleep would be one potential explanation for the decrement in pharyngeal dilator activity seen at that time. However, the importance of noradrenaline (norepinephrine) in the control of upper airway muscles awake and asleep and in the pathogenesis of OSAS remains unclear, as this neuromodulatory system has been less thoroughly studied than the serotonergic one. As a result, further studies are needed of both modulatory systems and of the interaction between the two (124, 137–143).

Finally, the importance of variability in chemoresponsiveness (responses to hypoxia and hypercapnea) in the pathogenesis of obstructive sleep apnea has been argued for years. It seems clear that there are no consistent differences in chemoresponsiveness between apnea patients and controls particularly when nonhypercapneic patients are considered (144–146). Small differences in these responses also seem to play little role in the development of obstructive apnea, although they may be important in the pathogenesis of central apnea and Cheyne-Stokes respirations (145–150). Whether subtle abnormalities in ventilatory control stability contribute to the waxing and waning of ventilation characteristic of OSAS is debatable, with some data suggesting that apnea patients do demonstrate such instability (151). However, the true importance of these observations is unclear at this time with upper airway anatomy or motor control remaining the predominant focus of pathophysiological studies.

PERPETUATING MECHANISMS

Once a person develops OSAS, there are a number of events that perpetuate upper airway collapse, which are discussed in this section (152). First, the repetitive collapse of the upper airway and the vibration associated with snoring could lead to edema formation on the basis of mechanical trauma (153). Edema in the upper airway could reduce luminal area, thereby contributing to the propensity for collapse. Several studies support this concept. Recently, Anastassov et al. have confirmed the presence of such edema in the upper airway of OSAS patients using histological techniques (154). Furthermore, using cephalometrics, Mortimore and Douglas (81) measured the size of the posterior air space of apneic subjects before and after CPAP therapy. An increase in the posterior air space in these persons was observed after treatment with CPAP, which they speculated to result from resolution of edema. In addition, as discussed previously, edema could affect mucosal neural processes such as the negative pressure reflex. As stated previously, Mortimore and Douglas demonstrated an increase in this reflex in apnea patients after CPAP treatment, and they speculated that decreased edema was the explanation (81). Thus trauma-induced upper airway edema could negatively impact on pharyngeal patency in a variety of ways.

Second, trauma or injury to upper airway dilator muscles has been proposed as a potential perpetuating event in sleep apnea. In theory, the upper airway muscles of apneic persons could respond to their increased workload in one of several ways. They could become stronger, more trained muscles or they could deteriorate secondary to fatigue, overuse, or eccentric contraction (Fig 4.8). There are some data supporting these possibilities. In bulldogs with sleep apnea, Petrof et al. described a 'pharyngeal myopathy of the loaded upper airway' (155) characterized by a greater proportion of fast fibers in the dilator muscles compared to control animals and a higher proportion of histologically abnormal

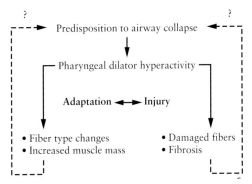

Fig 4.8 A proposed model for the possible role of activity-induced upper airway muscle remodeling and injury in the pathogenesis of OSA. Predisposed anatomy leads to compensatory dilator activity. This hyperactivity leads to muscle structure changes that may be adaptive or injurious. A vicious cycle may be produced if adaptive muscle changes further narrow the pharynx or if injury to dilators compromises their ability to maintain airway patency. (From Petrof BJ, Hendricks JC, Pack AI. Does upper airway muscle injury trigger a vicious cycle in obstructive sleep apnea. A hypothesis. Sleep 1996; 19[6]:465–471.)

fibers, consistent with an overuse myopathy. In addition, quantitative MR imaging studies in these bulldogs by Schotland et al. also demonstrated edema and fibrosis in the upper airway muscles (156). Petrof et al. have argued that eccentric contraction (muscle lengthening during active contraction) is likely to produce damage, with myositis and myocyte necrosis having been demonstrated in animal models of such eccentric contraction (157). Thus, animal studies suggest that upper airway muscle damage is possible with sleep apnea.

Human studies examining upper airway muscle histology are somewhat limited. Series et al. (78) examined the musculus uvulae of snorers and apneic patients undergoing uvulopalatopharyngoplasty (UPPP), finding snorers to have a higher proportion of fast IIa fibers, higher protein content, and higher levels of anaerobic enzymes, consistent with adaptation to increased load and hypoxia. In addition, in a recent study Friberg et al. (158) reported muscle fiber type differences between normal subjects, snorers, and apneic persons. These authors observed significantly increased hypertrophied or atrophied fibers in the palatopharyngeus muscle of apnea patients compared to normal control (158). Moreover, they demonstrated a significant correlation between the degree of morphological muscle abnormality and the severity of obstructed breathing. These authors speculated that the vibration trauma of habitual snoring could initiate a local muscle lesion, which they believe most likely to be neurogenic in origin. This concept is supported by a previous study of Edstrom et al. (159), who provide some evidence for a neurogenic lesion in the palatopharyngeus muscle of OSAS patients not encountered in controls (159). Therefore, current data suggest that both trauma and injury may occur in the upper airway of apnea patients.

In comparison to injury, there is less evidence of upper airway muscle fatigue in the apnea patient population. The normal human genioglossus has been demonstrated to be susceptible to fatigue by Scardella et al. (160), with muscle endurance deteriorating as the force of contraction increased. Evidence for pharyngeal dilator fatigue in OSAS is currently lacking. However, careful studies have not been conducted to date.

A third potential mechanism of perpetuation in OSAS is sleep deprivation. The recurrent arousals experienced by OSAS patients virtually always lead to sleep fragmentation, diminished sleep quality, and ultimately longstanding sleep deprivation. Although the impact of sleep deprivation on pharyngeal muscle control and mechanics has been minimally studied, there are several suggestive observations. Leiter et al. (161) observed substantially diminished genioglossal responsiveness to carbon dioxide in normal subjects after sleep deprivation. In addition, Series et al. (162) compared the effect of sleep deprivation with that of sleep fragmentation on upper airway collapsibility (Pcrit) and reported sleep fragmentation (as OSAS patients typically experience) to significantly increase collapsibility (i.e., less negative Pcrit). As a result, muscle activation may be affected by diminished or fragmented sleep. Whether increasing the total sleep time of OSAS patients would lead to a less vulnerable airway has not yet been tested. Therefore, the role of sleep fragmentation in perpetuating sleep apnea remains unresolved.

Fourth, changing craniofacial structure could perpetuate apnea. Retrognathia has been noted in many studies to be associated with OSAS, with most investigators believing this to be an inherited trait that increases susceptibility to OSA. However, Lugaresi et al. (163) have speculated that the chronic activation of the protrusion muscles of the tongue may lead to mandibular remodeling and the gradual development of retrognathia. This type of chronic skeletal remodeling would be analogous to the changes in chest wall shape that can occur in emphysema patients. Changes in mandibular shape have been demonstrated previously in primates after changes in the route of airflow (oral versus nasal) (164, 165). The authors concluded that changes in the inclination of the mandibular plane are controlled by the balance of suprahyoid and orofacial muscles. This observation in primates lends some support to the possibility that mandibular remodeling could occur in humans with OSAS. However, this remains completely speculative.

Finally, obese persons with OSAS often experience an inability to lose weight despite attempts at dietary and activity modifications. As a result, apnea continues. Although weight loss is commonly unsuccessful in many obese patient groups, apneic subjects may have particular difficulty. This lack of weight loss is a frequent clinical observation despite an often substantial increase in activity after adequate therapy for the OSAS (e.g., CPAP). Studies on untreated apneic patients have shown substantial energy expenditure during sleep, presumably from the metabolic cost of repetitive arousals with the huge associated respiratory effort (166). In addition, during these apneic events pulsatile growth hormone (GH) secretion has been observed, which may contribute to increased lipolysis. These two factors are presumably offset in untreated apneic persons by extremely low physical activity levels during wakefulness. Thus, after successful treatment of OSAS, despite a possible increase in physical activity during wakefulness, net weight loss may remain difficult owing to the reduced energy consumption during sleep (diminished respiratory work) and the loss of pulsatile GH secretion (diminished lipolysis) (167–169). Therefore, body fat may represent another mechanism perpetuating airway compromise and apneic events (17, 170).

EPIDEMIOLOGICAL FACTORS

OBESITY

Given the foregoing discussion, clearly both anatomical and physiological abnormalities play a role in the pathogenesis of OSAS. The mechanisms by which specific epi-

demiological factors exert their influence on these variables are beginning to be understood. Obesity is clearly an important risk factor for OSAS, although the mechanism for this increased risk is somewhat unclear (169, 171). From the standpoint of anatomy, as previously stated, there exists controversy as to whether OSAS patients have increased fat deposition around the upper airway as compared to weight-matched controls (34–37, 172). The preponderance of evidence suggests preferential deposition of fat in the parapharyngeal soft tissues, leading to a compromised upper airway lumen. In addition, Schwartz et al. (38) demonstrated a correlation between the change in Pcrit and the change in body mass index (BMI) of persons undergoing weight loss, suggesting that the loss of adiposity made the upper airway less vulnerable to collapse (Fig. 4.9). Alterations in physiology with obesity are somewhat less clear. Although morbidly obese persons can clearly have abnormalities of ventilatory control, as stated above, these are unlikely to be playing a major role in the pathogenesis of OSAS. Therefore, the majority of the available evidence in OSAS patients suggests that obesity influences pharyngeal anatomy, leading to a more vulnerable upper airway, although further studies are ongoing.

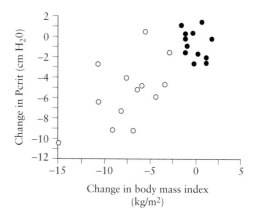

Fig 4.9 The relationship between change in BMI with change in collapsing pressure (Pcrit). As a person loses weight, the upper airway becomes less prone to collapse, whereas people who maintain constant weight do not see a major change in collapsibility. (From Schwartz AR, Gold AR, Schubert N, et al. Effect of weight loss on upper airway collapsibility in obstructive sleep apnea. Am Rev Respir Dis 1991; 144[3 Pt 1]:494–498.)

Sex

Male sex is also an important risk factor for the development of OSAS. Depending on the study, men have between a twofold and fivefold increased risk of OSAS compared to weight-matched women (1, 173–176). Although the mechanisms explaining this gender effect are poorly understood, a number of observations are of interest. First, suggestive data exist implicate that androgens as a cause of this increased risk of OSAS whereas, conversely, estrogens may reduce OSAS risk. Several studies indicate that hypogonadal men rarely have sleep apnea yet can develop OSAS with androgen replacement (177, 178). Therefore, androgens may, in some yet to be defined way, lead to increased pharyngeal collapsibility (179). Estrogen or progesterone may, on the other hand, protect women from the development of apnea (180–187). This concept is supported by several observations. First, women have been observed to have greater genioglossus muscle activation than men, with this muscle activity declining with falling progesterone levels (follicular versus luteal menstrual phase, postmenopausal versus premenopausal status) (72, 73, 188) (Fig. 4.10). Second, estrogen plus progesterone replacement in post-

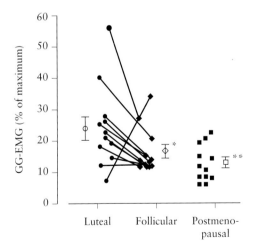

*Fig 4.10 Individual baseline peak phasic genioglossus EMG (GG-EMG) values. Mean values ± standard errors are also provided. *p = 0.05 versus luteal phase, **p < 0.01 versus luteal phase. (From Popovic RM, White DP. Upper airway muscle activity in normal women: influence of hormonal status. J Appl Physiol 1998; 84[3]:1055–1062.)*

menopausal women increased upper airway muscle activation. Third, postmenopausal women have a greater prevalence of sleep apnea than premenopausal ones (1). On the other hand, progesterone or estrogen plus progesterone administration to apnea patients often has little effect on apnea frequency. As a result, the role of gender specific hormones in the pathogenesis of sleep apnea remains unclear,

Second, a number of studies have assessed upper airway anatomy in men versus women with the prediction being that women would have a larger airway, thereby protecting them from collapse. However, most such studies have demonstrated a smaller upper airway luminal size in women or one of similar size when normalized for body surface area (189). However, careful assessment of gender influences on pharyngeal soft tissues has not been completed to date.

Preliminary data from our laboratory suggest that women have a considerably shorter pharyngeal airway (hard palate to epiglottis) than age-matched men even when normalized for body height. As several studies have indicated that increasing airway length may predispose to collapse (190, 191), this shorter airway in women may prove to be protective. However, these observations remain preliminary, with no clearly established gender anatomical differences being defined at this time.

Finally, numerous studies have assessed both waking and sleeping ventilatory control in men versus women with most focusing on the hypoxic and hypercapnic ventilatory responses. However, most such studies have found little difference between the sexes, particularly when controlled for body size (192). In addition, small differences in these responses have not been shown to seriously affect the frequency of apnea. As a result, we cannot, at this time, implicate gender influences on ventilatory control as an important explanation for the male predominance in OSAS. Therefore, the cause for this epidemiological observation (increased prevalence of apnea in male subjects) remains largely unexplained.

Age

Aging represents an important risk for the development of apnea, as many studies have shown progressive increases in the prevalence of OSAS, at least up to the sixth or seventh decade, independent of body mass index (1, 193–206). The few studies that have addressed pathophysiological explanations have not reached clear conclusions regarding either anatomical or physiological factors that predispose to an increased risk of apnea with aging. Burger et al. (207) actually found an increase in size of the upper airway with increasing age, the opposite of what might be expected. These investigators speculated that the reason for this unexpected finding was due to their inclusion criteria, as they studied only extremely healthy elderly people (207). They also reported no clear differences in dilator muscle activation or upper airway collapsibility in elderly subjects, although the methods used to assess these variables could be questioned. As a result, the explanation for the increased prevalence of apnea with aging remains unresolved (208–216).

CONCLUSIONS

The pathogenesis of obstructive sleep apnea is becoming increasingly understood, although much work remains. Convincing evidence supports deficient upper airway anatomy in afflicted patients, which requires increased neuromuscular activity during wakefulness as a compensatory response. The mechanism driving this response is still poorly defined. The neurochemical and physiological changes that occur at sleep onset, leading to a loss of muscle activity and subsequent pharyngeal collapse, are the subject of ongoing investigation, but they may relate to diminished reflex pharyngeal control and a loss of the neuromuscular compensation present during wakefulness. However, further studies are needed to better define both the physiology and the neurobiology of this disorder. Only with a clear understanding of the basic mechanisms of structural and functional abnormalities in OSAS are new therapies likely to emerge.

REFERENCES

1. Young T, Palta M, Denysly J, et al. The occurrence of sleep-disordered breathing among middle-aged adults. N Engl J Med 1993; 32:1230–1235.

2. Findley LJ, Unverzagt ME, Suratt PM. Automobile accidents involving patients with obstructive sleep apnea. Am Rev Respir Dis 1988; 138(2):337–340.

3. Aldrich CK, Aldrich MS, Aldrich TK, et al. Asleep at the wheel. The physician's role in preventing accidents 'just waiting to happen.' Postgrad Med 1986; 80(5):233–235, 238, 240.

4. Kimoff RJ. Sleep fragmentation in obstructive sleep apnea. Sleep 1996; 19(9 Suppl):S61–156.

5. Haponik E, Smith P, Bohlman M, et al. Computerized tomography in obstructive sleep apnea: correlation of airway size with physiology during sleep and wakefulness. Am Rev Respir Dis 1983; 127:221.

6. Schwab RJ, Gupta KB, Gefter WB, et al. Upper airway and soft tissue anatomy in normal subjects and patients with sleep-disordered breathing. significance of the lateral pharyngeal walls. Am J Respir Crit Care Med 1995; 152(5 Pt 1): 1673–1689.

7. Schwab RJ. Properties of tissues surrounding the upper airway. Sleep 1996; 19(10 Suppl):S170–S174.

8. Schwab RJ, Pack AI, Gupta KB, et al. Upper airway and soft tissue structural changes induced by CPAP in normal subjects. Am J Respir Crit Care Med 1996; 154(4 Pt 1): 1106–1116.

9. Schwab RJ. Upper airway imaging. Clin Chest Med 1998; 19(1):33–54.

10. Mezzanotte WS, Tangel DJ, White DP. Waking genioglossal electromyogram in sleep apnea patients versus normal controls (a neuromuscular compensatory mechanism) J Clin Invest 1992; 89:1571–1579.

11. Bixler EO, Vgontzas AN, Ten Have T, et al. Effects of age on sleep apnea in men: I. Prevalence and severity. Am J Respir Crit Care Med 1998; 157(1):144–148.

12. Partinen M, Telakivi T. Epidemiology of obstructive sleep apnea syndrome. Sleep 1992; 15(6 Suppl):S1–S4.

13. Partinen M. Epidemiology of obstructive sleep apnea syndrome. Curr Opinion Pulmonary Med 1995; 1(6):482–487.

14. Teschler H, Berthon Jones M, Wessendorf T, et al. Influence of moderate alcohol consumption on obstructive sleep apnoea with and without AutoSet nasal CPAP therapy. Eur Respir J 1996; 9(11):2371–2377.

15. Bray GA. Health hazards of obesity. Endocrinol Metab Clin North Am 1996; 25(4):907–919.

16. Bresnitz EA, Goldberg R, Kosinski RM. Epidemiology of obstructive sleep apnea. Epidemiol Rev 1994; 16(2):210–227.

17. Shinohara E, Kihara S, Yamashita S, et al. Visceral fat accumulation as an important risk factor for obstructive sleep apnoea syndrome in obese subjects. J Intern Med 1997; 241(1):11–188.

18. Leiter JC, Doble EA, Knuth SL, et al. Respiratory activity of genioglossus. Interaction between alcohol and the menstrual cycle. Am Rev Respir Dis 1987; 135(2):383–386.

19. Aldrich MS, Shipley JE, Tandon R, et al. Sleep-disordered breathing in alcoholics: association with age. Alcohol Clin Exp Res 1993; 17(6):1179–1183.

20. Vitiello MV, Prinz PN, Personius JP, et al. History of chronic alcohol abuse is associated with increased nighttime hypoxemia in older men. Alcohol Clin Exp Res 1987; 11(4):368–371.

21. Vitiello MV, Prinz PN, Personius JP, et al. Nighttime hypoxemia is increased in abstaining chronic alcoholic men. Alcohol Clin Exp Res 1990; 14(1):38–41.

22. Vitiello MV, Prinz PN, Personius JP, et al. Relationship of alcohol abuse history to nighttime hypoxemia in abstaining chronic alcoholic men. J Stud Alcohol 1990; 51(1):29–33.

23. Guilleminault C, Silvestri R, Mondini S, et al. Aging and sleep apnea: action of benzodiazepine, acetazolamide, alcohol, and sleep deprivation in a healthy elderly group. J Gerontol 1984; 39(6):655–661.

24. Remmers JE, deGroot WJ, Sauerland EK, et al. Pathogenesis of upper airway occlusion during sleep. J Appl Physiol 1978; 44(6):931–938.

25. Horner RL, Shea SA, McIvor J, et al. Pharyngeal size and shape during wakefulness and sleep in patients with obstructive sleep apnoea. Q J Med 1989; 72(268):719–735.

26. Schwab RJ, Gefter WB, Hoffman FA, et al. Dynamic upper airway imaging during awake respiration in normal subjects and patients with sleep-disordered breathing. Am Rev Respir Dis 1993; 148:1375–1400.

27. Hoffstein V, Weiser W, Haney R. Roentgenographic dimensions of the upper airway in snoring patients with and without obstructive sleep apnea. Chest 1991; 100(1):81–85.

28. Hoffstein V, Zamel N, Phillipson EA. Lung volume dependence of pharyngeal cross-sectional area in patients with obstructive sleep apnea. Am Rev Respir Dis 1984; 130(2):175–178.

29. Bradley TD, Brown IG, Zamel N, et al. Differences in pharyngeal properties between snorers with predominantly central sleep apnea and those without sleep apnea. Am Rev Respir Dis 1987; 135(2):387–391.

30. Rivlin J, Hoffstein V, Kalbfleisch J, et al. Upper airway morphology in patients with idiopathic obstructive sleep apnea. Am Rev Respir Dis 1984; 129(3):355–360.

31. Bradley TD, Brown IG, Grossman RF, et al. Pharyngeal size in snorers, nonsnorers, and patients with obstructive sleep apnea. N Engl J Med 1986; 315(21):1327–1331.

32. Davies RJ, Stradling JR. The relationship between neck circumference, radiographic pharyngeal anatomy, and the obstructive sleep apnoea syndrome. Eur Respir J 1990; 3(5):509–514.

33. Gozal D. Sleep-disordered breathing and school performance in children. Pediatrics 1998; 102(3 Pt 1):616–620.

34. Mortimore IL, Marshall I, Wraith PK, et al. Neck and total body fat deposition in nonobese and obese patients with sleep apnea compared with that in control subjects. Am J Respir Crit Care Med 1998; 157(1):280–283.

35. Horner RL, Mohiaddin RH, Lowell DG, et al. Sites and sizes of fat deposits around the pharynx in obese patients with obstructive sleep apnoea and weight matched controls. Eur Respir J 1989; 2(7):613–622.

36. Shelton KE, Woodson H, Gay SB, et al. Adipose tissue deposition in sleep apnea. Sleep 1993; 16(8 Suppl):S103; discussion S103–5.

37. Shelton KE, Woodson H, Gay S, et al. Pharyngeal fat in obstructive sleep apnea. Am Rev Respir Dis 1993; 148(2):462–466.

38. Schwartz AR, Gold AR, Schubert N, et al. Effect of weight loss on upper airway collapsibility in obstructive sleep apnea. Am Rev Respir Dis 1991; 144(3 Pt 1):494–498.

39. Isono S, Remmers JE, Tanaka A, et al. Anatomy of pharynx in patients with obstructive sleep apnea and in normal subjects. J Appl Physiol 1997; 82(4):1319–1326.

40. Rothen HU, Sporre B, Engberg G, et al. Atelectasis and pulmonary shunting during induction of general anaesthesia—can they be avoided? Acta Anaesthesiol Scand 1996; 40(5):524–529.

41. Rothen HU, Sporre B, Engberg G, et al. Influence of gas composition on recurrence of atelectasis after a reexpansion maneuver during general anesthesia. Anesthesiology 1995; 82(4):832–842.

42. Rothen HU, Sporre B, Engberg G, et al. Re-expansion of atelectasis during general anaesthesia: a computed tomography study. Br J Anaesth 1993; 71(6):788–795.

43. Reber A, Engberg G, Sporre B, et al. Volumetric analysis of aeration in the lungs during general anaesthesia. Br J Anaesth 1996; 76(6):760–766.

44. Issa FG, Sullivan CE. Upper airway closing pressures in snorers. J Appl Physiol 1984; 57(2):528–535.

45. Issa FG, Sullivan CE. Upper airway closing pressures in obstructive sleep apnea. J Appl Physiol 1984; 57(2):520–527.

46. Isono S, Shimada A, Utsugi M, et al. Comparison of static mechanical properties of the passive pharynx. Am J Respir Crit Care Med 1998; 157(4 Pt 1):1204–1212.

47. Morrison DL, Launois SH, Isono S, et al. Pharyngeal narrowing and closing pressures in patients with obstructive sleep apnea. Am Rev Respir Dis 1993; 148(3):606–611.

48. Smith PL, Wise RA, Gold AR, et al. Upper airway pressure-flow relationships in obstructive sleep apnea. J Appl Physiol 1988; 64(2):789–795.

49. Gleadhill I, Schwartz A, Wise R, et al. Upper airway collapsibility in snorers and in patients with obstructive hypopnea and apnea. Am Rev Respir Dis 1991; 143:1300–1303.

50. Sforza E, Petian C, Weiss T, et al. Pharyngeal critical pressure in patients with obstructive sleep apnea syndrome. Clinical implications. Am J Respir Crit Care Med 1999; 159(1):149–157.

51. Schwartz AR, Smith PL, Wise RA, et al. Effect of positive nasal pressure on upper airway pressure-flow relationships. J Appl Physiol 1989; 66(4):1626–1634.

52. Schwartz AR, Smith PL, Wise RA, et al. Induction of upper airway occlusion in sleeping individuals with subatmospheric nasal pressure. J Appl Physiol 1988; 64(2):535–542.

53. Rodenstein DO, Dooms G, Thomas Y, et al. Pharyngeal shape and dimensions in healthy subjects, snorers, and patients with obstructive sleep apnoea. Thorax 1990; 45(10):722–727.

54. Leiter JC. Upper airway shape: is it important in the pathogenesis of obstructive sleep apnea? Am J Respir Crit Care Med 1996; 153(3):894–898.

55. Jager L, Gunther E, Gauger J, et al. Fluoroscopic MR of the pharynx in patients with obstructive sleep apnea. AJNR 1998; 19(7):1205–1214.

56. Abbey NC, Block AJ, Green D, et al. Measurement of pharyngeal volume by digitized magnetic resonance imaging. Effect of nasal continuous positive airway pressure. Am Rev Respir Dis 1989; 140(3):717–723.

57. Abbey NC, Block AJ, Green D, et al. A method for measuring pharyngeal volumes using magnetic resonance imaging in subjects who snore with and without nasal CPAP. Progr Clin Biol Res 1990; 345:283–288; discussion 289–290.

58. White DP. Sleep-related breathing disorder. Pathophysiology of obstructive sleep apnoea. Thorax. 1995; 50(7):797–804.

59. Von Lunteren E, Strohl KP. The muscles of the upper airway. Clin Chest Med 1986; 7:171–195.

60. Tangel DJ, Mezzanotte WS, Sandberg EJ, et al. Influences of NREM sleep on the activity of tonic vs. inspiratory phasic muscles in normal men. J Appl Physiol 1992; 73(3):1058–1066.

61. Horner RL, Innes JA, Holden HB, et al. Afferent pathway(s) for pharyngeal dilator reflex to negative pressure in man: a study using upper airway anaesthesia. J Physiol (Lond) 1991; 436:31–44.

62. Horner RL, Innes JA, Holden HB, et al. Afferent pathway(s) for pharyngeal dilator reflex to negative airway pressure in man: a study using upper airway anesthesia. J Physiol 1991; 436:31–34.

63. Wheatley JR, White DP. The influence of sleep on pharyngeal reflexes. Sleep 1993; 16(8 Suppl):S87–89.

64. Wheatley JR, Tangel DJ, Mezzanotte WS, et al. Influence of sleep on response to negative airway pressure of tensor palatini muscle and retropalatal airway. J Appl Physiol 1993; 75(5):2117–2124.

65. Wheatley JR, Mezzanotte WS, Tangel DJ, et al. Influence of sleep on genioglossus muscle activation by negative pressure in normal men. Am Rev Respir Dis 1993; 148(3):597–605.

66. White DP, Edwards JK, Shea SA. Local reflex mechanisms: influence on basal genioglossal muscle activation in normal subjects. Sleep 1998; 21:719–728.

67. Onal E, Lopata M, O'Connor T. Diaphragmatic and genioglossal electromyogram responses to isocapnic hypoxia in humans. Am Rev Respir Dis 1981; 124:215–217.

68. McEvoy RD, Popovic RM, Saunders NA, et al. Effects of sustained and repetitive isocapnic hypoxia on ventilation and genioglossal and diaphragmatic EMGs. J Appl Physiol 1996; 81(2):866–875.

69. Smith PL, Haponik EF, Bleecker ER. The effects of oxygen in patients with sleep apnea. Am Rev Respir Dis 1984; 130(6):958–963.

70. Onal E, Lopata M, O'Connor TD. Diaphragmatic and genioglossal electromyogram responses to CO_2 rebreathing in humans. J Appl Physiol 1981; 50(5):1052–1055.

71. Schwartz AR, Thut DC, Brower RG, et al. Modulation of maximal inspiratory airflow by neuromuscular activity: effect of CO_2. J Appl Physiol 1993; 74(4):1597–1605.

72. Popovic RM, White DP. Influence of gender on waking genioglossal electromyogram and upper airway resistance. Am J Respir Crit Care Med 1995; 152(2):725–731.

73. Popovic RM, White DP. Upper airway muscle activity in normal women: influence of hormonal status. J Appl Physiol 1998; 84(3):1055–1062.

74. Begle RL, Badr S, Skatrud JB, et al. Effect of lung inflation on pulmonary resistance during NREM sleep. Am Rev Respir Dis 1990; 141(4 Pt 1):854–860.

75. Series F, Cormier Y, Lampron N, et al. Influence of lung volume in sleep apnea. Thorax 1989; 44(1):52–57.

76. Mezzanotte WS, Tangel DJ, White DP. Waking genioglossal electromyogram in sleep apnea patients versus normal controls (a neuromuscular compensatory mechanism). J Clin Invest 1992; 89(5):1571–1579.

77. Hendricks JC, Petrof BJ, Panckeri K, et al. Upper airway dilating muscle hyperactivity during non-rapid eye movement sleep in English bulldogs. Am Rev Respir Dis 1993; 148(1):185–194.

78. Series F, Cate C, Simoneau JA, et al. Physiologic, metabolic and muscle fiber type characteristics of musculus uvulae in sleep apnea hypopnea syndrome and in snorers. J Clin Invest 1995; 95:20–25.

79. Deegan PC, McNicholas WT. Pathophysiology of obstructive sleep apnoea. Eur Respir J 1995; 8(7):1161–1178.

80. Deegan PC, Nolan P, Cavey M, et al. Effects of positive airway pressure on upper airway dilator muscle activity and ventilatory timing. J Appl Physiol 1996; 81(1):470–479.

81. Mortimore IL, Douglas NJ. Palatal muscle EMG response to negative pressure in awake sleep apneic and control subjects. Am J Respir Crit Care Med 1997; 156(3 Pt 1):867–873.

82. Horner RL, Innes JA, Morrell MJ, et al. The effect of sleep on reflex genioglossus muscle activation by stimuli of negative airway pressure in humans. J Physiol (Lond) 1994; 476(1):141–151.

83. Shea SA, Edwards JK, White DP. Effects of sleep-wake transitions and REM sleep on genioglossal response to upper airway negative pressure. Am J Resp Crit Care Med 1998; 157:A653.

84. Basner RC, Ringler J, Schwartzstein RM, et al. Phasic electromyographic activity of the genioglossus increases in normals during slow-wave sleep. Respir Physiol 1991; 83(2):189–200.

85. Wiegand L, Zwillich CW, White DP. Collapsibility of the human upper airway during normal sleep. J Appl Physiol 1989; 66:1800–1808.

86. Wiegand L. Sleep and resistive loading influences on human upper airway collapsibility. Progr Clin Biol Res 1990; 345:157–166.

87. Parisi RA, Santiago TV, Edelman NH, et al. Genioglossal and diaphragmatic EMG responses to hypoxia during sleep. Am Rev Respir Dis 1988; 138(3):610–616.

88. Wiegand L, Zwillich CW, Wiegand D, et al. Changes in upper airway muscle activation and ventilation during phasic REM sleep in normal men. J Appl Physiol 1991; 71:488–497.

89. Kimura H, Niijima M, Edo H, et al. The effect of hypoxic depression on genioglossal muscle activity in healthy subjects and obstructive sleep apnea patients. Sleep 1993; 16(8 Suppl):S135–S136.

90. Kimura H, Niijima M, Edo H, et al. Differences in the response of genioglossal muscle activity to sustained hypoxia between healthy subjects and patients with obstructive sleep apnea. Respiration 1994; 61(3):155–160.

91. Okabe S, Hida W, Kikuchi Y, et al. Upper airway muscle activity during sustained hypoxia in awake humans. J Appl Physiol 1993; 75(4):1552–1558.

92. Okabe S, Chonan T, Hida W, et al. Role of chemical drive in recruiting upper airway and inspiratory intercostal muscles in patients with obstructive sleep apnea. Am Rev Respir Dis 1993; 147(1):190–195.

93. Worsnop C, Kag A, Pierce R, et al. Activity of respiratory pump and upper airway muscles during sleep onset. J Appl Physiol 1998; 85(3):908–920.

94. Rowley JA, Williams BC, Smith PL, et al. Neuromuscular activity and upper airway collapsibility. Mechanisms of action in the decerebrate cat. Am J Respir Crit Care Med 1997; 156(2 Pt 1):515–521.

95. Weiner D, Mitra J, Salamone J, et al. Effect of chemical stimuli on nerves supplying upper airway muscles. J Appl Physiol 1982; 52(3):530–536.

96. Okabe S, Hida W, Kikuchi Y, et al. Upper airway muscle activity during REM and non-REM sleep of patients with obstructive apnea. Chest 1994; 106(3):767–773.

97. Tangel DT, Mezzanotte WS, White DP. The influence of sleep on tensor palatini EMG and upper airway resistance in normal subjects. J Appl Physiol 1991; 70:2574–2581.

98. Mezzanotte WS, Tangel DJ, White DP. Influence of sleep onset on upper-airway muscle activity in apnea patients versus normal controls. Am J Respir Crit Care Med 1996; 153(6 Pt 1):1880–1887.

99. Kuna ST, Smickley JS. Superior pharyngeal constrictor activation in obstructive sleep apnea. Am J Respir Crit Care Med 1997; 156(3 Pt 1):874–880.

100. Kuna ST, Smickley JS, Vanoye CR. Respiratory-related pharyngeal constrictor muscle activity in normal human adults. Am J Respir Crit Care Med 1997; 155(6):1991–1999.

101. Neill AM, Angus SM, Sajkov D, et al. Effects of sleep posture on upper airway stability in patients with obstructive sleep apnea. Am J Respir Crit Care Med 1997; 155(1):199–204.

102. Koenig JS, Thach BT. Effects of mass loading on the upper airway. J Appl Physiol 1988; 64(6):2294–2299.

103. Oksenberg A, Silverberg DS, Arons E, et al. Positional vs. nonpositional obstructive sleep apnea patients: anthropomorphic, nocturnal polysomnographic, and multiple sleep latency test data. Chest 1997; 112(3):629–639.

104. Matsuzawa Y, Hayashi S, Yamaguchi S, et al. Effect of prone position on apnea severity in obstructive sleep apnea. Intern Med 1995; 34(12):1190–1193.

105. Pevernagie DA, Shepard JW Jr. Effects of body position on upper airway size and shape in patients with obstructive sleep apnea. Acta Psychiatry Belg 1994; 94(2):101–103.

106. Pevernagie DA, Stanson AW, Sheedy PF 2nd, et al. Effects of body position on the upper airway of patients with obstructive sleep apnea. Am J Respir Crit Care Med 1995; 152(1):179–185.

107. Kavey NB, Blitzer A, Gidro-Frank S, et al. Sleeping position and sleep apnea syndrome. Am J Otolaryngol 1985; 6(5):373–377.

108. Katz A, Dinner DS. The effect of sleep position on the diagnosis of obstructive sleep apnea: a word of caution. Clev Clin J Med 1992; 59(6):634–636; discussion 636.

109. Wasicko MJ, Hatt DA, Parisi RA, et al. The role of vascular tone in the control of upper airway collapsibility. Am Rev Respir Dis 1990; 141(6):1569–1577.

110. Olson LG, Ulmer LG, Saunders NA. Mechanical properties of the rabbit upper airway during hypoxia and hypercapnia. Respir Physiol 1991; 83(3):333–342.

111. Olson LG, Ulmer LG, Saunders NA. Pressure-volume properties of the upper airway of rabbits. J Appl Physiol 1989; 66(2):759–763.

112. Olson LG, Strohl KP. Non-muscular factors in upper airway patency in the rabbit. Respir Physiol 1988; 71(2):147–155.

113. Shepard JW Jr, Pevernagie DA, Stanson AW, et al. Effects of changes in central venous pressure on upper airway size in patients with obstructive sleep apnea. Am J Respir Crit Care Med 1996; 153(1):250–254.

114. Ray CS, Sue DY, Bray G, et al. Effects of obesity on respiratory function. Am Rev Respir Dis 1983; 128(3):501–506.

115. Collins LC, Heberty PD, Walker JF, et al. The effect of body fat distribution on pulmonary function tests. Chest 1995; 107(5):1298–1302.

116. Collins DV, Cutillo AG, Armstrong JD, et al. Large airway size, lung size, and maximal expiratory flow in healthy nonsmokers. Am Rev Respir Dis. 1986; 134(5):951–955.

117. Nahmias J, Kirschner M, Karetzky MS. Weight loss and OSA and pulmonary function in obesity. NJ Med 1993; 90(1):48–53.

118. Van de Graaff WB. Thoracic traction on the trachea: mechanisms and magnitude. J Appl Physiol 1991; 70:1328–1363.

119. Van de Graaff WB. Thoracic influence on upper airway patency. J Appl Physiol 1988; 65:2124–2131.

120. Smith PL, Elsile DW, Podszus T, et al. Electrical stimulation of upper airway musculature. Sleep 1996; 19(10 Suppl):S284–S287.

121. Garcia-Colunga J, Awad JN, Miledi R. Blockage of muscle and neuronal nicotinic acetylcholine receptors by fluoxetine (Prozac). Proc Natl Acad Sci USA 1997; 94(5):2041–2044.

122. Garcia-Colunga J, Miledi R. Serotonergic modulation of muscle acetylcholine receptors of different subunit composition. Proc Natl Acad Sci USA 1996; 93(9):3990–3994.

123. Vertes RP, Kucsis B. Projections of the dorsal raphe nucleus to the brainstem: PHA-L analysis in the rat. J Comp Neurol 1994; 340(1):11–26.

124. Horner RL. Motor control of the pharyngeal musculature and implications for the pathogenesis of obstructive sleep apnea. Sleep 1996; 19(10):827–853.

125. Kubin L, Tojima H, Davies RO, et al. Serotonergic excitatory drive to hypoglossal motoneuron in the decerebrate cat. Neurosci Lett 1992; 139:243–248.

126. Kubin L, Kimura H, Tojima H, et al. Suppression of hypoglossal motoneurons during the carbachol-induced atonia of REM sleep is not caused by fast synaptic inhibition. Brain Res 1993; 611(2):300–312.

127. Kubin L, Reignier C, Tojima H, et al. Changes in serotonin level in the hypoglossal nucleus region during carbachol-induced atonia. Brain Res 1994; 645(1–2):291–302.

128. Kubin L, Tojima H, Reignier C, et al. Interaction of serotonergic excitatory drive to hypoglossal motoneurons with carbachol-induced, REM sleep-like atonia. Sleep 1996; 19(3):187–195.

129. Aldes LD, Marco LA, Chronister RB, Serotonin-containing axon terminals in the hypoglossal nucleus of the rat. An immuno-electronmicroscopic study. Brain Res Bull 1989; 23(3):249–256.

130. Hilaire G, Morin D, Lajard AM, et al. Changes in serotonin metabolism may elicit obstructive apnoea in the newborn rat. J Physiol (Lond) 1993; 466:367–381.

131. Okabe S, Kubin L. Role of 5HT1 receptors in the control of hypoglossal motoneurons in vivo. Sleep 1996; 19(10 Suppl):S150–S153.

132. Richard CA, Harper RM. Respiratory-related activity in hypoglossal neurons across sleep-waking states in cats. Brain Res 1991; 542:167–170.

133. Hanzel DA, Proia NG, Hudgel DW. Response of obstructive sleep apnea to fluoxetine and protriptyline. Chest 1991; 100(2):416–421.

134. Kopelman PG, Elliott MW, Simonds A, et al. Short-term use of fluoxetine in asymptomatic obese subjects with sleep-related hypoventilation. Int J Obes Relat Metab Disord 1992; 16(10):825–830.

135. Slamowitz DA, Shea SA, Edwards JK, et al. Serotonergic and cholinergic influences on pharyngeal muscles (Abstract). Sleep 1998; 21:418C.

136. Veasey SC, Panckeri KA, Hoffman EA, et al. The effects of serotonin antagonists in an animal model of sleep-disordered breathing. Am J Respir Crit Care Med 1996; 153(2):776–786.

137. Manaker S, Tischler LJ, Bigler TL, et al. Neurons of the motor trigeminal nucleus project to the hypoglossal nucleus in the rat. Exp Brain Res 1992; 90(2):262–270.

138. Gorea E, Davenne D, Lanfumey L, et al. Regulation of noradrenergic coerulean neuronal firing mediated by 5–HT2 receptors: involvement of the prepositus hypoglossal nucleus. Neuropharmacology 1991; 30(12A):1309–1318.

139. Aldes LD. Topographically organized projections from the nucleus subceruleus to the hypoglossal nucleus in the rat: a light and electron microscopic study with complementary axonal transport techniques. J Comp Neurol 1990; 302(3):643–656.

140. Ennis M, Aston-Jones G. Potent inhibitory input to locus caeruleus from the nucleus prepositus hypoglossi. Brain Res Bull 1989; 22(5):793–803.

141. Aldes LD, Shaw B, Chronister RB, et al. Catecholamine-containing axon terminals in the hypoglossal nucleus of the rat: an immuno-electronmicroscopic study. Exp Brain Res 1990; 81(1):167–178.

142. Aldes LD, Chronister RB, Shelton C 3rd, et al. Catecholamine innervation of the rat hypoglossal nucleus. Brain Res Bull 1988; 21(2):305–312.

143. Aldes LD, Chapman ME, Chronister RB, et al. Sources of noradrenergic afferents to the hypoglossal nucleus in the rat. Brain Res Bull 1992; 29(6):931–942.

144. Appelberg J, Sundstrom G. Ventilatory response to CO_2 in patients with snoring, obstructive. Clin Physiol 1997; 17(5):497–507.

145. Wilcox I, Collins FL, Grunstein RR, et al. Relationship between chemosensitivity, obesity and blood pressure in obstructive sleep apnoea. Blood Press 1994; 3(1–2):47–54.

146. Wilcox I, McNamara SG, Dodd MJ, et al. Ventilatory control in patients with sleep apnoea and left ventricular. Eur Respir J 1998; 11(1):7–13.

147. Bradley TD, McNicholas WT, Rutherford R, et al. Clinical and physiologic heterogeneity of the central sleep apnea syndrome. Am Rev Respir Dis 1986; 134(2):217–221.

148. Bradley TD, Floras JS. Pathophysiologic and therapeutic implications of sleep apnea in congestive heart failure. J Cardiac Failure 1996; 2(3):223–240.

149. Naughton M, Benard D, Tam A, et al. Role of hyperventilation in the pathogenesis of central sleep apneas in patients with congestive heart failure [see comments]. Am Rev Respir Dis 1993; 148(2):330–338.

150. Naughton MT, Bradley TD. Sleep apnea in congestive heart failure. Clin Chest Med 1998; 19(1):99–113.

151. Hudgel DW, Gordon EA, Thanakitcharu S, et al. Instability of ventilatory control in patients with obstructive sleep apnea. Am J Respir Crit Care Med 1998; 158(4):1142–1149.

152. Pendlebury ST, Pepin JL, Veale D, et al. Natural evolution of moderate sleep apnoea syndrome: significant. Thorax 1997; 52(10):872–878.

153. Teculescu D. Can snoring induce or worsen obstructive sleep apnea? Med Hypotheses 1998; 50(2):125–129.

154. Anastassov GE, Trieger N. Edema in the upper airway in patients with obstructive sleep apnea syndrome. Oral Surg 1998; 86(6):644–647.

155. Petrof BJ, Pack AI, Kelly AM, et al. Pharyngeal myopathy of loaded upper airway in dogs with sleep apnea. J Appl Physiol 1994; 76(4):1746–1752.

156. Schotland HM, Insko EK, Panckeri KA, et al. Quantitative magnetic resonance imaging of upper airways musculature in an animal model of sleep apnea. J Appl Physiol 1996; 81(3):1339–1346.

157. Petrof BJ, Hendricks JC, Pack AI. Does upper airway muscle injury trigger a vicious cycle in obstructive sleep apnea? A hypothesis. Sleep 1996; 19(6):465–471.

158. Friberg D, Ansved T, Borg K, et al. Histological indications of a progressive snorers disease in an upper. Am J Respir Crit Care Med 1998; 157(2):586–593.

159. Edstrom L, Larsson H, Larsson L. Neurogenic effects on the palatopharyngeal muscle in patients with obstructive sleep apnoea: a muscle biopsy study. J Neurol Neurosurg Psychiatry 1992; 55(10):916–920.

160. Scardella AT, Kraweiw N, Petrozzino JJ, et al. Strength and endurance characteristics of the normal human genioglossus. Am Rev Respir Dis 1993; 148(1):179–184.

161. Leiter JC, Knuth SL, Bartlett D Jr. The effect of sleep deprivation on activity of the genioglossus muscle. Am Rev Respir Dis 1985; 132(6):1242–1245.

162. Series F, Roy N, Marc I. Effects of sleep deprivation and sleep fragmentation on upper airway collapsibility in normal subjects. Am J Respir Crit Care Med 1994; 150(2):481–485.

163. Lugaresi E, Cirignotta F, Montagna P. Pathogenic aspects of snoring and obstructive apnea syndrome. Schweiz Med Wochenschr 1988; 118(38):1333–1337.

164. Tomer BS, Harvold EP. Primate experiments on mandibular growth direction. Am J Orthod 1982; 82(2):114–119.

165. Harvold EP, Tomer BS, Vargervik K, et al. Primate experiments on oral respiration. Am J Orthod 1981; 79(4):359–372.

166. Stenlof K, Grunstein R, Hedner J, et al. Energy expenditure in obstructive sleep apnea: effects of treatment with continuous positive airway pressure. Am J Physiol 1996; 271(6 Pt 1):E1036–E1043.

167. Grunstein R, Wilcox I, Yang TS, et al. Snoring and sleep apnoea in men: association with central obesity and hypertension. Int J Obes Relat Metab Disord 1993; 17(9):533–540.

168. Grunstein RR. Metabolic aspects of sleep apnea. Sleep 1996; 19(10 Suppl):S218–S220.

169. Grunstein RR, Wilcox I. Sleep-disordered breathing and obesity. Baillieres Clin Endocrinol Metab 1994; 8(3):601–628.

170. Soultan Z, Wadowski S, Rao M, et al. Effect of treating obstructive sleep apnea by tonsillectomy and/or adenoidectomy on obesity in children. Arch Pediatr Adolesc Med 1999; 153(1):33–37.

171. Kilpatrick C. Obesity and the sleep apnoea syndrome. Aust NZ J Med 1982; 12(6):656.

172. Shelton KE, Gay SB, Hollowell DE, et al. Mandible enclosure of upper airway and weight in obstructive sleep apnea. Am Rev Respir Dis 1993; 148(1):195–200.

173. Young T. Analytic epidemiology studies of sleep-disordered breathing—what explains the gender difference in sleep-disordered breathing? Sleep 1993; 16(8 Suppl):S1–S2.

174. Young T, Hutton R, Finn L, et al. The gender bias in sleep apnea diagnosis. Are women missed because they have different symptoms? Arch Intern Med 1996; 156(21):2445–2451.

175. Redline S, Kump K, Tishler PV, et al. Gender differences in sleep-disordered breathing in a community-based sample. Am J Respir Crit Care Med 1994; 149(3 Pt 1):722–726.

176. Wittels EH. Obesity and hormonal factors in sleep and sleep apnea. Med Clin North Am 1985; 69(6):1265–1280.

177. White DP, Schneider BK, Santen RJ, et al. Influence of testosterone on ventilation and chemosensitivity in male subjects. J Appl Physiol 1985; 59(5):1452–1457.

178. Cistulli PA, Grunstein RR, Sullivan CE. Effect of testosterone administration on upper airway collapsibility during sleep. Am J Respir Crit Care Med 1994; 149(2 Pt 1):530–532.

179. Johnson MW, Anch AM, Remmers JE. Induction of the obstructive sleep apnea syndrome in a woman by exogenous androgen administration. Am Rev Respir Dis 1984; 129(6):1023–1025.

180. Guilleminault C, Quera-Salva MA, Partinen M, et al. Women and the obstructive sleep apnea syndrome. Chest 1988; 93(1):104–109.

181. Guilleminault C, Stoohs R, Clerk A, et al. Excessive daytime somnolence in women with abnormal respiratory efforts during sleep. Sleep 1993; 16(8 Suppl):S137–S138.

182. Kimura H, Tatsumi K, Kunitomo F, et al. Obese patients with sleep apnea syndrome treated by progesterone. Tohoku J Exp Med 1988; 156 Suppl:151–157.

183. Kimura H, Tatsumi K, Kunitomo F, et al. Progesterone therapy for sleep apnea syndrome evaluated by occlusion pressure responses to exogenous loading. Am Rev Respir Dis 1989; 139(5):1198–1206.

184. Ohshima H. Medroxyprogesterone acetate and sleep apnea. Jpn J Psychiatry Neurol 1987; 41(4):645–650.

185. Orr WC, Imes NK, Martin RJ. Progesterone therapy in obese patients with sleep apnea. Arch Intern Med 1979; 139(1):109–111.

186. Millman RP, Carlisle CC, McGarvey ST, et al. Body fat distribution and sleep apnea severity in women. Chest 1995; 107(2):362–366.

187. Cistulli PA, Barnes DJ, Grunstein RR, et al. Effect of short-term hormone replacement in the treatment of obstructive sleep apnoea in postmenopausal women. Thorax 1994; 49(7):699–702.

188. Wilhoit SC, Suratt PM. Obstructive sleep apnea in premenopausal women. A comparison with men and with postmenopausal women. Chest 1987; 91(5): 654–658.

189. Brooks LJ, Strohl KP. Size and mechanical properties of the pharynx in healthy men and women. Am Rev Respir Dis 1992; 146(6):1394–1397.

190. Woodson BT, Conley SF, Dohse A, et al. Posterior cephalometric radiographic analysis in obstructive sleep apnea. Ann Otol Rhinol Laryngol 1997; 106(4):310–313.

191. Woodson BT, Conley SF. Prediction of uvulopalatopharyngoplasty response using cephalometric radiographs. Am J Otol 1997; 18(3):179–184.

192. Aitken ML, Franklin JL, Pierson DJ, et al. Influence of body size and gender on control of ventilation. J Appl Physiol 1986; 60:1894–1899.

193. Ancoli-Israel S, Kripke DF, Mason W, et al. Sleep apnea and nocturnal myoclonus in a senior population. Sleep 1981; 4(4):349–358.

194. Ancoli-Israel S, Kripke DF, Mason W, et al. Comparisons of home sleep recordings and polysomnograms in older adults with sleep disorders. Sleep 1981; 4(3):283–291.

195. Ancoli-Israel S, Kripke DF, Mason W, et al. Sleep apnea and periodic movements in an aging sample. J Gerontol 1985; 40(4):419–425.

196. Ancoli-Israel S, Kripke DF, Mason W. Characteristics of obstructive and central sleep apnea in the elderly: an interim report. Biol Psychiatry 1987; 22(6):741–750.

197. Ancoli-Israel S. Epidemiology of sleep disorders. Clin Geriatr Med 1989; 5(2):347–362.

198. Ancoli-Israel S, Klauber MR, Kripke DF, et al. Sleep apnea in female patients in a nursing home. Increased risk of mortality. Chest 1989; 96(5):1054–1058.

199. Ancoli-Israel S, Kripke DF, Klauber MR, et al. Periodic limb movements in sleep in community-dwelling elderly. Sleep 1991; 14(6):496–500.

200. Ancoli-Israel S, Kripke DF, Klauber MR, et al. Sleep-disordered breathing in community-dwelling elderly. Sleep 1991; 14(6):486–495.

201. Ancoli-Israel S, Kripke DF. Prevalent sleep problems in the aged. Biofeedback Self Regul 1991; 16(4):349–359.

202. Ancoli-Israel S, Klauber MR, Butters N, et al. Dementia in institutionalized elderly: relation to sleep apnea. J Am Geriatr Soc 1991; 39(3):258–263.

203. Ancoli-Israel S, Kripke DF, Klauber MR, et al. Natural history of sleep-disordered breathing in community dwelling elderly. Sleep 1993; 16(8 Suppl):S25–S29.

204. Ancoli-Israel S, Coy T. Are breathing disturbances in elderly equivalent to sleep apnea syndrome? Sleep 1994; 17(1):77–83.

205. Ancoli-Israel S. Sleep problems in older adults: putting myths to bed. Geriatrics 1997; 52(1):20–30.

206. Redline S. Age-related differences in sleep apnea: generalizability of finding in older populations. In: Skung, ed. Sleep and respiration in aging adults. New York: Elsevier Publishing; 1991: 189–193.

207. Burger CD, Stanson AW, Sheedy PF, et al. Fast- computed tomography evaluation of age-related changes in upper airway structure and function in normal men. Am Rev Respir Dis 1992; 145(4 Pt 1):846–852.

208. Karacan I, Williams RL. Sleep disorders in the elderly. Am Fam Physician 1983; 27(3):143–152.

209. Johnston JE. Sleep problems in the elderly. J Am Acad Nurse Pract 1994; 6(4):161–166.

210. Hoch CC, Reynolds CF, Kupfer DJ, et al. Sleep-disordered breathing in normal and pathologic aging. J Clin Psychiatry 1986; 47(10):499–503.

211. Hoch CC, Reynolds CF, Houck PR. Sleep apnea in Alzheimer's patients and the healthy elderly. Sch Inq Nurs Pract 1987; 1(3):221–235.

212. Hoch CC, Reynolds CF, Kupfer DJ, et al. Stability of EEG sleep and sleep quality in healthy seniors. Sleep 1988; 11(6):521–527.

213. Hoch CC, Reynolds CF, Nebes RD, et al. Clinical significance of sleep-disordered breathing in Alzheimer's disease. Preliminary data. J Am Geriatr Soc 1989; 37(2):138–144.

214. Hoch CC, Reynolds CF, Monk TH, et al. Comparison of sleep-disordered breathing among healthy elderly in the seventh, eighth, and ninth decades of life. Sleep 1990; 13(6):502–511.

215. Hoch CC, Reynolds CF, Buysse DJ, et al. Sleep-disordered breathing in healthy and spousally bereaved elderly: a one-year follow-up study. Neurobiol Aging 1992; 13(6):741–746.

216. Hoch CC, Dew MA, Reynolds CF, et al. Longitudinal changes in diary- and laboratory-based sleep measures in healthy 'old old' and 'young old' subjects: a three-year follow-up. Sleep 1997; 20(3):192–202.

5 CLINICAL FEATURES OF OBSTRUCTIVE SLEEP APNEA SYNDROME

W Ward Flemons and William A Whitelaw

BACKGROUND

HISTORY

The remarkable thing about obstructive sleep apnea syndrome (OSAS) is that is should be so common and so obvious and yet have gone unrecognized until 1965, when it was described by Gastaut et al. (1). It makes us wonder what other diseases are sitting under our noses waiting to be discovered, and what defect of the human power to make associations was responsible for the oversight. Once the connection was made between snoring, apnea, and somnolence, it has been easy to find descriptions in history, art, and literature of people who probably had OSAS.

Students of sleep medicine are most familiar with the case of Joe in *The Pickwick Papers*, a character in whom so many clinical details are mentioned, making so characteristic a syndrome, that we must assume that Charles Dickens was acquainted with at least one person with the disease we would now call severe OSAS (2). The members of the Pickwick Club first meet Joe as they are getting into a coach to visit the house where Joe works as a servant. 'On the box sat a fat and red-faced boy, in a state of somnolency.' Somnolence was a prominent feature: 'Joe—damn that boy, he's gone to sleep again.' During a military exercise, 'everybody was excited except the fat boy, and he slept soundly as if the roaring of cannon were his ordinary lullaby. . . . Be good enough to pinch him, sir – in the leg, if you please; nothing else wakes him.' At night, sending him to deliver a message, his master instructs him to keep knocking loudly and continually on the door until it is opened, for fear he would otherwise go to sleep standing on the mat. Joe is also a loud snorer; 'the snoring of the fat boy penetrated in a low and monotonous sound from the distant kitchen.' Joe is a tremendous eater, frequently responsible for the disappearance of large pies and other delectables, and is great-

ly overweight. Descriptions in the text and the contemporary illustrations by Phiz show a large belly and a very thick neck. As to alcohol, Joe says, 'I likes a little bit something, if it's good' but there is no mention of him being a smoker. He seems to have had impaired cognition, 'the fat boy's perception being rather slow,' and he is referred to as 'young dropsy' an old term for edema. Two medical students demonstrate their sympathy and their profession's comprehension of the problem during a winter evening when they sit by the fire eating oysters and throwing the shells at the sleeping fat boy. A modern physician of course would have made a presumptive diagnosis of OSA with possible obesity-hypoventilation, polycythemia, cor pulmonale, and carbon dioxide (CO_2) retention.

Scrooge, who 'wakened himself one night with a prodigious snore' must have had sleep apnea too. It probably accounts for his bad temper which has made him so widely reviled, and for his hypnagogic hallucinations, the account of which takes up so much of *A Christmas Carol* (3). The heartwarming end of the story in which Scrooge has a sudden and permanent reform of character is completely implausible for the time but would have been just an ordinary medical fact if he had lived after the introduction of nasal continuous positive airway pressure (CPAP).

It is very unlikely that OSA was either new or uncommon in Dickens' time. Hippocrates mentioned sleep apnea, and Shakespeare very vividly describes an apneic event in *Henry IV* part 2 (4). This was not just a dramatic device but an episode drawn from the historical chronicle of Monstrelet, a contemporary witness of events in the English court. In Henry IV's case the evidence points more toward central apnea. On the other hand, Sir John Falstaff, the colourful low-life friend of Henry IV's son Prince Hal, clearly had OSAS. He was very fat, drank large quantities of wine, habitually dozed well into the afternoon, and one evening slept soundly through the commotion of a police raid on the lair of his gang of highwaymen. His friends find him after the sheriff goes away; Peto exclaims 'Falstaff! Fast asleep behind the arras and snoring like a horse,' and Prince Henry remarks 'Hark how hard he fetches breath.' (5).

If we can judge by the necks, waists, and chins of the characters in the original illustrations, the prevalence of OSAS must have been high in the population surveyed by Mr. Pickwick in his fact-finding travels around England in the mid-nineteenth century. It is even higher in the populations of characters drawn by Hogarth and by Rowlandson in the eighteenth century. In addition, if we can presume the diagnosis of OSAS in all the characters in history who were outstandingly bright and energetic in their youth but indulged the ease and comfort brought them by early success and became corpulent, inattentive, muddle-headed, and bad-tempered in middle age, the disease has been an important social problem for a very long time. According to Phillipson, even the giant that Jack killed was owed his reputation and his death to the effects of OSAS (6).

The diagnosis of OSAS in all of these historical examples has been inferred from clinical data alone because none of the patients ever had polysomnography. The accuracy of diagnosis of OSAS from physical appearance, complaints of somnolence, and reports of apneic events is reviewed in this chapter.

MODERN DEVELOPMENT

The initial reports of sleep apnea described very severe cases, typically in obese, middle-aged men, who came to clinical attention because of severe daytime sleepiness (7). In a series published in 1978, the main features were as follows 1) loud snoring (in all patients) that was embarrassing and annoying; 2) excessive daytime somnolence to the extent that patients described sudden, inappropriate, irresistible urges to sleep and 54% had a motor vehicle accident; 3) intellectual deterioration, including difficulty with concentrating, memory, and judgment; 4) personality changes, including patients who had consulted with psychiatrists about depression and anxiety; 5) impotence; 6) nocturnal enuresis; 7) morning headaches; 8) abnormal motor activity during sleep; 9) two women had a 'bird-like

face' and many men had a short neck; 10) 52% had hypertension.

These symptoms are still common in patients with severe sleep apnea; but with the advent of several useful therapies, improved accessibility to diagnostic facilities, and a large increase in clinical research, it is now recognized that the patients who are now seen in sleep clinics have a greater diversity of symptoms, physical characteristics, and risk factors than those described in early case series. It has been necessary to adapt clinical decision making so that patients who have treatable disease are diagnosed and offered therapy.

Coinciding with recognition of the clinical diversity of sleep apnea has been a marked advance in the understanding of the pathogenesis of sleep apnea. OSAS is caused by a critical narrowing of the upper airway, which impedes normal airflow (8). The narrowest points in the pharynx during sleep are at the level of the soft palate and the hypopharynx (9). The main outward anatomical features that increase the likelihood of upper airway narrowing during sleep are obesity and craniofacial structure. Narrowing of the nasopharynx at any level predisposes to pharyngeal narrowing (9).

⊙━ Key points box 5.1

Practice points

1. The clinical features of sleep apnea have probably been known about for over 300 years, described by Dickens and Shakespeare; however, medical recognition of the disorder is very recent.

2. Initial medical reports of sleep apnea patients focused on nocturnal symptoms of loud snoring, abnormal movements during sleep, and enuresis as well as daytime symptoms of excessive sleepiness, personality changes, and intellectual deterioration.

3. It is now recognized that patients currently seen in sleep clinics for assessment of possible sleep apnea have a wider diversity of symptoms, physical characteristics, and risk factors than patients who were initially described.

THE CLINICAL PROBLEM

People are not really separated into those who 'have sleep apnea' and those who 'do not have sleep apnea.' Most people probably have occasional obstructive events in sleep. Some have runs of events only when they are tired or ill, some have them more regularly only during certain parts of the night, and others have events that recur frequently through the whole night. All degrees of average frequency of events—from zero to 150 per hour—can be found in a general population.

Obstructive events by themselves are not necessarily a disease. The disease associated with OSAS is primarily an impairment of central nervous system function that may show itself mainly as somnolence, fatigue, difficulty concentrating, irritability, or poor memory. With worsening OSAS the degree of central nervous system impairment is assumed to increase continuously from negligible to incapacitating. In some cases the importance of the central nervous system impairment is outweighed by some other consequence of OSAS such as cor pulmonale. The significance to patients of smaller degrees of somnolence or loss of mental clarity can depend a great deal on their occupation, on their expectations of mental performance, and on their insight. There are, of course, many causes besides OSAS of fatigue, somnolence, and impaired cognition. There seems also to be wide inter-personal variation in the degree of impairment caused by a given degree of OSAS (events per hour). The methods to quantify fatigue, somnolence, or impairment of cognitive function are very rough. The correlation between the number of obstructed breathing events at night and daytime impairment is very poor.

DIAGNOSTIC PROCESS

What the clinician wants to do once the question of OSAS has been raised is to identify patients who would benefit from diagnosis and treatment of OSAS and those who would not. In this chapter we discuss the contribution of clinical data to the process of diagnosis and determining whether in fact patients are clinically improved with therapy.

One approach would be simply to treat all patients in whom the question of OSAS has been raised, and to continue the treatment only in those who improved. There are several difficulties with this. First is the cost to patients and to the health care system of treatment trials in patients who do not have OSAS. Second is the lack of a precise, reliable measurement of the outcome variable, which is somnolence or fatigue. Third is the problem of interpreting the result of a single, unblinded test of treatment in one person. Fourth is the potential negative impact of the currently available treatments on some patients.

The usual approach tries to avoid some of the foregoing problems by a stepwise process. Data from the history and physical examination are used to sort out patients who either have a very low likelihood of having an apnea-hypopnea index (AHI) high enough to be of significance or who are so likely to have a high AHI of significance that further testing is pointless. Use of clinical assessment for this purpose is discussed later under 'Diagnosis of OSAS'. Data from the history and physical examination or ancillary tests (blood gases, hemoglobin) and from questionnaires can be used to identify patients who have no obvious impairment in their cognition, cardiorespiratory system, or quality of life that could be attributed to OSAS and therefore could not benefit from treatment specific for OSAS. It is important to understand how patients describe the impact of OSAS on their lives so an appropriate history can be taken to assess this. This use of clinical information is discussed under 'Using Clinical Features to Assess the Impact of OSAS on Patients.'

In some patients who complain of somnolence, fatigue, or cognitive impairment, clinical data may point so strongly to a diagnosis other than OSAS (myxedema, narcolepsy, or depression) that the most economical route to the final treatment decision may bypass testing for OSAS.

The remaining patients then undergo a diagnostic test that gives values for AHI and nocturnal oxygen levels. With the results of that test in hand, the clinician decides whether to recommend a course of treatment. This decision is based on two factors. One is an estimate of the likelihood that the patient has an important health deficit and an estimate of the long-term consequences of leaving the condition untreated. The other is the degree of confidence that the somnolence or other health deficit is in fact related to the AHI and not caused by something else. The higher the AHI and the greater the estimated impairment or long-term risk, the stronger is the inclination to recommend treatment. As with all the other steps in the process, there are no cut-off levels. The outcome of initial treatment is then used to refine the diagnosis. If the expected improvement in alertness does not occur after a treatment that does improve sleep apnea, there is reason to doubt a cause-and-effect relation between the sleep apnea and the symptoms and therefore this would indicate the importance of reassessing the problem.

Research on symptoms and signs in patients referred to sleep centers can give useful answers to several kinds of questions: 1) key clinical data can be combined in algebraic formulas that place patients into categories of risk or probability that they will have a positive result on a test for sleep apnea; 2) scores from 'quality of life' questionnaries can be used to evaluate the impact that sleep apnea has had on a patient's life; 3) epidemiological studies can give information about prognostic factors; and 4) outcome trials can give information about what clinical information helps to predict a patient's response to therapy. This chapter review's the first two of these.

USING SENSITIVITY, SPECIFICITY, PREDICTIVE VALUES AND LIKELIHOOD RATIOS TO ASSIST IN CLINICAL DECISION MAKING

CLINICAL DECISION MAKING

There are many reasons for patients to be assessed for sleep apnea. They may be disabled by daytime sleepiness. They may be asymptomatic but have a bed partner who is worried because they stop breathing while asleep. They may have another problem, such as impotence, hypertension, or headaches that could be attributed to sleep apnea. To avoid ordering unnecessary tests and at the same time avoid missing treatable cases, the clinician would like to use simple clinical data to exclude some patients from testing but at the same time be sure of ordering tests on all those in whom there is a reasonable chance of doing some good.

The process of making clinical decisions is complex to understand and to model. One theory proposes that there are probability thresholds that define when a clinician will act (10,11). When the probability of a disease is low enough, further testing is not warranted (the do-not-treat, do-not-test threshold). On the other hand, the probability of the disease may be so high that further testing is not warranted before a decision is made to initiate treatment (the treatment threshold). Between these two extremes lies an intermediate probability of disease that warrants further testing, which may revise the probability either upward past the treatment threshold or downward past a threshold where no further testing is warranted. The

threshold levels can be determined mathematically if certain information is available, including the outcomes of treated and untreated disease and the operating characteristics and potential complications of the diagnostic test or tests. In sleep apnea this information is generally not available, and thus the level of disease probability at which thresholds are set depends on individual clinicians' experience, hunches, and partial evidence in the literature.

In the assessment of the clinical features of a patient who may possibly have sleep apnea, the decision that clinicians are faced with depends on the setting in which they practice. In primary care or an otolaryngology practice the required decision is usually whether or not to refer the patient to a sleep center. In a sleep center the decision is whether the patient requires immediate treatment, polysomnography, or a portable home recording or whether her or she can be discharged without any testing. The threshold that has to be crossed is the 'do something' threshold (for primary care, refer the patient; for a sleep center, treat or order some testing). Below this threshold a clinician should feel reasonably secure in the decision to do nothing. Where the threshold between doing something and doing nothing lies on the spectrum of the probability that a patient has sleep apnea will be influenced by an estimate of the impact that sleep apnea is having on the patient's quality of life (that is, on his or her job, family, safety, and the severity of their symptoms) as well as by the presence or absence of coexisting illness. For example, in an otherwise healthy patient who attends a sleep clinic primarily because of bothersome snoring and perhaps some suspected apnea events based on observations by the bed partner, a clinician may be prepared to accept a 'do something' threshold of 30% or higher. However, if the same patient had a history of hypertension and coronary artery disease, the clinician would demand much more certainty that the patient did not have sleep apnea and thus the 'do something' threshold may need to be 5% or even lower (Fig. 5.1 A, B). The clinician will determine the threshold that seems appropriate for each given patient. Knowing the probability that a patient may or may not have sleep apnea assists in clinical decision making.

SENSITIVITY AND SPECIFICITY, PREDICTIVE VALUES, AND LIKELIHOOD RATIOS

In clinical medicine, diagnostic tests are performed to determine if a target disorder is present. Often there is a reference or gold standard test that, in an ideal setting,

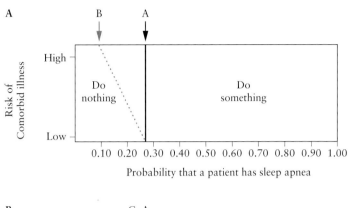

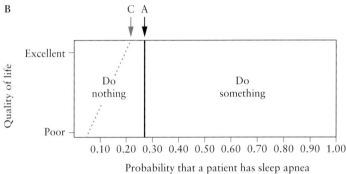

*Fig 5.1 The 'Do something' threshold in a healthy patient with an excellent quality of life **A** is set arbitrarily by the clinician but may be lowered by an increasing risk of comorbid illness **B** and/or by a reduced quality of life **C**.*

would be performed on any patient suspected of having the disorder in question and that would separate patients perfectly into those who have and those who do not have the disease. The reference standard test may not be available, may be costly, or may carry a risk for morbidity or mortality. In such circumstances surrogate diagnostic tests are evaluated for their ability to substitute for the reference standard.

A test result can be the answer to a question about medical history or a physical examination observation or the result of a laboratory test. Thus, we could ask what is the sensitivity and specificity of the symptom of snoring for the diagnosis of sleep apnea or of the findings of obesity, retrognathia, neck size, or tongue size. In what follows, 'diagnostic test' will refer to any clinical information (symptom, physical characteristic, or laboratory test).

The 'operating characteristics' of tests are often summarized as sensitivity (the proportion of patients with disease who have a positive test result, the 'true positive' rate) and specificity (the proportion of patients without disease who have a negative result, the 'true negative' rate). Using sensitivity and specificity to describe the utility of a diagnostic test has some limitations since these parameters indicate the probability that the test result will be positive *if the patient has the disease* or the probability that the test will be negative *if the patient does not have the disease*. Clinicians cannot apply these numbers directly, because they do not know whether or not the patient has the disease. What the physician wants to know is the probability that the patient actually has the disease if the test is positive. This is called the positive predictive value of the test. The sensitivity and specificity are given by analyzing the vertical columns in a 2 × 2 table, such as Figure

5.2A, whereas the positive and negative predictive values are obtained by analyzing the horizontal rows. Sensitivity, specificity, prevalence (or pretest probability), and predictive values provide valuable information about a diagnostic test; however, it can be a challenge to interpret several different numbers that describe the operating characteristics of a test. A superior approach is to calculate a single number, the likelihood ratio (LR), that directly relates how good a test is for increasing or decreasing the probability of disease. For a given level of diagnostic test result, a LR reflects the proportion of patients with disease compared to those without. It is possible to calculate LRs for multiple levels of a diagnostic test result. This is an advantage over the approach of sensitivity and specificity, which requires dichotomizing a diagnostic result into positive or negative. If a patient undergoes a test and gets a result associated with a LR of 2, this indicates the patient is twice as likely to have the disease in question as he or she was prior to having the test. If the test result was

associated with an LR of 0.5, the patient is half as likely to have the disease. Generally LRs of < 0.2 and > 10 have a very large impact on changing the probability of disease. The information about clinical features for diagnosing sleep apnea has been summarized in Table 5.1 using LRs. Those readers who prefer a more detailed discussion about the difference between sensitivity and specificity, predictive values, and LRs may go on to the following discussion; those who prefer to avoid a detailed mathematical discussion can proceed to the section 'Using Clinical Features to Predict it a Patient Has Sleep Apnea.'

A	RS +ve	RS −ve	
DT +ve	180	100	280
DT −ve	20	700	720
	200	800	1000

B	RS +ve	RS −ve	
DT +ve	360	72	432
DT −ve	40	528	568
	400	600	1000

Fig 5.2 Hypothetical example comparing a reference standard test (RS) to a surrogate diagnostic test (DT). In this example, the prevalence is 200/1000 or 20% in 2a and 40% in 2b.

⚬→ Key points box 5.2

Practice points

1. Clinicians are faced with trying to decide whether a particular patient has features suggestive enough of sleep apnea that they warrant investigation and possible treatment. These decisions are usually based on selected clinical features that predict a positive diagnosis of sleep apnea and on how much the disorder appears to be affecting the patient's life.
2. The diagnostic utility of particular patient features can be summarized by their sensitivity and specificity, but a superior method is to use likelihood ratios.
3. Likelihood ratios can be calculated for multiple levels of a test result (or a clinical characteristic) and, in a single number, can more fully describe its diagnostic utility.

CALCULATION OF SENSITIVITY AND SPECIFICITY, PREDICTIVE VALUES, AND LIKELIHOOD RATIOS

The calculation of sensitivity, specificity, and predictive values is easiest to understand by examining a 2 × 2 table (Fig. 5.2A). In this hypothetical example, 180 of the 200 patients who have a disease defined by a positive reference standard (RS) test have a positive diagnostic test (sensitivity 90%) and 700/800 of those who do not have the disease have a negative test (specificity 88%). The positive and negative predictive values are obtained by analyzing the horizontal rows in the table. The positive predictive value is 180/280 or 64%. The negative predictive value is 20/720 or 3%.

The predictive value of a test (also known as the posttest probability) depends not only on sensitivity and specificity but also on the pretest probability of disease. This is illustrated in Figure 5.2B. The pretest probability of disease has increased from 20% to 40%. The sensitivity in Figure 5.2A of 90% and the specificity of 88% remains the same in Figure 5.2B (sensitivity = 360/400 = 90%; specificity = 528/600 = 88%). The posttest probability of disease given a positive diagnostic test result (positive predictive value) in Figure 5.2A is 180/280 or 64% and for a negative result (negative predictive value) is 20/720 or 3%. The corresponding posttest probabilities for Figure 5.2B are 83% (360/432) and 7% (40/568).

In the example of Figure 5.2A even though the sensitivity and specificity are quite high, the probability that a patient has the target disorder in question given a positive diagnostic test result is only 64%. Why is that? Based on Bayes' theorem, the posttest probability of disease depends on sensitivity and specificity but also on the prevalence (sometimes referred to as the a priori probability) of disease.

In the population shown in Figure 5.2A the prevalence of the disease is 20% (number of positive reference tests/total number of patients). In the population shown in Figure 5.2B the prevalence is 40%. The posttest probabilities (horizontal calculations) are therefore different. It is always true that the probability that a patient whose test is positive actually has the disease is higher if the pretest probability is higher. Conversely, if the pretest probability is lower and the test result is negative, the posttest probability is lower.

The pretest probability is essentially the percentage of patients in the set of patients being considered who actually have the disease or, in other words, the prevalence of the disease in the patient population under consideration. To attach a meaning to a positive test result, it is clearly necessary to know the prevalence or pretest probability. This can be measured simply by doing the reference diagnostic test on a population of patients and thus determining the percentage of patients with the disease. As long as future patients are drawn from the same population, this pretest probability is valid.

A second way of determining pretest probability is simply to take an estimate made by experienced clinicians. In so doing, of course, it is necessary to assume that the clinicians in question have a broad enough experience to enable them to give an accurate value for the likelihood that the patients do have the disease and that their experience is drawn from a similar population of patients.

Young et al. have shown the prevalence of an AHI ≥ 15 in the general adult population (age 30 to 60 years) to be 4.0% in women and 9.1% in men (12). These rates would be appropriate to use in a primary care setting. In populations of patients currently being referred to sleep centers because of sleep-related complaints, the prevalence of sleep apnea is much higher, approximately 40–60%.

The likelihood that a patient has sleep apnea is different for snorers and nonsnorers, but by how much? These important questions are addressed in a later section. Estimates of disease probability can be used as a starting point and can be modified by knowing certain key clinical characteristics of a patient.

A different kind of difficulty with using sensitivity and specificity for clinical decision making is that it requires that the test result be categorized simply as either positive or negative. Many disorders including OSAS are not either/or categories. Instead, there is a continuous gradation in the test result (such as respiratory disturbance index (RDI)) from zero to a large number, where the higher the value the more likely it is that a patient suffers from the disorder or has a significant health impairment. A great deal of information is lost by calling the test result positive or negative. This limitation can be partly avoided by classifying test results into multiple categories such as 'negative,' 'mild,' 'moderate,' or 'severe.' In that case, posttest probabilities for each category are calculated using LRs. As an example, a LR of 2.0 indicates that a patient with a positive diagnostic test is twice as likely to have the disease. A LR of 1 indicates that the diagnostic test result has not changed the pretest probability of disease. LRs of less than 1 change the pretest probability to a lower value whereas ratios greater than 1 change the pretest probability to a higher value.

Mathematically, when using LRs to convert pretest to posttest probabilities, the pretest probability estimate has to be converted to an odds expression (pretest odds = pretest probability / 1 − pretest probability) multiplied by the LR to obtain the posttest odds, which can then be converted back to a probability statement (posttest probability = posttest odds/posttest odds + 1). This process can be greatly simplified with the use of a nomogram (Fig. 5.3). Figure 5.4 demonstrates the relationship between some common pretest probabilities,

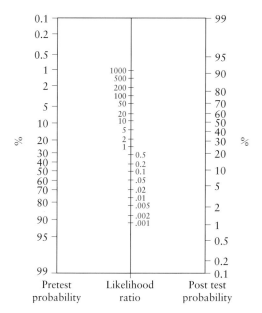

		RS +ve		RS −ve		Likelihood Ratio
		# of Pts	Proportion	# of Pts	Proportion	
	< 5	13	$\frac{13}{400} = .033$	339	$\frac{339}{600} = .565$	$\frac{.033}{.565} = 0.06$
DT	5 – 10	27	$\frac{27}{400} = .068$	189	$\frac{189}{600} = .315$	$\frac{.068}{.315} = 0.2$
Result	11 – 20	53	$\frac{53}{400} = .133$	33	$\frac{33}{600} = .055$	$\frac{.133}{.055} = 2.5$
	21 – 40	129	$\frac{129}{400} = .323$	31	$\frac{31}{600} = .052$	$\frac{.323}{.052} = 6.8$
	> 40	178	$\frac{178}{400} = .445$	8	$\frac{8}{600} = .013$	$\frac{.445}{.013} = 34.2$
		400		600		

Fig 5.5 *The calculation of likehood ratios.*

LRs, and posttest probabilities. Figure 5.5 demonstrates how LRs are calculated. Consider the same hypothetical test as in Figure 5.2B but instead of categorizing the diagnostic test as positive or negative, the test results are reported on multiple levels.

Fig 5.3 *A nomogram for converting pretest to posttest probability (probabilities listed as percentages), using likehood ratios. To use the nomogram, anchor a straight edge at the pretest probability and direct it through the appropriate likehood ratio. The intersection of the straight edge with the thrid (right) line produces the probability result. (Reprinted with permission from Fagan TJ. Nomogram for Bayes' Theorum. N Engl J Med 1975; 293:257.)*

Pretest Probability	Likelihood Ratios					
	0.2	0.5	1.5	2.0	5.0	10.0
5%	1.0	2.6	7.3	9.5	20.8	34.5
10%	2.2	5.3	14.3	18.2	35.7	52.6
15%	3.4	8.1	20.9	26.1	46.9	63.8
20%	4.8	11.1	27.3	33.3	55.6	71.4
30%	7.9	17.6	39.1	46.2	68.2	81.1
40%	11.8	25.0	50.0	57.1	76.9	87.0
50%	16.7	33.3	60.0	66.7	83.3	90.9
60%	23.1	42.9	69.2	75.0	88.2	93.8
70%	31.8	53.8	77.8	82.4	92.1	95.9
80%	44.4	66.7	85.7	88.9	95.2	97.6

Fig 5.4 *Post-test probabilities for combinations of pretest probability and likelihood ratios.*

> **⊶ Key points box 5.3**

Practice Points

1. A clinician needs to know, given a certain level of a diagnostic test or clinical feature, what the probability is that a patient has sleep apnea; this is referred to as the posttest probability or the predictive value.

2. When using sensitivity and specificity or likelihood ratios to estimate the posttest probability of disease, it is necessary to have an estimate of the a priori (or pretest) probability of disease.

3. In most sleep centers, approximately 40–60% of referred patients have sleep apnea, which is the estimate that can be used as the a priori probability. In a primary care setting it is more appropriate to use estimates based on the prevalence of disease in the general population, which is 4% for women and 9% for men (based on a defining criterion AHI ≥ 15).

4. Likelihood ratios close to 1 do not change the probability of disease, indicating poor diagnostic utility. Likelihood ratios < 0.2 and > 10 substantially alter the probability of disease.

A LR captures the utility of a diagnostic test in a single number, which is a distinct advantage over using the approach of sensitivity and specificity. If the only information available about a diagnostic test is its sensitivity and specificity, these numbers can be converted into LRs. The LR for a positive diagnostic test result = sensitivity/1 – specificity; conversely, the LR for a negative result is 1 – sensitivity/specificity.

USING CLINICAL FEATURES TO PREDICT IF A PATIENT HAS SLEEP APNEA

A clinician who understands which clinical features are useful for distinguishing between patients with sleep apnea and those without, and who knows how useful each clinical feature (or combination of features) is, which are best summarized through LRs, and how to use LRs to modify an estimate of the probability that a patient may have sleep apnea, has the necessary information to make rational choices about 'doing something' or 'doing nothing' (Fig. 5.1). For example, in a patient with a low pretest probability of disease (the clinician estimates there is less than a 20% chance the patient has sleep apnea) who has few of the key clinical characteristics, it is possible to show that the risk of sleep apnea is low (less than 5–8%) and thus it is justifiable not to pursue further diagnostic testing. There are a few cautions about the information that will be quoted in the subsequent section. Research on the clinical aspects of sleep apnea has largely been conducted in sleep centers, where patients are mostly middle-aged men. Theoretically, the only difference between a primary care setting and a sleep center should be the prevalence of the disease. Since sensitivity, specificity, and LRs are not influenced by prevalence, the results from sleep centers should be applicable to the primary care setting. However, referral bias to tertiary care sleep centers may affect some of the reports published to date, in that some of the patients who did not have obvious sleep apnea may have been screened out in the primary care setting and were not referred. The current clinical prediction rules for sleep apnea that have been published have not been validated in the primary care setting. Neck circumference, when measured in studies on sleep apnea patients, has consistently been shown to be the strongest predictor of the disorder (13). This has also been found in a primary care setting of 1001 patients (14), suggesting that results

generated from sleep centers do have some applicability for clinical decision making in primary care. An additional concern about the generalizability of these results is that the patient populations studied to date have been predominantely Caucasian. It is not clear whether the approach is applicable to other racial groups.

In this section we review what is known about individual clinical characteristics as they apply to estimating the likelihood of sleep apnea. Then we address the issue of combining clinical characteristics of patients into approaches called clinical prediction rules. Since many of the individual characteristics of sleep apnea patients may influence the chance they could have other clinical characteristics, it is incorrect to combine the LRs. For example, if a patient was a frequent snorer (LR of 1.4) and had a waist circumference more than 110 cm (LR of 3.2), only one of these characteristics should be used to modify the probability that the patient has sleep apnea (rather than multiplying 1.4 × 3.2 to establish a combined LR of 4.5). Clinical features should only be combined using mathematical approaches that develop a clinical prediction rule (see below).

INDIVIDUAL CLINICAL FEATURES
Nocturnal Symptoms

■ **Snoring.** Snoring is the hallmark symptom of sleep apnea because it reflects the basic pathophysiology underlying the disorder, critical narrowing of the upper airway. In population surveys 25% of men and 15% of women are habitual snorers (snore almost every or every night) (15). The prevalence of snoring increases progressively with age; 60% of men and 40% of women between the ages of 41 and 65 years of age habitually snore (16). Snoring can be quantified either by frequency (how many times per week) or by intensity. When it is quantified by asking patients how often they snore, or how often they snore loudly, the information is only modestly helpful for making a clinical decision, since LRs range only from 0.5 to 1.7 (17) (Table 5.1). Some investigators have found even less diagnostic utility from asking patients about snoring frequency (18, 19). Thus, even though snoring is thought of as a 'hallmark' symptom of sleep apnea, its diagnostic utility is limited. The reasons for this may be because patients tend to underreport their symptom of snoring (especially if their bed partners do not assist in answering the question) and because subjective report-

Table 5.1 Diagnosis of sleep apnea likelihood ratios (LR) for symptoms and physical characteristics

Symptom or Physical Characteristic	Level	LR
Nocturnal		
Snoring frequency[17*]	< 3 nights per week	0.4
	≥ 3 nights per week	1.4
Loud, disruptive snoring frequency[17*]	< 3 nights per week	0.5
	≥ 3 nights per week	1.7
Snoring intensity[21]	Extremely loud	3.6
	Louder than talking	1.3
	As loud as talking	0.5
	Slightly louder than heavy breathing	0.3
Partner's report of choking or gasping[17*]	< 1 night per month	0.5
	1–8 nights per month	1.1
	≥ 3 nights per week	1.9
Partner's report of apneas[19,22]	Yes	1.4, 1.5
	No	0.2, 0.5
Nocturia[24]	Yes	1.5
	No	0.6
Daytime		
Excessive daytime sleepiness[19]	Yes, against the person's will	1.4
	Yes, but willingly	1.2
	None	0.8
Weight gain over previous 2 years[17*]	< 10 pounds	0.8
	≥ 10 pounds	1.4
Impotence[18]	Yes	3.2
	No	0.9
Physical Examination		
Pharyngeal examination[19]	Abnormal	1.4
	Normal	0.8
Hypertension[17*, 22, 24]	Yes	1.6, 2.2, 2.4
	No	0.4, 0.6, 0.8
Body mass index[17*]	< 25 (kg/m^2)[17*]	0.3
	25–30 (kg/m^2)[17*]	0.7
	> 30 (kg/m^2)[17*, 24]	2.0, 2.3
Waist circumference[17*]	< 90 cm	0.3
	90–110 cm	1.1
	> 110 cm	3.2
Waist: hip ratio[17*]	< 0.8	0.2
	0.8–1.0	1.0
	> 1.0	2.8

Table 5.1 (*cont.*)

Symptom or Physical Characteristic	Level	LR
Neck circumference[17]*	< 38 cm	0.5
	38–44 cm	1.1
	> 44 cm	4.1
Clinical Prediction Rule		
Sleep apnea clinical score (SACS)[17]	< 5.0	0.3
	5–10.0	1.1
	10.1–15.0	2.2
	> 15.0	5.2

* LRs calculated from the original, unpublished data of this study.

ing of snoring (even by trained observers) correlates relatively poorly with objective measurements (20).

It appears to be more useful diagnostically to quantify snoring on the basis of intensity, since there is a greater range of possible LRs (21) (Table 5.1). It is not known whether combining questions about frequency and intensity would improve the usefulness of reported snoring in discriminating between patients with and those without sleep apnea.

■ **Witnessed Apneas.** An obvious question to patients and their bed partners is one about observed apneas made by the partner and reported to the patient. Inquiring about the frequency of apneas observed by the partner has about the same diagnostic utility as asking about snoring frequency (19, 22). Bed partners seldom give accurate information about frequency of recurrent hypopneas. Even trained medical personnel seem unable to make an accurate diagnosis of sleep apnea by clinical observation of breathing during sleep (23). At least three groups have found similar results in a sleep center setting (Table 5.1). When constructing clinical prediction rules this symptom is often replaced in the model by the symptom of reports of nocturnal choking or gasping. Both questions 1) a question of how frequently apneas are observed and 2) a question about how frequently there are reports of nocturnal choking or grasping. Both questions appear to be equivalent and are likely interchangeable for the purpose of diagnosis.

■ **Nocturnal Choking or Gasping.** This symptom is not asked as frequently in studies of sleep apnea as the question of apnea events. It is more useful to ask patients if their bed partner reports to them that they choke or gasp during the night than it is to simply ask the patients if they wake up experiencing these symptoms. In our study of clinical predictors we found bed partner reports to the patients of their choking or gasping slightly more useful than reported apneas and have included it in a clinical prediction rule (17).

Spells in which patients have attacks of dyspnea or choking that wake them from sleep may result in referral to a sleep clinic; however, it is not always possible to be sure of the diagnosis. Ordinary sleep apnea can waken patients, who are likely to report it as being wakened by snoring. We assume they become alert enough to register events only after the airway has opened and they are in the middle of a postapneic snore.

Occasional sleep apnea patients describe very dramatic episodes in which they come wide awake and find they cannot breathe at all because their airway is completely closed. They are unable to open it for some time in spite of violent efforts, sometimes jump out of bed and take a few steps or throw themselves on the floor. They may make small stridorous sounds. After what seems like a very long time the airway opens suddenly and they are fine. We suspect these episodes can be explained by a sequence of events that we have observed in numerous sleep apnea patients during polysomnography. At the beginning of an obstructive apnea, esophageal pressure tracings show recurrent negative inspiratory deflections, which increase in amplitude as the apnea goes on. Toward the end of the apnea, expiratory muscles come into play and make positive deflections in pleural pressure in expiration. The upper airway remains closed in inspiration, but some air is expelled with each of these expiratory efforts. The volume of gas in the lungs goes down, partly through gas exchange and partly through expiratory efforts, and it may get very close to residual volume. We postulate that when the patient wakes up in this circumstance, the elastic recoil of the respiratory system is exerting a substantial negative subglottic pressure, which may be enough to overpower the dilator capability of upper airway muscles. A similar imbalance may keep the airway closed in inspiration as the patient frantically makes huge inspiratory efforts with the thoracic cage muscle. Being at residual volume makes it difficult to generate significant positive pressure to open the airway in expiration. The blockage can continue until either a change in posture or incoordination between thoracic and upper airway muscle changes the balance of collapsing and dilating forces on the airway. We have seen rare patients who had similar attacks in the day and in whom the epiglottis was seen at endoscopy during sleep to be very loosely coupled to the base of the tongue. In such cases the epiglottis may fall over the larynx, occlude the airway, and be held in place by inspiratory suction, and protrusion of the tongue may fail to pull the epiglottis from the laryngeal orifice.

Patients with Cheyne-Stokes breathing sometimes come awake during the hyperpneic phase, find themselves taking unusually deep breaths, and report dyspnea.

Laryngospasm, perhaps set off by gastroesophageal reflux, is suspected when stridor, a change in voice, a story of heartburn, or a sensation of acid in the throat is reported. Patients with laryngospasm are usually extremely frightened, often feel they are going to die, and are unable to breathe properly for much longer (often several minutes) than patients with sleep apnea. In addition, they are usually unable to vocalize while they are struggling to breathe and are quite specific, when asked, that the source of their dyspnea is related to a 'blockage in the throat.'

Some patients describe sleep paralysis with an emphasis on inability to breathe. Nocturnal panic attacks are considered if the symptoms take a long time to subside and there are other features of panic besides the dyspnea. Dyspnea in the night caused by pulmonary edema is usually recognized by the timing and time course of the event and the appropriate clinical setting.

- **Insomnia.** Sleep maintenance insomnia is often mentioned as a symptom of obstructive apnea and of Cheyne-Stokes breathing. As an independent predictor of OSAS it has not been shown to be helpful, but infrequently patients may have it as their major symptom.

- **Other Nocturnal Symptoms.** Several other nocturnal symptoms may be reported by patients or their bed partners, such as nocturia, enuresis, frequent arousals, and diaphoresis. The exact prevalence of these symptoms in patients with sleep apnea is not known; however, in our experience they have not been shown to discriminate between patients with and without sleep apnea, nor do they correlate with severity of the AHI. One group of investigators have found that nocturia is more common in sleep apnea patients than in heavy snorers (24) (Table 5.1). In one study, impotence was reported more frequently in sleep apnea patients (18).

- **Patient or Partner Reports.** In general, reports by patients about what goes on when they are asleep are all second-hand and ought to be less reliable than first-hand accounts from bed partners. The importance of first-hand reports has not been assessed in studies of diagnostic accuracy for sleep apnea. However, when we developed a clinical prediction rule for sleep apnea we systematically asked patients and their bed partners to fill out identical questionnaires. We then evaluated the diagnostic utility of their responses and found no circumstances under which the partner's reports were more accurate (17). It is possible that this reflects the difficulty in recording the patient's history by questionnaire, and perhaps qualitative methods of recording bed partners' observations would be more valid.

Physical Characteristics and Examination

- **Obesity.** The body mass index (BMI), the most commonly reported measurement of obesity, is calculated by dividing a patient's weight in kilograms (kg) by the square of his or her height in meters (kg/m^2). Overweight may be defined as a body weight greater than 120% of ideal (25), which corresponds to a BMI greater than 27. Using these definitions approximately

24% of men and 27% of women in the United States are overweight (26). A relationship exists between obesity and sleep apnea, especially upper body obesity (android obesity or increased waist:hip ratio) (27). There are several ways to characterize obesity: skin fold thickness, BMI, waist circumference, waist:hip ratio, and neck circumference. We have previously attempted to measure skin fold thickness in a population of patients referred for assessment of sleep apnea but found the measurements variable and difficult to reproduce in very obese subjects (17). All of these anthropomorphic variables are highly correlated with each other and thus can not be combined to predict sleep apnea. Several investigators have found that neck circumference correlates most closely with the AHI, but others report measurements such as the waist circumference to be superior (13, 17). The diagnostic utility of neck circumference is summarized in the next section. Waist circumference and waist:hip ratio appear to discriminate between sleep apnea and non–sleep apnea patients slightly better than the BMI does (Table 5.1).

■ **Neck Circumference.** Many studies have confirmed that patients with sleep apnea have larger than average necks, usually assessed by measuring neck circumference at the level of the cricoid membrane. Patients with sleep apnea also have a smaller internal diameter of the pharyngeal airway, especially the distal part, suggesting that sleep apnea patients have 'thick necks,' caused in part by excess fat deposition (28,29). Practically speaking, the neck circumference and the AHI are continuous variables so although there is a definite relationship between them, there is no single threshold value that can be used by itself on which to base a firm clinical decision. As discussed in the section on clinical prediction rules, some general statements can be made about how to use information on neck circumference. Patients with small neck circumferences (< 37 cm) are at low risk of having sleep apnea and, conversely, patients with quite large neck circumferences (> 48 cm) are at a substantially higher risk.

■ **Craniofacial or Neck Anatomy.** Certain anatomical abnormalities seem to predispose to sleep apnea and we would therefore expect them to be useful for assessing the probability that a patient has sleep apnea. Through cephalometry, computed tomographic (CT) scanning, or magnetic resonance (MR) imaging it has been demonstrated that some patients with OSAS have retrognathia, micrognathia, tonsillar hypertrophy, macroglossia, fat deposition, certain facial configurations, and inferior displacement of the hyoid (30,31). Small case series give limited information about how to utilize the measurements for clinical decision making. Some patients have recognizable pathological abnormalities of craniofacial anatomy that can be described by clinical examination. However, it is hard to know what to make of clinical features of the pharynx since the observations are not anchored in quantifiable, reproducible measurements that would permit them to be standardized and applied by one clinician in the same way as another. One group reported the results of an examination of the posterior oropharynx, rating it abnormal if 1) it appeared to be narrow and small; 2) the uvula was bulky, long, and rested on the base of the tongue during phonation; or 3) the tonsils were large enough to compromise the pharyngeal orifice (19). This method of rating the examination of the pharynx was not particularly helpful for diagnosing sleep apnea (Table 5.1). There has been no evaluation of cephalometry, CT scanning, or MR imaging on large populations of patients suspected of having sleep apnea to determine their ability to discriminate between patients with and without the disorder. One report has been published of clinical measurements of craniofacial anatomy, including palatal height, that appear to discriminate very well between sleep apnea patients and non–sleep apnea patients who had been seen at a tertiary care sleep center. Before such findings can be applied for diagnosis it is necessary to study them in a broader population of patients. The generalizeability of the findings is not clear because the prevalence of disease was very high (85%), and the majority of the small number of non–sleep apnea patients were not clinically suspected of having the disorder (32).

■ **Hypertension.** A link between sleep apnea and hypertension has been consistently demonstrated in many studies (33). The difficulty with using the presence or absence of hypertension to predict whether a patient has sleep apnea is that many patients assessed at a sleep center are normotensive because of drug therapy. Patients must therefore be rated hypertensive if their diastolic or systolic pressures are above threshold values (typically 95 torr and 160 torr, respectively) or if they are on antihypertensive therapy irrespective of their current blood pressure. In our studies we have also scored patients as 'positive' for hypertension if they had previously been on treatment but had stopped it. With these criteria we have found LRs for the presence of hypertension to be approximately 2.4 and for the absence of hypertension to be 0.8 (17).

Daytime Symptoms

■ **Excessive Daytime Sleepiness.** Although sleep apnea is the most common cause of excessive daytime sleepiness (EDS), it has not been found to be very useful as a clinical feature to discriminate between patients with and without the disorder. Many studies have found that severity of EDS and sleep apnea do not correlate (13); the few that have found a correlation report only modest associations reflected in LRs close to 1.0 (Table 5.1). This lack of relationship between EDS and sleep apnea is likely because many other sleep disorders also cause EDS and because there are, to date, a lack of well-validated systematic methods for quantifying EDS.

■ **Other Daytime Symptoms.** Sleep apnea is reported to be associated with many symptoms other than EDS, such as fatigue, memory impairment, personality changes, morning nausea, morning headaches, automatic behavior, and depression (34). Although these features may be important in assessing the impact of sleep apnea on a patient and the effectiveness of therapy, there has been no systematic study of the capacity of these features to predict the presence or absence of OSAS.

Combined Features

■ **Subjective Clinical Impression.** When the ability of experienced sleep physicians to predict the result of a polysomnogram (i.e., whether the AHI will be above a given threshold value) without using clinical prediction rules is formally tested, the sensitivity and specificity of subjective clinical impression are only approximately 60% (19). LRs have been calculated for several levels of clinical estimates of the probability that patients may have sleep apnea and range from 0.5 to 3.7 (17). This indicates that the judgments of experienced physicians are superior to individual clinical

characteristics but are not as good as a clinical prediction rule for estimating the probability that a patient has sleep apnea in a sleep clinic setting.

■ **Clinical Prediction Rules.** Many clinical features of patients may individually help to predict the result of diagnostic testing, but it is not possible to determine which clinical features are 'most' predictive, and in what combination, without using multivariate statistical techniques. Valid combinations of features that are individually predictive are called clinical prediction rules and are developed by analyzing a large sample of the population in whom the diagnosis is considered, and in whom a diagnostic test is then carried out. In order to develop useful rules that are applicable to patient populations other than the study population, this type of research should be conducted on unbiased samples of patients who represent a broad spectrum of disease severity and in whom the diagnostic result can be clearly defined. Thus, the sample should be a consecutive series of patients, all of whom undergo the diagnostic test regardless of the investigators' level of 'diagnostic suspicion.' The relationship of each clinical feature that is believed to have some ability to predict the diagnostic result is first evaluated by univariate statistical analysis. Those clinical features with statistically significant relationships can then be combined using multivariate statistics into a core group of clinical features that independently predict the diagnostic outcome of interest. This multivariate analysis is often accomplished by multiple regression analysis, either linear or logistic. Not only does this approach allow for a grouping of key clinical features, it also allows the relative weight or importance of each of the clinical features to be determined. The result, calculated from a clinical prediction rule, can be treated just like any diagnostic test result, and its usefulness can be defined by its sensitivity and specificity or by LRs.

In general, most reports of sleep apnea clinical prediction rules have shown relationships between the AHI and several physical characteristics, findings on examination, and symptoms. Since many of these variables are highly correlated, it is possible to generate several different models that have similar diagnostic performance. There are important similarities in many of the reports of sleep apnea clinical prediction rules. All investigators have included some type of anthropomorphic measurement in addition to bed partner reports of nocturnal breathing disturbances (snoring, apneas, choking or gasping respirations) (13). Other variables, such as age, gender, and hypertension, have been incorporated into some rules in varying ways. The reasons for the variability among the studies are likely related to the different types of populations studied and the different statistical techniques employed.

These clinical prediction rules are thus clinical tests that provide an estimate of the likelihood that a patient has or does not have sleep apnea as defined by some arbitrary AHI cut-off. The sensitivity for these rules can be quite high (78%–95%) if the cut-offs for positive results are appropriately set; but specificity tends to be relatively low (41%–63%) (13). These rules could therefore be used with confidence to exclude sleep apnea in some patients but could not be used with confidence to confirm the diagnosis. LRs for one clinical prediction rule have been calculated and range from 0.25 for a low clinical score to 5.17 for a high clinical score (Table 5.1) (17). All of the published clinical prediction rules for sleep apnea have been constructed from populations of patients referred to a sleep laboratory or clinic setting where the prevalence of sleep apnea is high (approximately 45–55%). A study of a population of referred patients among whom the prevalence of an AHI ≥ 10 was 45% and of AHI ≥ 20 was 30% found that if the clinical score was low, only 17% had an

AHI ≥ 10 and only 8% had an AHI ≥ 20. These numbers would be even lower if the prevalence or pretest probability of sleep apnea was lower, as in a primary care setting. Whether these numbers fall below the 'do something' threshold is a decision each clinician would have to make depending on other important clinical characteristics (Fig. 5.1).

Clinical prediction rules are very useful in highlighting which variables do and which do not predict the AHI. The determination of a sleep apnea clinical score can be made quite simply through the use of a table. This sleep apnea clinical score can then be used to place the patient in one of three probability groups; low, intermediate, or high. The clinical data needed to determine this clinical score are the patient's neck circumference, whether or not the patient has a history of hypertension, habitual snoring, or partner reports that the patient has frequent choking or gasping respirations while asleep. Full details of how the prediction rule operates are given in the original article (17). As shown in Figure 5.6, as the neck circumference increases, so does the probability that the patient has sleep apnea. The probability also increases progressively if the patient has one, two, or all three clinical features (hypertension, habitual snoring, partner reports of choking or gasping). For example, a patient with a neck

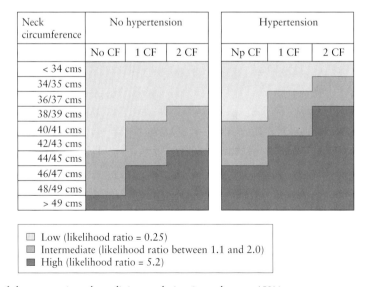

Fig 5.6 Probability of sleep apnea in a sleep clinic population (prevalence = 45%).

circumference of 42 cm would have a low probability of sleep apnea in the absence of any of the other three clinical features. If he or she were hypertensive the probability would be intermediate, and if he or she was also a habitual snorer, the probability of sleep apnea would be high.

0→ Key points box 5.4

Practice points

1. Many clinical features of sleep apnea patients recorded by questionnaire have likelihood ratios close to 1 and thus low diagnostic utility (Table 5.1).

2. Anthropomorphic measurements such as neck circumference, waist circumference, or body mass index have greater diagnostic utility than most other clinical features, such as daytime somnolence, snoring frequency, or reported apneas.

3. Sleep apnea clinical prediction rules, by combining several features, have a greater range of likelihood ratios than individual features alone. They may reduce the probability of disease in some patients to a level that a clinician can decide not to test or treat a patient for sleep apnea with a high degree of confidence.

4. Clinical features alone are usually not capable of increasing the likelihood that a patient has sleep apnea to such a level that some type of diagnostic testing, such as unattended monitoring or full polysomnography, can be avoided.

Other Features

■ **Family History.** There is no doubt that an inheritance factor is present in some patients with OSAS, as there is with obesity. A familial pattern of sleep apnea has been reported independent of obesity (35). Nonobese subjects seem to have components of craniofacial structure, narrowed upper airways, and enlarged uvulae that are inherited (36). No systematic studies have specifically addressed how much of a contribution family history might make to estimating risk of sleep apnea in a particular patient when considering other diagnostic features. In developing a clinical prediction rule for estimating the probability of sleep apnea, a family history was not identified as contributing to the model; however, this could be related to underdiagnosis in affected family members (17).

■ **Age, Sex, and Race.** The prevalence of sleep apnea increases with age, is at least twice as high in men than in women, and appears to be higher in some minority populations, especially blacks (37). Age and sex have been incorporated into some clinical prediction rules but not into others (13). So far it is not clear what the strongest clinical predictors of sleep apnea will be in non-Caucasian populations.

Special Clinical Scenarios

■ **Endocrine Disorders.** The prevalence of sleep apnea in various endocrine disorders has not been well characterized. There are pathophysiologic explanations to indicate that sleep apnea is common in several disorders, notably hypothyroidism and acromegaly and possibly Cushing syndrome (38). Hypothyroidism is by far the most common of these disorders (prevalence of 0.5% of the general population), in comparison, acromegaly has an estimated prevalence of 0.005%. Symptoms of hypothyroidism overlap considerably with the symptoms of OSAS. The precision of diagnosis of hypothyroidism from clinical features alone is no better for hypothyroidism than for OSAS. Hypothyroidism can cause OSAS, and in cases in which the two diseases are found together, the OSAS can sometimes be cured by administration of thyroxine (38). Therefore, some authors have recommended that thyroid stimulating hormone (TSH) levels be measured in all patients referred to sleep clinics with suspected OSAS. The costs and benefits of such a policy are not very clear and will likely vary depending on the patient referral population. It is uncommon to diagnose clinically important hypothyroidism when routinely screening sleep apnea patients in a sleep clinic (39). In a series of 200 cases referred to our clinic in which TSH determination was routinely ordered on all patients, we found no examples of previously undiagnosed hypothyroidism. Thus, we do not routinely screen for hypothyroidism in our clinic population.

■ **Pulmonary Hypertension.** Patients with few symptoms to suggest OSAS are sometimes referred because they have been found to have pulmonary hypertension. The prevalence of pulmonary hypertension in OSAS has been estimated to be approximately 15–20%; however the hypertension in most cases is mild (40). The prevalence of right heart failure in one consecutive series of sleep apnea patients was 12%. The sleep apnea patients with right heart failure also had daytime hypoxemia and abnormal pulmonary function, suggesting that several factors contribute to the development of pulmonary hypertension and eventual right ventricular failure (41). When the diagnosis of pulmonary hypertension is based on echocardiography, it may be important to check for its presence by more direct measurement. It is reasonable, however, to conduct a test for sleep apnea, which is found often enough to make the test worthwhile. It is unclear what percentage of sleep apnea patients who have pulmonary hypertension will have a clinically important reduction in pulmonary artery pressures with treatment for their sleep apnea. Additional causes for pulmonary hypertension should always be investigated.

■ **Polycythemia.** It is very unusual in our experience for patients with OSAS, to have polycythemia, even in those patients with severe nocturnal oxygen desaturation. In general, other explanations for the polycythemia are much more likely. It makes sense to look for other causes before performing a sleep test.

■ **Nocturnal Cardiac Dysrhythmias.** There are numerous anecdotal reports of dysrhythmias in association with OSAS with bradydysrythmias probably the most common (42). A study of the prevalence of dysrhythmias in a general OSAS referral population found it to be no different from that in a control group (43). Such studies cannot exclude the possibility that occasional patients may have dysrhythmias precipitated by apneas or by nocturnal hypoxemia, which is probably more likely in patients with severe sleep apnea (44). Support for such a hypothesis in clinical practice would come from treatment trials in individual patients.

■ **Hypercarbia.** Carbon dioxide retention is uncommon in pure OSAS without some accompanying problem that promotes CO_2 retention, such as chronic obstructive pulmonary disease (COPD), morbid obesity, alco-

holism, or chronic intoxication with benzodiazepines. Drug-induced OSAS may be part of the mechanism. Postoperative patients occasionally develop CO_2 retention that resolves when a narcotic antagonist is given, even when the dose of narcotic is quite small. A mechanism for this unusual sensitivity to narcotics in some of these cases may be that it precipitates severe OSAS or high upper airway resistance in susceptible people.

When patients have CO_2 retention attributed to a major respiratory disease, such as weak muscles or COPD, it is very often due to a combination of factors. Mild OSAS or high upper airway resistance in sleep that would be unimportant in a normal person can make a crucial difference when the respiratory system is just barely compensating. In such cases, use of CPAP for a breathing problem during sleep may make a substantial improvement in daytime CO_2 levels.

■ **Heart Failure.** The risk factors for OSAS overlap with those for coronary heart disease, and many patients with heart failure have periodic breathing in sleep (45). In many cases this is classified as Cheyne-Stokes breathing, or central apnea, but it is often hard to be sure that upper airway narrowing is not playing some role in pathogenesis of the unstable breathing pattern. There are no certain theoretical or practical ways of separating such patients completely into those with central versus obstructive apnea. Objective improvement in oxygen saturation or AHI, and or in both, symptomatic improvement in the individual patients may be the only way to assess the usefulness of CPAP in these patients.

■ **Suspected Multiple Sleep Disorders.** Patients with a story that suggests another sleep disorder in combination with OSAS are common. Examples are symptoms of OSAS with a delayed phase sleep disorder, shift work, or restless legs or periodic leg movements in sleep, depression, or sleep deprivation from overwork.

In these cases it is very difficult to know what contribution the OSAS alone is making to somnolence or fatigue, except by treating OSAS and observing the outcomes.

■ **Elderly Patients.** There are little data on clinical diagnosis of OSAS in elderly patients. It seems likely that 1) clinical prediction rules for a high respiratory distress index (RDI) established in studies of a population with mean age of 55 to 60 years will turn out to be less accurate when applied to elderly patients, 2) success rates of treatment will be lower, and 3) estimates of impairment attributable to OSAS will be less exact than in younger people. Estimates of the prevalence of OSAS in the elderly suggest it is higher than in the general population (46) and the clinical consequences may be different (37).

⌐ Key points box 5.5

Practice Points

1. Although there appears to be an important inherited component of sleep apnea, the presence or absence of a family history has not been formally studied to determine its degree of diagnostic utility.

2. Sleep apnea is more common in certain endocrine disorders, such as hypothyroidism, Cushing syndrome, and acromegaly; however, it is not clear whether these disorders, especially hypothyroidism, should be screened for in patients referred for suspected sleep apnea.

3. In selected patients sleep apnea may contribute to, or be primarily responsible for, pulmonary hypertension, polycythemia, hypercarbia, cardiac dysrhythmias, or heart failure. There are no systematic studies that have shown whether clinical features can indicate what contribution sleep apnea may be making to the overall clinical scenario; therefore, some type of objective testing would be necessary.

4. Sleep apnea is more common in the elderly, and current clinical prediction rules may not be as diagnostically useful in this population.

USING CLINICAL FEATURES TO ASSESS THE IMPACT OF SLEEP APNEA ON PATIENTS

Patients are referred for assessment of possible sleep apnea because of one or more symptoms. Clinicians, primarily interested in establishing a diagnosis, may focus more on the clinical features that predict that the patient may have sleep apnea or some other type of sleep disorder and therefore may not appreciate the impact that the disease process may be having on the patient. Understanding this aspect better may influence clinical decision making (Fig. 5.1) and will be important in understanding the response of the patient to any subsequent trials of therapy. It may be challenging to obtain accurate reports from sleep apnea patients about the impact that the disease is having on their lives for several reasons. If they have had OSAS for years, they may have slowly adapted to the chronic state of poor quality of sleep, daytime sleepiness, and lack of energy and now consider their current state to be 'normal' for them. They may have a job that demands maximal alertness, which masks their underlying sleepiness. However, an impressive effect of sleep apnea on quality of life as well as an improvement after CPAP therapy has been documented in population surveys and in clinic populations, (47–51).

To determine the broad impact of a disorder on a patient, a clinician can use one of a number of quality of life indices. There are several well-validated and widely used instruments, such as the SF-36 or the Sickness Impact Profile (SIP). These are commonly referred to as 'generic' instruments, since they were designed to be used in large samples of people with different illnesses. However, they may not adequately capture the impact of a particular disease on a specific patient since the questions are nonspecific. For example, the SF-36 does not have any questions on sleep quality or daytime somnolence. For sleep apnea patients there are now two disease-specific instruments that have been published that capture the pertinent aspects of the impact of the disorder (48, 49). In developing one of these instruments we (48), had sleep apnea patients rate a series of items or statements about their quality of life to determine which aspects were most troublesome. We surveyed 113 randomly selected patients (88 men, 25 women) who had been diagnosed at our institution as having sleep apnea. Each patient was asked, for each item, if it was a problem (yes or no) and, if yes, how important this problem was to the patient. This allowed us to rank the items according to frequency (how many patients answered yes) and importance (mean importance using a five point Likert scale from 0 to 4). The highest rated items are included in Table 5.2. We found that although men and women may have rated the

Table 5.2 Items ranked by sleep apnea patients as having the most impact on their quality of life

Item	Frequency[a]	Mean Importance[b]	Male rank	Female rank
Normal Daily Routine				
Having to push yourself to remain alert	73	3.21	3	1
Decreased ability to concentrate	78	3.00	2	2
Having to fight to stay awake	71	3.22	1	9
Decreased ability to remember things	66	3.18	4	6
A decrease in your motivation to do exercise and leisure type activities	65	3.21	5	5
Having to force yourself to go to work, school, etc.	58	3.25	7	3
Giving what energy you have to accomplish only work-related activities	53	3.45	6	7
Social Interactions				
Being told that your snoring disturbs your spouse's or partner's sleep	80	2.96	1	4
Being told that your snoring was bothersome or irritating to your spouse or partner	79	2.95	2	3
Less interest in socializing	58	3.13	3	1
Wanting to be left alone	50	3.04	6	2
A decrease in sexual intimacy	41	3.24	5	8
Emotional State				
Frustration	66	3.30	3	2
Irritability	70	3.10	2	3
A feeling of depression or being down	64	3.33	1	1
Impatience	56	3.10	4	5
A decreased ability to cope with everyday issues	53	3.17	6	4
Symptoms				
Daytime:				
Decreased energy	80	3.28	1	1
Excessive fatigue	71	3.47	2	2
Difficulty in staying awake while reading	78	2.93	3	4
Ordinary activities require an extra effort to perform or complete	65	3.18	5	3
Falling asleep if not stimulated or active	61	3.10	6	5
Fighting the urge to fall asleep while driving	58	2.94	4	6
Nocturnal:				
Waking up often (more than twice) during the night	77	3.06	1	1
Restless sleep	69	3.17	2	2
Concern about the times you stop breathing at night	52	3.22	4	3
Waking up at night feeling like you were choking	50	3.02	3	4

Table 5.2 (*cont.*)

* Reproduced in part from Flemons W, Reimer M. Development of a sleep apnea quality of life index. Am J Respir Crit Care Med 1998; 158: 494–503.

a Frequency: Frequency with which respondents picked the item as a problem that was affecting their quality of life as a result of suffering with sleep apnea

b Mean Importance: Each item was ranked on a five item Likert scale from 0 (not important) to 4 (very important).

Table 5.3 Most troublesome symptoms attributed to sleep apnea ranked in order of the frequency selected

Symptom	Frequency Selected
1. Decreased energy	57%
2. Waking up in the morning feeling unrefreshed and tired	56%
3. Excessive fatigue	55%
4. Difficulty with a dry or sore mouth or throat upon awakening	29%
5. Waking up often (more than twice) during the night	29%
6. Feeling that ordinary activities require an extra effort to perform or complete	27%
7. Falling asleep if not stimulated or active	25%
8. Falling asleep at inappropriate times or places	22%
9. Waking up more than once per night (on average) to urinate	22%
10. Fighting the urge to fall asleep while driving	22%

importance of the items slightly differently (women rated them on average more important than men), there were only a few differences in their ranking of the items (ranking was done on the basis of the frequency × mean importance product). Very little difference also was seen in ranking of items by patients with different sleep apnea severity levels. We used this information to assist in constructing the final version of the Sleep Apnea Quality of Life Index (SAQLI) (48). We have created four domains in the SAQLI that feature different areas of impact on the quality of life that sleep apnea may be having. These four domains are normal daily routine, social interactions, emotional functioning, and symptoms. All domains are scored using a seven item Likert scale with higher numbers reflecting a better quality of life (lower impact of the disease). In general, we find that symptoms are consistently rated as having a larger impact on patients than the other domains and improve more with effective therapy, such as CPAP. In the SAQLI, patients are asked to select the five symptoms that are the most troublesome to them from a list of over 20 symptoms. The symptoms that are selected most commonly are listed in Table 5.3.

Using well-validated quality of life indices to assess the impact of sleep apnea on patients will assist clinical decision making and help to determine, in a quantifiable way, if patients have improved with therapy.

⊶ Key points box 5.6

Practice points

1. It is important to assess the impact of sleep apnea on a patient's life, since this will dictate, to some extent, whether a trial of therapy is indicated and what impact the treatment has had. This is best done with a well-validated quality of life index.

2. Generic quality of life indices such as the SF-36 are useful to compare the impact of sleep apnea on patients with other types of chronic disorders. Improvements in several domains of the SF-36 have been demonstrated after CPAP therapy.

---

3. Disease-specific questionnaires, such as the Sleep Apnea Quality of Life Questionnaire (SAQLI) or the Functional Status Outcomes Questionnaire, more closely capture the unique impact of sleep apnea on patients' lives and can assist in clinical decision making as well as assessment of the benefit of treatment.

4. The most common symptoms that sleep apnea patients indicate are important to them are decreased energy, excessive fatigue, and unrefreshing sleep.

REFERENCES

1. Gastaut H, Tassinari CA, Duron B. Etude polygraphique des manifestations episodique (hypnic et respiratores), diurnes et nocturne, du syndrome de Pickwick. Rev Neurol 1965; 112:568–579.

2. Charles Dickens. The Pickwick Papers, 1836.

3. Charles Dickens. A Christmas Carol, 1843.

4. William Shakespeare. Henry IV part 2. Act IV, scene 11, 1599.

5. William Shakespeare. Henry IV part 1. Act II, scene IV, 1599.

6. Phillipson EA. Pickwickian, obesity-hypoventilation, or fee-fi-fo-fum syndrome. Am Rev Respir Dis 1980; 121: 781–782.

7. Guilleminault C, van den Hoed J, Mitler MM. Clinical overview of the sleep apnea syndromes. In: Guilleminault C, Dement WC, eds. Sleep apnea syndromes. New York: Alan R. Liss; 1978:1–12.

8. Badr MS. Pathophysiology of upper airway obstruction during sleep. Clin Chest Med 1998; 19:21–32.

9. Douglas NJ, Pollo O. Pathogenesis of obstructive sleep apnoea/hypopnoea syndrome. Lancet 1994; 344: 653–655.

10. Sackett DL, Haynes RB, Guyatt GH, et al. Clinical epidemiology: a basic science for clinical medicine. Boston: Little, Brown; 1991.

11. Pauker SG, Kassirer JP. The threshold approach to clinical decision making. N Engl J Med 1980; 302: 1109–1117.

12. Young T, Palta M, Dempsey J, et al. The occurrence of sleep-disordered breathing in middle-aged adults. N Engl J Med 1993; 328:1230–1235.

13. Flemons WW, McNicholas WT. Clinical prediction of the sleep apnea syndrome. Sleep Med Rev 1997; 1:19–32.

14. Stradling JR, Crosby JH. Predictors and prevalence of obstructive sleep apnoea and snoring in 1001 middle aged men. Thorax 1991; 46:85–90.

15. Lugaresi E, Cirignotta F, Coccagna G, et al. Some epidemiological data on snoring and cardiocirculatory disturbances. Sleep 1980; 3:221–224.

16. Lugaresi E, Cirignotta F, Montagna P, et al. Snoring: pathogenic, clinical, and therapeutic aspects. In Kryger MH, Roth T, Dement WC (eds) Principles and practice of sleep medicine, 2nd ed. Philadelphia: W.B. Saunders; 1994:621–1629.

17. Flemons WW, Whitelaw WA, Brant R, et al. Likelihood ratios for a sleep apnea clinical prediction rule. Am J Respir Crit Care Med 1994; 150:1279–1285.

18. Hoffstein V, Szalai JP. Predictive value of clinical features in diagnosing obstructive sleep apnea. Sleep 1993; 16:118–122.

19. Viner S, Szalai JP, Hoffstein V. Are history and physical examination a good screening test for sleep apnea? Ann Intern Med 1991; 115:356–359.

20. Hoffstein V, Mateika S, Anderson D. Snoring: is it in the ear of the beholder? Sleep 1994; 17:522–526.

21. Kump K, Whalen C, Tishler PV, et al. Assessment of the validity and utility of a sleep-symptom questionniare. Am J Respir Crit Care Med 1994; 150:735–741.

22. Crocker BD, Olson LG, Saunders NA, et al. Estimation of the probability of disturbed breathing during sleep before a sleep study. Am Rev Respir Dis 1990; 142:14–18.

23. Haponik EF, Smith PL, Meyers DA, et al. Evaluation of sleep-disordered breathing. Is polysomnography necessary? Am J Med 1984; 77:671–677.

24. Rauscher H, Popp W, Zwick H. Model for investigating snorers with suspected sleep apnea. Thorax 1993; 48:275–279.

25. Williamson D. Descriptive epidemiology of body weight and weight change in U.S. adults. Ann Intern Med 1993; 119:646–649.

26. Van Itallie TB. Health implications of overweight and obesity in the United States. Ann Intern Med 1985; 103:983–988.

27. Grunstein RR, Wilcox I, Yang TS, et al. Snoring and sleep apnea in men—association with central obesity and hypertension. Int J Obesity 1993; 17:533–540.

28. Katz I, Stradling J, Slutsky AS, et al. Do patients with obstructive sleep apnea have thick necks? Am Rev Respir Dis 1990; 141:1228–1231.

29. Mortimore IL, Marshall I, Wraith PK, et al. Neck and total body fat deposition in nonobese and obese patients with sleep apnea compared with that in control subjects. Am J Respir Crit Care Med 1998; 157:280–283.

30. Kuna ST, Remmers JE. Neural and anatomic factors related to upper airway occlusion during sleep. Med Clin North Am 1985; 69:1221–1240.

31. Schwab RJ. Upper airway imaging. Clin Chest Med 1998; 19:33–54.

32. Kushida CA, Efron B, Guilleminault C. A predictive morphometric model for the obstructive sleep apnea syndrome. Ann Intern Med 1997; 127:581–587.

33. Fletcher EC. The relationship between systemic hypertension and obstructive sleep apnea: facts and theory. Am J Med 1995; 98:118–128.

34. Guilleminault C. Obstructive sleep apnea. The clinical syndrome and historical perspective. Med Clin North Am 1985; 69:1187–1203.

35. Redline S, Tishler PV, Tosteson TD, et al. The familiar aggregation of obstructive sleep apnea. Am J Respir Crit Care Med 1995; 151:682–687.

36. Mathur R, Douglas NJ. Family studies in patients with the sleep apnea-hypopnea syndrome. Ann Intern Med 1995; 122:174–178.

37. Strohl KP, Redline S. Recognition of obstructive sleep apnea. Am J Respir Crit Care Med 1996; 154:279–289.

38. Rosenow F, McCarthy V, Caruso AC. Sleep apnoea in endocrine diseases. J Sleep Res 1998; 7:3–11.

39. Kapur VK, Koepsell TD, deMaube J, et al. Association of hypothyroidism and obstructive sleep apnea. Am J Resper Crit Care Med 1998; 158:1379–1383.

40. Kessler R, Chaouat A, Weitzenblum E, et al. Pulmonary hypertension in the obstructive sleep apnoea syndrome: prevalence, causes and therapeutic consequences. Respir J 1996; 9:787–794.

41. Bradley TD, Rutherford R, Grossman RF, et al. Role of daytime hypoxemia in the pathogenesis of right heart failure in the obstructive sleep apnea syndrome. Am Rev Respir Dis 1985; 131:835–839.

42. Shepard JW Jr. Hypertension, cardiac arrhythmias, myocardial infarction, and stroke in relation to obstructive sleep apnea. Clin Chest Med 1992; 13:437–458.

43. Flemons WW, Remmers JE, Gillis A. Sleep apnea and cardiac arrhythmias: is there a relationship? Am Rev Resp Dis 1993; 148:618–621.

44. Becker HF, Koehler U, Stammnitz A, et al. Heart block in patients with sleep apnoea. Thorax 1998; 53 (Suppl 3):S29–532.

45. Naughton MT, Bradley TD. Sleep apnea in congestive heart failure. Clin Chest Med 1998; 19:99–114.

46. Ancoli-Israel S, Kripke DF, Klauber MR, et al. Sleep-disordered breathing in community-dwelling elderly. Sleep 1991; 14:486–495.

47. Jenkinson C, Stradling J, Petersen S. Comparison of three measures of quality of life outcome in the evaluation of continuous positive airway pressure therapy for sleep apnoea. J Sleep Res 1997; 6:199–204.

48. Flemons WW, Reimer MA. Development of a disease-specific quality of life questionnaire for sleep apnea. Am J Respir Crit Care Med 1998; 158:494–503.

49. Weaver TE, Laizner AM, Evans LK, et al. An instrument to measure functional status outcomes for disorders of excessive sleepiness. Sleep 1997; 20:835–843.

50. Finn L, Young T, Palta M, et al. Sleep-disordered breathing and self-reported general health status in the Wisconsin sleep cohort study. Sleep 1998; 21:701–706.

51. Engleman HM, Kingshott RN, Wraith PK, et al. Randomized placebo-controlled crossover trial of CPAP for mild sleep apnea/hypopnea syndrome. Am J Respir Crit Care Med 1999; 159:461–469.

6 OBSTRUCTIVE SLEEP APNEA SYNDROME: SCREENING AND DIAGNOSIS

Daniel I Loube and Kingman P Strohl

INTRODUCTION

The current definitive test for the diagnosis of obstructive sleep apnea syndrome (OSAS) is the 12 channel polysomnogram (PSG) which is performed in a sleep laboratory or sleep center (1). Patients may experience inconvenience in having to travel to an unfamiliar place and setting to have a PSG. Patient discomfort may result from the extensive monitoring equipment that must be applied or worn during the examination. The total costs to a health-care system for PSG may be considered to be relatively high in view of the expected prevalence of OSAS in adults, which was 2% to 4% in a cohort of middle-aged workers in the United States (2). These characteristics of OSAS as diagnosed with a technician-attended, in-laboratory PSG suggest the need for surrogate tests.

Screening is performed in disease states by two distinct methods. Clinical screening refers to the method of employing a surrogate test, rather than a definitive test, for a patient for whom there is a clinical reason to test for the presence or absence of a disease. Possible justifications for a surrogate test are characteristics of the definitive test that are undesirable, including associated patient inconvenience, discomfort, morbidity, or mortality. An additional and often important justification for a surrogate test is cost, especially if the more costly definitive test is used to diagnose a disease that is as common as OSAS.

Population screening refers to the method of evaluating large groups of patients for the presence of a disease. One objective of population screening is to detect disease earlier, thereby preventing cumulative excess morbidity and mortality due to the natural progression of the untreated disease (3). Another objective of population screening is to extend diagnostic techniques to populations of patients who would otherwise not be assessed. The objectives of

population screening are satisfied by application of these principles of disease management to the diagnosis of OSAS. Untreated OSAS is known to result in a decreased quality of life and impaired vigilance (4). Although ongoing data collection and analysis from the Sleep Heart Health Study and other large prospective studies are required to fully determine the association of untreated OSAS and cardiovascular morbidity and mortality, a number of completed studies demonstrate the independent association of OSAS and hypertension (5). Some data suggest that untreated OSAS will increase in severity over time (6). The presence of undiagnosed OSAS may not be considered by health care professionals owing to the nonspecific nature of its symptoms. Population screening for OSAS has utility not only in a cohort at increased risk for OSAS, such as patients from an obesity clinic, but also in populations who present with a somewhat lesser risk for OSAS and atypical clinical features, such as postmenopausal women.

This chapter provides a synopsis and review of the surrogate tests for the diagnosis of OSAS, which include clinical impression by history and physical examination, questionnaires, morphometric measurements, awake imaging techniques, and nocturnal testing, such as oximetry and monitoring limited to cardiopulmonary variables. The accepted definitive test for OSAS, 12 channel PSG, is discussed, including the definitions for obstructive respiratory events and the criteria for a PSG diagnosis of OSAS. Application of newer technologies, techniques, and modifications in the protocol for the performance and analysis of nocturnal 12 channel PSG is reviewed and includes consideration of at-home and unattended studies. Finally, the integration of testing into a disease management program for OSAS is considered with an emphasis on the impact of screening methods on cost and outcome.

LIMITATIONS OF CLINICAL IMPRESSIONS

The common symptoms of untreated OSAS are found frequently both in the general population and in patients examined in outpatient clinics. Hence, reports of snoring and sleepiness begin a recognition strategy rather than provide a diagnosis. Kapuniai et al. (7) demonstrated that the complaints by a bed partner of both witnessed apnea and loud snoring had 78% sensitivity and 67% specificity, with a positive predictive value of 64%, for the presence of OSAS as diagnosed by an apnea-hypopnea index (AHI) > 10 events/hour on PSG. False-positive results might be due to the observation by the bed partner of the normal phenomenon of the occurrence of an occasional central sleep apnea as the patient falls asleep or transitions from non–rapid eye movement (NREM) sleep to REM sleep. The use of a bed partners report for the diagnosis of OSAS has known validity, as the correlation of bed partner and patient reports of OSAS symptoms determined by Kump et al. (8) was in the modest to excellent range.

In a study by Hoffstein and Szalai (9) evaluating a patient population with a high probability of OSAS, an expert health care provider subjective impression, based on history and physical examination alone, correctly identified only approximately 50% of OSAS patients. In a patient group with a low predicted probability of OSAS, a clinical impression suggestive of OSAS was very sensitive but not specific, resulting in the authors' conclusion that approximately 20% of patients referred to a sleep disorders center for evaluation could be reliably determined not to have OSAS on the basis of clinical impression alone.

Isolated qualitative observations from physical examination have not proven useful in distinguishing OSAS from non-OSAS patients. Although hypertension is associated with untreated OSAS, the strength of this association is not sufficient to use in isolation as a predictor for the occurrence of OSAS (10). Obesity is associated with OSAS, but the predictive value of body mass index (BMI, weight/height^2) alone is useful in selected populations, such as middle-aged American men referred for the evaluation of snoring. Obesity is a less useful predictor in community-based populations, including surveys of younger adults (11).

Qualitative observations of upper airway abnormalities in OSAS patients include a high-arched palate, large tongue, tonsillar hypertrophy, redundant soft palatal tissue, and retrognathia or micrognathia. No systematic studies have demonstrated the clinical utility of these qualitative findings in the identification of OSAS patients. The predictive value of quantitative upper airway assessment is discussed below.

VALUE OF QUESTIONNAIRES

EXCESSIVE DAYTIME SLEEPINESS

The Epworth Sleepiness Scale (ESS) is a simple questionnaire measuring the general level of daytime sleepiness by determining the probability of falling asleep in a variety of situations (Table 6.1) (12). An early study by the originator of the ESS suggested that it was useful in distinguishing simple snorers from OSAS patients, but a number of subsequent studies have not found this finding to be generalizeable (13). This limited utility of the ESS and other sleepiness scales to predict the presence of OSAS in individual patients may be due to the weak correlation between subjective and objective measures of daytime sleepiness. Another confounding factor is the widespread nature of excessive daytime sleepiness due to chronic, partial sleep deprivation, circadian rhythm abnormalities, substance abuse, and the occurrence of additional sleep disorders other than OSAS.

Identifying functional endpoints for excessive sleepiness is one strategy to avoid these pitfalls. The concept is that active sleepiness is the trait of consequence for OSAS, so that important work or social activities that are interrupted by sleepiness have greater meaning in regard to a need for medical management. One functional consequence of excessive daytime sleepiness is a motor vehicle crash. The prevalence of motor vehicle crashes is increased in OSAS patients compared to the general population (14). The likelihood ratio for the diagnosis of OSAS increases in a linear fashion with the frequency of reported episodes of falling asleep while driving (8). This consequence of excessive daytime sleepiness is not specific for OSAS and can frequently occur with primary disorders of daytime sleepiness, such as narcolepsy. It should be noted that the prevalence of narcolepsy is some one hundredth that for OSAS and that the occurrence of any car crash due to falling asleep should trigger an evaluation for the cause or causes for excessive sleepiness.

Table 6.1 Epworth Sleepiness Scale (a subjective measure of daytime sleepiness)

How likely are you to doze off or fall asleep in the following situations, in contrast to feeling just tired? This refers to your usual way of life in recent times. Even if you have not done some of these things recently, try to work out how they would have affected you. Use the following scale to choose the most appropriate number for each situation:

0 = would *never* doze
1 = *slight* chance of dozing
2 = *moderate* chance of dozing
3 = *high* chance of dozing

Situation	Chance of Dozing
Sitting and reading	_____
Watching TV	_____
Sitting, inactive in a public place (e.g. theater or a meeting)	_____
As a passenger in a car for an hour without a break	_____
Lying down to rest in the afternoon when circumstances permit	_____
Sitting and talking to someone	_____
Sitting quietly after a lunch without alcohol	_____
In a car, while stopped for a few minutes in the traffic	_____

MORPHOMETRIC MEASUREMENTS

Truncal, also called abdominal, obesity is a risk factor for OSAS and can be quantified by measuring neck size, performing skin fold thickness measurements, and comparing various measures of upper and lower body proportions. The predictive value of truncal obesity alone is not sufficient to distinguish OSAS from non-OSAS patients, but it does account for a 10% improvement in the predictive ability of a multiple question screening survey (8).

Kushida et al. (15), who combined factors for obesity and factors for craniofacial dysmorphism, developed a sophisticated morphometric model for OSAS prediction. Craniofacial measurements are obtained with the use of calipers to measure palatal height, intermolar distance and 'overjet,' an index for retrognathia. In a population of predominantly Caucasian subjects with suspected OSAS, this model had 97% sensitivity and 100% specificity using an AHI ≥ 5 from PSG as the criterion for OSAS (15). Despite the accuracy of this screening model, its clinical utility is limited by the inability to predict the illness severity of OSAS and the need for treatment. Further studies are indicated to evaluate this model's accuracy in other populations, especially different racial groups and those with a lower expected occurrence rate of OSAS. The feasibility of the widespread application of this OSAS screening method may be hampered by the requirement for exact craniofacial measurements.

CLINICAL PREDICTION: INTEGRATION OF MULTIPLE FACTORS

A number of studies have formulated pretest diagnostic criteria for OSAS based on the integration of the common symptoms and signs. The factors used in these formulas often include witnessed apnea, snoring, nocturnal choking, excessive daytime sleepiness, motor vehicle accidents, male sex, obesity, and hypertension (16); symptoms are also graded in respect to frequency or chronicity. An additional factor that has utility in predicting OSAS occurrence is alcohol use (17). Without the application of detailed craniofacial measurements as described above, the optimal sensitivity and specificity of these multiple factor clinical predictors has not exceeded 80%. Results approaching optimal sensitivity and specificity for multiple factors can be obtained with the use of as few as four factors (18). These multiple factor models have treated the AHI as a dichotomous variable, either being below or above a certain number of events/hour of sleep. Given the variable relationship between AHI and symptoms, these pretest probabilities do not convey severity and need for treatment.

Certain populations are less likely to be accurately screened for the presence of OSAHS with the current multiple factor predictor profiles. Women underreport OSAS symptoms compared to men, and postmenopausal women with OSAS are less likely to be obese than men of a similar age (19). A very limited number of studies evaluate the occurrence of OSAS in non-Caucasian populations, and even fewer studies have applied multiple factor predictive models to these populations. The application to children, to the elderly, and to neuromuscular disease remains to be done.

POPULATION SCREENING

SCREENING FOR THE POSSIBILITY OF OSAS

Only 5–10% of all OSAS patients in the United States have been diagnosed to date, and the percentage of undiagnosed patients may be even higher in countries where lesser resources are available for health care expenditures (20). Extending the potential for OSAS diagnosis may be especially important to specific populations because of the possible additive risk of OSAS to preexistent increased mortality rates. A retrospective study of 3200 OSAS patients by Lavie et al. (21) suggested that only those OSAS patients with underlying cardiovascular or pulmonary disease were at risk for OSAS-related mortality. Other studies have suggested that the prevalence of OSAS is greatly increased in populations of patients who have had myocardial infarction. Prospective studies are required to validate or refute the association between

OSAS and myocardial infarction, but in lieu of these data, some experts believe efforts to diagnose and treat OSAS should be focused on this and other populations with potential increased risk of cardiopulmonary morbidity and mortality.

Other diseases with potential increased morbidity, or mortality, or both, due to untreated OSAS include diabetes mellitus, hypertension, stroke, and carotid artery disease (22). Few studies have evaluated the predictive value of clinically derived observations compared to PSG in the diagnosis of high-risk populations for OSAS other than those referred to either sleep disorders centers or obesity clinics.

A recent study of patients examined at general medical visits to urban primary care clinics utilized a patient-based survey shown in Table 6.2 to allow for stratification into groups at high and low risk for OSAS. In a subset of 100 patients who received unattended PSG, the high-risk group had an OSAS prevalence, as defined by an AHI ≥ 15 events/hour, of 50% and the low-risk group had a 2% prevalence. This study suggests that patient-based techniques can be used outside the sleep center to identify patients at increased risk for OSAS in general medical practice. Studies are under way to evaluate the next step, in other words, deciding whom to evaluate with diagnostic tests or initiate treatment (23).

SCREENING FOR OSAS IN THE TRANSPORTATION INDUSTRY

Another population for whom OSAS screening seems indicated is transportation industry professionals, including airline pilots, bus drivers, and truck drivers. Although all drivers and pilots must maintain sustained vigilance while operating a vehicle, professionals are required to do so on a daily and sustained basis and are at increased risk for the consequences of untreated sleep disorders leading

Table 6.2 Results of a positive summary score for a high risk of OSAS[a]

	Sensitivity	Specificity	Positive Predictive Value	Negative Predictive Value
AHI > 5	89%	23%	89%	77%
AHI > 15	92%	50%	52%	93%
AHI > 30	65%	65%	20%	93%

[a] High risk is any combination of chronic persistent snoring with observed pauses, chronic sleepiness (including drowsy driving on a regular basis), and cardiovascular risk factors of obesity (BMI > 30) or a history of hypertension, or any combination of these.

to decreased vigilance and moving vehicle accidents. This increased risk of accidents has health implications for the general public, who are also potentially endangered by impaired transportation professionals. Of particular concern for transportation professionals is OSAS, since this is a common sleep disorder for which it is well established that both subjective and objective measures of vigilance demonstrate decrements, especially when the disorder goes unrecognized and untreated.

Some studies suggest the prevalence of OSAS to be higher for truckers than for the general adult population, possibly due to an increased propensity for obesity in that population (24). A recent study of 80 long-haul truckers in the United States and Canada detected OSAS in only two drivers, which would be consistent with the prevalence in a middle-aged, predominantly male cohort (25). In this study sleep deprivation appeared to be most closely associated with impaired vigilance while driving. Thus, it is unlikely that much benefit would be gained from an intensive effort of OSAS screening in this population, although screening for impaired vigilance from any cause, including sleep deprivation, substance abuse, or untreated sleep disorders, is advisable. Vigilance and wakefulness tests include the Multiple Sleep Latency Test, Maintenance of Wakefulness Test, Performance Vigilance Test, and numerous driving simulators. None of these

---

☞ Key points box 6.1

Clinical Impressions

■ Expert clinical assessment by history and physical examination alone has inadequate power to distinguish OSAS from non-OSAS patients.

■ Subjective and objective measures of daytime sleepiness correlate weakly.

■ Subjective measures of daytime sleepiness alone are of limited utility to identify OSAS patients.

■ Written survey screening for OSAS has not exceeded sensitivity and specificity of 80% in a population of suspected OSAS patients.

■ Truncal obesity and craniofacial abnormalities may provide a powerful predictor of the presence of OSAS.

---

tests is specific for untreated OSAS, although many of these may deserve consideration as methods to assess the adequacy of OSAS treatment response.

ASSESSMENT OF THE UPPER AIRWAY

DIRECT VISUALIZATION

Patients with OSAS have qualitative, characteristic anatomical abnormalities discussed above. A semiquantitative method of grading the patency of the oropharynx is the Mallampati score, used by anesthesiologists to predict the difficulty of endotracheal intubation. A number of studies demonstrate inconsistencies between observers performing this assessment (26), and no peer-reviewed studies have demonstrated utility of the Mallampati score to predict the presence or severity of OSAS.

ENDOSCOPY

Fiberoptic endoscopy of the pharynx may be useful in delineating individual patient anatomical abnormalities that predispose to the occurrence of OSAS but has not proven useful as a screening method to distinguish OSAS from non-OSAS patients (27). The Mueller maneuver, a forced inspiratory effort with the mouth closed and nose occluded, likewise does not aid the endoscopist in identifying OSAS patients, although there may be utility in identifying potential responders to site-specific pharyngeal surgery.

IMAGING

Cephalometric radiographs are images of the lateral head and neck soft tissue and bony structures. Cephalometric measurements assess structures in the anteroposterior dimension but do not provide an assessment of lateral measurements. Studies by Schwab et al. (28) suggest that pharyngeal collapse in OSAS patients is due to changes predominantly in the lateral dimension; hence cephalometry will not detect these changes. In aggregate, OSAS patients differ from snoring but otherwise asymptomatic OSAS patients with respect to a number of cephalometric measurements (29). However, these measurements have not been shown to be useful as clinical predictors of OSAS, which may be a consequence of the wide degree of variability in the head and neck anatomy of non-OSAS patients. An advantage of cephalography is a relatively low cost; disadvantages are the requirements for standardized technique and specialized equipment, including head calipers.

Computerized tomographic (CT) and magnetic resonance (MR) imaging of the pharynx may detect the exact anatomical sites of obstruction in OSAS patients but have not yet been studied as a screening or diagnostic tool for OSAS. Disadvantages of CT and MR imaging are the relatively high price and radiation exposure for CT.

Acoustical pharyngometry is the analysis of reflected sound waves to determine pharyngeal volume and cross-sectional areas. OSAS patients demonstrated decreased pharyngeal airway volume compared to non-OSAS patients; however, the predictive value of this technique has not been well studied to date (30). Its advantages are ease of obtaining measurements, relatively low cost, and avoidance of radiation. Disadvantages include variation in measurements with tongue and palate position and inability to assess anatomical structures above the tip of the soft palate.

ASSESSMENTS BY OXIMETRY

Transcutaneous oximetry allows measurement of arterial oxygen saturation (SaO_2) by sensing the difference in absorption spectra between oxyhemoglobin and deoxyhemoglobin. In the range of SaO_2 from 70–100%, accuracy is ± 5% in comparison with a standard co-oximeter and diverges to a greater magnitude at saturations < 70% (31). As an estimate of PO_2, SaO_2 is not very accurate when it is measured on the flattened, right-hand portion of the oxyhemoglobin desaturation curve, especially in younger and nonobese adults, who have relatively elevated total body oxygen stores, compared to older or obese patients. A finger probe is worn overnight by a suspected OSAS patient, and continuous SaO_2 measurements are stored in a recorder for analysis at a later time.

Some studies evaluating the utility of oximetry to diagnose OSAS have shown a sensitivity as low as 50% but a specificity as high as 95% (32). Other studies have demonstrated the reverse, including a study by Series et al. (33) with a sensitivity of 98% and specificity of 48%. The variability of these results may be due to the contrasting demographics of the populations studied and the different criteria used to define desaturation events. Frequently described criteria for distinguishing OSAS patients from non-OSAS patients include ≥ 15 desaturation events/hour with a SaO_2 decrease ≥ 4% or ≥ 1% recording time with SaO_2 ≤ 90%.

Confounders leading to false-positive results for the presence of OSAS on nocturnal oximetry are the occurrence of other conditions such as chronic alveolar hypoventilation due to emphysema or neuromuscular disease or non hypercapnic central sleep apnea with Cheyne-Stokes breathing. False-negative oximetry results can occur in younger and less obese patients in whom desaturation does not occur despite changes in PO_2 or inpositional OSAS patients who do not sleep in the supine position during the course of the night's recording. Advantages of nocturnal oximetry recording are that it is quite inexpensive in comparison to PSG and is simple to apply and interpret. The cost savings for nocturnal oximetry compared to PSG in one study was found to be $4290 per 100 patients, but 17% of these patients had other treatable sleep disorders, such as upper airway resistance syndrome or periodic limb movements not detected by this technique (34). Nocturnal oximetry recording for the diagnosis of OSAS is most likely to be useful in patients with a high pretest probability of OSAS based on clinical screening, for which this test is used to confirm the heightened clinical suspicion (Fig. 6.1).

OBJECTIVE ASSESSMENT OF SNORING

Sophisticated nocturnal snore recording and analysis in small numbers of patients demonstrate that OSAS patients have a larger high frequency sound component compared to simple snorers, which allows for some discrimination of these patient groups (Fig. 6.2) (35). The amplitude of measured snoring alone recorded for the entire night does not allow for the discrimination of OSAS patients from simple snorers, but it does add to the accuracy of a predictive linear equation for OSAS diagnosis, which integrates patient reported apnea and snoring severity (36). Technical problems with snore analysis for the diagnosis of OSAS include variance in sound recording with patient position, ambient room noise, and the wide spectrum of sounds produced by OSAS patients, which would include choking and gasping. The use of the quantitative analysis of snoring alone to identify OSAS patients cannot be recommended at this time based on the paucity of studies demonstrating its efficacy. The integration of snoring analysis with cardiorespiratory monitoring is discussed below.

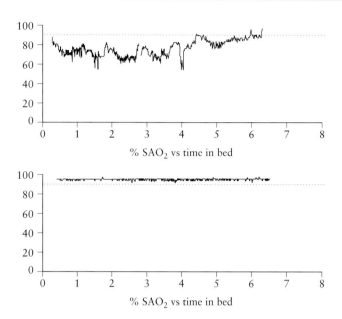

Fig 6.1 *Six hours of nocturnal pulse oximetry recordings for a patient with severe OSAS in the upper panel and for a patient with UARS in the lower panel. Note that the UARS patient did not demonstrate obvious nocturnal oxygen desaturation by pulse oximetry recording.*

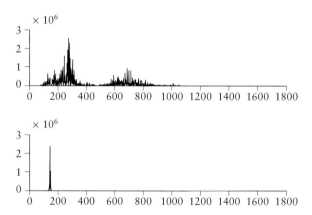

Fig 6.2 *Snore recording profiles of an OSAS patient (upper panel) and a primary snorer (lower panel). The snore from the sleep apnea patient demonstrates increased decibel amplitudes in the lower sound frequencies compared to the snore from a patient with primary snoring. Investigators have used snoring characteristics as a method of identifying OSAS patients (35).*

ASSESSMENTS UTILIZING HEART RATE VARIABILITY

Frequency domain analysis of heart rate variability allows for the noninvasive assessment of autonomic nervous system function. The signal from a pulse oximeter can be analyzed with commercially available software to provide heart rate variability data. The low frequency band, in the range of 0.04 to 0.16 Hz, is considered to be reflective of baroreflex dynamics, and the high frequency band, in the range of 0.15 to 0.4 Hz, reflective of vagal cardiac tone. The ratio between low and high frequency spectral power when modified for respiratory variability was three to four times greater in OSAS patients than in normals both in wakefulness and in sleep (37). These findings are consistent with other studies that demonstrate elevated sympathetic tone in OSAS patients compared to normals. The predictive value of heart rate variability alone to distinguish individual OSAS patients from normals has not been assessed to date, although one recent study has demonstrated its utility in a multifactorial model (38). Potential technical confounders for heart rate variability analysis include adjusting for respiratory cycle variables and individual patient factors, such as age, sex, and use of cardiac medication. It is likely that the technical ease of acquiring heart rate variability data and the increased sophistication of electrocardiographic signal analysis will lead to further and more detailed investigation of this modality to diagnose OSAS patients.

CARDIORESPIRATORY MONITORING WITHOUT THE ELECTROENCEPHALOGRAM

Cardiorespiratory monitoring allows for the quantification of obstructive respiratory events and assesses basic hemodynamic responses to these events without the added rigorous technical requirement of electroencephalogram (EEG) placement and maintenance of signal quality. Typical cardiorespiratory monitoring systems include measurement of oronasal airflow, chest wall and abdominal effort, electrocardiography (ECG), and oxyhemoglobin saturation. Additional measurements included in these systems may be body position, snoring sounds, leg movement, and eye movement. Cardiorespiratory monitoring studies are typically unattended by a technician and are usually portable systems well suited to use outside the sleep center.

ACCURACY
Cardiorespiratory monitoring is less accurate than PSG in determining the number of obstructive respiratory events per hour of sleep because of uncertainty of the total duration of reported sleep, leading to potential discrepancy in the calculation of the AHI. However, the recording of sleep quality and duration was shown not to have signifi-

cant impact on the ability to diagnose OSAS in a study of 200 patients by Whittle et al. (39).

Cardiorespiratory monitoring typically does not detect other sleep disorders, which may occur concomitant with or independently of OSAS, such as movement disorders. It may be difficult to differentiate between nonobstructive nocturnal respiratory events and breath-holding during wakefulness with cardiorespiratory monitoring. Upper airway resistance syndrome (UARS), characterized by very subtle hypopneas or chest–abdominal wall asynchrony terminated by arousals, is difficult to accurately diagnose with standard PSG and is likely to be missed with cardiorespiratory monitoring (40). This type of monitoring is indicated for patients with a high pretest probability of OSAS based on validated screening algorithms discussed above, for whom the diagnosis of OSAS must be confirmed and the severity estimated for possible use in directing treatment options. However, one recent study suggested that, compared to PSG, diagnosis of OSAS with a cardiorespiratory monitoring system resulted in significantly decreased compliance with continuous positive airway pressure (CPAP) treatment 2 years after diagnosis. A few of the proprietary cardiorespiratory monitoring systems have been validated in multiple studies performed by single investigator groups, some funded by the equipment manufacturers, but the majority are poorly validated. It is recommended that potential purchasers review the literature pertaining to these individual systems and seek objective verification of accuracy compared to 12 channel polysomnography. Validation of the clinical utility of any testing device will depend on the influence of local factors, such as experience, patient population, and cost.

COST FACTORS IN TESTING FOR OSAS
Few studies have examined basic issues of cost, and no studies have been published of cost-effectiveness in the work-up of OSAS. One recent study compared the 'costs' of PSG for all suspected OSAS patients to initial screening with cardiorespiratory monitoring to identify severe OSAS patients for treatment and preclude PSG in that subgroup (39). Costs were lower with the cardiorespiratory monitoring approach by £46 per patient; however, 15% of the patients with non severe, suspected OSAS did not receive PSG after cardiorespiratory monitoring, because they denied excessive daytime sleepiness. If these patients were to receive PSG, the costs between the two diagnostic approaches would be nearly equal. More

studies are required to delineate and validate potential cost-saving approaches to OSAS diagnosis incorporating cardiorespiratory monitoring and PSG.

The problem in evaluation of costs is inherently one of cost effectiveness. Certainly, the use of a portable device that is taken to a patient's home will be less expensive than center-based PSG with regard to overhead costs, equipment costs, and similar factor. There are, however, issues of cost of travel, personnel, and retesting that are potentially important to consider. If a clinical screening test costs a third that of PSG, our estimate is that some 70–80% of the time clinical screening tests have to make a difference in clinical management for true savings to a system to occur; otherwise the retesting and uncertainty with portable monitoring may be cost prohibitive.

> **⊶ Key points box 6.2**
>
> **OSAS screening studies**
> - Fiberoptic endoscopy during wakefulness does not allow the distinction of OSAS from non-OSAS patients.
> - Nocturnal pulse oximetry, snore, and heart rate variability recording and analysis are promising screening tools for OSAS but have not been sufficiently validated either alone or in combination to allow for advocating widespread use in the diagnosis of OSAS without PSG.
> - Cardiorespiratory monitoring may not detect some non-OSAS sleep disorders but is accurate in identifying patients with severe OSAS.

POLYSOMNOGRAPHY

TECHNIQUE

Twelve channel PSG includes recording and analysis of the following parameters: EEG, electro-oculogram (EOG), electromyogram (EMG), oronasal airflow, chest wall effort, body position, snore microphone, ECG, and oxyhemoglobin saturation. The duration of a diagnostic PSG is typically at least 6 hours. The 6 hour minimum duration of a diagnostic nocturnal polysomnogram (NPSG) is preferred, which allows for the assessment of variability related to sleep stage and position with respect

to the frequency of obstructive respiratory events and the occurrence of other types of nocturnal events, such as periodic limb movements (41).

DEFINITIONS

Until recently, there has not been any well-organized effort to standardize the criteria for the recording and analysis of obstructive respiratory events. The lack of standardized methodology may have enhanced the disparity among the approacher of various clinical centers to the diagnosis and treatment of OSAS patients. The definition for hypopnea has been especially variable from sleep center to sleep center. A recent consensus group has proposed the following definitions for the recognition and scoring of nocturnal obstructive respiratory events. These criteria are relatively simple to apply and should allow for a uniform and common-sense approach to OSAS diagnosis. Based on the American Sleep Disorders Association criteria for measurements, definitions, and severity ratings of the Sleep Related Breathing Disorders Task Force Report, (42), apnea is defined as the cessation of airflow ≥ 10 s and hypopnea is defined as a recognizable, transient reduction, but not a complete cessation of, breathing ≥ 10 s. A $\geq 50\%$ decrease in the amplitude of a validated measure of breathing must be evident or a $< 50\%$ amplitude reduction that is associated with either an oxygen desaturation of $\geq 3\%$ or an arousal. Obstructive apneas and hypopneas are typically distinguished from central events by the detection of respiratory efforts during the event (42).

A respiratory effort–related arousal (RERA) is an event characterized by increasing respiratory effort for ≥ 10 s leading to an arousal from sleep, but which does not fulfill the criteria for hypopnea or apnea. A RERA is detected with nocturnal esophageal catheter pressure measurement, which demonstrates a pattern of progressive negative esophageal pressures (Pes) terminated by a change in pressure to a less negative pressure level associated with an arousal (43). As discussed below, novel techniques are available that may allow for increased technical ease in the detection of RERAs.

The respiratory disturbance index (RDI) is defined as the number of obstructive apneas, hypopneas, and RERAs/hour averaged over the course of at least 2 hours of sleep as determined by PSG.

At the present time, the recommendations are that there is no added clinical value in differentiating apneas from hypopneas because apneas and hypopneas have a similar pathophysiology and both usually end in arousal and often in desaturation (44). Similarly, with the exception of AHI, respiratory PSG parameters were the same for UARS and OSAS patients when BMI and sex were controlled for (40). These findings suggest that the inclusion of apneas, hypopneas, and RERAs in a single index, the RDI, is appropriate.

REPRODUCIBILITY

The respiratory measures from PSG in patients with moderate or severe OSAS (AHI > 15 events/hour) are very reproducible on a night-to-night basis. Patients with milder OSAS demonstrate variability in the AHI which may result in a false-negative rate as high as 50% using an OSAS definition of an AHI ≥ 5 events/hour (45). This discrepancy in the AHI can be due to night-to-night variability in time spent in the supine position. Supine position leads to a marked increase in the AHI in approximately 35% of OSAS patients (46) and suggests the need for the inclusion of position monitoring in both PSG and cardiorespiratory studies. Reporting the total AHI and supine AHI separately allows for the recognition of the subset of patients with positional with OSAS who might otherwise be undiagnosed. Additional potential causes for the lack of night-to-night reproducibility of the AHI are variable alcohol and drug use, sleep stage distribution variation due to prior sleep debt and acclimatization to the PSG testing environment, and fluctuation in the severity of rhinitis due to allergy or upper respiratory infections. Factors leading to the lack of reproducibility of AHI over months are weight change

---

┌───┐
│ ⊶ **Key points box 6.3**   │
│   │
│ **Polysomnography**   │
│ ■ The lack of consistency between sleep │
│   centers on the definition for hypopnea │
│   has hampered standardization in the   │
│   reporting of PSG results for OSAS   │
│   patients.   │
│ ■ The reproducibility of PSG is very   │
│   good for patients with moderate and   │
│   severe OSAS but may demonstrate   │
│   variability in patients with mild   │
│   OSAHS due to night-to-night   │
│   variability in sleep posture and other │
│   factors.   │
└───┘

and the progression in severity, independent of weight change, over time.

ESOPHAGEAL PRESSURE (PES) MANOMETRY AS A SURROGATE FOR UPPER AIRWAY INSTABILITY

Patients with UARS typically have complaints of excessive daytime sleepiness and snoring and do not have OSAS on evaluation with PSG using oronasal thermistor to measure airflow (47). For UARS patients, Pes manometry demonstrates progressive negative pressures followed by frequent arousals or micro-arousals. The prevalence of UARS in an asymptomatic population is unknown, but studies estimate that approximately 10–15% of all patients examined in sleep disorders centers with snoring and excessive daytime sleepiness have UARS (48).

The gold standard for the diagnosis of UARS, Pes measurement, requires the use of an esophageal catheter. Few clinical sleep centers measure Pes routinely, possibly owing to associated patient discomfort, or added technical requirements and expense. There are few studies that demonstrate morbidity associated with UARS, other than excessive daytime sleepiness. Thus, another plausible explanation for the infrequent application of Pes measurement is that many physicians do not believe UARS requires treatment. Twelve channel PSG with oronasal thermocouple airflow measurement has not been demonstrated to be an adequate technique to distinguish UARS patients from normals. Data from the Walter Reed Army Medical Center suggest that 31% of patients who did not have OSAS but did have crescendo snoring and a total arousal index > 20 events/hour, which is suggestive of UARS, did not have UARS when Pes manometry was performed (49). As discussed below, there are promising novel techniques for the diagnosis of UARS patients. Until these newer techniques are validated in studies with larger patient numbers, Pes manometry should still be used to evaluate patients with suspected UARS.

OTHER TECHNIQUES

INADEQUACY OF THERMISTOR MEASUREMENT OF ABSOLUTE OR RELATIVE AIRFLOW

To date, the predominant technique for assessing oronasal airflow during sleep has been the thermocouple or thermistor. These sensors function by detecting an increase in the temperature of expired air. The sensor is positioned to sample air expired nasally and through the mouth. The detection of airflow by thermal sensors provides qualitative information that is not well correlated with breath amplitude. Therefore, a relative reduction in amplitude of this signal cannot be used to reliably indicate the presence of a hypopnea. Thermistors have been shown to have poor accuracy in recording hypopneas in awake subjects under ideal conditions (50). Owing to the nature of the signal, it is unlikely that any further research on thermal sensors would yield acceptable data on accuracy or precision. Hence, newer techniques are described below that aid in the detection of obstructive respiratory events.

NASAL PRESSURE AS AN INDEX OF UPPER AIRWAY RESISTANCE TO AIRFLOW

Nasal pressure transduction is the measurement of nasal airflow using a nasal cannula connected to a 2 cm H_2O pressure transducer to produce a simple flow waveform that can be analyzed for contour characteristics. Using this recording technique, nasal pressure waveform contours were qualitatively graded as normal, intermediate, or flattened (flow limited) (Fig. 6.3). In a recent study of 14 patients, this semi quantitative analysis of nasal pressure waveform contour allowed for 9 OSAS patients to be distinguished from 5 non-OSAS patients (51). Nasal pressure transduction is more sensitive but less specific for the detection of hypopneas than thermistor measured airflow as compared to the gold standard, pneumotachometer-derived airflow. Nasal pressure transducers could supplant thermistors as the standard technique for measuring airflow as a component of PSG; however, no studies to date indicate that this technique is adequate to detect RERAs accurately. The advantages of nasal pressure transduction over thermistor use as a part of PSG or cardiorespiratory monitoring need to be elucidated further to justify the effort and expense of replacing the widely used thermistor.

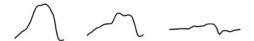

Fig 6.3 The progressive pattern (normal, intermediate, flattened) of airflow contour limitation, as measured by nasal pressure signal transduction and other techniques, is suggestive of increasing pharyngeal obstruction in OSAS patients.

CRITICAL CLOSING PRESSURES AS MEASURED DURING SLEEP

The critical pressure (Pcrit) is the pressure for which maximal inspiratory airflow occurs during sleep. It is measured by applying a gradation of airway pressures through a nasal mask and assessing airflow characteristics with a pneumotachometer. Investigators at Johns Hopkins University propose that in normal patients the Pcrit is negative, that is, the pharynx remains open during sleep unless negative pressure is applied through the nose. In contrast, OSAS patients will have a positive Pcrit, which requires the application of positive airway pressure for the pharynx to remain open during sleep (52). However, the clinical utility of Pcrit remains unclear, as a recent study by Sforza, et al. (53) determined that in OSAS patients, only 3% of the variability in directly measured upper airway resistance was attributable to Pcrit, whereas neck circumference, BMI, Pes measurements, and the AHI all were stronger predictors. Although individual increases in Pcrit may predispose to pharyngeal collapse, upper airway obstruction in OSAS patients likely requires a combination of factors. Additional studies are needed to determine whether adding Pcrit measurement to multiple factor predictive equations will aid in the effective screening and diagnosis of OSAHS patients.

FORCED OSCILLATORY MEASURES OF AIRWAY PATENCY DURING SLEEP

This technique estimates pharyngeal resistance during sleep using the measurement of reflected random noise within the frequency range of 4 to 32 Hz. A single study with a small number of patients suggests that forced oscillation may be a more accurate measure of upper airway resistance during sleep than Pes, nasal pressure transduced waveform analysis, or Pcrit (54). Further study is required to determine whether this technique is a reliable and easily applied tool for the diagnosis of OSAS.

RELATIVE MOTION OF THE RIB CAGE AND ABDOMEN BY INDUCTANCE PLETHYSMOGRAPHY

Quantitative respiratory inductance plethysmography (RIP) measurements are based on the detection of changes in volume of the chest and abdomen over the breathing cycle. The sum of these measurements has been demonstrated to provide an estimate of tidal volume if calibration is maintained (55). Assessment of the degree of asynchrony between chest and abdomen by RIP during sleep allows detection of hypopneas, which has been demonstrated to be clinically useful to measure ventilation quantitatively in OSAS patients. However, Whyte et al. (56) demonstrated that there is difficulty in maintaining the calibration of RIP when it is used as a measure of tidal volume over the course of a night of sleep in normal subjects. Berg et al. (50) found that RIP, nasal pressure transduction, and use of oronasal thermistor are not adequate in comparison to the direct measurement of minute ventilation when these are utilized to detect hypopneas.

Measures derived from RIP signals do not allow for the accurate distinction of apneas from hypopneas in the absence of an airflow measurement (55). However, there are no data to suggest different long- or short-term outcomes for patients with predominantly apneas as compared to hypopneas. An RIP-derived measure, the ratio of peak inspiratory flow to mean flow compared for wakefulness and sleep, allowed for the accurate distinction of UARS patients from non-UARS patients in a recent small study when breaths were analyzed prior to arousals. Randomly selected breaths from total sleep were not accurate for the identification of UARS patients (43).

'AUTOMATIC' TREATMENT WITH CONTINUOUS POSITIVE AIRWAY PRESSURE

Some newer CPAP machines contain electronic systems designed to analyze surrogates of airflow or respiratory effort to allow for continuous adjustment of pressures based on the detection or resolution of obstructive respiratory events. Automatic CPAP allows for the titration of CPAP without the immediate involvement of a technologist. Recent studies suggest that some automatic CPAP systems are effective in determining the optimal CPAP setting for most OSAS patients; however, few studies have evaluated the diagnostic capabilities of these systems. An exception to this lack of validation is the AutoSet CPAP, which was evaluated in the diagnostic mode in four studies with simultaneous nocturnal polysomnography (PSG). Overall, correlations were robust for the apnea index (mean number of apneas/hour) and AHI (mean number of apneas and hypopnea/hour) in studies by Bradley et al. (57), Gugger et al. (58), and Kiely et al. (59), but for patients with an AHI < 15 there was poor agreement between AutoSet and PSG. In approximately 10% of OSAHS patients, large magnitude discrepancies between the AHIs were attributed to inadequate airflow due to increased oral breathing and displaced nasal pressure transducer position. A recent study by Rees et al. (60) of 20 patients with severe OSAS determined that the AutoSet underdetected hypopneas during sleep by 41% and that 20% of the apneas and hypopneas detected occurred during wakefulness. Based on the data available for the current obstructive event sensing algorithm for AutoSet, it is likely that patients with severe OSAS can be accurately identified from a population of patients with suspected OSAS. Whether mild or moderate OSAHSS patients can be identified from patients with other sleep disorders with AutoSet™ or any other system remains to be determined. Evaluation of the diagnostic capabilities of each of these individual automatic CPAP systems will be important, as cost constraints and commercial forces tend to promote the application of this technology over that of diagnostic PSG or cardiorespiratory monitoring.

⊙╼ Key points box 6.4

Other techniques in OSAS diagnosis

- Oronasal thermistor provides poor accuracy for recording hypopneas.
- Promising alternative methods to detect residual obstructive respiratory events include nasal pressure, quantitative respiratory inductive plethysmography, and critical closing pressure measurements.
- The diagnostic mode of some automatic CPAP systems is accurate in identifying severe OSAS patients.

VENUE FOR DIAGNOSTIC SLEEP STUDIES

LABORATORY VERSUS HOME STUDIES

In many countries technology is now widely available that allows for the transfer of the relatively large amounts of information included in a PSG or cardiorespiratory sleep study over telephone lines and by satellite. This technology permits the collection and analysis of PSG or cardiorespiratory studies at centralized hubs. These hubs may be used to increase the efficiency of and decrease costs associated with performing OSAHS diagnosis and screening or may allow for the extension of recording capabilities to more remote sites.

There may be minimal differences in the technical quality of a PSG or cardiorespiratory study recorded in a sleep laboratory located in a hospital or freestanding clinic compared to that recorded in a patient's home, if the same recording systems are used and the same acuity of on-site technical attendance is maintained (61). In reality, cost constraints typically dictate that home studies will be either unattended by a technician or continuously monitored by a technician from a centralized hub. Unattended PSG from the Sleep Heart Health Study was deemed technically inadequate in 5% of all patients studied, and sleep staging and arousal data were not reliable in 25% of these PSGs (62). The determination of whether this failure rate for unattended studies is acceptable depends on cost considerations and the availability of repeat testing. The seemingly intuitive notion that patients prefer to be studied at home is subject to question, as Fry et al. (63) found that patients preferred to be studied in a sleep center due to minor inconveniences and apprehension regarding acquisition of data at home.

SLEEP APNEA DISEASE MANAGEMENT: SCREENING AND DIAGNOSIS

The objectives of a disease management program are to contain costs without compromising quality of care. The tools to assist managed care decision makers to develop strategic plans for disease management are clinical management plans and outcomes research. The development and implementation of a clinical management plan is a continuous process, guided by ongoing performance improvement monitoring. The starting point for a disease management program are expert, peer-reviewed clinical studies that address the specific disease of interest in a population as similar as possible to the target population. It is of great importance to carefully define the characteristics of the target population, as this will be the group for whom the disease management program will be made available and outcomes measured and tracked.

Typically, one of the two objectives is chosen as the primary goal. Either lower costs are sought with preservation or improvement of quality of care or higher costs are accepted in exchange for improved patient outcomes. Conflict of interest in a disease management program arises when costs

related to maximizing the health of the individual patient results in less availability of resources for maximizing the health of the overall target population.

COST ANALYSIS FOR SLEEP APNEA DIAGNOSIS

A recent study by Chervin et al. (64) estimated and compared the costs and utility of 12 channel PSG, cardiorespiratory monitoring, and empirical treatment of OSAS patients with CPAP. Using cost analysis of a hypothetical cohort of OSAS patients over 5 years after initial evaluation, the incremental charges for PSG were $13,400 versus $9200 for cardiorespiratory monitoring or empirical treatment. The cost utility of PSG over the alternatives compared favorably with that of other procedures for which society judges the added utility per dollar spent to be worthwhile. Modeling assumptions that qualify the findings of this study include a 100% CPAP adherence rate and robust quality of life benefits with effective treatment of OSAS. Of note, CPAP adherence was determined by two recent CPAP outcome studies to be only approximately 35–40% (4,65), although adherence rates of 70% were observed in several older studies in which patients were closely supervised (66). The quality of life benefits of OSAS treatment are well documented in patients with severe OSAS, although recent studies (69) of patients with less than severe OSAS report varied strengths of association with improvement in these measures.

Using a decision tree to compare the costs of two clinical pathways, in this case cardiorespiratory monitoring and PSG, involves multiplying the probability of each outcome by its cost and adding the results at each branch. If the probability of OSAS is increased in a specific population, the added costs required to establish the diagnosis of sleep disorders other than OSAS are minimized, thus favoring the use of cardiorespiratory monitoring as a cost-saving measure. However, if the probability of OSAS is decreased in a specific population, the added costs required to establish the diagnosis of sleep disorders other than OSAS are maximized, as the cost of the initial cardiorespiratory monitoring must be added to that of a PSG. Thus, the overall cost effectiveness of a screening tool such as cardiorespiratory monitoring must be individualized to the population being treated with respect to the resources available and the goals of therapy. The key question is whether the objective is only to treat OSAS, or is it to provide treatment for the patient's complaint, no matter what the causative underlying sleep disorder. Managed care organizations attempting to closely control costs may find it difficult to resist establishing formidable logistical barriers to receiving a PSG after a patient has already completed cardiorespiratory monitoring, whose results were not suggestive of OSAS (67).

SLEEP APNEA DIAGNOSIS IN THE INDIVIDUAL PATIENT'S INTEREST

For patients who present with the signs and symptoms of an untreated sleep disorder, such as excessive daytime sleepiness, the most cost effective clinical approach may be evaluation by a physician familiar with a broad range of sleep disorders (including insomnia), primary disorders of daytime sleepiness (such as narcolepsy), insufficient sleep, nocturnal movement disorders, parasomnias, and nocturnal breathing disorders. Clinical algorithms that encompass this manner of triage of patients with sleep complaints are contained in the indications for polysomnography and related procedures published by the American Sleep Disorders Association (68). Accurate clinical assessment allows for the triage of patients to the appropriate clinical pathways, which are characterized by various types and complexity of diagnostic evaluation and disease specific treatment plans.

An example of the utility of an accurate clinical assessment is a patient who is referred for the evaluation of excessive daytime sleepiness and mild snoring that is not disruptive to a bed partner. Upon further evaluation it becomes evident that the cause of this patient's excessive daytime sleepiness is chronic, conditioned insomnia and that the report of snoring is related to seasonal allergies that are inadequately treated. This patient does not require PSG or other diagnostic sleep testing for possible sleep-disordered breathing. The costs associated with the evaluation and treatment of this example patient are only those associated with office visits and medication for allergic rhinitis rather than unnecessary screening tests for OSAS.

From the individual patient's viewpoint, full PSG remains the preferred technique to diagnose and assess the severity OSAS. The risk of misdiagnosis is less likely with PSG than with screening tests, and repeat testing with increasingly complex diagnostic methods is avoided. The application of various screening techniques for the diagnosis of OSAS requires vigorous validation efforts in more heterogeneous patient cohorts than have been studied to date.

SLEEP APNEA DIAGNOSIS IN THE POPULATION'S INTEREST

As discussed in other sections of this chapter, recommendations on the resources which should be designated to diagnose OSAS and other sleep disorders must await data from studies that more fully delineate and characterize the consequences of these untreated conditions. Similarly, the medical and economic benefits of treating sleep disorders, especially OSAS, must be well established before exact monetary values can be attributed to the untreated condition and resources allotted for treatment in a fashion that is cost effective.

Based on the studies to date, it is likely that patients with occupations that put them at high risk for accidents caused by excessive sleepiness should be screened for impaired vigilance, including that caused by common sleep disorders, such as untreated OSAS. It is also likely that patients with severe pulmonary and cardiovascular disease from any cause (21) may be at increased risk for death from untreated OSAS. Thus, patients in these groups are appropriate for OSAS screening efforts. The high prevalence of OSAS (approximately 30–40%) in obesity clinics or in an American urban general medicine clinic population suggests that these groups of patients may also benefit from OSAS screening if treatment benefits justify this.

Will most populations benefit from treating OSAS patients on the basis of the results of screening tests, rather than the gold standard PSG? Probably not at this time, considering the range of sensitivities and specificities of OSAS screening tests described in this chapter and the considerable costs and inadequate treatment responses to widely available treatments, such as pharyngeal surgeries (efficacy approximately 30–50%) or CPAP (adherence 30–70%) (22). To conclude the chapter on a positive note, it is likely that ongoing efforts directed at designing and validating more accurate screening tests and more effective treatments for OSAS will result in lower costs and wider availability of these to the individual patient and to the population as a whole.

ACKNOWLEDGEMENT

Supported in part by the United States Veterans Administration and by a Sleep Academic Award (HL 05387)

REFERENCES

1. Standards of Practice Committee of the American Sleep Disorders Association. Practice parameters for the indications for polysomnography and related procedures. Sleep 1997; 20:406–422.

2. Young T, Palta M, Dempsey J, et al. The occurrence of sleep-disordered breathing in middle-aged adults. N Engl J Med 1993; 328: 1230–1235.

3. Baumel MJ, Maislin G, Pack AI. Population and occupational screening for obstructive sleep apnea: are we there yet? Am J Respir Crit Care Med 1997; 155:9–14.

4. Redline S, Adams N, Strauss ME, et al. Improvement of mild sleep-disordered breathing with CPAP compared with conservative therapy. Am J Respir Crit Care Med 1998; 157:858–865.

5. Young T, Peppard P, Palta M, et al. Population-based study of sleep-disordered breathing as a risk factor for hypertension. Arch Intern Med 1997; 157:1746–1752.

6. Bixler EO, Vgontzas AN, Ten Have T, et al. Effects of age on sleep apnea in men: I. Prevalence and severity. Am J Respir Crit Care Med 1998; 157:144–148.

7. Kapuniai LE, Andrew DJ, Crowell DH, et al. Identifying sleep apnea from self-reports. Sleep 1988; 11:430–436.

8. Kump K, Whalen C, Tishler PV, et al. Assessment of the validity and utility of a sleep-symptom questionnaire. Am J Respir Crit Care Med 1994; 150: 735–741.

9. Hoffstein V, Szalai JP. Predictive value of clinical features in diagnosing obstructive sleep apnea. Sleep 1993; 16: 118–122.

10. Maislin G, Pack AI, Kribbs LR, et al. A survey screen for prediction of apnea. Sleep 1995; 18:158–166.

11. Redline S, Strohl KP. Recognition and consequences of obstructive sleep apnea hypopnea syndrome. Clin Chest Med 1998; 19; 1–19.

12. Johns MW. A new method for measuring daytime sleepiness: the Epworth sleepiness scale. Sleep 1991; 14:540–545.

13. Benbadis SR, Mascha E, Perry MC, et al. Association between the Epworth sleepiness scale and multiple sleep latency testing in a clinical population. Ann Intern Med 1999; 130:289–292.

14. Teran-Santos J, Jimenez-Gomez A, Cordero-Guevara J. The association between sleep apnea and the risk of traffic accidents. N Engl J Med 1999; 340:847–851.

15. Kushida CA, Efron B, Guilleminault C. A predictive morphometric model for the obstructive sleep apnea syndrome. Ann Intern Med 1997; 127: 581–587.

16. Redline S, Strohl KP. Recognition of obstructive sleep apnea. Am J Respir Crit Care 1996; 154:279–289.

17. Stradling JR, Crosby JH. Predictors and prevalence of obstructive sleep apnoea and snoring in 1001 middle-aged men. Thorax 1991; 46:85–90.

18. Flemons WW, Whitelaw WA, Brant R, et al. Likelihood ratios for a sleep apnea clinical prediction rule. Am J Respir Crit Care Med 1994; 1279–1285.

19. Redline S, Kump K, Tishler PV, et al. Gender differences in sleep-disordered breathing in a community. Am J Respir Crit Care Med 1994; 149:722–726.

20. Young T, Evans L, Finn L, et al. Estimation of the clinically diagnosed proportion of sleep apnea syndrome in middle-aged men and women. Sleep 1997; 20:705–706.

21. Lavie P, Herer P, Peled R, et al. Mortality in sleep apnea patients: a multivariate analysis of risk factors. Sleep 1995; 18:149–157.

22. Strollo PJ, Rogers RM. Obstructive sleep apnea. N Engl J Med 1996; 334: 99–104.

23. Netzer N, Stoohs R, Netzer C, et al. Sleep-related symptoms in a primary care population. Am J Respir Crit Care Med 1998 157:A852.

24. Stoohs RA, Bingham LA, Itoi A, et al. Sleep and sleep-disordered breathing in commercial long-haul truck drivers. Chest 1995; 107:1275–1282.

25. Mitler MM, Miller JC, Lipsitz JJ, et al. The sleep of the long-haul truck driver. N Engl J Med 1997; 337:755–761.

26. Tse JC, Rimm EB, Hussain A. Predicting difficult endotracheal intubation in surgical patients scheduled for general anesthesia: a prospective blind study. Anesth Analg 1995; 81:254–258.

27. Schwab RJ. Upper airway imaging. Clin Chest Med 1998; 19:33–54.

28. Schwab RJ, Gupta KB, Gefter WB, et al. Upper airway and soft tissue anatomy in normal subjects and patients with sleep-disordered breathing. Significance of the lateral pharyngeal walls. Am J Respir Crit Care Med 1995; 152:1673–1689.

29. Jamieson A, Guilleminault C, Partinen M, et al. Obstructive sleep apneic patients have craniomandibular abnormalities. Sleep 1986; 9:469–477.

30. Rivlin J, Hoffstein V, Kalbfleisch J, et al. Upper airway morphology in patients with idiopathic obstructive sleep apnea. Am Rev Respir Dis 1984; 129:355–360.

31. Legrand TS, Peters JI. Pulse oximetry: advantages and pitfalls. J Respir Dis 1999; 20:195–206.

32. Gyulay S, Olson LG, Hensley MJ, et al. A comparison of clinical assessment and home oximetry in the diagnosis of obstructive sleep apnea. Am Rev Respir Dis 1993; 147: 50–53.

33. Series F, Marc I, Cormier Y, et al. Utility of nocturnal home oximetry for case finding in patients with suspected sleep apnea hypopnea syndrome. Ann Intern Med 1993; 119:449–453.

34. Epstein LJ, Dorlac GR. Cost-effectiveness analysis of nocturnal oximetry as a method of screening for sleep apnea-hypopnea syndrome. Chest 1998; 113:97–103.

35. Fiz JA, Abad J, Jane R, et al. Acoustic analysis of snoring sound in patients with simple snoring and obstructive sleep apnoea. Eur Respir J 1996; 9:2365–2370.

36. Van Brunt DL, Lichstein KL, Noe SL, et al. Intensity pattern of snoring sounds as a predictor for sleep-disordered breathing. Sleep 1997; 20:1151–1156.

37. Khoo MC, Berry RB, Asyali MA, et al. Spectral indices of cardiac autonomic function in obstructive sleep apnea. Sleep. 1999; 22: 443–451.

38. Keyl C, Lemberger P, Pfeifer M, et al. Heart rate variability in patients with daytime sleepiness suspected of having sleep apnoea syndrome: a receiver-operating characteristic analysis. Clin Sci (Colch) 1997; 92:335–343.

39. Whittle AT, Finch SP, Mortimore IL, et al. Use of home sleep studies for diagnosis of the sleep apnoea/hypopnoea syndrome. Thorax 1997; 52: 1068–1073.

40. Loube DI, Andrada TF. Comparison of nocturnal respiratory parameters in upper airway resistance and obstructive sleep apnea syndrome patients. Chest 1999; 115:1519–1524.

41. Loube DI, Gay P, Strohl KP, et al. Indications for positive airway pressure treatment of adult obstructive sleep apnea syndrome. Chest 1999; 115:863–866.

42. Report of a Task Force of the American Academy of Sleep Medicine. Sleep-related breathing disorders in adults: recommendations for syndrome definition and measurement techniques in clinical research. Sleep 1999; 22:667–689.

43. Loube DI, Andrada TF. Upper airway resistance syndrome: detection with respiratory inductive plethysmography. Chest 1999; 115:1333–1337.

44. Gould GA, Whyte KF, Rhind GB, et al. The sleep hypopnea syndrome. Am Rev Respir Dis 1988; 137:895–898.

45. Chediak AD, Acevedo-Crespo JC, Seiden DJ. Nightly variability in the indices of sleep-disordered breathing in men being evaluated for impotence with consecutive night polysomnograms. Sleep 1996; 19:589–592.

46. Oksenberg A, Silverberg DS, Arons E, et al. Positional vs nonpositional obstructive sleep apnea patients: anthropomorphic, nocturnal polysomnographic, and multiple sleep latency test data. Chest 1997; 112:629–639.

47. Guilleminault C, Stoohs R, Clerk A, et al. A cause of excessive daytime sleepiness: the upper airway resistance syndrome. Chest 1993; 104:781–787.

48. Guilleminault C, Stoohs R, Kim Y, et al. Upper airway sleep-disordered breathing in women. Ann Intern Med 1994; 122:493–501.

49. Nicolas JM, Loube DI, Andrada TF, et al. Prevalence of upper airway resistance syndrome in patients referred for presumed sleep-disordered breathing. Am J Resper Crit Care Med 1998; 157:A651.

50. Berg S, Haight JSJ, Yap V, et al. Comparison of direct and indirect measurements of respiratory airflow: implications for hypopneas. Sleep 1997; 20: 60–64.

51. Hosselet JJ, Norman RG, Ayappa I, et al. Detection of flow limitation with a nasal cannula/pressure transducer system. Am J Respir Crit Care Med 1998; 157: 1461–1467.

52. Sforza E, Petiau C, Weiss T, et al. Pharyngeal critical pressure in patients with obstructive sleep apnea syndrome. Am J Respir Crit Care Med 1999; 159:149–157.

53. Schwartz AR, Gold AR, Schubert N, et al. Effect of weight loss on upper airway collapsibility in obstructive sleep apnea. Am Rev Respir Dis 1991; 144: 494–498.

54. Badia JR, Farre R, Montserrat JM, et al. Forced oscillation technique for the evaluation of severe sleep apnoea/hypopnoea syndrome: a pilot study. Eur Respir J 11: 1128–1134.

55. Cantineau JP, Escourrou P, Sartene R, et al. Accuracy of respiratory inductive plethysmography during wakefulness and sleep in patients with obstructive sleep apnea. Chest 1992; 102: 1145–1151.

56. Whyte KF, Gugger M, Gould GA, et al. Accuracy of respiratory inductive plethysmograph in measuring tidal volume during sleep. J Appl Physiol 1991; 71: 1866–1871.

57. Bradley PA, Mortimore IL, Douglas NJ. Comparison of polysomnograph with ResCare Autoset in the diagnosis of the sleep apnoea/hypopnoea syndrome. Thorax 1995; 50: 1201–1203.

58. Gugger M, Mathis J, Bassetti C. Accuracy of an intelligent CPAP machine with in-built diagnostic abilities in detecting apnoeas: a comparison with polysomnography. Thorax 1995; 50: 1199–1201.

59. Kiely JL, Delahunty C, Mathews S, et al. Comparison of a limited computerized diagnostic system (ResCare Autoset) with polysomnography in the diagnosis of suspected sleep apnoea syndrome. Eur Respir J 1996; 9: 2360–2364.

60. Rees K, Wraith PK, Berthon-Jones M, et al. Detection of apnoeas, hypopnoeas and arousals by the AutoSet in the sleep apnoea/hypopnoea syndrome. Eur Respir J 1998; 12: 764–769.

61. White DP, Gibb TJ, Wall JM, et al. Assessment of accuracy and analysis time of a novel device to monitor sleep and breathing in the home. Sleep 1995; 18: 115–126.

62. Quan SF, Howard BV, Iber C, et al. The Sleep Heart Health Study: design, rationale, and methods. Sleep 1997; 20: 1077–1085.

63. Fry JM, DiPhillipo MA, Curran K, et al. Full polysomnography in the home. Sleep 1998; 15: 635–642.

64. Chervin RD, Murman DL, Malow BA, et al. Cost-utility of three approaches to the diagnosis of sleep apnea: polysomnography, home testing, and empirical therapy. Ann Intern Med 1999; 130: 496–505.

65. Engleman HM, Kingshott RN, Wraith PK, et al. Randomized placebo-controlled crossover trial of continuous positive airway pressure for mild sleep apnea/hypopnea syndrome. Am J Respir Crit Care Med 1999; 159: 461–467.

66. Rolfe I, Olson LG, Saunders NA. Long-term acceptance of continuous positive airway pressure in obstructive sleep apnea. Am Rev Respir Dis 1991; 144: 1130–1133.

67. Johnson SF. Sleep medicine as preventative medicine. In: Sleep disorders. Poceta JS, Mitler MM, Totowa, NJ, Humana Press; 1998: 199–24.

68. Chesson AL, Ferber RA, Fry JM, et al. The indications for polysomnography and related procedures. American Sleep Disorders Association 1997; 20: 423–487.

69. Engleman HM, Martin SE, Deary IJ, Douglas NJ. Effect of CPAP therapy on daytime function in patients with mild sleep apnea/hypopnea syndrome. Thorax 1997; 52: 114–119.

PART THREE
MANAGEMENT

MANAGEMENT OPTIONS IN OBSTRUCTIVE SLEEP APNEA SYNDROME

Patrick Lévy and Jean-Louis Pépin

INTRODUCTION

In the last decade, obstructive sleep apnea syndrome (OSAS) has been identified as a common clinical condition. Recent epidemiological studies have confirmed a high prevalence of the disease in middle-aged adults (1). OSAS is associated with significant neuropsychological impairment (2, 3) and a high cardiovascular morbidity, for which causal relationships are postulated (4). Since 1981, nasal continuous positive airway pressure (CPAP) has been the first-line therapy (5). However, there are important side effects related to CPAP use (6) and, although there is no doubt that CPAP is nearly the only therapeutic possibility in severe OSAS, other alternatives are highly desirable in moderate OSAS. This is even more important in situations such as snoring or mild OSAS. The upper airway resistance syndrome (UARS), which is associated with an abnormal increase in upper airway resistance during sleep and which results in day time sleepiness (7), although it is still discussed as a specific entity, is also part of the spectrum of disease in which CPAP is not the only therapeutic choice (8).

The treatment of OSAS and other abnormal increases in upper airway resistance during sleep should achieve three goals: 1) to alleviate symptoms; 2) to reduce morbidity; and 3) to decrease mortality. There is, however, an additional goal that has become increasingly important in recent years—namely, to improve quality of life (9). Consequently, the choice of a particular treatment for a given patient should induce the lowest possible level of side effects while achieving the same rate of success for the three goals listed above. If we use these criteria for assessing different modes of treatment, it is obvious that the morbidity associated with the different clinical situations has to be clearly established.

Thus, we have tried to define the spectrum of severity and have attempted to define a strategy of management in each of these clinical situations through specific algorithms.

DEFINITIONS

OSAS has been recently redefined (10). To be diagnosed as having OSAS, the individual patient must fulfill several criteria. There should be excessive daytime sleepiness that is not better explained by other factors or two or more of 'minor' symptoms (choking or gasping during sleep, recurrent awakenings from sleep, unrefreshing sleep, daytime fatigue, impaired concentration) plus an overnight monitoring demonstrating five or more obstructed breathing events per hour of sleep. These events may include any combination of obstructive apneas, hypopneas, or respiratory effort–related arousals (RERAs).

A RERA has been defined as a sequence of breaths characterized by increasing respiratory effort leading to an arousal from sleep, but which does not meet the criteria for an apnea or hypopnea. There is a pattern of progressively more negative esophageal pressure, terminated by a sudden change in pressure to a less negative level and an arousal lasting 10s or longer.

The use of an event frequency of five per hour as a minimal threshold value was based on epidemiological data that suggest minimal health effects, such as hypertension, sleepiness, and motor vehicle accidents (2, 11), may be observed at an apnea-hypopnea index (AHI) threshold of 5. Additionally, limited data from intervention studies suggest treatment associated improvements in vitality, mood, and fatigue in subjects with AHIs between 5 and 30 (9) and improvements in sleepiness and neurocognitive function in subjects with AHI levels of 5 to 15 (12, 13). It should be noted, however, that all of these data were acquired with relatively insensitive methods for detecting hypopneas and without any reference to RERAs. Thus, this threshold may be partly inadequate depending on the methods used in the assessment of airflow.

Defining the severity of OSAS is essential when establishing a treatment strategy. According to the American Academy of Sleep Medicine (AASM) task force (10), a severity level should be specified for two components, namely, the severity of daytime sleepiness and the objective level of respiratory disturbance on overnight monitoring. The rating of severity for the syndrome should be based on the most *severe* component. Sleepiness has been defined as mild, moderate, severe. The severity of sleep-related obstructive breathing events has been rated as follows: Mild, 5 to 15 events/hour; moderate: 15 to 30 events/hour; severe: greater than 30 events/hour.

There are currently no adequate prospective studies that have validated severity criteria for sleepiness. The data to justify a severity index based on event frequency are derived from the Wisconsin Sleep Cohort data, which show an increased risk of hypertension that becomes substantial at an AHI of approximately 30 (11). At present no data are available to indicate an appropriate distinction between mild and moderate degrees of obstructed breathing events during sleep. The recommended level of 15 reflected a consensus opinion of the Task Force. Here again, the methods of assessment of airflow are critical.

SEVERE OBSTRUCTIVE SLEEP APNEA SYNDROME

Since 1981, CPAP has progressively become the reference treatment in OSAS (5). Only very few alternatives should be discussed. Very occasionally, upper airway surgery can be considered in severe OSAS. There are still very limited data to consider the stimulation of the hypoglossal nerve as an option. Finally, oral appliances are usually considered as less effective in severe OSAS.

CONTINUOUS POSITIVE AIRWAY PRESSURE

As mentioned above, CPAP remains the first line therapy in OSAS. However, a key consideration is compliance. A few studies coming mainly from the United States (14–16) have demonstrated a low compliance and an irregular use of CPAP. However, most of the other studies using cumulative time meters have found a high rate of compliance

(65–80%) (17–20) and acceptance (about 15% of patients refusing this treatment after a single night's use in the laboratory [18, 19]). This high rate of compliance remained to be firmly established when monitoring the effective compliance (time spent at the effective pressure ±1 or 2 cm H_2O). However, the differences observed in compliance may merely reflect the respective efficacy of technical and medical follow-up evaluations in the different countries. In a very recent study, we have demonstrated that the effective compliance to treatment is significantly higher in Europe, which may be related to the educational support provided by the home care delivery network (21). However, there are significant side effects for a majority of patients using CPAP (6, 22). The reason for a high compliance despite these side effects (daily use between 5 and 6 hours [6, 21]) is obviously the clinical benefit obtained: only 1% of the patients had no subjective benefit induced by their therapy (6).

UPPER AIRWAY SURGERY

Snoring and OSA are associated with recurrent sleep-induced narrowing or collapse of the pharyngeal airway at the level of the oropharynx or hypopharynx. The patency of this floppy segment is critically dependent upon upper airway anatomy and function.

Anatomical factors that predispose to upper airway narrowing during sleep are craniofacial skeletal abnormalities, or increased tongue size, redundant pharyngeal soft tissues or a combination of these. The more frequent modifications in cranial structure are nasal abnormalities, such as deviated nasal septum, retroposition of the mandible associated with posterior displacement of the tongue, and inferior position of the hyoid bone. The tongue and pharyngeal soft tissues (soft palate, tonsils, adenoids), are usually larger than in normal subjects, and these abnormalities are worsened by fat deposition and oedema induced by vibration injury or repeated upper airway collapse. Finally, upper airway size is also dependent upon lung volume, and therefore smaller lung volume may also contribute to reduced upper airway size in obese subjects. However, upper airway anatomical abnormalities explain the major part of the variance in AHI only in young and lean subjects (23). In obese and older patients other factors, such as changes in upper airway collapsibility, ventilatory instability, fragmented sleep, and abnormalities in upper airway muscle function, are predominant. As upper airway anatomical abnormalities seem to play an important pathophysiological role in young and lean patients, these subjects probably represent the best candidates for surgical therapy.

The objectives of the uvulopalatopharyngoplasty (UPPP) procedure are to enlarge the oropharyngeal airway and to reduce the collapsibility of this particular segment of the upper airway. The results of the procedure have been summarized in a meta-analysis done by Sher et al. (24). For many authors the acceptable criteria for a good response are defined as a 50% drop in (AI) or AHI and the consequent achievement of an AI value of < 10 or an AHI of < 20. When this last criterion was taken into account (24), the response rate in the meta-analysis attained 41% (137/337 patients). Nonresponders had a higher baseline AI and AHI. The percentage of patients who reached a 50% decrease in AHI and a postoperative AHI < 20 was much higher in patients with retropalatal collapse or narrowing than in patients with retrolingual collapse (46% versus 5%, respectively). Moreover, among the patients with retropalatal narrowing, the best results were obtained in the group of subjects with the lower baseline AHI. Thus, when an imaging or endoscopic technique has undoubtedly shown retrolingual narrowing while awake or, more so, a retrolingual collapse during apneas, UPPP should be avoided. In summary, in OSAS patients, UPPP indications should be restricted to patients with mild or moderate disease and evidence of retropalatal narrowing. It should also be remembered that, by increasing mouth leaks, UPPP may compromise CPAP therapy and reduce the maximal level of pressure that can be tolerated (25).

Two different treatment philosophies coexist in the literature concerning maxillofacial surgery for OSAS. The Stanford group (26) has designed a step-by-step surgical approach tailored to the specific anatomical abnormalities encountered in each patient.

The goal is to avoid a full maxillomandibular advancement osteotomy (MMO), at least in a subgroup of patients, beginning with a limited mandibular osteotomy (with or without hyoid myotomy and suspension, and with or without UPPP). In this procedure MMO is performed as the second or third step. Conversely, other groups proceed (27, 28) directly to MMO. If necessary, a further chin advancement by genioplasty or an additional advancement of the palatal plate or a palatorrhaphy is performed (28). In 249 patients reported by Riley et al. (26) the success rate of a limited mandibular osteotomy

(reduction of AHI by more than 50% and AHI less than 20/hour) was 61%. The likelihood of response tended to diminish with increasing preoperative AHI severity, the nonresponders being more obese and having more severe mandibular deficiency than the responders. The reproducibility of such satisfactory results remains, however, conflicting. Thus, we (29) and others (30), using this phase I surgery, were unable to achieve success rates of more than 25%. Conversely, MMO is highly effective (75–90% of rate of success) in all studies (26–30). It should be remembered, however, that this surgery is not without side effects and represents a major procedure that requires well-informed and well-motivated subjects. Furthermore, although there is no reliable predictive factor of success, maxillofacial surgery seems more effective in nonobese and young subjects

IS THERE ANY OTHER TREATMENT THAT CAN BE ENVISAGED IN SEVERE OSA?

Oral appliances are often recommended as an alternative therapy in moderate sleep apnea (see below). Pharmacological treatment in OSAS, although still very limited or in development, may also apply to moderate OSAS (see below).

Electrical stimulation of muscles and nerves has been tried by various investigators to treat sleep-disordered breathing. Several types of approaches have been tried: surface electrodes, muscular electrodes (on the surface of muscles and intramuscular), and nerve electrodes placed directly on the twelfth nerve in order to open the collapsing upper airway during sleep. When electrodes were placed on the skin with the goal of stimulating the geniohyoid and genioglossus muscles, the results were disappointing. Although positive results were initially reported with this procedure in OSAS (31), further studies indicated that upper airway dilators needed a high stimulus intensity that consistently led to sleep fragmentation, even when applied chronically (32). Direct stimulation of the twelfth nerve was then considered. With twelfth nerve stimulation, coordination with the thoracic muscles is mandatory, and this problem has been handled by measurement of intrathoracic pressure changes using either a transsternal or an intercostal pressure sensor. From the preliminary reports, it appears that several technical points are still unsolved and that the rate of response is variable when using a unilateral stimulation (33, 34). However, it seems unlikely that bilateral stimulation will be a viable approach for safety reasons.

○┄ Key points box 7.1

Management options in severe OSAS

1. Nasal CPAP is the definite treatment of choice.

2. Other treatment options should only be considered where CPAP fails or is not tolerated.

3. Measures to advance the mandible can benefit some severe cases:

    (i) oral appliances

    (ii) Maxillomandibular advancement osteotomy and variations thereof—usually considered only in young, lean, and highly motivated patients.

4. Surgery to the upper airway such as UPPP and radiofrequency ablation should not be considered in severe cases, unless as a last resort.

Radiofrequency (RF) has been recently proposed as a treatment of snoring and potentially of OSAS. This procedure generates thermal ablation, which involves passing an electrical current through an electrode to induce a thermal lesion. The important factors that affect heating and thermal lesions are current intensity (in watts), time (in seconds), and electrode size and length. An increase in any of these factors will increase tissue heating. RF thermal ablation has previously been used in the treatment of cancer, benign liver tumors, benign prostate adenoma, and Wolf-Parkinson-White syndrome. In clinical research, RF thermal ablation has mainly been used by the Stanford group (35–37) in patients with snoring, UARS or mild OSAS. However, using RF at the base of the tongue could be envisaged in severe OSAS. A recent study by Powell et al. (37) included 18 OSAS men with a mean respiratory disturbance index (RDI) of 39.5 ± 32.7 events hour of sleep and a mean AI of 22 ± 33 events/hour. At the end of the study, they had a mean RDI of 17.8 ± 15.6 events/hour and a mean AI of 4.1 ± 6.2 events/hour. This clearly indicates that some patients remained uncured. However, the authors considered these preliminary results as indicating that, for some patients, RF may be an alternative to nasal CPAP or to traditional surgical techniques.

MODERATE OSAS AND UARS

Several epidemiological, pathophysiological, and clinical questions arise when defining moderate sleep apnea and UARS. There are still some questions about the effective health risk associated with snoring without any apnea or hypopnea (38), although a continuum has been proposed from snoring to sleep apnea (39). In contrast, specific criteria are needed to diagnose UARS. The original definition (7) included a clinical complaint (daytime sleepiness with or without ± abnormal multiple sleep latency tests [MSLT]), flow limitation (detected by esophageal pressure [Pes] monitoring), and increased respiratory efforts with arousal just following the peak negative Pes. Although these criteria seem not to be always appropriate (nearly 30% of the women with UARS having a normal arousal index despite significant respiratory efforts [40]), this is a clear situation different from 'simple snoring,' in which the upper airway resistance may be slightly or moderately increased without sufficient respiratory efforts to produce microarousals or generate daytime somnolence. Whether UARS represents a distinct clinical entity is still controversial (10). If we recognize a continuum between snoring and apnea, the prevalence of UARS in the general population might be higher than that of OSAS. However, the percentage of UARS among a population of snorers remains unknown.

The evaluation of moderate sleep apnea (see above) is also complex, as the magnitude of overnight oxygen desaturation and the duration of the disease are difficult to assess. This affects the validity of both inter- and intra-individual comparisons. Another factor that influences the evaluation is night-to-night variability, which is more pronounced in persons with mild apnea, especially in the elderly (41). Therefore, a definition of moderate sleep apnea syndrome cannot rely only on the number of apneas, hypopneas, and RERAs. The best compromise could be the combination of the three following criteria: 1) AHI less than 30; 2) moderate sleepiness (i.e., Epworth Sleepiness Scale between 9 and 12); and 3) absence of any cardiovascular morbidity related to OSAS.

Thus, from a clinical point of view, the end points of the treatment should be to alleviate snoring in simple snorers and to alleviate snoring, RERAs, and daytime somnolence in patients with UARS. In moderate OSAS, elimination of apneas, hypopneas, and RERAs should be obtained together with the suppression of snoring and excessive daytime sleepiness.

CPAP TREATMENT

Only few data are available with regard to CPAP use in UARS and patients with mild apnea. Actually, the only results published at the present time concern snorers with excessive daytime sleepiness. These patients presumably had UARS, but the authors did not provide polygraphic data to establish UARS with the usual criteria (19, 42, 43). Rauscher et al. (42) studied 118 consecutive snoring patients. Half of them reported significant daytime sleepiness. Only 19% of these 59 hypersomnolent patients accepted nasal CPAP for ongoing home therapy. The pressure needed to abolish snoring was 7.3 ± 1.6 cm H_2O, which reduced the number of arousals from 20 ± 10 to 5 ± 3. Although compliance was low (2.8 ± 1.5 hour), the treatment resulted in a significant reduction in sleepiness score. The long-term acceptance and mean rate of use was studied by Krieger et al. (43) in nonapneic snorers and persons with mild apnea (RDI less than 15). The acceptance was greater than 60% at 3 years, with a mean rate of daily use of CPAP at 5.6 ± 1.4/day. However, although it actually resulted in significant improvements when compared to placebo, the compliance in persons with mild apnea was significantly lower in the study by Engleman et al. (less than 3 hours) (13). These conflicting results illustrate that further studies are needed to firmly establish CPAP compliance in these subsets of patients. However, it is clearly in these patients that alternative treatments are highly desirable. As with other investigators, our clinical experience has led us to less and less propose CPAP as the primary treatment in patients with mild to moderate OSAS.

PHARMACOLOGICAL TREATMENT

A huge number of drugs have been tested in OSAS with very little success (44, 45). Theophylline, almitrine, and other ventilatory stimulants have virtually no effect. Nicotine has been recently tested using transdermal application without significant effects on either sleep-disordered breathing or snoring (46).

Sleep apnea is more prevalent in men, and testosterone has known effects on ventilatory control. Therefore, hormonal therapy has been tested in OSAS (47). The reduction in androgen activity among male patients with OSAS resulted in no changes in sleep architecture or ventilatory responses to hypoxia and hypercapnia. Moreover, the reduction in sleep-disordered breathing obtained both during non–rapid eye movement (NREM) and REM sleep was nonsignificant. These drugs are not currently used in the management of snoring and sleep apnea.

Hormone replacement has also logically been tested in postmenopausal women, as women appear to be more susceptible to snoring and sleep-disordered breathing after the menopause. Short-term hormone replacement (estrogen either alone or in combination with progesterone over 50 days) demonstrated only a small and clinically insignificant reduction in RDI during REM sleep with no change in the overall RDI (48).

Protriptyline is probably the drug that has been used most commonly for treating OSAS. Most studies report protriptyline to be effective in 50–70% of cases of OSAS (49, 50), but its usefulness is limited by anticholinergic side effects. Fluoxetine, a specific serotonin agonist acting as a serotonin reuptake inhibitor, is comparable to protriptyline as both reduce the percentage of REM sleep and decrease RDI by about 50%. Only half of the patients have a definite beneficial response to one or both of these medications (51). These drugs should be used mainly in REM-related OSAS, if at all.

On the whole, until now, pharmacological treatment has demonstrated little effect on apnea and hypopnea. The brainstem neurons represent, however, a potentially important pharmacological target (52). The ultimate goal of pharmacological approaches for snoring and OSAS is the prevention of sleep-related suppression of pharyngeal muscle activity and the subsequent alleviation of sleep-related airway narrowing and closure. Although it is difficult to selectively target the proper neuronal structures, both increase in upper airway muscle activity and induced changes in sleep structure might be of interest. From that perspective, phase II studies are currently being conducted that suggest that an active drug may be available within the next 2 to 3 years. Whether these drugs will be effective in mild, moderate, or severe sleep-disordered breathing remains to be determined.

WEIGHT LOSS

Approximately 60–70% of OSAS patients are obese—that is, exhibiting a body mass index (BMI) of more than 28 kg/m^2 or a body weight in excess by more than 20% of the ideal weight (53). The relationship between obesity and OSAS is still unclear, but obesity is accepted as one of the most commonly recognized risk factors. Obesity appears to be largely determined by genetic factors that influence metabolic rate, fat storage, and eating behavior and is associated with autonomic, endocrine, and hypo-thalamic functional abnormalities. This is particularly true with regard to regional fat distribution (54), which may be of particular relevance to the pathogenesis of OSAS, in which upper body obesity may be a relatively greater risk factor than is total body fat. Weight loss has definite effects and results in improvement, or occasionally disappearance, of sleep-related breathing disorders in many patients (55). There is also a strong influence of weight reduction on snoring frequency and intensity. Both may result from the decrease of pharyngeal collapsibility obtained with weight loss (55). Furthermore, weight loss is associated not only with a reduction in RDI and upper airway collapsibility but also with a nearly complete elimination of apnea when the critical pressure (Pcrit) reflecting the collapsibility is lowered below -4 cm H_2O (56). As with other treatment modalities, it is important to reassess patients fully after weight loss and ensure that there is none or little residual disordered breathing. Some patients will have an important reduction in weight and a parallel cure of sleep apnea, but no improvement may be observed in other patients despite dramatic weight loss. Weight loss is difficult to achieve but even more difficult to maintain. However, in all cases, weight loss should be encouraged in obese OSAS patients. Moreover, other modalities of treatment may either require some weight loss (i.e., maxillofacial surgery) or be more easily applied due to the changes in compliance and resistance of the upper airway secondary to weight reduction (i.e., nasal CPAP). Weight loss also has beneficial effects on snoring.

SLEEP POSTURE

It has been long recognized that snoring patients snore most loudly in the supine position. Similarly, it has been well proven that a large proportion of unselected patients with a diagnosis of OSAS demonstrate a different rate of apneic events in the lateral than in the supine position (57–62). Positional sleep apnea syndrome has been defined as an AHI during the time in supine sleep that is two or more times the AHI during sleep in the lateral position (62). Up to 60% of 184 unselected cases of OSAS investigated in a sleep laboratory were reported to meet this criterion (63). A tennis ball sewn into the pyjama top at the midthoracic level was one of the first means used to prevent sleep in supine position. Two other different strategies have been used—namely, sleep position training using posture alarm (PA) device (58) and use of the retain-ing tongue device (RTD) to prevent tongue retrolapse when the patient sleeps in the supine position (64).

The positional factor is likely to be more important in patients with mild to moderate OSAS. Thus, positional treatment would be of interest in many of these patients. However, the long-term efficacy and tolerance of these positional devices are questionable.

ORAL APPLIANCES

Oral appliances are commonly used by dentists for correcting various types of dental malocclusion. In the last decade, however, several devices have been specifically designed to treat snoring and sleep apnea (65). The term 'oral appliances' defines devices inserted into the mouth to modify the position of the mandible, the tongue, and other structures in the upper airway for the purpose of relieving snoring or sleep apnea. The goal of therapy with oral appliances is to modify the position of upper airway structures to enlarge the airway, reduce the resistance, and presumably reduce the upper airway collapsibility. The effects on upper airway muscle function may also be important due to the changes in direction of muscle fibers.

A high proportion of patients show improvement whatever the type of device. In most studies, improvement in snoring has been inferred from the reports of patients or bed partners (66–68). A significant reduction in snore frequency and intensity can, however, be demonstrated objectively (69).

The effects on AHI have been widely studied, including several comparisons with nasal CPAP. Overall, oral appliances have been found to be less effective on breathing abnormalities and sleep structure than nasal CPAP but better accepted by the patients (70–72).

Side effects of treatment with OA have also been reported. Excessive salivation and transient discomfort after awakening are commonly experienced with initial use and may hinder early acceptance of the device (68, 72). Later complications are essentially represented by temporomandibular joint discomfort and changes in dental occlusion. These complications were relatively uncommon. However, when looking at unselected OSAS patients, we have found that nearly 40% of them exhibit significant side effects preventing continuing use of the device, such as significant dental or temporomandibular joint problems (unpublished data). Compliance has been evaluated on the basis of the patients' reports and in a limited number of studies. The main question remains about long-term compliance. The principal reasons for discontinuing the treatment are side effects and lack of efficacy.

When summarizing the indications, we can follow the recommendations of ASDA (68). Oral appliances are indicated for use in patients with primary snoring or mild OSAS who do not respond to or are not appropriate candidates for treatment with behavorial measures, such as weight loss or sleep-position change. Patients with moderate to severe OSAS should have an initial trial of nasal CPAP because greater efficacy has been shown with this intervention than with the use of oral appliances. Upper airway surgery should also be considered in this subgroup of patients. Oral appliances are indicated for patients with moderate to severe OSAS who are intolerant of or refuse treatment with nasal CPAP or who refuse or are not suitable candidates for upper airway surgery. Finally, UARS represents a situation in which oral appliances might have beneficial effects. However, no data are available at the present time.

Upper Airway Surgery

Upper airway surgery is still largely employed in the treatment of snoring and mild sleep apnea syndrome. The main characteristic of studies reporting the effects of surgery on OSAS and snoring is the lack of objective assessment, particularly regarding frequency and intensity of snoring (73). Moreover, if success is defined by a normalization of sleep structure, an RDI of less than 10 per hour, and a reduction of at least 50%, a quantitative evaluation is difficult in the literature. In fact, most series do not provide enough data to establish the effects of surgery on sleep (73). It would be critical to provide objective data on sleep and snoring when evaluating UPPP in this subset of patients.

Many studies have attempted to select good responders to UPPP. Indeed, the extension of upper airway collapse to the hypopharynx is associated with a poor outcome of UPPP. Many techniques have been proposed to predict the most likely anatomical level of obstruction in the pharynx. This has been done using pharyngeal endoscopy (74), pharyngeal pressure (75), or fluoroscopy (76). As a whole, none of these techniques seems capable of predicting the responders to UPPP (77).

When looking at the indications for UPPP, there is a general agreement that UPPP has virtually no place in severe OSAS (78). In moderate OSAS, the results are still contradictory. However, there are recent data demonstrating that the efficacy may also be poor in improving RDI as well as snoring frequency and intensity (79). Although frequently a dissociation exists between subjective and objective results (80, 81), the objective results are poor in persons with mild apnea in terms of RDI, with only 50% being good responders; the latter are also those who exhibit an enlargement of their upper airway at the velopalatal level (82).

Moreover, in UARS, skeletal changes that potentially increase upper airway resistance have been reported (40). In approximately 50% of women with features of UARS, it was observed that a narrow *ogival* palate with a triangular chin and a variable dental overjet occurred. A class II malocclusion was present in nearly all of these subjects (*141/156*). In this group of women with UARS, the subjects without these anatomical features had marked obesity with a BMI of more than 35 kg/m^2. Therefore, surgery dedicated to the correction of bony abnormalities would seem to be preferable to UPPP alone in UARS. However, there are no published data at the present time regarding the efficacy of maxillofacial surgery in UARS. Guilleminault et al. (53) have suggested that nasal CPAP might not be a long-term treatment of this syndrome and that other means of treatment, such as surgery, may have to be considered.

Using the definitions suggested above for asymptomatic snoring, moderate OSAS and UARS, and severe OSAS, we suggest the following management strategy based on the treatment options already discussed.

Severe OSAS

In cases of severe OSA, there is no doubt that CPAP remains the first line treatment. Maxillo facial surgery can be considered as a potential alternative in a limited number of young, non-obese, and well-motivated subjects. Whether hypoglossal nerve stimulation may play a role in the future is still doubtful at the present time. In cases of CPAP intolerance, if upper airway surgery is not possible, oral appliances can be evaluated as these can possibly work even in some cases of severe OSAS.

Mild to Moderate OSAS

Moderate OSAS and UARS remain difficult to define. We suspect that RDI does not reflect adequately the severity

Management options in mild and moderate OSAS

1. Although nasal CPAP has been shown to provide objective benefits to patients with mild to moderate OSAS, compliance is relatively poor.
2. Weight loss improves OSAS, but is difficult to achieve.
3. Sleep posture measures may benefit patients with predominantly supine OSAS.
4. Oral appliances are a reasonable alternative to CPAP in mild cases, and possibly in UARS, although there are no reports of efficacy in UARS.
5. Surgery, such as UPPP, can be considered in selected patients with mild OSAS, but it is more suited to nonapneic snoring patients. The role of UPPP in patients with UARS is unclear.
6. Various pharmacological agents have been evaluated in OSAS, with generally disappointing results.

of the disease. A combination of low RDI, moderate daytime sleepiness or tiredness, and absence of related cardiovascular morbidity may define moderate OSAS. In this condition, the following management strategy can be suggested:

1. A CPAP trial is recommended in the first instance, at least to establish whether CPAP, in normalizing sleep and respiration, leads to the relief of the symptoms attributed to sleep-disordered breathing. It should be remembered, however, that a significant placebo effect has been demonstrated when initiating CPAP treatment (83).
2. Either initially, or in cases of primary or secondary failure of CPAP (patients refusing CPAP or becoming noncompliant), oral appliances should be tried.
3. UPPP should probably no longer be recommended in OSAS. Maxillofacial surgery needs further evaluation in this specific condition but has to be considered in terms of cost-benefit ratio.

Nonapneic Snoring

In cases of simple snoring, the following step can be reasonably proposed:

1. Sleeping positioning measures and weight loss, where appropriate.
2. Use of oral appliance.
3. Surgical procedures. It might appear surprising that UPPP is not considered as the first line therapy. However, this recommendation reflects the lack of objective results on snoring intensity and frequency.

CONCLUSIONS

In the past decade, we have identified with increasing frequency patients with respiratory sleep disorders that differ from the classical description of severe OSAS. Snoring and moderate OSAS and UARS have to be considered differently from severe OSAS when choosing a strategy of treatment. However, the morbidity in less severe sleep-disordered breathing remains largely unknown. Thus, symptoms (e.g., excessive daytime sleepiness and its related consequences) are critical when recommending treatment. The clinician may also suggest that moderate OSAS is a suitable setting for prospective studies using untreated groups of patients, which would be unethical in severe OSAS. Thus, future management strategies may more strongly rely on objective and controlled evaluations of different modalities of therapy.

REFERENCES

1. Young T, Palta M, Dempsey J, et al. The occurrence of sleep-disordered breathing among middle-aged adults. N Engl J Med 1993; 328: 1230–1235.
2. Kim HC, Young T, Matthews CG, et al. Sleep-disordered breathing and neuropsychological deficits. Am J Respir Crit Care Med 1997; 157: 1813–1819
3. Naegele B, Thouvard V, Pepin JL, et al. Effect of nCPAP on deficits of cognitive executive functions in patients with sleep apnea syndrome. Sleep 1998; 21: 392–397.
4. Young T, Peppard P, Palta M, et al. Population-based study of sleep-disordered breathing as a risk factor for hypertension. Arch Intern Med 1997; 157: 1746–1752.
5. Sullivan CE, Berthon-Jones M, Issa FG, et al. Reversal of obstructive sleep apnea by continuous positive airway pressure applied through the nose. Lancet 1981; 1:862–865.

6. Pépin JL, Leger P, Veale D, et al. Side effects of nasal continuous positive airway pressure in sleep apnea syndrome (study of 193 patients in two French sleep centers). Chest 1995; 107: 375–381.

7. Guilleminault C, Stoohs R, Clerk A, et al. A cause of excessive daytime sleepiness: the upper airway resistance syndrome. Chest 1993; 104: 781–787.

8. Levy P, Pepin JL, Mayer P, et al. Management of snoring, upper airway resistance syndrome and moderate sleep apnea syndrome. Sleep 1996; 19:s100–s110.

9. Redline S, Adams N, Strauss M, et al. Improvement of mild sleep-disordered breathing outcomes with CPAP compared with conservative therapy. Am J Respir Crit Care Med 1998; 157: 858–865.

10. American Academy of Sleep Medicine Task Force. Sleep-related breathing disorders in adults: recommendations for syndrome definition and measurement techniques in clinical research. Sleep 1999; 22: 667–689.

11. Young T, Finn L, Hla KM, et al. Snoring as part of a dose-response relationship between sleep-disordered breathing and blood pressure. Sleep 1996; 19: S202–S205.

12. Engleman HM, Martin SE, Dreary IJ, et al. Effect of CPAP therapy on daytime function on patients with mild sleep apnoea/hpopnoea syndrome. Thorax 1997; 52: 114–119.

13. Engleman HM, Kingshott RN, Wraith PK, et al. Randomized placebo-controlled crossover trial of CPAP for mild sleep apnea/hypopnea syndrome. Am J Respir Crit Care Med; 1999; 159: 461–467.

14. Kribbs NB, Pack AI, Kline LR, et al. Objective measurement of patterns of nasal CPAP use by patients with obstructive sleep apnea. Am Rev Respir Dis 1993; 147: 887–895.

15. Reeves-Hoche MK, Meck R, Zwillich CW. Nasal CPAP: an objective evaluation of patient compliance. Am J Respir Crit Care Med 1994; 149: 149–154.

16. Engleman HM, Martin SE, Douglas NJ. Compliance with CPAP therapy in patients with the sleep apnoea/hypopnea syndrome. Thorax 1994; 49: 263–266.

17. Waldhorn RE, Herrick TW, Nguyen MC, et al. Long-term compliance with nasal continuous positive airway pressure therapy of obstructive sleep apnea. Chest 1990; 97: 33–38.

18. Rolfe I, Olson LG, Saunders NA. Long-term acceptance of continuous positive airway pressure in obstructive sleep apnea. Am Rev Respir Dis 1991; 144: 1130–1133.

19. Krieger J. Long-term compliance with nasal continuous positive airway pressure (CPAP) in obstructive sleep apnea patients and non-apneic snorers. Sleep 1992; 15: s42–s46.

20. Stokes Dickins QS, Jenkins NA, MRAD R, et al. Nasal continuous positive airway pressure in the treatment of obstructive sleep apnea. Op Tech Otolaryngol Head Neck Surg 1991; 2: 91–95.

21. Pépin JL, Krieger J, Rodenstein D, et al. Effective compliance during the first 3 months of continuous positive airway pressure: a European prospective study of 121 patients. Am J Respir Crit Care Med 1999; 160: 1124–1129.

22. Hoffstein V, Viner S, Mateika S, et al. Treatment of obstructive sleep apnea with nasal continuous positive airway pressure: patient compliance, perception of benefits and side effects. Am Rev Respir Dis 1992; 145: 841–845.

23. Mayer P, Pépin JL, Bettega G, et al. Relationship between body mass index, age and upper airway measurements in snorers and sleep apnea patients. Eur Resp J 1996; 9: 1801–1809.

24. Sher AE, Schechtman KB, Piccirillo JF. The efficacy of surgical modifications of upper airway in adults with obstructive sleep apnea syndrome. Sleep 1996; 19: 156–177.

25. Mortimore IL, Bradley PA, Murray JAM. Uvulopalato-pharyngoplasty may compromise nasal CPAP therapy in sleep apnea syndrome. Am J Respir Crit Care Med 1996; 154: 1759–1762.

26. Riley RW, Powell NB, Guilleminault C. Obstructive sleep apnea syndrome: a review of 306 consecutively treated surgical patients. Otolaryngol Head Neck Surg 1993; 108: 117–125.

27. Waite PD, Wooten V, Lachner J, et al. Maxillomandibular advancement surgery in 23 patients with obstructive sleep apnea syndrome. J Oral Maxillofac Surg 1989; 47: 1256–1261.

28. Hochban W, Conradt R, Brandenburg U, et al. Surgical maxillofacial treatment of obstructive sleep apnea. Plast Reconstr Surg 1997; 99: 619–628.

29. Bettega G, Pépin JL, Veale D, et al. Obstructive sleep apnea syndrome: 51 patients treated by maxillo-facial surgery. Am J Respir Crit Care Med 2000; 162: 641–645.

30. Bittencourt LR, Palombini LO, Morgado P, et al. Clinical and polysomnographic (PSG) findings in surgically treated patients with obstructive sleep apnea (OSA). Am J Respir Crit Care Med 1997; 155: A677.

31. Miki H, Hida W, Choan T, et al. Effects of submental stimulation during sleep on upper airway patency in patients with OSAS. Am Rev Respir Dis 1989; 140: 1285–1289.

32. Guilleminault C, Powell N, Bowman B, et al. The effect of electrical stimulations on obstructive sleep apnea syndrome. Chest 1995; 107: 67–73.

33. Eisele DW, Smith PL, Alam DS, et al. Direct hypoglossal nerve stimulation in obstructive sleep apnea. Arch. Otolaryngol Head Neck Surg 1997; 123: 57–61.

34. O'Hearn DJ, Schneider H, LeBlanc K, et al. Effects of unilateral hypoglossal stimulation on upper airway function. Am J Respir Crit Care Med 1998; 157: A284.

35. Powell NB, Riley RW, Troell RJ, et al. Radiofrequency volumetric tissue reduction of the palate in subjects with sleep-disordered breathing. Chest 1998; 113: 1163–1174.

36. Li K, Powell NB, Riley RW, et al. Radiofrequency volumetric tissue reduction for treatment of turbinate hypertrophy: a

pilot study. Otolaryngol Head Neck Surg 1998; 119: 569–573.

37. Powell NB, Riley RW, Guilleminault C. Radiofrequency tongue base reduction in sleep-disordered breathing: a pilot study. Otolaryngol Head Neck Surg 1999; (in press).

38. Strollo PJ, Sanders MH. Significance of treatment of nonapneic snoring. Sleep 1993; 5: 403–408.

39. Lugaresi E, Mondini S, Zucconi M, et al. Staging of heavy snorers disease: a proposal. Bull Europ Physiopathol Respir 1983; 19: 590–594.

40. Guilleminault C, Stoohs R, Kim Y, et al. Upper airway sleep-disordered breathing in women. Ann Intern Med 1995; 122: 493–501.

41. Mosko SS, Dickel MJ, Ashurst J. Night-to-night variability in sleep apnea and sleep-related periodic leg movements in the elderly. Sleep 1988; 11: 340–348.

42. Rauscher H, Formanek D, Zwick H. Nasal continuous positive airway pressure for nonapneic snoring? Chest 1995; 107: 58–61.

43. Krieger J, Kurtz D, Petiau C, et al. Long-term compliance with CPAP therapy in obstructive sleep apnea patients and in snorers. Sleep 1996, 19: 5136–5143.

44. Strohl KP, Cherniack NS, Gothe B. Physiologic basis of therapy for sleep apnea. Am Rev Respir Dis 1986; 134: 791–802.

45. Hudgel DW, Thanakitcharu S. Pharmacologic treatment of sleep-disordered breathing. Am J Respir Crit Care Med 1998; 158: 691–699.

46. Davila DG, Hurt RD, Offord KP, et al. Acute effects of transdermal nicotine on sleep architecture, snoring, and sleep-disordered breathing in nonsmokers. Am J Respir Crit Care Med 1994; 150: 469–474.

47. Stewart DA, Grunstein RR, Berthon-Jones M, et al. Androgen blockade does not affect sleep-disordered breathing or chemosensitivity in men with obstructive sleep apnea. Am Rev Respir Dis 1992; 146: 1389–1393.

48. Cistulli PA, Barnes DJ, Grunstein RR, et al. Effect of short-term hormone replacement in the treatment of obstructive sleep apnoea in postmenopausal women. Thorax 1994; 49: 699–702.

49. Brownell LG, West P, Sweatman P, et al. Protriptyline in obstructive sleep apnea: a double-blind trial. N Engl J Med 1982; 307: 1037–1042.

50. Smith PL, Haponik EF, Allen RP, et al. The effects of protriptyline in sleep-disordered breathing. Am Rev Respir Dis 1982; 127: 8–13.

51. Hanzel DA, Proia NG, Hudgel DW. Response of obstructive sleep apnea to fluoxetine and protriptyline. Chest 1991; 100: 416–421.

52. Horner R. Is there a rationale in modulating brainstem neurons in obstructive sleep apnea and is it clinically relevant? Sleep 1999, in press.

53. Guilleminault C. Clinical features and evaluation of obstructive sleep apnea. In: Kryger MH, Roth T, Dement WC, eds. Principles and practice of sleep medicine. Philadelphia: WB Saunders; 1983: 552–558.

54. Bouchard C. Genetic aspects of human obesity. In: Björntorp P, Brodoff BN, eds. Obesity. Philadelphia: JB Lippincott; 1992: 343–351.

55. Suratt PM, McTier R, Findley LJ, et al. Changes in breathing and the pharynx after weight loss in obstructive sleep apnea. Chest 1987; 92: 631–637.

56. Schwartz AR, Gold AR, Schubert N, et al. Effect of weight loss on upper airway collapsibility in obstructive sleep apnea. Am Rev Respir Dis 1991; 144: 494–498.

57. Cartwright R. Effect of sleep position on sleep apnea severity. Sleep 1984; 7: 110–114.

58. Cartwright R, Lloyd S, Lilie J, et al. Sleep position training as treatment for sleep apnea syndrome: a preliminary study. Sleep 1985; 8: 87–94.

59. McEvoy RD, Sharp DJ, Thornton AT. The effects of posture on obstructive sleep apnea. Am Rev Respir Dis 1986; 133: 662–666.

60. Phillips BA, Okeson J, Paesani D, et al. Effect of sleep position on sleep apnea and parafunctional activity. Chest 1986; 90: 424–429.

61. George CF, Millar TW, Kryger MH. Sleep apnea and body position during sleep. Sleep 1988; 11: 90–99.

62. Cartwright RD, Diaz F, Lloyd S. The effects of sleep posture and sleep stage on apnea frequency. Sleep 1991; 14: 351–353.

63. Lloyd S, Cartwright RD. Physiologic basis of therapy for sleep apnea. Am Rev Respir Dis 1987; 136: 525–526.

64. Cartwright RD, Ristanovic R, Diaz F, et al. A comparative study of treatments for positional sleep apnea. Sleep 1991; 14: 546–552.

65. Lowe AA. Dental appliances for the treatment of snoring and/or obstructive sleep apnea: In: Kryger M, Roth T, Dement W, eds. Principles and practice of sleep medicine, 2nd ed. Philadelphia: WB Saunders; 1994: 722–735.

66. Eveloff S, Rosenberg CL, Carlisle CC, et al. Efficacy of a Herbst mandibular advancement device in obstructive sleep apnea. Am J Respir Crit Care Med 1994; 149: 905–909.

67. Schmidt-Nowara W, Lowe A, Wiegand L, et al. Oral appliances for the treatment of snoring and obstructive sleep apnea: a review. Sleep 1995; 18: 501–510.

68. American Sleep Disorders Association. Practice parameters for the treatment of snoring and obstructive sleep apnea with oral appliances. Sleep 1995; 18: 511–513.

69. O'Sullivan R, Hillman DR, Mateljan R, et al. Mandibular advancement splint: an appliance to treat snoring and obstructive sleep apnea. Am J Respir Crit Care Med 1995; 151: 194–198.

70. Clark G, Blumenfeld L, Yoffe N, et al. A cross-over study comparing the efficacy of continuous positive airway pressure with anterior mandibular positioning devices on patients with obstructive sleep apnea. Chest 1996; 109: 1477–1483.

71. Ferguson K, Ono T, Lowe A, et al. A randomised cross-over study of an oral appliance versus nasal continuous positive airway pressure in the treatment of mild–moderate obstructive sleep apnea. Chest 1996; 109: 1269–1275.

72. Ferguson K, Ono T, Lowe A, et al. A short-term controlled trial of an adjustable oral appliance versus nasal continuous positive airway pressure in the treatment of mild to moderate obstructive sleep apnea. Thorax 1997; 52: 362–368.

73. Rodenstein DO. Assessment of uvulopalatopharyngoplasty for the treatment of sleep apnea syndrome. Sleep 1992; 15: S56–S62.

74. Launois SH, Feroah TR, Campbell WN, et al. Site of pharyngeal narrowing predicts outcome of surgery for obstructive sleep apnea. Am Rev Respir Dis 1993; 149: 182–189.

75. Shepard JW, Thawley SE. Localization of upper airway collapse during sleep in patients with obstructive sleep apnea. Am Rev Respir Dis 1990; 141: 1350–1355.

76. Pépin JL, Ferretti G, Veale D, et al. Somnofluoroscopy, computerised tomography, and cephalometry in the assessment of the upper airway in obstructive sleep apnoea. Thorax 1992; 47: 150–156.

77. Pépin JL, Veale D, Mayer P, et al. Critical analysis of the results of surgery in the treatment of snoring, upper airway resistance syndrome (UARS), and obstructive sleep apnea (OSA). Sleep 1996; 19: S90–S100.

78. Walker EB, Frith RW, Harding DA, et al. Uvulopalatopharyngoplasty in severe idiopathic obstructive sleep apnoea syndrome. Thorax 1989; 44: 205–208.

79. Miljeteig H, Mateika S, Haight JS, et al. Subjective and objective assessment of uvulopalatopharyngoplasty for treatment of snoring and obstructive sleep apnea syndrome. Am J Respir Crit Care Med 1994; 150: 1286–1290.

80. Janson C, Hillerdal G, Larsson L, et al. Excessive daytime sleepiness and fatigue in nonapnoeic snorers: improvement after UPPP. Eur Respir J 1994; 7: 845–849

81. De Backer W, Van de Heyning P. Is the role of UPPP in nonapnoeic snorers underestimated? Eur Respir J 1994; 7: 843–847.

82. Langin T, Pépin JL, Pendlebury S, et al. Upper airway changes in snorers and moderate sleep apnea sufferers after uvulopalatopharyngoplasty (UPPP). Chest 1998; 113: 1595–1603.

83. Jenkinson C, Davies RJO, Mullins R, et al. Comparison of therapeutic and subtherapeutic nasal continuous positive airway pressure for obstructive sleep apnoea: a randomised prospective parallel trial. Lancet 1999; 353: 2100–2105.

NASAL CONTINUOUS POSITIVE AIRWAY PRESSURE THERAPY FOR OBSTRUCTIVE SLEEP APNEA SYNDROME

Walter T McNicholas

INTRODUCTION

Nasal continuous positive airway pressure (CPAP) was first described as a therapy for obstructive sleep apnea syndrome (OSAS) in 1981 (1), and it represented a major advance in the management of the syndrome. Prior to this development, tracheostomy was often required to control severe cases of OSAS, and a testament to the efficacy of CPAP is that tracheostomy is now very rarely required. Although CPAP is highly effective in controlling sleep apnea, the device is cumbersome, and compliance data demonstrate only moderately satisfactory compliance. Nonetheless, nasal CPAP has become the most widely prescribed treatment for moderate to severe forms of OSAS and has transformed the lives of many patients (2).

MECHANISMS OF ACTION OF CPAP

The stability and patency of the upper airway are dependent upon the action of oropharyngeal dilator and abductor muscles, which normally are activated in a rhythmic fashion during each inspiration. The upper airway is subjected to collapse when the force produced by these muscles, for a given cross-sectional area of the upper airway, is exceeded by the negative airway pressure generated by inspiratory activity of the diaphragm and intercostal muscles. Upper airway obstruction can occur if the suction pressure is too high or if the counteracting forces of the dilating muscles are too weak for any given suction pressure (3). The upper airway muscles of OSAS patients contract more forcefully during wakefulness than the muscles of normal subjects (4), which is likely a mechanism to compensate for the structurally narrowed upper airways that is a typical finding in these patients (5). CPAP application is associated with relaxation of the upper airway dilator muscles during both wakefulness and sleep, which

appears to be mediated by upper airway reflex mechanisms (6).

Application of CPAP is immediately associated with a fall in genioglossus muscle contraction, a finding not seen when isolated expiratory positive airway pressure (EPAP) is applied (Fig. 8.1). This effect of CPAP is abolished in the presence of local upper airway anesthesia, which supports the effect being mediated by upper airway reflex mechanisms (Fig. 8.2). The general concept, therefore, is that CPAP acts principally as a pneumatic splint to prevent collapse of the pharyngeal airway. Incremental levels of CPAP result in progressive increase of upper airway size (primarily in the lateral direction) and thinning of the lateral pharyngeal walls with little effect at the level of the soft palate and tongue (7). This enlargement likely reflects a combined effect of positive intrapharyngeal pressure and also the fact that CPAP increases end expiratory lung volume, an action that is also associated with a reflex increase in the size of the pharyngeal lumen.

EFFECTS OF NASAL CPAP

SLEEP-RELATED EFFECTS

A schematic outline of the effects of nasal CPAP is given in Figure 8.3. Since CPAP immediately counteracts the physical forces that lead to the development of upper airway obstruction in sleep, the beneficial effects of treatment are often obvious after the first night's treatment with effective pressure levels (8). Breathing is normalized, and consequently respiratory effort diminishes. The cyclical oscillations of oxygen saturation (SaO_2), heart rate, and blood pressure in association with obstructive apneas are abolished, and snoring also disappears. Sleep architecture improves, and the percentages of slow wave deep (SWS) and rapid eye movement (REM) sleep increase, particularly in severe cases (9). In the early days

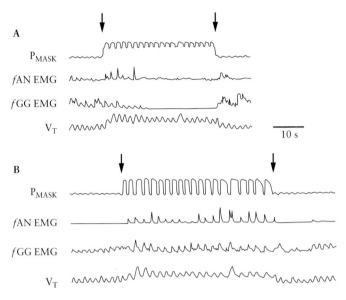

Fig 8.1 *Records from a normal subject demonstrate the effects of nasal CPAP while awake. Panel A, CPAP applied at 12 cm H_2O (between arrows) Panel B, EPAP applied at 12 cm H_2O (between arrows). P mask, Mask pressure; AN EMG, integrated ala nasi electromyogram; GG EMG, integrated genioglossus EMG; V_T, tidal volume. (From Deegan PC, Nolan P, Carey M, et al. Effects of positive airway pressure on upper airway dilator muscle activity and ventilatory timing. J Appl Physiol 1996; 81:470–479.)*

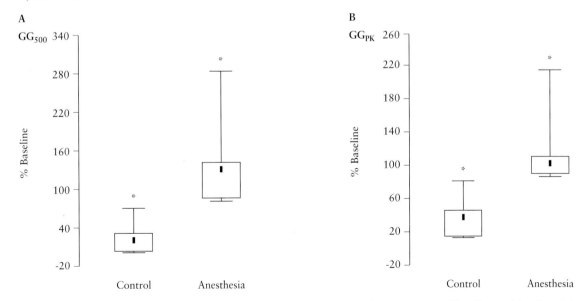

Fig 8.2 *Comparison of genioglossus electromyographic activity, expressed as percentage of baseline activity, for trials of 9 cm H_2O CPAP before (control) and after upper airway anesthesia. The median (small box), 25–75% quartiles (large box), and range (bars) are shown. *p < 0.05 for both comparisons (Wilcoxon rank sum test). GG_{500} = 500 ms into breath; GG_{Pk} = peak inspiratory activity. (Based on data from Deegan et al. [6].)*

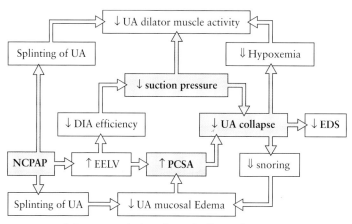

Fig 8.3 *Diagrammatic representation of the potential physiological effects of nasal CPAP (NCPAP) in patients with OSAS. UA, Upper airway; DIA, diaphragm; EELV, end expiratory lung volume; PCSA, pharyngeal cross-sectional area; EDS, excessive daytime sleepiness.*

of therapy, there tends to be a rebound of REM sleep, which later falls back to a normal level. Patients tend to be less restless in bed, and the frequency of micro-arousals greatly decreases (10). Because of increased respiratory efforts, arousals, and sympathetic surge, OSAS is associated with increased sleep energy expenditure, which is normalized by CPAP treatment (11). Some patients, particularly those with heart failure, may show a persistence of central apneas or hypopneas (12). This pattern may also be seen in some OSAS patients treated with too high pressure levels.

Effects of CPAP on Daytime Function and Quality of Life

Patients with OSAS principally complain of daytime sleepiness, whereas the bed partner is usually more affected by the snoring and restless sleep. The precise basis of the daytime sleepiness associated with OSAS is unclear, but the frequency of micro-arousals appears to be the best predictor (13). Many reports have documented improvements in daytime sleepiness with CPAP. Early reports tended to be retrospective, cross-sectional, or uncontrolled in design (14–17), whereas more recent studies have been randomized, prospective, and controlled (18–21). Studies have documented reductions in subjective sleepiness of greater than 50% as measured by the Epworth Sleepiness Scale, in addition to improvements in measures of attention and concentration. Most of these

reports have focused on patients with severe disease, but several recent reports have also documented significant improvements in these variables among patients with relatively mild OSAS (19, 20).

Several reports have also demonstrated significant improvements in objective measures of sleepiness, such as Multiple Sleep Latency Test (MSLT) and Maintenance of Wakefulness Test (MWT) with CPAP therapy, both at the severe end of the disease spectrum (17, 18) and also among patients with relatively mild OSAS (20). The degree of improvement in MSLT appears to correlate with the hourly use of CPAP at night. These findings, particularly from randomized controlled studies, provide strong support for the use of CPAP therapy in patients with moderate to severe OSAS, but the objective findings of benefit among patients with mild OSAS indicate support for the use of CPAP even among less severely affected patients. OSAS has also been reported to have adverse effects on sleep quality and daytime alertness on the bed partner. A recent report from this department has demonstrated improved subjective sleep quality and daytime well-being in the bed partners of OSAS patients treated with CPAP (22).

As a consequence of excessive daytime sleepiness, OSAS patients have more road traffic accidents than the general population (23–25), an increased risk that has been estimated to be about seven times that of the general population (23). However, the increased accident risk is largely removed after successful therapy with CPAP (24,25), and one study has reported a five-fold reduction in accident rate with long-term CPAP therapy compared to the pre-CPAP figures (24). Indeed, it has been suggested that the rate of accidents of OSAS patients using CPAP may even become less than that in the general population. The prevalance of work and domestic accidents is also reduced with CPAP, as is the number of in hospital days related to accidents (24).

Other reports have focused on neuropsychological effects of CPAP therapy and have demonstrated improvements in indices of depression and mood (26), although some neuropsychological deficits appear to persist, perhaps reflecting hypoxic brain damage (27). Improvements in vigilance, driving simulator performance, memory, and cognitive function have all been reported with CPAP. Several measures of quality of life, including the Short Form 36 (SF-36) and Functional Limitations Profile (FLP), have been shown to be impaired in patients with OSAS, and CPAP therapy produces a significant improvement in these measures, particularly at the severe end of the disease spectrum.

OSAS can also be associated with a large variety of somatic symptoms, including headache, heartburn, nocturia, impaired libido, and sweating (28), all of which may benefit from CPAP therapy (Table 8.1). Previous reports indicate that gastroesophageal reflux (GOR) may induce respiratory abnormalities during sleep, seems to be common in OSAS patients, and appears to benefit from CPAP therapy (29). Plasma renin activity and aldosterone levels are reduced, and atrial natriuretic peptide (ANP) levels are elevated in OSAS (30), resulting in increased nocturnal diuresis (31), which may lead to nocturnal polyuria and enuresis. These disturbances are normalized with CPAP in OSAS with resultant benefit to nocturia and enuresis.

EFFECTS OF CPAP ON CARDIOVASCULAR MORBIDITY AND MORTALITY

OSAS has been reported to be associated with a variety of cardiovascular complications, particularly hypertension, but also ischemic heart disease and cerebrovascular accidents (32–35). There appears to be a higher prevalence of coronary artery disease and myocardial ischemia with OSAS than in control populations. However, other reports dispute the independent association of snoring and OSAS with adverse vascular events as either unproven or of doubtful

significance. The report by Wright et al. (36) commented that most of the existing studies were poorly designed, and only weak or contradictory evidence was found of an association with cardiac arrhythmias, ischemic heart disease, cardiac failure, systemic or pulmonary hypertension, and stroke. A recent report from this department has shown that OSAS patients are at high risk of future cardiovascular disease from factors other than OSAS, particularly obesity, hyperlipidemia, diabetes mellitus, and thyroid disease (37). These comorbid risk factors may help explain some of the difficulties in identifying a potential independent risk from OSAS.

An obvious way to evaluate the potential association of OSAS with cardiovascular disease would be to assess the impact of CPAP therapy, but studies are generally lacking in this regard. Although the evidence is now reasonably strong that OSAS predisposes to hypertension (35, 38), the impact of CPAP therapy on blood pressure levels is less clearcut, and there is a great need for controlled studies to evaluate the impact of CPAP on cardiovascular morbidity. In most of the studies of the effects of CPAP on blood pressure, the subjects acted as their own controls, which is far from ideal. At present, there is only one placebo-controlled trial in a small group of OSAS patients (39) and in this study to changes were observed in 24 hour blood pressure. However, there was a significant decrease in nocturnal blood pressure levels in the subgroup of patients who did not show the normal drop in nocturnal blood pressure before CPAP therapy was instituted ('nondippers'). It has been suggested that this category of patients may be most at risk for cardiovascular complications. Other reports have also demonstrated beneficial effects of CPAP on hypertension (40, 41). One report showed a fall in blood pressure levels with CPAP, independent of weight change, and an associated fall in elevated catecholamine levels (41), suggesting that OSAS is an important cofactor in the pathogenesis and possibly the maintenance of hypertension in these patients. Norepinephrine secretion and sympathetic nerve activity have been reported to decrease during CPAP therapy (42), and the decrease correlates with the average hours of CPAP use per night (43). OSAS patients have impaired cardiovascular autonomic responses that can be normalized by CPAP therapy (44). Thus, there appears to be reasonable evidence of beneficial effects of CPAP on factors recognized to contribute to the development and progression of hypertension.

Table 8.1 Summary of symptom changes before and after institution of long-term CPAP therapy

Question: Do you (have)	95% C.I. Pre	95% C.I. Post	Wilcoxon p value
Snoring	2.5–2.9	0.4–0.9	< 0.0001
Witnessed apneas	1.5–1.8	0.1–0.5	< 0.0001
Excessive daytime fatigue	1.3–1.7	0.4–0.9	< 0.0001
Epworth score (units)	14.0–17.6	3.8–6.3	< 0.0001
Difficulty in concentration	0.7–1.1	0.4–0.8	< 0.05
Memory	0.7–1.1	0.4–0.8	n.s.[c]
Orientation on awakening	0.3–0.7	0.1–0.5	n.s.
Frequent waking during the night	0.8–1.3	0.5–0.9	< 0.05
Difficulty in getting a full night's sleep	0.7–1.2	0.4–0.8	< 0.005
Poor sleep quality	1.3–1.7	0.4–0.8	< 0.0001
Awaken at night with a choking feeling	0.3–0.7	0.0–0.3	< 0.05
Restless sleep	0.6–1.1	0.3–0.6	< 0.05
Restless legs while asleep	0.3–0.7	0.1–0.5	n.s.
Sleepwalking	0.0–0.1	0.0–0.1	n.s.
Depression	0.4–0.8	0.2–0.6	n.s.
Nocturnal sweating[a]	0.3–0.7	0.2–0.4	0.05
Hypnagogic hallucinations	0.2–0.6	0.1–0.3	< 0.01
Heartburn	0.4–0.8	0.1–0.4	< 0.01
Heartburn in bed	0.2–0.6	0.0–0.3	< 0.01
Awaken with heartburn	0.1–0.5	0.0–0.1	< 0.01
Get up at night to pass urine	1.1–1.5	0.4–0.8	< 0.0001
Daily frequency of passing urine (times)	1.5–1.9	1.5–2.0	n.s.
Nightly frequency of passing urine (times)	1.3–1.9	0.8–1.4	< 0.05
Blocked nose	0.8–1.3	0.5–0.9	< 0.01
Headache on rising in the morning[b]	0.1–0.5	0.0–0.2	< 0.05
Awaken with severe headache at night	0.0–0.2	0.0–0.1	n.s.
Headache after daytime nap	0.0–0.3	0.0–0.2	n.s.
Reduction in hearing	0.3–0.6	0.2–0.6	n.s.
Ankle swelling	0.2–0.5	0.1–0.4	n.s.
Smoking habit (yes = 1, no = 0)	0.1–0.3	0.1–0.3	n.s.
Weekly alcohol consumption (units)	6.4–13.6	7.8–16.3	n.s.
Regular exercise (yes = 1, no = 0)	0.2–0.5	0.3–0.6	n.s.
Change rooms from partner (yes = 2, no = 1)	1.2–1.6	0.9–1.4	< 0.05

[a] Bad enough to require a change of clothing or bedclothes.

[b] Without having consumed alcohol.

[c] n.s., Not significant.

From Kiely JL, Murphy M, McNicholas WT. Subjective efficacy of nasal CPAP in the obstructive sleep apnoea syndrome: a prospective controlled study. Eur Respir J 1999; 13:1086–1090)

Answer scores based on a three point scale (0, 1, 2) as indicated in text, except snoring (four point scale) and unless otherwise indicated in the table. Patients without partners answered 0 (not applicable) to the last question in the table.

Nocturnal cardiac rhythm disturbances have been reported to be common in patients with OSAS but also in control subjects (45, 46). A recent report from this department has shown that CPAP therapy is associated with resolution of nocturnal cardiac rhythm disturbances within 24–48 hours of instituting therapy (47), which provides supportive evidence of a real association between OSAS and cardiac dysrhythmias.

In a small group of OSAS patients on long-term CPAP therapy, hospitalization days due to cardiovascular and pulmonary disease were reduced by 80%, as compared to the period preceding CPAP treatment (48). Although it is far from clear-cut, there is some evidence that overall survival is diminished in severe OSAS patients and that survival is improved by CPAP (49, 50). The excess of mortality associated with OSAS was prevented as effectively with CPAP as with tracheostomy (49).

EFFECTS OF CPAP ON DAYTIME GAS EXCHANGE

The majority of patients with OSAS have normal awake blood gases, but particular categories may be associated with awake hypoxemia and hypercapnia, particularly those with associated severe obesity or coexisting chronic lung disease such as chronic obstructive pulmonary disease (COPD). Long-term CPAP treatment has been reported to be associated with improved awake PaO_2 levels in a subgroup of OSAS patients with daytime hypoxemia (51), together with improvements in ventilatory drive among patients (52). Patients with both COPD and OSAS may be better managed with bilevel positive airway pressure (BiPAP), since this modality provides a degree of assisted ventilation over and above that achieved with regular CPAP. A minority of OSAS patients display hypercapnia during wakefulness, and the associated abnormal ventilatory drives have been shown to improve within 2 weeks of CPAP therapy, with concomitant normalization of arterial CO_2 tension (41).

PATIENT SELECTION CRITERIA

The current management of moderate to severe OSAS is largely dependent on nasal CPAP. However, although CPAP is highly effective in controlling sleep apnea, the device is cumbersome, and compliance data demonstrate only moderately satisfactory compliance (53). These considerations have prompted many clinicians and health care funding agencies to address the question of which patients with

---

Key points box 8.1

Effects of nasal CPAP

- The beneficial effects of CPAP on sleep quality and awake performance are often evident after the first night's treatment.
- There is now overwhelming evidence of benefit in terms of decreased daytime sleepiness, improved vigilance, concentration, memory, and cognitive function in addition to general measures of quality of life.
- Many somatic symptoms, including headache, heartburn, nocturia, sweating, and impaired libido, also improve after CPAP.
- Driving accidents are up to 10 times more common in patients with OSAS, but the excess risk can be largely abolished by CPAP.
- CPAP benefits hypertension in OSAS, particularly at night, but only limited data are available on the impact on other aspects of cardiovascular morbidity, such as ischemic heart disease and arrhythmias.
- There are only limited and inconclusive data on the impact of CPAP on mortality.

OSAS should be treated. The high prevalence of OSAS has generated alarm in some funding agencies because of the potential cost implications of investigation and treatment, and the recent report of Wright et al. that challenged the clinical significance of sleep apnea syndrome and the need for active therapy in most cases (36) has further added to this debate. However, on the other hand, recent reports that have demonstrated objective benefits with CPAP even among patients with mild OSAS (19, 20) have provided support for the view that even patients with mild disease can benefit from active therapy. Thus, restrictive definitions of eligibility may deny potentially effective therapy to many patients.

SHOULD THERE BE A SPECIFIC AHI THRESHOLD TO JUSTIFY CPAP?

Some health care funding agencies have imposed an arbitrary apnea-hypopnea index (AHI) threshold to determine funding of CPAP therapy. This approach is unjustified for several reasons. First, the AHI is only one measure of severity of OSAS, and such thresholds would deny effective therapy to patients with relatively low AHI levels but prominent daytime sleepiness. Second, objective benefits have been demonstrated with CPAP even in patients with a relatively low AHI, as indicated above (19,20). Thus, there is no particular AHI threshold that allows the prescriber to determine a likely clinical benefit from CPAP. Furthermore, specific AHI thresholds would deny CPAP to patients with disorders such as the upper airway resistance syndrome (UARS), in which a clinically significant AHI is not found on polysomnography, but in which patients may benefit from CPAP therapy, possibly owing to relief of recurring arousals resulting from elevated upper airway resistance. Finally, AHI correlates poorly with subjective severity of OSAS, particularly as determined by the level of daytime sleepiness (54).

The above considerations indicate that the choice of therapy is best left to the responsible clinician, but also emphasize the importance of appropriate training and expertise of those clinicians who are actively involved in treating patients with OSAS in order that the most appropriate treatment choice is made for each individual patient.

NASAL CPAP VERSUS OTHER THERAPIES

In severe cases, nasal CPAP is the treatment of choice, unless there is a specific correctable anatomical lesion, such as enlarged tonsils. In moderately severe cases, most patients are best managed by CPAP, but alternative options can be considered, such as an oral appliance or mandibular advancement by surgery. Mild cases can often be the most difficult to treat but do offer a choice of therapy. Weight loss, alcohol avoidance, relief of nasal obstruction (if present), and measures to improve sleep hygiene may be sufficient in some cases and have been shown to be effective in improving the severity of OSAS and associated symptoms (55). Uvulopalatopharyngoplasty (UPPP) can also be considered in mild cases of OSAS, although it is better reserved for non apneic snorers (56).

Oral appliances may also be effective, but they require considerable expertise and may not represent a significant cost-saving compared with CPAP, particularly if the device is individually molded and fitted to the patient.

However, reports suggest that these appliances are better tolerated than CPAP and are likely to particularly benefit patients with mild OSAS. The American Sleep Disorders Association has issued practice guidelines which state that oral appliances are indicated for mild OSAS and for moderate to severe OSAS if CPAP is not accepted and surgery is inappropriate (57). One review indicated that the cure rate with oral appliances in OSAS is about 50% and that there is a high likelihood of failure when the AHI is greater than 40 (58). In three controlled studies (59–61), CPAP was compared to oral appliances in patients suffering from moderate OSAS (AHI about 25/hour). Although CPAP was uniformly effective at correcting OSAS and was more effective than oral appliances at relieving excessive daytime sleepiness, the pressure device was not accepted by about one third of patients. Oral appliances corrected OSAS in 48–55% of patients across the three studies, of whom nearly all accepted the treatment. Approximately 85% of the patients with moderate OSAS preferred oral appliances to CPAP. A mandibular repositioning device was prospectively studied in mild to moderate OSAS patients who proved intolerant to CPAP. Nearly two thirds of the patient were considered as (partial) responders, and 55% of the patients continued to use the device after 3 years (62).

Although the beneficial effects of CPAP therapy are well established in moderate and severe OSAS, the demonstration of significant benefits with CPAP in mild OSAS poses a significant challenge to those involved in the therapy of OSAS by suggesting that the indications for CPAP therapy in OSAS may be much wider than previously thought. In particular, one study (19) that showed CPAP to be superior to an intensive regimen of conservative therapy challenges conventional practice in this regard.

PRESSURE GENERATING SYSTEMS

Although there are different types of positive airway pressure devices available to treat OSAS, the basis of each system is to deliver a sufficient level of pressure to the oropharyngeal airway to prevent obstruction during sleep. There have been major developments in technology since CPAP was first described in 1981. In early systems, the pressure generators and nasal masks were generally custom-made for each individual patient, and the initial systems contained separate inspiratory and expiratory

---

⊶ Key points box 8.2

Treatment criteria

- Some health care funding agencies have proposed minimum AHI thresholds to determine funding for CPAP therapy, which might appear justified by some critical reviews.

- However, benefits from CPAP therapy in mild OSAS have been demonstrated in controlled trials, and CPAP has also been shown to be superior to an intensive regimen of conservative therapy.

- Furthermore, symptoms such as sleepiness correlate poorly with the AHI.

- Thus, the decision to treat with CPAP is best left to a suitably qualified sleep specialist rather than following arbitrary guidelines.

- CPAP is the treatment of choice in moderate and severe OSAS but other modalities, such as oral appliances, can be considered in mild to moderate cases.

- Oral appliances are not as effective as CPAP in controlling OSAS but appear to be better tolerated.

---

limbs (1). Later systems were modified to include a single circuit with a standard leak in the form of a small hole in order to prevent reinhalation of CO_2.

CPAP

Early devices had fixed speed motors in which the pressure was generated by a fan system and pressure adjustment was by means of a blow-off valve. These systems had high flow rates (up to 200 L/min), which made them noisy, and pressure overshoot occurred during expiration. This feature resulted in increased work of breathing (63), which made the device uncomfortable. Modern machines have better pressure-flow characteristics and provide feedback control of pressure with a microprocessor. The pressure is adjusted by altering the motor speed, and airway pressure changes are minimal between inspiration and expiration (64). Modern machines also are more effective than earlier devices in ensuring the maintenance of pre-

scribed pressure at high altitude or in the presence of air leak (64). The flow rates can vary between less than 10 L/min and greater than 50 L/min according to the absence or presence of mouth air leak. In general, modern CPAP machines may be interchanged without readjustment of pressure levels. Furthermore, these machines are considerably quieter than earlier models; noise levels are such that sleep should not be significantly disturbed. However, part of the noise generated by CPAP systems does not come from the device itself but relates to air leaks around the nasal mask.

Ramp Feature

A delay timer function has been added to most commercial CPAP systems to allow the applied pressure to gradually build up to the therapeutic level, thereby facilitating sleep onset. The time interval is selected by the patient and is generally between 5 and 20 min. Although this feature undoubtedly makes the device more comfortable when initially started, there are no data to show that the ramp function improves overall patient compliance. In fact, it could be argued that repeated actuation of the ramp function throughout the night might lead to suboptimal pressures during much of the sleeping period. Nonetheless, in clinical practice, most patients report a preference for the ramp feature rather than the immediate delivery of a full therapeutic pressure level.

Bilevel Positive Airway Pressure

BiPAP is a modification described in 1990 (65) whereby the pressure delivered can be varied between inspiration and expiration. The device is generally calibrated to deliver a lower pressure during expiration (EPAP) than during inspiration (IPAP), based on the principle that collapsing forces in the upper airway are higher during inspiration than expiration. However, BiPAP seems to be less effective than CPAP in maintaining upper airway patency, and it has been reported that the upper airway has a smaller cross-sectional area during BiPAP as compared to CPAP (66). This finding may be explained by reports that EPAP is important in the maintenance of upper airway patency (65), and lowering EPAP levels can lead to a reduction of pharyngeal dimensions during expiration that extends into the subsequent inspiratory phase, thus facilitating upper airway collapse.

These considerations indicate that BiPAP should not be a first choice therapy for OSAS but should be reserved for patients who have difficulty tolerating standard CPAP, particularly when the pressure generated during expiration appears to be a contributing factor in poor compliance. However, a BiPAP device can also act as a pressure-support ventilator, and thus it may be appropriate in OSAS patients with associated respiratory insufficiency, such as may occur in severe COPD.

AUTO-CPAP

Automatically adjusting CPAP devices (auto-CPAP) have been developed over the past 5 years or so and probably represent the greatest advance in CPAP technology since the original description in 1981. Auto-CPAP machines can be used to help determine the optimum pressure for use with a standard CPAP machine or alternatively can be used for long-term home therapy. These machines are designed to continuously adjust the applied pressure to the 'optimal' level throughout the night (67). This design makes intuitive sense since the concept of a single ideal level of positive pressure for any individual patient is overly simplistic. Upper airway resistance is dependent on multiple factors, such as body position, sleep stages, sleep deprivation, body weight, and fluctuations of nasal congestion (68,69), any or all of which may change within a single night or between nights. For example, it has been demonstrated that sleeping upright or in the lateral position can reduce the therapeutic level of CPAP by nearly 50% in non-REM (NREM) sleep (70). Alcohol intake can also depress the tone and contractility of the upper airway muscles and thus result in higher pressure requirements to maintain upper airway patency. Therefore, a single level of pressure throughout the night will likely result in a situation in which the pressure is excessive for parts of the night, but it may be insufficient at other times and under particular circumstances such as after alcohol consumption.

Several studies have confirmed that auto-CPAP devices are at least as effective as manually determined pressure in correcting the abnormal respiratory events (71, 72), and the immediate effects on sleep are similar to manual titration, including the reduction of microarousals and improvement of excessive daytime sleepiness.

Depending on the particular device, auto-CPAP devices use pressure or flow signals, or both, to detect apneas, hypopneas, or flow limitation. Snoring is detected as high frequency changes in pressure, which are considered as reflecting the acoustic vibrations of snoring. Most machines are regulated by an algorithm based on detection of apneas and hypopneas alone or in combination with snoring. Other algorithms include inspiratory flow limitation derived from the shape of the inspiratory flow–time relation. OSAS can be distinguished from central sleep apnea (CSA) from the calculated airway conductance.

Although it is more expensive, auto-CPAP devices greatly simplify CPAP initiation, since a single optimum pressure no longer needs to be calculated. Furthermore, patient follow-up is also simplified as repeat titration over subsequent years of therapy is no longer required. Auto-CPAP may be particularly useful in patients intolerant of higher pressures or in patients in whom the ideal pressure is highly variable. At present, there is insufficient evidence that auto-CPAP has enough advantages over traditional fixed CPAP in unselected OSAS patients to justify the additional cost. In one study the hourly rate of use has been shown to be higher with auto-CPAP than with standard CPAP (7.1 versus 5.7 hours), despite the fact that the mean mask pressure was not lower than the fixed CPAP (67). The long-term benefits of auto-CPAP have not been determined, and less expensive constant CPAP should still be considered as the standard home therapy for the majority of patients. However, it is likely that auto-setting CPAP machines will become increasingly popular over the coming years, and they may replace the standard fixed pressure machines in the future, particularly if the price is reduced toward that of the standard CPAP machines.

MASK SELECTION

The selection of a comfortable mask, which provides an effective seal against the face to minimize air leaks, is a critically important aspect of CPAP therapy in OSAS. This aspect should be addressed at the initial institution of CPAP therapy, and it has a major impact on the ongoing success of therapy. Mask fitting is a highly skilled process. It is best performed by a trained and experienced technologist or nurse practitioner. As the technology of nasal masks has evolved greatly over the years, there are now a large variety of masks available. Adequate time is essential for proper fitting and patient education, and careful attention to this aspect of therapy will have a significant benefit in terms of treatment efficacy, side effects, and compliance.

<table>
<tr><td>

⊶ Key points box 8.3

Choice of device

- *CPAP:* The device consists of a servo-controlled turbine in which the pressure is altered by adjusting the motor speed. Flow rates vary and may increase considerably in the presence of mouth leak, which may increase local side effects.
- *BiPAP:* This device varies pressure between inspiration and expiration and may be indicated in a few patients who find the expiratory positive pressure uncomfortable. In patients with coexisting respiratory insufficiency, BiPAP may be particularly effective by acting partly as an assisted ventilator.
- *Auto-CPAP:* This device varies the pressure delivered constantly throughout the night based on feedback from airway sensors to continuously provide the optimum pressure required to prevent upper airway obstruction. The device usually delivers a lower mean pressure than standard CPAP, which may be more comfortable, and greatly simplifies CPAP initiation and subsequent patient follow-up. However, auto-CPAP is considerably more expensive and, thus, cannot be justified on a routine basis at present.

</td></tr>
</table>

The earliest CPAP devices utilized masks that had to be individually molded onto the nose, a technique that is still occasionally used in very difficult cases. However, commercial masks are generally prescribed as they are more comfortable and, because of the very wide choice available, a mask can usually be found to fit nearly every face. Most are nasal masks held in position by straps around the head that cover the nose and leave the mouth free. They have a skirt and buttress design that allows the mask to fit and seal well over the nose without too much tightening of the straps, thereby reducing the pressure on the skin. One particular nasal interface uses two soft cushions that plug into the nasal orifices, mounted on a bridge. Since this particular type exerts no pressure on the bridge of the nose, it is particularly helpful for patients who develop pressure sores on the bridge of the nose with the standard nasal mask.

Leakage of air through the mouth can occur, which reduces the effective pressure delivered to the oropharyngeal airway. Mouth leak also increases the likelihood of nasal side effects in addition to increasing the noise of the device since the flow rate is automatically increased by the pressure generator in an effort to correct the loss of pressure at the level of the pharynx. Mouth leak can usually be overcome by using either a chin strap or a full facemask that covers both nose and mouth. The pressure required to maintain upper airway patency using a full facemask appears to be similar to that with a nasal mask (73). Potential problems with the full facemask include coughing and vomiting. In addition, the risks associated with failure of the device may be greater.

INITIATION OF CPAP THERAPY

Effective therapy with CPAP is critically dependent on adequate pressures being delivered to the pharynx throughout the night to prevent apneas and hypopneas and also to eliminate snoring. On the other hand, there is evidence that too high pressures are detrimental, not only by increasing the prevalence of side effects but also by predisposing to the development of central apnea. Therefore, titration is the process of balancing the desire to eliminate all obstructive events by increasing pressure against the desire to minimize side effects by using the lowest possible effective pressure. During progressive increase in applied pressure levels, apneas change to hypopneas, and further increases in pressure result in hypopneas changing to a pattern of inspiratory flow limitation with persistence of high negative pleural pressure during inspiration. Finally, when the optimum level of pressure is applied, a regular breathing pattern ensues with only small pleural pressure swings consistent with normal respiration (74).

There is no clear consensus on the criteria for optimum CPAP titration, although the elimination of apneas, hypopneas, and snoring in all sleep stages and all sleep positions would be the most widely used. However, this approach may be suboptimal in some cases since some patients might have persistent elevation of upper airway resistance with associated sleep fragmentation and consequent persistence of excessive daytime sleepiness. Therefore, since sleep fragmentation is an important consequence of OSAS, an effective CPAP could also be considered as one that not only eliminates apneas and snoring but also normalizes the number of electroencephalographic (EEG) arousals and restores normal sleep architecture. This requirement raises the question of whether sleep staging should be performed in conjunction with CPAP titration, as has been recommended by some author (2). However, the logistics of performing full polysomnography in conjunction with CPAP titration are beyond the resources of many sleep centers.

Some sleep centers also record esophageal pressure during titration and advocate that the endpoint of titration should be to obtain the lowest possible esophageal pressure. However, this approach is invasive and consequently not widely used. Furthermore, the contour of inspiratory flow tracing from a CPAP system can be used to infer the persistence of elevated upper airway resistance and flow limitation. Optimizing the flow contour could therefore be a way to determine the optimal pressure (75), particularly since the flow contour correlates well with the lowest esophageal pressure during CPAP titration (74). Finally, respiratory resistive impedance measured by forced oscillations has been proposed for automatic and noninvasive monitoring of upper airway obstruction and for CPAP titration (76).

The optimal pressure varies among patients and is usually between 5 and 15 cm H_2O. Fewer than 1% of patients require a pressure higher than 15 cm H_2O. Patients requiring higher pressure tended to be characterized by a greater degree of obesity, more severe sleep apnea, and more collapsible pharynx (77). In patients who cannot tolerate the optimal CPAP level, treatment can be started at a lower pressure, such as 2–3 cm H_2O below the optimal pressure. Under such conditions, patients usually derive at least partial benefit from CPAP and usually improve further over subsequent weeks and months (78).

METHODS OF CPAP TITRATION

MANUAL TITRATION DURING POLYSOMNOGRAPHY

The traditional gold standard for CPAP titration has been the process of manual titration in the sleep laboratory in association with full overnight polysomnography (PSG). This technique requires the full resources of a sleep laboratory, including the continuing presence of a

sleep technologist. Therefore, because of the high costs involved together with the demands on equipment for diagnostic purposes, cheaper and shorter procedures have been sought and developed over the years.

SPLIT-NIGHT POLYSOMNOGRAPHY

CPAP is sometimes implemented in the second half of the diagnostic night (a so-called split-night study). However, the first and second parts of a PSG are not identical, and split-night protocols may be inappropriate when REM sleep does not occur in the first part of the study (78). This approach is appropriate where resources are limited, but cannot be regarded as ideal for several reasons. First, the patient does not know in advance of the sleep study whether CPAP will be the appropriate management for the presenting symptoms, yet he or she will require some level of introduction to CPAP therapy in addition to basic mask fitting in advance of the study to allow CPAP titration, if it is found appropriate during the study. Thus, careful explanation and education are required to prevent possible frustration and disappointment on the part of the patient should CPAP not be selected as ongoing therapy. Second, 'on the spot' diagnostic and therapeutic decisions are required midway through the sleep study by the technologist in attendance, which necessitates considerable skill and experience to make the correct call. Finally, the shorter period available in the latter part of the study night for CPAP titration may compromise the selection of optimum pressure. The level of pressure chosen from split-night studies appears to underestimate the optimum level of pressure when compared to full-night studies.

PREDICTION EQUATIONS

Various groups have made efforts to predict the optimum CPAP levels in advance of therapy by using regression models based on anthropometric and PSG information. A prediction equation based on neck circumference, AHI, body mass index and (BMI) accounted for three quarters of the variability in pressure in one study (79). In a prospective study from the same center, this equation predicted the optimal pressure within 1 cm H_2O in 20 of 26 patients (80). However, other reports have found prediction equations to be less useful (81). Overall, it seems reasonable that the predicted CPAP value from such equations could be used to facilitate manual titration by providing a starting pressure level to commence titration. However, it is generally accepted that prediction formulas should not be substituted for objective titration studies.

GRADUAL HABITUATION

Some centers also provide the patient with a CPAP device set at a low pressure (usually about 5 cm H_2O) for several nights' use at home prior to formal titration of optimum pressure levels. This approach allows time for the patient to get used to the system at a more comfortable pressure level, and the REM rebound effect often seen during early CPAP therapy may be reduced. However, a full-night titration is subsequently required to titrate optimum CPAP levels, which makes this method at least as labor intensive as traditional titration. Although this refinement has some merit, few data are available to indicate that the method is superior to standard titration. Furthermore, it could be argued that the introduction of CPAP therapy at a pressure at which sleep-disordered breathing is not being effectively controlled might provide a disappointing introduction to CPAP therapy for many patients.

CPAP TITRATION WITH LIMITED SIGNALS AND UNATTENDED OR HOME TITRATION

Several groups have attempted to find an effective and safe method to titrate CPAP in the unsupervised home environment using simpler recordings than PSG. This approach has been prompted by the need to cater for the very large numbers of patients with OSAS who come to sleep centers and also by the need to control costs. Waldhorn and Wood (82) titrated CPAP in the patient's home using a four channel recorder that measured heart rate, thoracic impedance, oxygen saturation (SaO$_2$), and pressure at the mask. The long-term compliance with CPAP therapy initiated in this fashion appeared to be as good as after conventional titration and the cost was reported to be much lower (82). Another study found a good agreement between CPAP levels determined at full-night PSG performed in the sleep laboratory setting and a system that recorded SaO$_2$, pulse, chest and abdominal motion, and body position (83). However, the lack of EEG recording limits the utility of such titration strategies, since sleep quality is unknown. Furthermore, the lack of technician supervision during home titration means that leads that become displaced during the night are not replaced. Nonetheless, it is likely that home titration of CPAP therapy will become increasingly common,

and it is presently being formally evaluated by several international scientific societies.

AUTOMATIC TITRATION

Auto-CPAP devices not only can be used to treat OSAS on an ongoing basis but can also be used to help determine the single optimum pressure to be used in standard CPAP devices over a single or several nights' titration, either in the sleep laboratory or in the patient's home. In general, the optimal CPAP determined automatically and manually by experienced technicians is similar, although the autosetting device may predict a slightly higher fixed pressure (72). In one study, failure of a self-titrating prototype necessitated subsequent manual resetting in a quarter of OSAS patients (84). In another study, unattended auto-CPAP titration was associated with undesirable cardiorespiratory complications (including central apneas and high-grade arrhythmia) in 6 of 21 patients, all of

---

⊶ Key points box 8.4

Initiation of CPAP

- Optimum CPAP titration is a balance of the desire to eliminate all obstructive events by increasing pressure against the desire to minimize side effects by using the lowest effective pressure.

- Manual titration during polysomnography is regarded as the gold standard but is expensive and time consuming.

- Prediction equations based on AHI, neck circumference, and weight may facilitate CPAP titration but do not replace the need for objective studies.

- Split-night studies are used in many centers but are hampered by the fact that sleep architecture differs between the first and second parts of the night.

- Unattended or home titration using limited recording signals are labor and cost efficient but have a higher failure rate than conventional titration.

whom had underlying cardiorespiratory disorders (85). Therefore, unattended auto-CPAP titration is not advisable in patients with significant daytime cardiorespiratory disorders. Automatic titration does not appear to reduce acceptance or subsequent compliance with CPAP when compared with manual titration (86, 87).

SIDE EFFECTS OF CPAP THERAPY

Side effects are common with CPAP therapy but are rarely serious. Most side effects are minor, and their main consequence is poor compliance. Optimizing the comfort and fit of the nasal mask have a major impact on the likelihood of side effects, which emphasizes the importance of adequate expertise of the personnel responsible for initiation of therapy. Furthermore, side effects usually occur early on after institution of therapy, and close patient follow-up evaluation in the initial weeks of therapy is very important. This goal is usually best achieved by providing telephone contact numbers to each patient together with an early appointment for outpatient follow-up review.

The most common adverse effects related to the nasal mask are local pressure effects that can cause irritation or ulceration of the bridge of the nose, and air leaks, which can cause eye irritation. Refitting of the nasal mask or switching to a different type of mask that covers only the nasal orifice can often correct these problems. Nose and throat problems occur in about 40% of patients using CPAP and include dry mouth, rhinorrhea, sneezing, nasal congestion, and pain (88–90). Air leak through the mouth is an important mechanism contributing to dry mouth and nasal side effects. Such mouth leaks lead to a higher airflow through the nose and can result in a large increase in nasal mucosal blood flow and resistance (91). In most cases, heated humidification is successful in controlling these problems, but if nasal congestion and blockage are the principal concerns, an intranasal steroid spray may be more appropriate. There is evidence that UPPP may compromise subsequent nasal CPAP therapy (92), and it has been reported that, after UPPP, patients have mouth air leak at lower levels of pressure and also tolerate higher pressures badly. Furthermore, long-term compliance with CPAP appears to be lower in patients after UPPP. These considerations underline the importance of avoiding UPPP in patients whose OSAS severity may justify CPAP therapy.

Major side effects are very rare and have been described as single case reports. These include pneumocephalus, massive epistaxis, atrial arrhythmia, bacterial meningitis, subcutaneous emphysema after facial trauma, and pneumopericardium after cardiac surgery. One patient developed suffocation during application of CPAP when a large and floppy epiglottis was blown downward by the positive pressure and occluded the hypopharynx.

COMPLIANCE

After the initial CPAP titration, about 80% of patients accept CPAP as ongoing therapy (93, 94). Problems and side effects are generally encountered during the first few weeks of therapy, which may adversely affect compliance. This experience further emphasizes the importance of close patient follow-up evaluation and support in the early weeks of therapy. About 10% of patients abandon CPAP after initial acceptance, usually during the first few months of home therapy. The major reasons for refusal or discontinuation of CPAP therapy are lack of perceived benefit and the obvious drawbacks of the system, such as discomfort, claustrophobia, and the noise of the system (95). Patients' subjective reports are unreliable in determining compliance with therapy; self-reports usually overestimate the actual use by about 1 hour per night on average (95–97). Objective compliance data can be obtained from the built-in time-counter, which records the cumulative machine run time, or from an additional microprocessor, which records both machine run time and the time spent at effective pressure. These data indicate that the patient is wearing the mask and that the prescribed pressure is being delivered. Compliance can be improved by follow-up support in which education, symptom treatment, and equipment monitoring are provided (98).

Several cross-sectional studies of long-term compliance in large groups of patients followed for at least 1 year have reported an average of 5 to 6.5 hours of nightly use (53, 90, 99), although some reports have described fewer hours of nightly use (53). Long-term compliers apply CPAP on more than 90% of nights, and their rate of use does not appear to decrease over time (100). Such compliance levels compare favorably with levels reported for the treatment of other chronic diseases, such as asthma and hypertension. Compliance with CPAP is only weakly correlated with indices of OSAS severity at diagnosis

(101) and cannot reliably be predicted before prescription. Thus, objective evaluations of use should be obtained regularly in all patients when possible.

The fact that patients use their CPAP device for only part of the night raises the possible benefit of adding other modalities of therapy to CPAP in patients with moderate to severe OSAS. Prior to the widespread use of CPAP, there was considerable interest in pharmacological therapy, and a number of agents have been shown to have limited beneficial effects in this disorder (102–104). Pharmacological therapy largely fell out of favor once CPAP use became widespread, because of the realization that CPAP was a much more effective form of therapy. However, if patients spend significant periods of each night without CPAP, the addition of one or more pharmacological agents might provide some additional benefit during that part of the night when the CPAP mask has been removed. Further study will be required to establish if such additional therapy provides significant clinical benefit. The limited compliance with CPAP should also be taken into account when comparing the relative efficacy of CPAP with other forms of therapy that might be somewhat less effective but better tolerated, such as oral prostheses.

CESSATION OF CPAP THERAPY

While continuing long-term CPAP is highly effective in controlling OSAS, this therapy does not provide a cure. Thus, interruption of CPAP is soon followed by the return of sleep apnea, although a carry-over effect of CPAP has been described in several studies. Respiratory efforts, assessed by esophageal pressure recordings, have been shown to be lower during the first night off CPAP in patients established on long-term therapy (105). Furthermore, there is some evidence that indices of OSAS are less severe during the first few hours of sleep (106) or during the first night off CPAP (107). Mechanisms that may contribute to this short-term carryover benefit include stabilization of the upper airway as a consequence of the removal of sleep deprivation (108) and an increase in pharyngeal volume as a result of the reduction in mucosal edema (109, 110). An improved reflex response of upper airway dilator muscles to negative pressure, which has been described after CPAP therapy, could also play a role (111). However, withdrawal of CPAP for even a single night has been reported to result in the reappearance of abnormal sleep latencies as determined by MSLT, even though the subjects concerned indicated no subjective sleepiness (106). After several years of regular CPAP use, a small proportion of patients can be successfully weaned from CPAP, without recurrence of sleep apnea, and substantial weight loss is the most likely reason (93, 94, 99).

FUTURE DIRECTION

Nasal CPAP is firmly established as the principal modality of therapy in OSAS. However, most patients dislike the cumbersome nature of the apparatus and the fact that continuing therapy is required to maintain the effect. The development of auto-CPAP devices should make CPAP somewhat easier to tolerate, particularly since recent reports have indicated that average pressures are lower with auto-CPAP (111,112). Furthermore, auto-CPAP should simplify CPAP initiation and subsequent follow-up support. Thus, a gradual shift towards auto-CPAP devices is likely to occur over the coming years. Recent evidence has emerged to support a beneficial effect of CPAP in certain nonrespiratory disorders in which sleep-related breathing abnormalities have been described. There is growing evidence of benefit in congestive heart failure complicated by either OSAS or Cheyne-Stokes breathing syndrome (113, 114), although not all categories of patients may benefit to the same extent (115). Intriguing recent developments have been the description of disordered breathing during sleep in patients with preeclampsia and the recent report that short-term nasal CPAP results in lowered nocturnal blood pressure levels in these patients (116). Whether these early reports indicate a clinically useful role for CPAP in the management of these disorders remains to be seen.

REFERENCES

1. Sullivan CE, Issa FG, Berthon-Jones M, et al. Reversal of obstructive sleep apnoea by continuous positive airway pressure applied through the nares. Lancet 1981; 1:862–865.

2. American Thoracic Society. Indications and standards for use of nasal continuous positive airway pressure (CPAP) in sleep apnea syndromes. Am J Respir Crit Care Med 1994; 150:1738–1745.

3. Issa FG, Sullivan CE. Upper airway closing pressures in obstructive sleep apnea. J Appl Physiol 1984; 57:520–527.

4. Mezzanotte WS, Tangel DJ, White DP. Waking genioglossal electromyogram in sleep apnea patients versus normal controls (a neuromuscular compensatory mechanism). J Clin Invest 1992; 89:1571–1579.

5. Collard P, Rombaux P, Rodenstein DO. Why should we enlarge the pharynx in obstructive sleep apnea? Sleep 1996; 19:S85–S87.

6. Deegan PC, Nolan P, Carey M, et al. Effects of positive airway pressure on upper airway dilator muscle activity and ventilatory timing. J Appl Physiol 1996; 81:470–479.

7. Kuna ST, Bedi DG, Ryckman C. Effect of nasal airway positive pressure on upper airway size and configuration. Am Rev Respir Dis 1988; 138:969–975.

8. Lamphere J, Roehrs T, Wittig R, et al. Recovery of alertness after CPAP in apnea. Chest 1989; 96:1364–1367.

9. Issa FG, Sullivan CE. The immediate effects of nasal continuous positive airway pressure treatment on sleep pattern in patients with obstructive sleep apnea syndrome. Electroencephalogr Clin Neurophysiol 1986; 63:10–17.

10. Collard P, Dury M, Delguste P, et al. Movement arousals and sleep-related disordered breathing in adults. Am J Respir Crit Care Med 1996; 154:454–459.

11. Stenlof K, Grunstein R, Hedner J, et al. Energy expenditure in obstructive sleep apnea: effects of treatment with continuous positive airway pressure. Am J Physiol 1996; 271:1036–1043.

12. Marrone O, Stallone A, Salvaggio A, et al. Occurence of breathing disorders during CPAP administration in obstructive sleep apnoea syndrome. Eur Respir J 1991; 4:660–666.

13. Bennett LS, Langford BA, Stradling JR, et al. Sleep fragmentation indices as predictors of daytime sleepiness and nCPAP response in obstructive sleep apnea. Am J Respir Crit Care Med 1998; 158:778–786.

14. Sullivan CE, Issa FG, Berthon-Jones M, et al. Home treatment of obstructive sleep apnoea with continuous positive airway pressure applied through a nose mask. Bull Eur Physiopathol Respir 1984; 20:49–54.

15. McEvoy RD, Thornton AT. Treatment of obstructive sleep apnea syndrome with nasal continuous positive airway pressure. Sleep 1988; 7:313–325.

16. Hoffstein V, Viner S, Mateika SC, et al. Treatment of obstructive sleep apnea with nasal continuous positive airway pressure: patient compliance, perception of benefits, and side effects. Am Rev Respir Dis 1992; 145:841–845.

17. Sforza E, Krieger J. Daytime sleepiness after long-term continuous positive airway pressure treatment in obstructive sleep apnea syndrome. J Neurol Sci 1992; 110:21–26.

18. Engleman HM, Martin SE, Deary IJ, et al. Effect of continuous positive airway pressure treatment on daytime function in sleep apnoea/hypopnoea syndrome. Lancet 1994; 343:572–575.

19. Redline S, Adams N, Strauss ME, et al. Improvement of mild sleep-disordered breathing with CPAP compared with conservative therapy. Am J Respir Crit Care Med 1998; 157:858–865.

20. Engleman HM, Martin SE, Deary IJ, et al. Effect of CPAP therapy on daytime function in patients with mild sleep apnoea/hypopnoea syndrome. Thorax 1997; 52:114–119.

21. Jenkinson C, Davies RJO, Mullins R, et al. Comparison of therapeutic and subtherapeutic nasal continuous positive airway pressure for obstructive sleep apnoea: a randomised propsective parallel trial. Lancet 1999; 353:2100–2105.

22. Kiely JL, McNicholas WT. Bed partners assessment of nasal continuous positive airway pressure therapy in obstructive sleep apnea syndrome. Chest 1997; 111:1261–1265.

23. Teran-Santos J, Jimenez-Gomez A, Cordero-Guevara J. The association between sleep apnea and the risk of traffic accidents. N Engl J Med 1999; 340:881–883.

24. Krieger J, Meslier N, Lebrun T, et al. Accidents in obstructive sleep apnea patients treated with nasal continuous positive airway pressure. A prospective study. Chest 1997; 112:1561–1566.

25. Findley L, Smith C, Hooper J, et al. Treatment with nasal CPAP decreases automobile accidents in patients with sleep apnea. Am J Respir Crit Care Med 2000; 161:857–859.

26. Derderian SS, Bridenbaugh RH, Rajagopal KR. Neuropsychological symptoms in obstructive sleep apnea improve after treatment with nasal continuous positive airway pressure. Chest 1988; 94:1023–1027.

27. Bedard MA, Montplaisir J, Malo J, et al. Persistent neuropsychological deficits and vigilance impairment in sleep apnea syndrome after treatment with continuous positive airway pressure. J Clin Exp Neuropsychol 1993; 15:330–341.

28. Kiely JL, Murphy M, McNicholas WT. Subjective efficacy of nasal CPAP in the obstructive sleep apnoea syndrome: a prospective controlled study. Eur Respir J 1999; 13:1086–1090.

29. Kerr P, Shoenut JP, Millar T, et al. Nasal CPAP reduces gastroesophageal reflux in obstructive sleep apnea syndrome. Chest 1992; 101:1539–1544.

30. Follenius M, Krieger J, Krauth MO, et al. Obstructive sleep apnea treatment: peripheral and central effects on plasma renin activity and aldosterone. Sleep 1991; 14:211–217.

31. Krieger J, Follenius M, Sforza E, et al. Effects of treatment with nasal continuous positive airway pressure on atrial natriuretic peptide and arginine vasopressin release during sleep in patients with obstructive sleep apnoea. Clin Sci (Colch) 1991; 80:443–449.

32. Shepard JW, Jr. Hypertension, cardiac arrhythmias, myocardial infarction, and stroke in relation to obstructive sleep apnoea. Clin Chest Med 1992; 13:437–458.

33. Schafer H, Koehler U, Ploch T, et al. Sleep-related myocardial ischemia and sleep structure in patients with obstructive sleep apnea and coronary heart disease. Chest 1997; 111:387–393.

34. Good DC, Henkle JQ, Gelber D, et al. Sleep-disordered breathing and poor functional outcome after stroke. Stroke 1996; 27:252–259.

35. Lavie P, Herer P, Hoffstein V. Obstructive sleep apnoea syndrome as a risk factor for hypertension: population study. Br Med J 2000; 320:479–482.

36. Wright J, Johns R, Watt I, et al. Health effects of obstructive sleep apnoea and the effectiveness of continuous positive airways pressure: a systematic review of the research evidence. Br Med J 1997; 314:851–860.

37. Kiely JL, McNicholas WT. Cardiovascular risk factors in patients with obstructive sleep apnoea syndrome. Eur Respir J 2000; 16:128–133.

38. Young T, Peppard P, Palta M, et al. Population-based study of sleep-disordered breathing as a risk factor for hypertension. Arch Intern Med 1997; 157:1746–1752.

39. Engleman HM, Gough K, Martin SE, et al. Ambulatory blood pressure on and off continuous positive airway pressure therapy for the sleep apnea/hypopnea syndrome: effects in "non-dippers." Sleep 1996; 19:378–381.

40. Akashiba T, Minemura H, Yamamoto H, et al. Nasal continuous positive airway pressure changes blood pressure "non-dippers" to "dippers" in patients with obstructive sleep apnea. Sleep 1999; 22:849–853.

41. Hedner J, Darpo B, Ejnell H, et al. Reduction in sympathetic activity after long-term CPAP treatment in sleep apnoea: cardiovascular implications. Eur Respir J 1995; 8:222–229.

42. Somers VK, Dyken ME, Clary MP, et al. Sympathetic neural mechanisms in obstructive sleep apnea. J Clin Invest 1995; 96:1897–1904.

43. Waravdekar NV, Sinoway LI, Zwillich CW, et al. Influence of treatment on muscle sympathetic nerve activity in sleep apnea. Am J Respir Crit Care Med 1996; 153:1333–1338.

44. Veale D, Pepin JL, Wuyam B, et al. Abnormal autonomic stress responses in obstructive sleep apnoea are reversed by nasal continuous positive airway pressure. Eur Respir J 1996; 9:2122–2126.

45. Hoffstein V, Mateika S. Cardiac arrhythmias, snoring, and sleep apnea. Chest 1994; 106:466–471.

46. Flemons WW, Remmers JE, Gillis AM. Sleep apnea and cardiac arrhythmias. Is there a relationship? Am Rev Respir Dis 1993; 148:618–621.

47. Harbison J, O'Reilly P, McNicholas WT. Cardiac rhythm disturbances in the obstructive sleep apnea syndrome: effects of nasal continuous positive airway pressure. Chest 2000; 118:591–595.

48. Peker Y, Hedner J, Johansson A, et al. Reduced hospitalization with cardiovascular and pulmonary disease in obstructive sleep apnea patients on nasal CPAP treatment. Sleep 1997; 20:645–653.

49. He J, Kryger MH, Zorick FJ, et al. Mortality and apnea index in obstructive sleep apnea. Experience in 385 male patients. Chest 1988; 94:9–14.

50. Lavie P, Herer P, Peled R, et al. Mortality in sleep apnea patients: a multivariate analysis of risk factors. Sleep 1995; 18:149–157.

51. Chaouat A, Weitzenblum E, Kessler R, et al. Five-year effects of nasal continuous positive airway pressure in obstructive sleep apnoea syndrome. Eur Respir J 1997; 10:2578–2582.

52. Lin CC. Effect of nasal CPAP on ventilatory drive in normocapnic and hypercapnic patients with obstructive sleep apnoea syndrome. Eur Respir J 1994; 7:2005–2010.

53. McNicholas WT. Compliance with nasal CPAP in obstructive sleep apnoea: how much is enough? Eur Respir J 1997; 10:969–970.

54. Deegan PC, McNicholas WT. Predictive value of clinical features for the obstructive sleep apnoea syndrome. Eur Respir J 1996; 9:117–124.

55. Montserrat JM, Ballester E, Hernandez L. Overview of management options for snoring and sleep apnoea. In: McNicholas WT, ed. Respiratory disorders during sleep. European Respiratory Monographs. Volume 3. Copenhagen: Munsgard Press; 1998: 144–178.

56. Lévy P, Bettega G, Pépin JL. Surgical management options for snoring and sleep apnoea. In: McNicholas WT, ed. Respiratory disorders during sleep. European Respiratory Monographs, Volume 3. Copenhagen: Munsgard Press; 1998:205–226.

57. Standards of Practice Committee, American Sleep Disorders Association. Practice parameters for the treatment of snoring and obstructive sleep apnea with oral appliances. Sleep 1995; 18:511–513.

58. Schmidt-Nowara W, Lowe A, Wiegand L, et al. Oral appliances for the treatment of snoring and obstructive sleep apnea: a review. Sleep 1995; 18:501–510.

59. Clark GT, Blumenfeld I, Yoffe N, et al. A crossover study comparing the efficacy of continuous positive airway pressure with anterior mandibular positioning devices on patients with obstructive sleep apnea. Chest 1996; 109:1477–1483.

60. Ferguson KA, Ono T, Lowe AA, et al. A randomized crossover study of an oral appliance vs nasal-continuous positive airway pressure in the treatment of mild-moderate obstructive sleep apnea. Chest 1996; 109:1269–1275.

61. Ferguson KA, Ono T, Lowe AA, et al. A short-term controlled trial of an adjustable oral appliance for the treatment of mild to moderate obstructive sleep apnoea. Thorax 1997; 52:362–368.

62. Menn SJ, Loube DI, Morgan TD, et al. The mandibular repositioning device: role in the treatment of obstructive sleep apnea. Sleep 1996; 19:794–800.

63. Demirozu MC, Chediak AD, Nay KN, et al. A comparison of nine nasal continuous positive airway pressure machines in maintaining mask pressure during simulated inspiration. Sleep 1991; 14:259–262.

64. Lofaso F, Heyer L, Leroy A, et al. Do turbines with servo-controlled speed improve continuous positive airway pressure generation? Eur Respir J 1994; 7:2077–2081.

65. Sanders MR, Kern N. Obstructive sleep apnea treated by independently adjusted inspiratory and expiratory positive airway pressures via nasal mask. Physiological and clinical implications. Chest 1990; 98:317–324.

66. Gugger M, Vock P. Effect of reduced expiratory pressure on pharyngeal size during nasal positive airway pressure in patients with sleep apnoea: evaluation by continuous computed tomography. Thorax 1992; 47:809–813.

67. Meurice JC, Marc I, Series F. Efficacy of auto-CPAP in the treatment of obstructive sleep apnea/hypopnea syndrome. Am J Respir Crit Care Med 1996; 153:794–798.

68. Pevernagie DA, Shepard JW Jr. Relations between sleep stage, posture and effective nasal CPAP levels in OSA. Sleep 1992; 15:162–167.

69. Miljeteig H, Hoffstein V. Determinants of continuous positive airway pressure level for treatment of obstructive sleep apnea. Am Rev Respir Dis 1993; 147:1526–1530

70. Neill AM, Angus SM, Sajkov D, et al. Effects of sleep posture on upper airway stability in patients with obstructive sleep apnea. Am J Respir Crit Care Med 1997; 155:199–204.

71. Lloberes P, Ballester E, Montserrat JM, et al. Comparison of manual and automatic CPAP titration in patients with sleep apnea/hypopnea syndrome. Am J Respir Crit Care Med 1996; 154:1755–1758.

72. Teschler H, Berthon-Jones M, Thompson AB, et al. Automated continuous positive airway pressure titration for obstructive sleep apnea syndrome. Am J Respir Crit Care Med 1996; 154:734–740.

73. Prosise GL, Berry RB. Oral-nasal continuous positive airway pressure as a treatment for obstructive sleep apnea. Chest 1994; 106:180–186.

74. Montserrat JM, Ballester E, Olivi H, et al. Time-course of stepwise CPAP titration. Behavior of respiratory and neurological variables. Am J Respir Crit Care Med 1995; 152:1854–1859.

75. Condos R, Norman RG, Krishnasamy I, et al. Flow limitation as a noninvasive assessment of residual upper-airway resistance during continuous positive airway pressure therapy of obstructive sleep apnea. Am J Respir Crit Care Med 1994; 150:475–480.

76. Farr, R, Rotger M, Montserrat JM, et al. A system to generate simultaneous forced oscillation and continuous positive airway pressure. Eur Respir J 1997; 10:1349–1353.

77. Miljeteig H, Hoffstein V. Determinants of continuous positive airway pressure level for treatment of obstructive sleep apnea. Am Rev Respir Dis 1993; 147:1526–1530.

78. Fanfulla F, Patruno V, Bruschi C, et al. Obstructive sleep apnoea syndrome: is the "half-night polysomnography" an adequate method for evaluating sleep profile and respiratory events? Eur Respir J 1997; 10:1725–1729.

79. Series F, Marc I, Cormier Y, et al. Required levels of nasal continuous positive airway pressure during treatment of obstructive sleep apnoea. Eur Respir J 1994; 7:1776–1781.

80. Hoffstein V, Mateika S. Predicting nasal continuous positive airway pressure. Am J Respir Crit Care Med 1994; 150:486–488.

81. Sforza E, Krieger J, Bacon W, et al. Determinants of effective continuous positive airway pressure in obstructive sleep apnea. Role of respiratory effort. Am J Respir Crit Care Med 1995; 151:1852–1856.

82. Waldhorn RE, Wood K. Attended home titration of nasal continuous positive airway pressure therapy for obstructive sleep apnea. Chest 1993; 104:1707–1710.

83. Montserrat JM, Alarcon A, Lloberes P, et al. Adequacy of prescribing nasal continuous positive airway pressure therapy for the sleep apnoea/hypopnoea syndrome on the basis of night time respiratory recording variables. Thorax 1995; 50:969–971.

84. Sharma S, Wali S, Pouliot Z, et al. Treatment of obstructive sleep apnea with a self-titrating continuous positive airway pressure (CPAP) system. Sleep 1996; 19:497–501.

85. Juhasz J, Schillen J, Urbigkeit A, et al. Unattended continuous positive airway pressure titration. Clinical relevance and cardiorespiratory hazards of the method. Am J Respir Crit Care Med 1996; 154:359–365.

86. Stradling JR, Barbour C, Pitson DJ, et al. Automatic nasal continuous positive airway pressure titration in the laboratory: patient outcomes. Thorax 1997; 52:72–75.

87. Teschler H, Farhat AA, Exner V, et al. AutoSet nasal CPAP titration: constancy of pressure, compliance and effectiveness at 8 month follow up. Eur Respir J 1997; 10:2073–2078.

88. Hoffstein V, Viner S, Mateika S, et al. Treatment of obstructive sleep apnea with nasal continuous positive airway pressure. Patient compliance, perception of benefits, and side effects. Am Rev Respir Dis 1992; 145:841–845.

89. Pepin JL, Leger P, Veale D, et al. Side effects of nasal continuous positive airway pressure in the sleep apnea syndrome. Study of 193 patients in two French sleep centers. Chest 1995; 107:375–381.

90. Meurice JC, Dore P, Paquereau, et al. Predictive factors of long term compliance with nasal continuous positive airway pressure treatment in sleep apnea syndrome. Chest 1994; 105:429–433.

91. Richards GN, Cistulli PA, Ungar RG, et al. Mouth leak with nasal continuous positive airway pressure increases nasal airway resistance. Am J Respir Crit Care Med 1996; 154:182–186.

92. Mortimore IL, Bradley PA, Murray JA, et al. Uvulopalatopharyngoplasty may compromise nasal CPAP therapy in sleep apnea syndrome. Am J Respir Crit Care Med 1996; 154:1759–1762.

93. Pieters T, Collard P, Aubert G, et al. Acceptance and long-term compliance with nCPAP in patients with obstructive sleep apnoea syndrome. Eur Respir J 1996; 9:939–944.

94. Pepin JL, Krieger J, Rodenstein D, et al. Effective compliance during the first 3 months of continuous positive airway pressure. A European prospective study of 121 patients. Am J Respir Crit Care Med 1999; 160: 1124–1129.

95. McArdle N, Devereux G, Heidarnejad H, et al. Long-term use of CPAP therapy for sleep apnea/hypopnea syndrome. Am J Respir Crit Care Med 1999; 159:1108–1114.

96. Kribbs NB, Pack AI, Kline LR, et al. Objective measurement of patterns of nasal CPAP use by patients with obstructive sleep apnea. Am Rev Respir Dis 1993; 147: 887–895.

97. Rauscher H, Formanek D, Popp W, et al. Self-reported vs measured compliance with nasal CPAP for obstructive sleep apnea. Chest 1993; 103:1675–1680.

98. Likar LL, Panciera TM, Erickson AD, et al. Group education sessions and compliance with nasal CPAP therapy. Chest 1997; 111:1273–1277.

99. Noseda A, Kempenaers C, Kerkhofs M, et al. Sleep apnea after 1 year domiciliary nasal-continuous positive airway pressure and attempted weight reduction. Potential for weaning from continuous positive airway pressure. Chest 1996; 109:138–143.

100. Fleury B, Rakotonanahary D, Hausser-Hauw C, et al. Objective patient compliance in long-term use of nCPAP. Eur Respir J 1996; 9:2356–2359.

101. Collard P, Pieters T, Aubert G, et al. Compliance with nasal CPAP in obstructive sleep apnea. Sleep Med Rev 1997; 1:33–44.

102. Mulloy E, McNicholas WT. Theophylline in obstructive sleep apnea: a double blind evaluation. Chest 1992; 101:753–757.

103. Rajagopal KR, Albrecht PH, Jabbari B. Effects of medroxy-progesterone acetate in obstructive sleep apnea. Chest 1986; 90:815–821.

104. Brownell LG, West P, Sweatman P, et al. Protriptyline in obstructive sleep apnea; a double blind trial. N Engl J Med 1982; 307:1037–1042.

105. Boudewyns A, Sforza E, Zamagni M, et al. Respiratory effort during sleep apneas after interruption of long-term CPAP treatment in patients with obstructive sleep apnea. Chest 1996; 110:120–127.

106. Hers V, Liistro G, Dury M, et al. Residual effect of nCPAP applied for part of the night in patients with obstructive sleep apnoea. Eur Resp J 1997; 10:973–976.

107. Kribbs NB, Pack AI, Kline LR, et al. Effects of one night without nasal CPAP treatment on sleep and sleepiness in patients with obstructive sleep apnea. Am Rev Respir Dis 1993; 147:1162–1168.

108. Series F, Roy N, Marc I. Effects of sleep deprivation and sleep fragmentation on upper airway collapsibility in normal subjects. Am J Respir Crit Care Med 1994; 150:418–485.

109. Mortimore IL, Kochhar P, Douglas NJ. Effects of chronic continuous positive airway pressure (CPAP) therapy on upper airway size in patients with sleep apnoea/hypopnoea syndrome. Thorax 1996; 51:190–192.

110. Ryan CF, Lowe AA, Li D, et al. Magnetic resonance imaging of the upper airway in obstructive sleep apnea before and after chronic nasal continuous positive airway pressure therapy. Am Rev Respir Dis 1991; 144:939–944.

111. Hudgel DW, Fung C. A long-term randomized, cross-over comparison of auto-titrating and standard nasal continuous airway pressure. Sleep 2000; 23:645–648.

112. Teschler H, Wessendorf TE, Farhat AA, et al. Two months auto-adjusting versus conventional nCPAP for obstructive sleep apnoea syndrome. Eur Respir J 2000; 15:990–995.

113. Naughton MT, Liu PP, Bernard DC, et al. Treatment of congestive heart failure and Cheyne-Stokes respiration during sleep by continuous positive airway pressure. Am J Respir Crit Care Med 1995; 151:92–97.

114. Malone S, Liu PP, Holloway R, et al. Obstructive sleep apnoea in patients with dilated cardiomyopathy: effects of continuous positive airway pressure. Lancet 1991; 338:1480–1484.

115. Kiely J, Deegan PC, Buckley A, et al. Efficacy of nasal continuous positive airway pressure in chronic heart failure: importance of underlying cardiac rhythm. Thorax 1998; 53:957–962.

116. Edwards N, Blyton DM, Kirjavainen GJ, et al. Nasal continuous positive airway pressure reduces sleep-induced blood pressure increments in preeclampsia. Am J Respir Crit Care Med 2000; 162:252–257.

9 UPPER AIRWAY SURGERY FOR OBSTRUCTIVE SLEEP APNEA SYNDROME

Aaron E Sher

RATIONALE AND STRATEGY FOR UPPER AIRWAY SURGERY

Upper airway surgical treatments for obstructive sleep apnea syndrome (OSAS) attempt to modify dysfunctional pharyngeal anatomy or bypass the pharynx (tracheotomy). Some modifications of the pharynx diminish the bulk of soft tissue structures that abut on the air column, place them under tension, or alter their spatial interrelationships. Modification of pharyngeal anatomy is achieved through ablating pharyngeal soft tissue, or indirectly, by modifying the facial skeleton from which the soft tissues are suspended.

For the estimated 2% of adult OSAS patients with specific space-occupying pathological lesions, surgical removal of these lesions is corrective. However, 98% of OSAS patients do not have pathology of this type. It is conceptualized that, in the latter, 'disproportionate anatomy' of the upper airway resulting from unfavorable anatomical features of the surrounding soft tissue structures and underlying maxillomandibular skeleton predisposes to OSAS. The configuration of the pharyngeal lumen is determined by the size and shape of soft tissue structures that abut it (such as faucial and lingual tonsils, tongue, soft palate) and their spatial orientation in relation to each other. The latter is determined by the orientation of underlying muscle planes established through their origins and insertions into the vertebral and craniofacial skeleton and will depend, ultimately, on the craniofacial skeletal characteristics of the patient (1–3).

The pharynx has properties associated with a collapsible biological conduit. Collapse occurs at a discrete (less than 1 cm) locus. Data derived from studies of the pharynx with awake endoscopy, awake endoscopy with Muller maneuver, asleep (drug-induced) endoscopy, asleep (natural and drug-induced) endoscopy with continuous positive airway pressure (CPAP), asleep fluoroscopy, computed tomographic (CT) scanning, and manometry suggest that the pattern of static pharyngeal narrowing or dynamic pharyngeal collapse is localized and patient specific (3–5). Observed failure of surgical procedures aimed at limited loci within the pharynx is assumed to result from residual or secondary airway compromise at a remote locus not addressed. A model considers the pharynx as consisting of two loci: 1) retropalatal: located posterior to the soft palate; and 2) retrolingual: located posterior to the vertical portion of the tongue. The pharynx is classified preoperatively as follows: 1) type I: only the retropalatal region is compromised; 2) type II: both retropalatal and retrolingual regions are compromised; and 3) type III: only the retrolingual region is compromised (6). Although awake endoscopy, awake endoscopy with Muller maneuver, asleep (drug-induced) endoscopy, asleep (natural and drug-induced) endoscopy with CPAP, asleep fluoroscopy, CT scanning, and manometry have been applied, awake lateral cephalometry and endoscopy are currently the most commonly applied methods of pharyngeal classification (2, 7).

UPPER AIRWAY SURGICAL PROCEDURES

Classic otorhinolaryngological techniques to enlarge the nasal or pharyngeal airways, such as nasal septal reconstruction, turbinate mucosal cauterization, turbinate outfracture, and tonsillectomy, frequently fail to correct OSAS in adults (7). Therefore, new surgical approaches have been developed to ablate pharyngeal soft tissue or modify the position of pharyngeal soft tissue structures through mobilization and repositioning of underlying skeletal structures.

SURGICAL PROCEDURES IN WHICH SOFT TISSUE IS ABLATED

Uvulopalatopharyngoplasty (UPPP) enlarges the retropalatal airway by excision of the tonsils (if present), trimming and reorientation of the posterior and anterior tonsillar pillars, and excision of the uvula and posterior portion of the palate (8) (Fig. 9.1).

Laser assisted uvulopalatoplasty (LAUP) enlarges the retropalatal airway by ablation of the uvula and posterior margin of the soft palate with carbon dioxide laser. Although tonsil ablation can be accomplished with laser, LAUP as reported frequently does not include tonsil abla-

tion. LAUP is generally performed under topical and local anesthesia in the physician's office (9) (Fig. 9.2A–D).

Uvulopalatopharyngo-glossoplasty (UPPGP) combines UPPP with limited resection of the tongue base, enlarging retropalatal and retrolingual portions of the airway (10, 11).

Laser midline glossectomy (LMG) *and linguolplasty* enlarge the retrolingual airway by laser extirpation of a 2.5 cm × 5 cm midline rectangular strip of posterior tongue and, in linguolplasty, additional lateral wedges. Laser lingual tonsillectomy, reduction of the aryepiglottic folds, and partial epiglottectomy are performed in selected patients (12, 13) (Fig. 9.3).

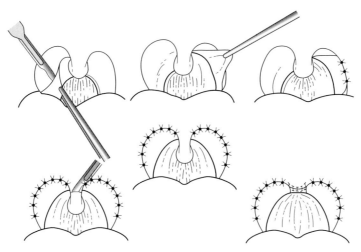

Fig 9.1 *UPPP. The tonsils are excised (if present), the anterior and posterior tonsillar pillars are trimmed and reoriented, and the uvula and posterior portion of the soft palate are excised. (Reproduced from Fujita S, Conway W, Zorick F, et al. Surgical correction of anatomical abnormalities in obstructive sleep apnea syndrome: uvulopalatopharyngoplasty. Otolaryngol Head Neck Surg 89:923–934, 1981, with permission from Mosby-Year Book, Inc.)*

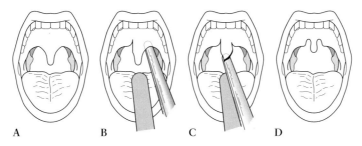

Fig 9.2 *LAUP. (A) Soft palate and uvula before LAUP is performed. (B) Transpalatal vertical incisions. (C) Partial uvula vaporization. (D) Soft palate and uvula after LAUP has been performed. (From Walker RP, Gopalsami C. Laser-assisted uvulopalatoplasty: Postoperative complications. Laryngoscope 1996;106:835. Reproduced with permission.)*

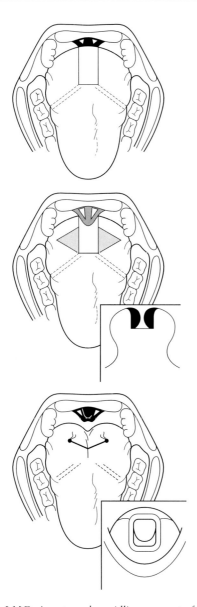

Radiofrequency tongue base ablation (RFTBA) enlarges the retrolingual airway by applying RF energy to the tongue base with a needle electrode. RFTBA is generally performed under topical and local anesthesia in the physician's office (14, 15).

Tongue base reduction with hyoepiglottoplasty (TBRHE) enlarges the retrolingual airway by excision of tongue base. The excision is performed through a transcervical incision. The neurovascular bundle is identified and protected. The hyoid is suspended from the mandible under tension. Unlike LMG and linguolplasty and RFTBA, which are performed transorally, TBRHE is performed through a cervical incision (16).

SURGICAL PROCEDURES IN WHICH SOFT TISSUE IS REPOSITIONED THROUGH SKELETAL ALTERATION

Transpalatal advancement pharyngoplasty (TPAP) enlarges the retropalatal airway by resection of the posterior hard palate with advancement of the soft palate in an anterior direction into the defect (17).

Mandibular advancement (MA) enlarges the retrolingual airway utilizing sagittal mandibular osteotomies to effect anterior mobilization of the insertion of the tongue at the genioid tubercle. There must be significant antecedent mandibular deficiency and dental malocclusion to permit the requisite degree of anterior movement of the mandible and mandibular teeth (18) (Fig. 9.4).

Maxillomandibular advancement (MMA) provides maximal enlargement of the retrolingual airway and some enlargement of the retropalatal airway. It permits significant mandibular advancement in patients lacking maxillomandibular disproportion. The maxilla and mandible are both advanced by means of Le Fort I maxillary and sagittal-split mandibular osteotomies. The degree of mandibular advancement achieved, if performed without maxillary advancement, would result in mandibular prognathism and dental malocclusion. The exception would be the patient with severe mandibular deficiency but normal maxillary development, who would then be a candidate for MA rather than MMA. Details of MMA depend on the patient's dental occlusion (19) (Fig. 9.5).

Genioglossal advancement (GA) places the tongue under anterior traction. It does so without altering dental occlusion and is achieved by performing limited parasagittal mandibular osteotomy and anterior

Fig 9.3 LMG. A rectangular midline segment of the posterior tongue is excised with a carbon dioxide laser. Lateral triangular wedges of tongue may be excised. (Reprinted with permission from Woodson BT, Fujita J: Laser midline glossectomy and lingualplasty for obstructive sleep apnea. In: Fairbanks DNF, Fujita S eds. Snoring and Obstructive Sleep Apnea, 2nd edn. New York, NY, Raven, 1994.)

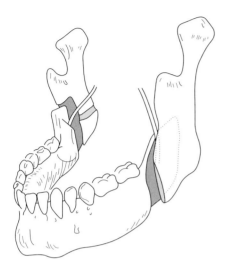

Fig 9.4 Mandibular Advancement. From: Bull Europ Physiopath Resp. 1983, 19,607–610 Powell N, Guilleminault C, Riley R, Smith L: Mandibular advancement & obstructive sleep apnea syndrome p 608.

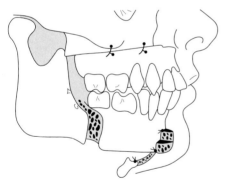

Fig 9.5 MMA. The maxilla and mandible are advanced simultaneously by means of LeFort I maxillary and sagittal-split mandibular osteotomies. (Reprinted with permission.)

advancement of the genioid tubercle (20) (Fig. 9.6). This procedure has undergone various modifications over time.

Hyoid myotomy and suspension (two variations, HM-1 and HM-2) tends to enlarge the retrolingual airway and exerts anterior traction on the tongue, hyoid, and suprahyoid musculature, with release of the infrahyoid muscles. Two techniques have been described: 1) sus-

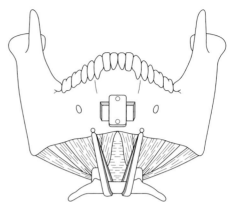

Fig 9.6 GA and HM-1. The genioid tubercle of the mandible is advanced through a limited parasagittal mandibular osteotomy. The hyoid bone is suspended from the anterior lower edge of the mandible by a fascial strip. (Reproduced from Riley RW, Powell NB, Guilleminault C: Obstructive sleep apnea and the hyoid. A revised surgical procedure. Otolaryngol Head Neck Surg 111: 717–721, 1994, with permission from Mosby-Year Book Inc.)

pension of the hyoid from the mandible by a fascial strip (HM-1); 2) suspension of the hyoid from the superior margin of the thyroid cartilage by permanent suture (HM-2) (20, 21) (Figs 9.6, 9.7).

SURGICAL PROCEDURE THAT BYPASSES THE PHARYNGEAL AIRWAY

Tracheotomy creates a percutaneous opening into the trachea. The tracheotomy is usually stented and maintained by inserting a rigid or semirigid hollow tube. The patient breathes through the tube when the external end is unplugged. Since the tracheotomy opens into the airway proximal to the pharynx, it bypasses the region of collapse. When the patient is awake, the external end of the tube is plugged. The tube is of sufficiently small diameter that, when plugged, it permits air to enter the trachea from the pharynx and larynx, passing around the tube. The increased resistance to airflow created by the presence of the plugged tube occupying a portion of the tracheal lumen can be decreased by using a tube that has distal ventilating holes through which air can flow. Alternatively, it may be possible to fashion a tracheostomy that does not require a cannula or utilize a stomal plug instead of cannula (22).

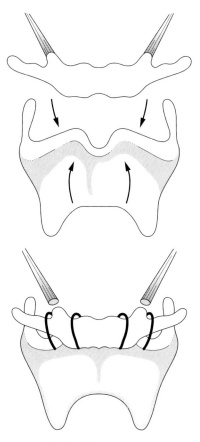

Fig 9.7 HM-2. The hyoid bone is suspended from the superior margin of the thyroid cartilage by a permanent suture. (Reproduced from Riley RW, Powell NB, Guilleminault C: Obstructive sleep apnea and the hyoid. A revised surgical procedure. Otolaryngol Head Neck Surg 111:717–721, 1994, with permission from Mosby-Year book, Inc.)

⊶ Key points box 9.1

Upper airway surgical procedures
Objective is to increase pharyngeal space
Procedures based on soft tissue ablation:

- Uvulopalatopharyngoplasty (UPPP) and variations thereof
- Tongue base reduction

Procedures based on skeletal alteration

- Advancement of the mandible ± maxilla
- Resection of the hard palate
- Hyoid suspension

Tracheotomy

- Bypasses the site of obstruction, but now rarely performed

SURGICAL OUTCOMES

The first portion of this section outlines surgical outcomes for individual procedures performed as the sole surgical intervention. The second portion outlines surgical outcomes of complex upper airway modifications, which consist of various permutations and combinations of individual surgical procedures. In series discussed in both sections, nasal surgery (including nasal septal reconstruction, nasal turbinate outfracture, nasal turbinate cauterization) and pharyngeal surgery (including tonsillectomy and adenoidectomy) may have been performed in individual patients as a concomitant or prior surgical modification, with the contribution of these procedures to the overall surgical outcome not determinable.

Authors of surgical case series have applied different criteria of improvement in polysomnography (PSG) variables to define surgical success. These are summarized as success criteria 1 through 4:

Criterion 1: Postoperative RDI is diminished by at least 50% from preoperative RDI.

Criterion 1A: Postoperative AI is diminished by at least 50% from preoperative AI.

Criterion 2: Postoperataive RDI is diminished by at least 50% from preoperative RDI to a level below 20 apneas and hypopneas/hour.

Criterion 2A: Postoperative AI is diminished by at least 50% from preoperative AI to a level below 10 apneas/hour.

Criterion 3: Postoperative RDI is diminished by at least 50% from preoperative RDI to a level below 10 apneas and hypopneas/hour.

Criterion 4: Postoperative RDI and AI are both decreased by 60% from preoperative values to postoperative AI less than 10 apneas/hour; or postoperative RDI is less than 15 apneas and hypopneas/hour and AI is less than 5 apneas/hour. These criteria will be referenced in the discussion that follows.

OUTCOMES OF INDIVIDUAL PROCEDURES

Uvulopalatopharyngoplasty

Short-term mean outcomes data for UPPP has been derived by metaanalysis of 37 papers, each of which reports on at least nine surgical subjects and assesses surgical outcomes through clear and unambiguous outcome measures (i.e., a preperative and postoperative polysomnogram) (7). The mean decrease in apnea index (AI) in more than 500 patients is 55% from a mean preoperative AI of 45 apneas/hour. The mean decrease in respiratory disturbance index (RDI) in approximately 500 patients is 38% from a mean preoperative RDI of 60 apneas and hypopneas/hour. In 14 papers (success criterion 1A) the response rate for 352 patients is 65%. In 16 papers (success criterion 1), the response rate for 375 patients is 53%. There is no significant preoperative difference between responders and nonresponders in terms of age, AI, RDI, minimum oxygen saturation, or body weight (7).

The preoperative pattern of pharyngeal narrowing or collapse is specified to be type I (retropalatal only), II (retropalatal and retrolingual), or III (retrolingual only) in each of 168 patients reported in 9 papers. Pharyngeal classification is achieved by application of one of the following techniques: awake fiberoptic endoscopy with or without Müller maneuver, asleep endoscopy with nasal CPAP, lateral cephalometry, airway manometry, or pharyngeal CT scan. The mean percentage decrease in AI for type I is 75% (from a mean preoperative AI of 39 apneas/hour), whereas for type II or III the mean percentage decrease in AI is 23% (from a mean preoperative AI of 60 apneas/hour). The mean decrease in RDI for type I is 33% (from a mean preoperative RDI of 57 apneas and hypopneas/hour), whereas for types II and III the mean percentage decrease in RDI is 7% (from a mean preoperative RDI of 65 apneas and hypopneas/hour). The percentage of patients attaining success criterion 2 or 2A is 52% for type I patients and 5% for type II or type III. If all patients (types I, II, and III) are combined, 43% achieve success criterion 2A and 39% achieve success criterion 2. If achievement of either of these criteria defines surgical success, 41% of patients respond to UPPP (7).

Efficacy of UPPP may diminish over time: 60% success (criterion 1) at mean of 6 months postoperatively to 50% at mean of 46 months postoperatively; 64% success (criterion 3) at mean of 6 months postoperatively to 48%

success at 48–96 months postoperatively; and 67% success (criterion 1) at 3–6 months postoperatively to 33% at mean of 88 months postoperatively. Weight gain has been implicated as an explanation for long-term recurrence in some but not all cases (23–25).

Surgical complications described in 640 patients for whom complications are delineated include velopharyngeal insufficiency (VPI) for greater than 1 month (2%), postoperative bleeding (1%), nasopharyngeal stenosis (1%), voice change (1%), successfully managed perioperative upper airway obstruction (0.3%, two cases), and death secondary to upper airway obstruction (0.2%, one case). However, since more than half of the papers do not comment on the presence or absence of postoperative complications, it is impossible to determine the true prevalence of complications in the entire population (7). In two series focusing on UPPP complications, the death rate from unsuccessfully managed upper airway obstruction is approximately 1% (26, 27). The prevalence of postoperative VPI is shown to be heavily dependent on the definition of VPI applied. Its prevalence 2 years after UPPP in 71 patients varies from 39% to 3% (39% with subclinical reflux of liquids, apparent only on nasal endoscopy; l6% with nasal reflux when the patient bends over a water fountain to drink water; 7% with subclinical nasal regurgitation [i.e., patients feeling bubbles in the nose after drinking gaseous drinks]; and 3% with mild nasal reflux for liquids) (28). One series of 91 patients reports complaints of dry throat and 'swallowing abnormalities' 1 year after UPPP in 31% and 10%, respectively (27).

Laser assisted Uvulopalatoplasty

Patients subjected to LAUP and evaluated postoperatively with PSG have a success rate ranging from 0 to 87% (criterion 1) and 0 to 48% (criterion 2) (9, 29–34). Two series demonstrate relatively similar success rates for patients with mild, moderate, and severe OSAS (32,33). In most reported case series, selection bias results from reporting preoperative PSG data on a small fraction of operated cases and postoperative PSG data on only a fraction of those who had had preoperative PSG. Although this represents a deficiency of the surgical literature for OSAS in general, the extreme measure to which it is true of LAUP reporting may result from a perception that LAUP is an operation appropriate for snoring only, not OSAS. Consequently, third party carriers often do not authorize preoperative or postoperative PSG when LAUP is contemplated or performed.

LAUP patients studied by PSG, videoendoscopy, and magnetic resonance (MR) imaging within 3 days after surgery demonstrate exacerbation of OSAS severity in the early postoperative period. In seven patients who had PSG at 48–72 hours after surgery, the mean preoperative RDI of 11 doubles to 22 apneas and hypopneas/hour, and the mean preoperative AI of 3 is multiplied by a factor of more than 4 to 14 apneas/hour. The pharyngeal cross-sectional area at 72 hours postoperatively is decreased by 48% from the preoperative cross-sectional area, resulting in a risk of postoperative airway compromise (35). This is particularly important, since LAUP is generally performed in the physician's office, and the patient is not observed during the first night of sleep, which occurs at home. Analysis of the dimensions and configuration of the pharynx before and after LAUP and UPPP in 10 patients (peroral photography of the oropharynx, nasopharyngoscopy of the velopharyngeal region, and lateral and frontal cephalometry with contrast enhancement) demonstrates that UPPP results in enlargement of the velopharyngeal space, but LAUP results in diminished velopharyngeal space. The authors conclude that LAUP may prove deleterious for OSAS patients (36).

Uvulopalatopharyngo-glossoplasty

Short-term success is reported to be 50% (N = 20, criterion 1) and 67% (N = 19, criterion 1A) (10, 11).

Laser Midline Glossectomy (LMG) and Linguolplasty

In patients in whom UPPP fails who are documented to have retrolingual narrowing by physical examination, radiographic evaluation, and fiberoptic endoscopy with Müller maneuver, rate of salvage by LMG (N = 12, criterion 1) is 42%. Patients with similar physical characteristics undergoing combined UPPP and LMG (or linguolplasty) have a success rate of 77% (N = 22, criterion 1). No permanent complications are reported (12, 13).

Radiofrequency Tongue Base Ablation

Radiofrequency ablation of tongue base tissue in 18 OSAS patients with previous unsuccessful surgery for OSAS and documented residual obstruction at the tongue base (mean preoperative RDI 40 apneas and hypopneas/hour) have a response rate of 39% (criteria 1 or 2) (14, 15).

Tongue Base Reduction with Hyoepiglottoplasty

There are no reports known to the author of TBRHE performed as a sole surgical maneuver, and TBRHE has been reported only in conjunction with other pharyngeal procedures.

Transpalatal Advancement Pharyngoplasty

TPAP performed after UPPP (N = 6) incrementally increases pharyngeal cross-sectional area and decreases pharyngeal collapsibility (compared to post-UPPP measurements). Overall clinical success of the combined procedure is 67% (N = 6; mean preoperative RDI 70/hour; success criterion 2) (17, 37).

Mandibular Advancement

Individual reports describe successful treatment of OSAS by mandibular advancement (MA) in patients with severe mandibular deficiency resulting from developmental or posttraumatic deformity or from temporomandibular joint ankylosis. These patients, described as having 'bird-like' facial profiles, have mandibular deficiency in the absence of significant maxillary deficiency. Although the reported cases are few in number, they are of historical significance for demonstrating that mandibular deficiency can result in OSAS and that mandibular advancement can result in resolution of OSAS. Whereas few OSAS patients are candidates for MA, these early reports resulted in the subsequent development of more widely applicable procedures to enlarge the retrolingual airway in OSAS patients who are not candidates for MA (18, 38).

Maxillomandibular Advancement

MMA applied as a primary surgical approach in nonobese, maxillomandibular deficient patients (who may have dolichofacial characteristics) has a response rate of 95% (N = 38; success criterion 2) and 100% (N = 7; success criterion 2). In a series in which patient selection is not fully described, success rate is 40% (N = 5; success criterion 2) (39–41).

Genioglossal Advancement

There are no reports known to the author of GA performed as a sole surgical maneuver, and GA has been reported only in conjunction with other pharyngeal procedures.

Hyoid Myotomy and Suspension

There are no reports known to the author of HM-1 or HM-2 performed as a sole surgical maneuver; HM-1 and HM-2 have been reported in conjunction with other pharyngeal procedures.

OUTCOMES OF PROCEDURES PERFORMED IN COMBINATION

Published reports have demonstrated outcomes of complex surgical modifications that incorporate two or more of several procedures (UPPP, GA, HM-1, HM-2, MMA, TBRHE), performed either in one surgical episode or in sequential episodes; as follows:

UPPP and GA
TRBHE and UPPP
GA and HM-1
GA and HM-2
UPPP and GA and HM-1
UPPP and GA and HM-2
UPPP and MMA
GA and MMA
GA and HM-1 and MMA
UPPP and GA and MMA
UPPP and GA and HM-1 and MMA

UPPP and GA

UPPP plus GA has a success rate of 78% (N = 9, success criterion 3), 69% (N = 35, success criterion 2), and 38% (N = 24, success criterion 2). Incomplete demographic data prevent rigorous comparison of the populations (21, 42, 43).

TRBHE and UPPP

TBRHE is performed on 10 patients (six with previous unsuccessful UPPP and three with concomitant UPPP). All patients lack craniofacial skeletal abnormalities on lateral cephalometry. The success rate is 80% (mean preoperative RDI 70 apneas and hypopneas/hour; criterion 2) (16).

GA and HM-1

GA plus HM-1 is performed in six patients with retrolingual collapse in the absence of retropalatal collapse with a response rate of 66% (criterion 2) (40).

GA and HM-2

Patients with retrolingual narrowing (in the absence of retropalatal narrowing) undergo GA plus HM-2 as an isolated surgical procedure with a response rate of 100% (N = 3, mean preoperative RDI 55 apneas and hypopneas/hour; criterion 2) (21).

UPPP and GA and HM-1

UPPP plus GA plus HM-1 achieves a success rate of 57% in a large series (N = 233, criterion 2). Patients with mild and moderately severe OSAS (RDI < 60 apneas and hypopneas/hour, lowest SaO_2 > 70%) have a success rate of 75%, whereas patients with severe OSAS have a success rate of 42% (40). Success rate (criterion 2) in 12 patients (mean RDI 49 apneas and hypopneas/hour) is 42% (44).

UPPP and GA and HM-2

The response rate is 73% (N = 11; mean preoperative RDI 80 apneas and hypopneas/hour; criterion 2) and 57% (N = 14; criterion 2) (21, 45).

Other Combinations (UPPP and GA and HM-1 and MMA; GA and HM-1 and MMA; UPPP and GA and MMA; UPPP and MMA; GA and MMA)

MMA performed as a salvage procedure after failed UPPP or GA (or both) and HM-1 has a salvage rate of 95% (N = 164; mean preoperative RDI 72 apneas and hypopneas/hour; criterion 2) and 100% (N = 3; mean preoperative RDI 74 apneas and hypopneas/hour; criterion 3) (42, 46). MMA performed with GA has a success rate of 100% (N = 40; 10 failures after prior UPPP; mean preoperative RDI 59 apneas and hypopneas/hour; criterion 4) (47). MMA performed alone (N = 5) has a success rate of 40%, whereas MMA performed in conjunction with one or more ancillary procedures (UPPP, GA, partial glossectomy) (N = 18) has a success rate of 78% (criterion 2) (41).

OUTCOMES OF TRACHEOTOMY

Early resolution of OSAS occurs in 83%, and delayed resolution occurs in the remainder as central apnea that appears immediately after tracheotomy resolves. Eighty-two to 100% of patients achieve resolution of excessive daytime sleepiness (N = 98) (19, 48, 49). Hypertension improves or resolves in 40% (48, 49). Hypercapnea, cor pulmonale, and cardiac arrhythmias improve or resolve (48). Patients who lose weight after tracheotomy tend to gain it back in 6 months (48). Complications include psychosocial problems, local granulation tissue (resulting in hemoptysis or obstruction), and recurrent bronchitis (48).

> ☞ **Key points box 9.2**
>
> **Surgical outcomes**
>
> *Classic UPPP*
>
> - Metaanalysis of 37 papers indicates a reduction in postoperative AHI of 38%
> - Results are best where the site of obstruction is retropalatal
> - Velopharyngeal insufficiency occurs postoperatively in at least 2% of cases
>
> *Laser-assisted UPP (LAUP)*
>
> - Reported success rates in OSAS are highly variable
> - OSAS severity may increase in the early postoperative days, probably due to a reduced velopharyngeal space
>
> *Other Procedures*
>
> - Mandibular ± maxillary advancement can be very effective in OSAS where these bones are deficient
> - Only limited reports are available on other procedures performed in isolation
> - Reports indicate superior results when several procedures are performed in combination

DISCUSSION

The role of upper airway surgery for OSAS is in evolution. The complex causation of sleep apnea has resulted in an array of treatment options. These modalities include behavioral approaches (weight reduction, postural conditioning), application of devices (intraoral devices, positive airway pressure devices), and surgical approaches (upper airway modification, tracheostomy, bariatric surgery). Etiological variability, differences in severity, comorbidity, and patient temperament make each patient a relatively unique clinical entity around which to customize a treatment strategy by choosing from and possibly combining treatment options. Although behavioral measures remain an integral part of the treatment program, patient ability to lose weight or alter sleep position is generally limited. Nasal CPAP is highly effective when applied under laboratory conditions, but the considerable issue of patient noncompliance was underestimated until the development of technology capable of objective assessment (50). Intraoral devices appear to have efficacy in some cases, and there is ongoing research into the objective assessment of patient compliance with these devices (51). Tracheotomy may remain the 'gold standard' of treatment (despite the obvious drawbacks) in that it ensures elimination of the pathological factor, transient airway obstruction, and its effectiveness is not dependent on patient compliance. However, the negative impact of tracheotomy is significant.

Surgical upper airway modification strives to eliminate OSAS without dependence on behavioral modification, mechanical devices, or tracheotomy. There is no single surgical procedure, short of tracheotomy, documented to consistently cure OSAS in all patients. On the other hand, published data suggest that current surgical techniques can potentially be applied in such a manner as to achieve surgical cure in most OSAS patients without resort to permanent tracheostomy. Patient selection, versatility in varied surgical approaches, and willingness to utilize more than one procedure when necessary appear to be important components of a successful surgical program.

A model of the upper airway in OSAS likens it to a simple collapsible tube. The tendency of the upper airway to collapse can be expressed quantitatively in terms of a critical pressure (Pcrit), which is the pressure surrounding the area of collapse. If atmospheric pressure is designated zero, airway collapse will occur whenever Pcrit is a positive number (indicating that it is higher than atmospheric pressure). Pcrit levels are higher during sleep than during wakefulness in both normal persons and OSAS patients. In normals, Pcrit rises from awake values that are more negative than -41 cm H_2O to sleep values of -13 cm H_2O (52–54). This means that, in normal subjects, atmospheric pressure is greater than Pcrit even during sleep, and the pharynx will not collapse. In OSAS patients, the spectrum of awake values of Pcrit is -40 cm H_2O to -17 cm H_2O, and Pcrit during sleep is $+ 2.5$ cm H_2O (52, 53, 55, 56). Although the pharyngeal airway of awake OSAS patients tends to be more collapsible than that of awake normal persons, Pcrit does not cross the critical line of zero (i.e., atmospheric pressure) except when the patient with OSAS has sleep onset and OSAS results (52). Patients who have varying degrees of partial pharyngeal collapse have intermediate, but negative, levels of Pcrit during sleep: -6.5 cm H_2O for asymptomatic snorers and -1.6 cm H_2O for patients with hypopneas but no apneas (52, 56). In general, Pcrit must be below -5 cm H_2O to eliminate sleep-disordered breathing (52). Pcrit for an OSAS patient can, alternatively, be defined as the lowest level of nasal CPAP at which airflow is maintained.

Examples of the decrement in Pcrit that can be achieved by nonsurgical interventions are -6 cm H_2O through the loss of 15% of body weight; -3 to -4 cm H_2O through proptriptyline treatment; and -4 to -5 cm H_2O through the avoidance of sleeping in the supine position (52). Pcrit decrement in response to upper airway surgery has been documented for UPPP and TPAP. When 13 patients underwent UPPP, Pcrit decreased from a level of 0 to a level of -3 cm H_2O ($p = 0.016$). In those patients who have greater than 50% decrease in RDI in REM sleep, Pcrit decreases from -1 to -7 cm H_2O ($p = 0.01$). The degree of improvement in sleep-disordered breathing is correlated significantly with the change of Pcrit ($0 = 0.001$), and the decrease in RDI is determined by the magnitude of the fall in Pcrit rather than by the initial level of Pcrit. No significant change in Pcrit is detected in nonresponders (4). Sequential performance of TPAP after UPPP results in incremental decrease in Pcrit to a level below that resulting from UPPP. Four patients underwent TPAP after previous UPPP. Mean post-UPPP Pcrit of 5 decreased after TPAP to -4 ($p < 0.01$). TPAP increases the retropalatal airway cross-sectional area by 321% compared to the post-UPPP cross-sectional area (29 to 95 cm^2, $p < 0.01$) (37). It is likely that each surgical procedure decreasing OSAS severity also decreases Pcrit, and that procedures performed concomitantly or in sequence result in incremental decreases in Pcrit. Further data are needed for verification. It is suggested that the application of Pcrit as an indirect measure of OSA treatment efficacy might prove valuable in patient selection, treatment selection, and treatment evaluation (52, 57).

UPPP was introduced in 1981 as the first surgical procedure specifically designed to treat OSAS. After an initial period of enthusiasm, UPPP fell into disfavor because of a failure rate exceeding 50%. However, analysis of UPPP failure and additional scientific data on the complex nature of OSAS suggested that UPPP addresses only one vulnerable site in the upper airway—the upper, or retropalatal, pharynx. UPPP failure was assumed to result from lack of modification of additional or secondary sites of pharyngeal obstruction in the lower, or retrolingual, pharynx. This was supported by documentation that OSAS resulting from retrolingual compromise secondary to extreme mandibular deficiency could be treated successfully by MA. This observation resulted in the development of new surgical procedures to modify the retrolingual pharynx of patients who do not have a major degree of mandibular deficiency and are, therefore, not candidates for MA. LMG (and linguolplasty)

and RFTBA result in ablation of a portion of the posterior tongue with laser or RF energy, whereas GA and HM-1 and HM-2 advance the tongue base in an anterior direction. Both procedures tend to augment the retrolingual airway. Both approaches achieve surgical salvage in some UPPP failures. There is uncertainty about the degree of contribution of HM-1 and HM-2 to the treatment protocol, as data by which to assess the relative efficacy of HM-1 and HM-2 and the efficacy and safety of HM-2 are limited. MMA moves both palate and tongue in an anterior direction, thus enlarging both the retropalatal and retrolingual airway. MMA serves to salvage patients in whom various combinations of UPPP, GA, HM-1 and HM-2, have failed, with a success rate of close to 100%.

The Stanford protocol was developed to systematically approach reconstruction of the upper airway based on the hypothesis that pharyngeal classification could serve as an effective basis for establishing a treatment plan for each patient (Fig. 9.8). The goal was to apply limited, regionally specific anatomical modification as phase 1 of surgical therapy (UPPP, GA, HM), the specific procedures selected in accordance with the pharyngeal classification based on fiberoptic endoscopy and lateral cephalometry. Patients were studied by polysomnography after completion of phase 1 surgery. If they demonstrated significant residual OSAS and elected to complete the surgical protocol, they were treated with phase 2 of the protocol: MMA. The goal of the protocol was to strive for cure of OSAS while minimizing the degree of surgical intervention. Response was defined as 50% decrease to postoperative RDI less than 20 apneas and hypopneas/hour and sleep parameters consistent with a night on CPAP. The response rate for phase 1 surgery was approximately 60% (75% for patients with mild and moderate OSA and 40% for patients with severe OSAS). The response rate for those patients who went on to phase II after phase I surgery failed was 95% (40). This protocol was amended when HM-2 was substituted for HM-1 (46). Exceptions to the Stanford protocol were made by the Stanford group for patients who, on initial presentation, demonstrated severe maxillomandibular disproportion with sequelae in addition to OSAS (such as dental malocclusion, temporomandibular joint syndrome, or cosmetic concerns). These patients were allowed to enter the protocol at phase 2 instead of phase 1. The response rate for those with severe skeletal deformity entering phase II without phase I was 100% (40). MMA was applied as a primary surgical approach, rather than 'in salvage' by other investigators.

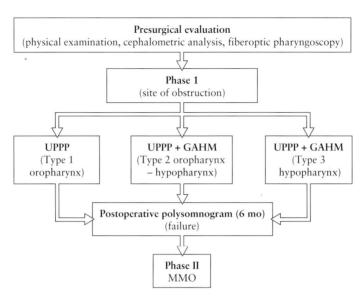

Fig 9.8 The Stanford Protocol. (Reproduced from Riley RW, Powell NB, Guilleminault C: Obstructive sleep apnea and the hyoid. A revised surgical procedure. Otolaryngol Head Neck Surg 111:717–721, 1994, with permission from Mosby-Year Book, Inc.)

Available data suggest that MMA may be highly effective and appropriate as the primary surgical approach in patients who are not obese and in whom the apparent cause of OSAS is maxillomandibular deficiency. On the other hand, in a less select group of patients, who frequently manifest varying degrees of obesity and relatively subtle degrees of maxillomandibular deficiency, neither phase I of the Stanford protocol nor primary MMA ensures a one-stop cure. When applied primarily to relatively unselected patient populations, both approaches have significant failure rates. Failure of each approach mandates secondary 'salvage' surgery through application of additional surgical methods not applied primarily. Application of 'salvage' procedures when necessary affords a high likelihood of cure. A recent study documents excellent results obtained by applying primary MMA and GA in 40 patients (only 10 of whom had prior failed UPPP) (47). TBRHE may provide another important option, but further experience is needed (16).

More work is needed to define which of these approaches minimizes morbidity and cost and maximizes success and patient satisfaction. It appears that the regimen of choice may be patient-specific with OSAS severity, degree of maxillomandibular deficiency, degree of obesity, and comorbidity all factoring into the decision-making process. If

comorbidity or patient preference precludes any of these surgical approaches, and nonsurgical options are unsuccessful or rejected, tracheotomy should be considered.

Although lateral cephalometry and fiberoptic endoscopy are widely applied for preoperative characterization of the pharyngeal airway, questions remain about the efficacy of these procedures. Both procedures are applied in the awake patient, whereas OSAS occurs in the sleeping patient. Both are generally applied sitting; however, the sleeping patient rarely assumes this position. Lateral cephalometry is not dynamic and views the airway in only two dimensions, whereas airway collapse in OSAS is dynamic and occurs in three dimensions. Nonetheless, pharyngeal classification into types I, II, and III by techniques that include fiberoptic endoscopy and lateral cephalometry permitted identification of two subgroups with markedly different rates of success with UPPP (52% for type I and 5% for types II and III) (7). It also provided the foundation for development of surgical strategies whereby surgical procedures were developed to 'salvage' UPPP failures and raise the overall surgical success rate. Several reports document OSAS cure rates close to 100% achieved through application of complex upper airway modification. Depending upon the complexity of anatomical compromise, one or multiple procedures may be required (16, 40, 46, 47). On the other hand, the pharyngeal classification system offers no explanation for failure of UPPP in 48% of patients classified as having type I. Investigators describe differing degrees of success in prognosticating UPPP outcome when fiberoptic endoscopy is used to characterize the pharyngeal airway preoperatively (7, 58–60). It is likely that there are nuances of pharyngeal anatomy or function not discerned by fiberoptic endoscopy or lateral cephalometry. These nuances may differ in patients classified type I in whom UPPP fails and those in whom it succeeds. However, it must also be considered that interpretation of endoscopic data, which is highly subjective, may vary from physician to physician, and even by the same physician at different times. Similarly, lateral cephalometry performed on the same patient may suggest different pharyngeal soft tissue relationships unless there is careful adherence to technique. Studies comparing fiberoptic endoscopy with pharyngeal manometry (awake and asleep) demonstrate disagreement between these techniques in identifying pharyngeal dynamics, as well as discrepancies in observation with the same technique in wakefulness and sleep (61–63). Alternatively, UPPP may not be sufficiently robust to consistently cure all type I patients, even if they are properly classified. The issue of inadequacy of UPPP as a surgical strategy versus inadequacy of the strategy for preoperative pharyngeal classification remains unresolved.

LAUP was introduced several years after UPPP and differs primarily in the magnitude of surgical modification and the nature of surgical instrument applied. UPPP routinely includes tonsillectomy unless the patient had had a prior tonsillectomy. Tonsillectomy is not generally performed as part of LAUP, although serial ablation of tonsil tissue with laser is possible, but cumbersome. Limited data suggest that OSAS of varying degrees of severity, from mild to severe, may respond to LAUP. Additional data are needed. It might be hypothesized that LAUP and UPPP should achieve similar results in previously tonsillectomized patients. On the other hand, in the absence of concomitant or prior tonsillectomy, LAUP might be expected to have lessened impact on OSAS, particularly if tonsils are of considerable volume. However, concerns have been voiced that the documented pattern of healing and scar formation in LAUP differs from that of UPPP and may be detrimental for OSAS. Although data suggest that LAUP may be effective across a spectrum of OSAS severity, care should be exercised in applying LAUP to patients with significant potential for postoperative airway obstruction. The airway is further compromised in the early postoperative period, and there is exacerbation of OSAS. This issue is of great importance because postoperative LAUP patients sleep at home unmonitored after surgery.

Criteria for surgical success and failure have evolved over the two decades since Fujita introduced UPPP, and this evolution is reflected in the criteria applied in the succession of papers on surgical treatment. Fujita established as the criterion for surgical success decrease in AI of at least 50% from its preoperative value. Current perceptions of pathophysiology of OSAS mandate a more restrictive criterion for success, one that takes into account not only apneas but also hypopneas and subobstructive events that result in arousal (64–69). The ideal definition of response may require development of a paradigm (applied preoperatively and postoperatively) that integrates parameters of sleep architecture, arousal, and excessive daytime sleepiness with measures of respiratory disturbance and oxygenation. Such a complex descriptor of disease severity might be designed in a manner akin to the tumor-mode-metastastis (TNM) tumor classification. Identification of which metrics and levels of severity best reflect thresholds of morbidity and mortality will be clarified by such investigations as the National Institutions of Health (NIH) Heart Health Study. However, the lack of uniform universal criteria for reporting surgical results poses difficulty in interpretation of surgical outcomes. There are steps under way to standardize reporting (70).

Analysis of the efficacy of individual surgical procedures is thwarted by the practice of many investigators to apply multiple procedures in various combinations in single operative sessions and assess the composite effect by postoperative PSG. The nature of the combination of procedures may vary from study to study, even in different studies performed by the same investigator. In many series, relevant upper airway surgery, such as nasal surgery and tonsillectomy, are performed sporadically and mentioned coincidentally but not formally tallied as part of the surgical intervention. This obscures their contribution to the overall surgical outcome. The tendency to perform multiple surgical maneuvers at one operative session results from the clinicians' desire to maximize the likelihood of success while minimizing exposure to anesthesia risk, patient inconvenience, and cost. However, this practice clearly compromises data interpretation. The difficulty is compounded by lack of standardization of surgical techniques for individual procedures performed by different surgeons, or even those performed by the same surgeon at different times.

Bias is frequently introduced by retrospective study design and nonrandom loss to follow-up study. This is most pointed in the LAUP literature. The number of patients exposed to the surgical procedure often exceeds the number having preoperative PSG. The number having preoperative PSG often exceeds the number having postoperative PSG. Although it is especially characteristic of the LAUP literature, this deficiency is commonly observed throughout the surgical literature. Studies are not randomized, and few have control groups. Sample size tends to be low, and statistical power is low. Papers do not present confidence bounds that might distinguish between statistical and clinical significance. Missing data and missing and inconsistent definitions are common. Most papers report only short-term follow-up results and infrequent repeat follow-up evaluations. Few papers associate PSG data with patient-based quality of life measures (71).

A patient's decision to pursue surgical treatment should follow full disclosure of the risks of untreated sleep apnea, the risks and benefits of nonsurgical modalities, and the risks and benefits of surgical modalities. It would appear prudent to suggest a trial of nonsurgical treatment in most cases, reserving surgical approaches for those patients who reject or undergo unsuccessful nonsurgical interventions. Patients with discrete upper airway pathology that is amenable to surgical correction would be exceptions to this policy, as might be apnea patients who have physical complaints (in addition to OSAS) related to surgically correctable maxillomandibular deficiency.

In general, multicenter studies of surgical treatments for sleep apnea would help to clarify the strengths and weaknesses of different approaches and determine the reproducibility of surgical outcomes in the hands of different surgical teams. The cost of effective treatment for OSAS will have to be compared to the cost of lack of treatment, both to the patient and to society as a whole. The relative costs of surgical and nonsurgical approaches will have to be compared with the relative benefit of each, to be defined through adequate outcomes assessment. Only in this way will the appropriate role for nonsurgical and surgical approaches be firmly established.

⚬━ Key points box 9.3

Summary points.

1. Successful surgical outcomes in OSAS are heavily dependent on:

   - Appropriate patient selection by careful preoperative evaluation – includes endoscopy and lateral cephalometry, and possibly other, more refined investigative techniques in the future.

   - Versatility of the surgical team in the varied surgical approaches available.

   - Willingness to utilise multiple procedures where appropriate (particularly illustrated by the Stanford Protocol where a phased surgical approach is undertaken).

2. Concern has been expressed that LAUP may have detrimental effects in OSAS, and this procedure is widely regarded as more appropriate for patients with a predominant snoring disorder.

3. The present literature on surgical management of OSAS is lacking in carefully controlled prospective clinical trials, which makes adequate interpretation of success rates difficult.

REFERENCES

1. Rojewski TE, Schuller DE, Clark RW, et al. Videoendoscopic determination of the mechanism of obstruction in obstructive sleep apnea. Otolaryngol Head Neck Surg 1984; 92(2): 127–131.

2. Sher AE. Obstructive sleep apnea syndrome: a complex disorder of the upper airway. Otolaryngol Clin North Am 1990; 23:593–608.

3. Shepard JW Jr, Gefter WB, Guilleminault C, et al. Evaluation of the upper airway in patients with obstructive sleep apnea. Sleep 1991; 14(4):361–371.

4. Schwartz AR, Schiebert N, Rothman W, et al. Effect of uvulopalatopharyngoplasty on upper airway collapsibility in obstructive sleep apnea. Am Rev Respir Dis 1992; 145:527–532.

5. Launois SH, Feroah TR, Campbell WN, et al. Site of pharyngeal narrowing predicts outcome of surgery for obstructive sleep apnea. Am Rev Respir Dis 1993; 147:182–189.

6. Fujita S. Midline laser glossectomy with lingualplasty: a treatment of sleep apnea syndrome. Op Tech Otolaryngol HNS 1991; 2:127–131.

7. Sher AE, Schechtman KB, Piccirillo JF. The efficacy of surgical modifications of the upper airway in adults with obstructive sleep apnea syndrome. Sleep 1996; 19(2): 156–177.

8. Fujita S, Conway W, Zorick F, et al. Surgical correction of anatomical abnormalities in obstructive sleep apnea syndrome: uvulopalatopharyngoplasty. Otolaryngol Head Neck Surg 1981; 89:923–934.

9. Kamami Y-V. Out-patient treatment of sleep apnea syndrome with CO2 laser: laser-assisted UPPP. J Otolaryngology 1994; 23(6):395–399.

10. Djupesland G, Schrader H, Lyberg T, et al. Palatopharyngoglossoplasty in the treatment of patients with obstructive sleep apnea syndrome. Acta Otolaryngol (Stockh) 1992; Suppl 492:50–54.

11. Miljeteig H, Tvinnereim M. Uvulopalatopharyngoglossoplasty (UPPGP) in the treatment of the obstructive sleep apnea syndrome. Acta Otolaryngol (Stockh) 1992; Suppl 492:86–89.

12. Fujita S, Woodson BT, Clark JK, et al. Laser midline glossectomy as a treatment for obstructive sleep apnea. Laryngoscope 1991; 101(8):805–809.

13. Woodson BT, Fujita S. Clinical experience with lingualplasty as part of the treatment of severe obstructive sleep apnea. Otolaryngol Head Neck Surg 1992; 107(1):40–48.

14. Powell NB, Riley RW, Troell RJ, et al. Radiofrequency volumetric reduction of the tongue: a porcine pilot study for the treatment of obstructive sleep apnea syndrome. Chest 1997; 111:1348–1355.

15. Powell NB, Riley RW, Guilleminault C. Radiofrequency tongue base reduction in sleep-disordered breathing: a pilot study. Otolaryngol Head Neck Surg 1999; 120:656–664.

16. Chabolle F, Wagner I, Blumen M, et al. Tongue base reduction with hyoepiglottoplasty: a treatment for severe obstructive apnea. Laryngoscope 1999; 109:1273–1280.

17. Woodson BT, Toohill RJ. Transpalatal advancement pharyngoplasty for obstructive sleep apnea. Laryngoscope 1993; 103:269–276.

18. Kuo PC, West RA, Bloomquist DS, McNeill RW. The effect of mandibular osteotomy in three patients with hypersomnia sleep apnea. Oral Surg 1979; 48(5):385–392.

19. Riley RW, Powell NB, Guilleminault C. Maxillofacial surgery and nasal CPAP. A comparison of treatment for obstructive sleep apnea syndrome. Chest 1990; 98(6):1421–1425.

20. Riley RW, Powell NB, Guilleminault C. Inferior mandibular osteotomy and hyoid myotomy suspension for obstructive sleep apnea: a review of 55 patients. J Oral Maxillofac Surg 1989; 47:159–164.

21. Riley RW, Powell NB, Guilleminault C. Obstructive sleep apnea and the hyoid. A revised surgical procedure. Otolaryngol Head Neck Surg 1994; 111:717–721.

22. Weitzman ED, Kahn E, Pollak CP. Quantitative analysis of sleep and sleep apnea before and after tracheostomy in patients with the hypersomnia-sleep apnea syndrome. Sleep 1980; 3:407–423.

23. Larsson LH, Carlsson-Nordlander B, Svanborg E. Four-year follow-up after uvulopalatopharyngoplasty in 50 unselected patients with obstructive sleep apnea syndrome. Laryngoscope 1994; 104:1362–1368.

24. Janson C, Gislason T, Bengtsson H, et al. Long-term follow-up of patients with obstructive sleep apnea treated with uvulopalatopharyngoplasty. Arch Otolaryngol Head Neck Surg 1997; 123:257–262.

25. Lu S-J, Chang S-Y, Shiao G-M. Comparison between short-term and long-term post-operative evaluation of sleep apnoea after uvulopalatopharyngoplasty. J Laryngol Otol 1995; 109: 308–312.

26. Esclamado RM, Glenn MG, McCulloch TM, et al. Perioperative complications and risk factors in the surgical treatment of obstructive sleep apnea syndrome. Laryngoscope 1989; 99:1125–1129.

27. Haavisto L, Suonpaa J. Complications of uvulopalatopharyngoplasty. Clin Otolaryngol 1994; 19:243–247.

28. Zohar Y, Finkelstein Y, Talmi YP, et al. Uvulopalatopharyngoplasty: evaluation of postoperative complications, sequelae, and results. Laryngoscope 1991; 101:775–779.

29. Krespi YP, Keidar AK, Khosh MM, et al. The efficacy of laser assisted uvulopalatopharyngoplasty in the management of obstructive sleep apnea and upper airway resistance syndrome. Op Tech Otolaryngol Head Neck Surg 1994; 5(4):235–243.

30. Walker RP, Grigg-Damberger MM, Gopalsami C, et al. Laser-assisted uvulopalatopharyngoplasty for snoring and obstructive sleep apnea: results in 170 patients. Laryngoscope 1995; 105:938–943.

31. Mickelson SA. Laser-assisted uvulopalatoplasty for obstructive sleep apnea. Laryngoscope 1996; 106:10–13.

32. Mickelson SA, Anoop A. Short-term objective and long-term subjective results of laser-assisted uvulopalatoplasty for obstructive sleep apnea. Laryngoscope 1999; 109:362–367.

33. Walker RP, Grigg-Damberger MM, Gopalsami C. Laser-assisted uvulopalatoplasty for the treatment of mild, moderate, and severe obstructive sleep apnea. Laryngoscope 1999; 109:79–85.

34. Walker RP, Grigg-Damberger MM, Gopalsami C. Uvulopalatopharyngoplasty versus laser-assisted uvulopalatoplasty for the treatment of obstructive sleep apnea. Laryngoscope 1997; 107:76–82.

35. Terris DJ, Clerk AA, Norbush AM, et al. Characterization of postoperative edema following laser-assisted uvulopalatoplasty using MRI and polysomnography: implications for the outpatient treatment of obstructive sleep apnea syndrome. Laryngoscope 1996; 106:124–128.

36. Finkelstein Y, Shapiro-Fernberg M, Stein G, et al. Uvulopalatopharyngoplasty vs. laser-assisted uvulopalatoplasty: anatomical considerations. Arch Otolaryngol Head Neck Surg 1997; 123:265–276.

37. Woodson BT. Retropalatal airway characteristics in uvulopalatopharyngoplasty compared with transpalatal advancement pharyngoplasty. Laryngoscope 1997; 107: 735–740.

38. Bear SE, Priest JH. Sleep apnea syndrome: correction with surgical advancement of the mandible. J Oral Surgery 1980; 38:543–549.

39. Hochban W, Conradt R, Brandenburg U, et al. Surgical maxillofacial treatment of obstructive sleep apnea. Plast Reconst Surg 1997; 99:619–626.

40. Riley RW, Powell NB, Guilleminault C. Obstructive sleep apnea syndrome: a review of 306 consecutively treated surgical patients. Otolaryngol Head Neck Surg 1993; 108(2): 117–125.

41. Waite PD, Wooten V, Lachner J, et al. Maxillomandibular advancement surgery in 23 patients with obstructive sleep apnea syndrome. J Oral Maxillofac Surg 1989; 47: 1256–1261.

42. Johnson NT, Chinn J. Uvulopalatopharyngoplasty and inferior sagittal mandibular osteotomy with genioglossus advancement for treatment of obstructive sleep apnea. Chest 1994; 105:278–283.

43. Lee NR, Givens CD Jr, Wilson J, et al. Staged surgical treatment of obstructive sleep apnea syndrome: a review of 35 patients. J Oral Maxillofac Surg 1999; 57:382–385.

44. Ramirez SG, Loube DI. Inferior sagittal osteotomy with hyoid bone suspension for obese patients with sleep apnea. Arch Otolaryngol Head Neck Surg 1996; 122:953–957.

45. Utley DS, Shin EJ, Clerk AA, et al. A cost-effective and rational surgical approach to patients with snoring, upper airway resistance syndrome, or obstructive sleep apnea syndrome. Laryngoscope 1997; 107:726–734.

46. Troell RJ, Powell JB, Riley RW. Hypopharyngeal airway surgery for obstructive sleep apnea syndrome. Semin Respir Criti Care Med 1998; 19(2):175–183.

47. Prinsell JR. Maxillomandibular advancement surgery in a site-specific treatment approach for obstructive sleep apnea in 50 consecutive patients. Chest 1999; 116: 1519–1529.

48. Conway WA, Victor LD, Magilligan DJ Jr, et al. Adverse effects of tracheostomy for sleep apnea. JAMA 1981; 246(4):347–350.

49. Guilleminault C, Simmons FB, Motta J, et al. Obstructive sleep apnea syndrome and tracheostomy. Long-term follow-up experience. Arch Intern Med 1981; 141:985–988.

50. Kribbs NB, Pack AI, Kline LR. Objective measurement of patterns of nasal CPAP use by patients with obstructive sleep apnea. Am Rev Respir Dis 1993; 147(4):887–895.

51. Ferguson KA. Oral appliance therapy for the management of sleep-disordered breathing. Semin Respir Crit Care Med 1998; 19(2):157–164.

52. Winakur SJ, Smith PL, Schwartz AR. Pathophysiology and risk factors for obstructive sleep apnea. Semin Respir Crit Care Med 1998; 19:999–1112.

53. Suratt PM, Wilhoit SC, Cooper K. Induction of airway collapse with subatmospheric pressure in awake patients with sleep apnea. J Appl Physiol 1984; 57:140–146.

54. Schwartz AR, Smith PL, Wise RA, et al. Induction of upper airway occlusion in sleeping individuals with subatmospheric nasal pressure. J Appl Physiol 1988; 64:535–542.

55. Horner Rl, Mohiaddin RH, Lowell DG, et al. Sites and sizes of fat deposits around the pharynx in obese patients with obstructive sleep apnoea and weight matched controls. Eur Respir J 1989; 2:613–622.

56. Gleadhill IC, Schwartz AR, Schubert N, et al. Upper airway collapsibility in snorers and in patients with obstructive hypopnea and apnea. Am Rev Respir Dis 1991; 143:1300–1303.

57. Sher AE. An overview of sleep-disordered breathing for the otolaryngologist. Ear Nose Throat J 1999; 78:694–708.

58. Aboussouan LS, Golish JA, Wood BG, et al. Dynamic pharyngoscopy in predicting outcome of uvulopalatopharyngoplasty for moderate and severe obstructive sleep apnea. Chest 1995; 107:946–951.

59. Doghramji K, Jabourian ZH, Pilla M, et al. Predictors of outcome for uvulopalatopharyngoplasty. Laryngoscope 1995; 105:311–314.

60. Petri N, Suadicani P, Wildschiodtz G, et al. Predictive value of Muller maneuver, cephalometry and clinical features for the outcome of uvulopalatopharyngoplasty. Acta Otolaryngol (Stockh) 1994; 114:565–575.

61. Woodson BT, Wooten MR. Comparison of upper airway evaluation during wakefulness and sleep. Laryngoscope 1994; 104:821–828.

62. Woodson BT, Wooten MR. Manometric and endoscopic localization of airway obstruction after uvulopalatopharyngoplasty. Otolaryngol Head Neck Surg 1994; 111:38–43.

63. Skatvedt O. Localization of site of obstruction in snorers and patients with obstructive sleep apnea syndrome: a comparison of fiberoptic nasopharyngoscopy and pressure measurements. Acta Otolaryngol (Stockh) 1993; 113:206–209.

64. Sher AE. Soft tissue surgery for obstructive sleep apnea syndrome. Semin Respir Crit Care Med 1998; 19:165–173.

65. He J, Kryger M, Zorick F, et al. Mortality and apnea index in obstructive sleep apnea. Experience in 385 male patients. Chest 1988; 94(1):9–14.

66. Guilleminault C, Stoohs R, Clerk A, et al. A cause of excessive daytime sleepiness: the upper airway resistance syndrome. Chest 1993; 104:781–787.

67. Miljeteig H, Mateika S, Haight JS, et al. Subjective and objective assessment of uvulopalatopharyngoplasty for treatment of snoring and obstructive sleep apnea. Am J Respir Crit Care Med 1994; 150:1286–1290.

68. Zorick F, Roehrs T, Conway W, et al. Effects of uvulopalatopharyngoplasty on the daytime sleepiness associated with sleep apnea syndrome. Bull Eur Physiopath Resp 1983; 19:600–603.

69. Boudewyns A, De Cock W, Willemen M, et al. Influence of uvulopalatopharyngoplasty on alpha-EEG arousals in non-apnoeic snorers. Eur Respir J 1997; 10:129–132.

70. American Academy of Sleep Medicine Task Force Sleep Related Breathing Disorders in Adults. Recommendations for syndrome definition and measurement techniques in clinical research. Sleep 1999; 5:667–689.

71. Schechtman KB, Sher AE, Piccirillo JF. Methodological and statistical problems in sleep apnea research: The literature on uvulopalatopharyngoplasty. Sleep 1995; 18(8):659–666.

10 PHARMACOLOGICAL THERAPY OF SLEEP APNEA

Jan Hedner and Ludger Grote

INTRODUCTION

Considering the extraordinarily high prevalence of sleep apnea (SA) and the profound impact of SA on daytime performance and cardiovascular function, there have been surprisingly few systematic attempts to identify an effective drug treatment. Moreover, currently available treatment modalities for SA have limitations. For instance, problems affecting nasal continuous positive airway pressure (CPAP) treatment include a sense of dryness in the mouth and throat, nasal congestion, claustrophobia, air leaks, and non-acceptance of using a machine. Upper airway surgery as a method has yet to overcome problems with unpredictable response and limited long-term success rate. Still, no drug to date has proven to have a short-term efficacy comparable with CPAP in large clinical trials.

The systematic search for a pharmacological treatment may be directed according to several different approaches. These include a selective increase of upper airway muscle activity during sleep, a modulation of central respiratory control, and an alteration of sleep patterns. Indirect approaches include a widening of the upper airway space, which may be achieved by treatment with anti-obesity agents. In addition, therapy may be directed toward the complications of SA by minimizing the damaging effects of hypoxemia by neuroprotective agents. Alternatively, the daytime sleepiness component of SA may be reduced, as demonstrated after use of the stimulating agent modafinil, or after suppression of arousals during sleep, which may be obtained by hypnotics.

A number of pertinent issues need to be considered when developing a drug treatment of SA. First, there are different subtypes of SA, each which may be selectively suitable for a particular form of pharmacological treatment. For example, while it may be appropriate to use a drug which stimulates respiration in one subgroup of SA, the same drug may worsen breathing during sleep in another subgroup. Second, there are no established animal models of SA useful for drug development. Finally, any drug development program is likely to be hampered by problems related to classification and quantification of SA and its complications. At the milder end of the disease spectrum, factors such as night-to-night variability may affect the assessment of treatment efficacy. In fact, there is no absolute consensus on the best way of measuring of treatment efficacy. Moreover, there is no absolute consensus on the best way of measuring the severity of SA and its complications or even whether it may be important to

---

⊶ Key points box 10.1

Potential pharmacological approaches to managing sleep apnea

Direct:	Stimulate upper airway muscle activity
	Modulate central respiratory control
	Alter sleep patterns (suppress REM sleep; arousals)
Indirect:	Anti-obesity agents (enlarge upper airway)
	Nasal decongestants (relieve nasal obstruction)
Treat complications:	Wake promoting agents (daytime sleepiness)
	Oxygen (apnea-associated hypoxemia)

develop disease-specific outcome measures in quality of life and daytime symptoms in patients with mild disease. However, such measurements are crucial because up to 15–20% of adults have mild degrees of SA, a situation which has been described as a serious potential public health problem (1).

For practical reasons, this chapter is subdivided into the pharmacological treatments used or evaluated in obstructive SA and central SA (CSA), respectively.

OBSTRUCTIVE SLEEP APNEA SYNDROME

TRICYCLIC ANTIDEPRESSANTS (IMIPRAMINE, PROTRIPTYLINE)

The first trials suggesting a beneficial effect of the non-sedating tricyclic antidepressant protriptyline on SA were published in the early 1970s (2). In fact, these studies aimed to investigate agents for treatment of the narcolepsy-cataplexy syndrome. The efficacy of protriptyline in SA is highly variable, depending on the selection of the study population and the type of outcome variable used. A 5–75% reduction in SA events was achieved after a daily dosage of 2.5–30 mg administered over 2–24 weeks in patients with OSAS (3–5). The overall effect appears to be in the order of 25–30%, but dramatic effects have been described in single patients. Most trials, often in non-placebo–controlled designs, have included fewer than 10 patients.

The mechanism of the protriptyline action in SA activity remains unclear. However, protriptyline is well known to reduce rapid eye movement (REM) sleep, a sleep stage that is commonly associated with increased apnea severity in patients with SA. Thus, reduction of REM sleep may account at least in part for the overnight apnea reducing effect of protriptyline (3). In general, the specific effects of certain drugs during this sleep stage is an important consideration in clinical drug studies in SA. However, the disproportionate improvement of symptoms associated with daytime somnolence after protriptyline administration in SA suggests that effects other than reduction of apneas may be of importance. For instance, masked or coexisting depression is not uncommon in OSAS patients, and it is possible that at least part of the protriptyline effect may be explained by its antidepressive properties. In addition, the REM sleep restriction in itself may be responsible for the reduction of daytime hypersomnolence, analogous to

what has been demonstrated in patients without apnea (6). The therapeutic effect of protriptyline on SA is not unique among tricyclic antidepressants. The less selective noradrenaline (norepinephrine) uptake inhibitor imipramine has been found to exert similar effects to protriptyline (7, 8). In fact, one report suggested the response may be even greater in central SA (8).

There is a need for larger, controlled, and prospective trials to better classify the effects of tricyclic agents in SA. Such trials could lead to a better identification of subgroups of patients that are particularly good responders to therapy. For instance, tricyclic antidepressive agents may be more useful in patients with highly REM-dependent SA. Also, patients with coexisting depression may be a specific target group. However, the relatively frequent side effects, including bladder atonia and impotence in men, constrain the use of tricyclic agents in SA. In fact, female patients with SA may constitute the preferable target group for treatment.

SEROTONERGIC AGENTS

The serotonin precursor L-tryptophan was early found to induce a moderate reduction of obstructive apnea (9), a finding that triggered a considerable interest in serotonergic agents and SA. New tools for investigation in this field have been provided by the subsequent development of selective serotonin reuptake inhibitors (SSRI). An open trial of fluoxetine (10) reported approximately 40% reduction of apnea hypopnea index (AHI), mainly during non-REM (NREM) sleep. The effect was comparable with that of protriptyline, although fluoxetine treatment was associated with significantly fewer side effects. Similarly, in a double-blind controlled study (11), another SSRI, paroxetine, caused an approximately 20% reduction of RDI during NREM sleep.

Central serotonergic transmission in certain animal experimental models of SA has attracted an increased interest. Stimulation of 5-HT2 receptors in the cat brainstem facilitated hypoglossal nerve activity, potentially consistent with an increased upper airway patency (12). Reciprocally, inhibition of 5-HT2 receptors led to a diminution of upper airway muscle activity in the English bulldog (13). In humans, it is interesting to note that paroxetine has been reported to reduce the frequency of apneas more than hypopneas (11). The unchanged number of hypopneas may reflect a shift from complete to partial airway occlusion episodes. In other words, if the airway is stabilized, some hypopneas will resolve. However, the partial resolution of apneas will result in the generation of new hypopneas, which would appear as a selective effect on apneas while the number of hypopneas remains unchanged. Consequently, upper airway stability appears to improve in response to a stimulation of serotonin transmission. It remains to be determined whether this effect is attributable to a specific subpopulation of serotonergic receptors and if the treatment effect may be enhanced with the introduction of specific serotonin subreceptor agonists. This may be resolved by future trials directed toward exploring the efficacy of such compounds.

Serotonergic agents may be preferable to tricyclic agents by virtue of an approximately similar efficacy but fewer side effects. Serotonergic agents appear to have a reasonable effect on SA during NREM sleep and to be less effective during REM sleep. The reduced NREM AHI suggests that the suppression of REM sleep time, which has been described after SSRI use cannot explain the effect on breathing during sleep. However, it remains a possibility that the positive effects on daytime function in patients with sleep apnea at least in part may be related to a reduced total exposure of REM-related apneas and hypopneas. Owing to limited overall efficacy and the lack of long-term data, general treatment in SA by these agents is not warranted unless treatment with nonpharmacological modalities such as CPAP are unsuccessful.

Sex Steroids

A protective effect of sex steroids against SA is suggested by an epidemiological preponderance in men versus women and an increased prevalence in postmenopausal versus premenopausal women. Experimental data have demonstrated a lower awake genioglossus electromyogram activity in postmenopausal than in premenopausal women. In support, estrogen and progesterone replacement in postmenopausal women resulted in a significant increase of muscle activity (14). Disappointingly, however, there was no clinically significant reduction in apneic events during sleep after hormone replacement therapy in postmenopausal women (15), use of antiandrogens in men (16), or administration of medroxyprogesterone (MPG) to male patients (17, 18) with SA.

In contrast to pure SA, MPG appears to have a beneficial effect in patients with breathing disorders and concomitant daytime hypercapnia. Hypercapnia in patients with the 'pickwickian syndrome' (in reality patients with the obesity hypoventilation syndrome) was reduced and recurred after withdrawal of MPG treatment (19). This beneficial effect, which also was demonstrated in other studies of patients with obesity and hypercapnia, appears to have an extended duration in women (20). It implies that MPG may be used successfully in hypercapnic conditions and in particular those associated with nocturnal hypoventilation. Although MPG may have a mild beneficial effect on sleep-disordered breathing and apnea, the more isolated effect of MPG on hypercapnic conditions is supported by a direct ventilatory stimulant effect, which has been demonstrated in several different animal models (21, 22).

The applicability of MPG in sleep and breathing disorders is clearly limited by potential side effects, which include impotence, breast discomfort, hirsutism, alopecia, and thromboembolic disease. However, target groups for treatment may be identified in ongoing and future trials in specific subgroups of patients with hypercapnic ventilatory failure. At present, the only role for MPG is in the management of SA patients with awake respiratory failure and noncompliance with CPAP or pressure support ventilation.

Theophylline

The ventilatory stimulating effects of theophylline may be attributed to blockade of the ventilatory depressant action of the endogenous neuromodulator adenosine. In addition, diaphragm contractility is increased by theophylline, whereas the effect on upper airway muscle function is uncertain. The widespread use of theophylline in patients with SA may have been inspired by data from studies suggesting an overall improvement in SA by up to 40% (23, 24). Other studies, in contrast, found no effect (25, 26). Most of these previous studies were not placebo controlled, and data on sleep quality were not presented. The discrepant findings may be explained by data from a subsequent long-term follow-up study of theophylline, which demonstrated that any potentially beneficial effect is lost with time in the majority of patients (23). One placebo controlled trial of theophylline in SA (27) found a significant reduction in obstructive events during sleep (–29%), but sleep quality was significantly worsened by theophylline. Indeed, theophylline has a prominent negative influence on sleep structure, with increased frequency of arousals as well as increased amount and latency of sleep stage 1, which may result in increased daytime sleepiness (28). The poorly documented beneficial effects in combination with consistent reports on sleep disturbances after theophylline use limits its usefulness in the routine treatment of SA patients.

ANTI-HYPERTENSIVE AGENTS

Systemic hypertension is common in patients with SA, and the importance of this condition for the maintenance of upper airway stability is not fully known. Although pharmacologically induced blood pressure elevation increased upper airway collapsibility in a dog model (29), experimentally induced nocturnal blood pressure increases in humans did not induce upper airway collapse during NREM sleep (30). In a simulation model of SA in the rat, SA activity decreased after hydralazine-induced blood pressure reduction (31). Taken together, it cannot be excluded that nocturnal blood pressure elevation *per se* may sustain apneic activity during sleep.

Some studies have dealt with the effects of antihypertensive agents on apnea frequency and severity in patients with SA. Both the angiotensin converting enzyme (ACE) inhibitor cilazapril and the beta-blocker metoprolol reduced apnea-hypopnea frequency by approximately 30% (32). Similarly, the alpha-2-adrenergic agonist clonidine reduced REM sleep related SA activity in six of eight patients, but no effects were seen in NREM sleep (33). Beneficial effects on SA have also been described for calcium channel blocking agents (34, 35). However, there are also data suggesting that antihypertensive treatment may result in an increase of SA (33, 34) and the effect of anti-hypertensive agents on SA therefore remains unclear. In fact, the decline in SA may be directly caused by blood pressure reduction, but it is also possible that the decline is a direct effect of the drug itself. Furthermore, it remains unclear whether any effect persists during long-term treatment with antihypertensive agents.

MEDICAL GASES: OXYGEN AND CARBON DIOXIDE

Only few studies have dealt with the effect of medical gases administered to patients with SA. This lack may in part be explained by the complexity of the administration form, although such studies are likely to bring interesting information into this area of research. Low flow oxygen partly reduced hypoxemia during sleep in SA but had no clinically significant impact on symptoms and frequency of apneic events (36). With higher oxygen flows the duration of apneas was extended, and a decrease in tonic genioglossal muscle electrical activity was observed (37). In another study dealing with extended nocturnal low flow oxygen administration for 30 days, there was a modest reduction in nocturnal apnea frequency and an increase in daytime PCO_2 (36). However, no change was found in sensitivity to chemical ventilatory stimuli or in daytime symptoms. The beneficial effect of oxygen, if any, has been attributed to an increased ventilatory drive resulting from an elevation of PCO_2. At present, however, there is not sufficient data to support a recommendation for nocturnal oxygen in the therapy of SA.

Inhalation of 3% CO_2 during sleep markedly increased upper airway inspiratory muscle activity and reduced SA dramatically, by approximately 80% (37). Despite these promising data, the effect of CO_2 on sleep quality has not been thoroughly investigated. It remains unclear whether the beneficial effect of CO_2 is related to an alteration of sleep, but data certainly suggest that the chemosensory

---

◦┐ Key points box 10.2

Principal pharmacological agents available for the management of OSAS

1. **Tricyclic antidepressants:** Suppress REM sleep and may increase upper airway muscle tone. Benefits limited by side effects, particularly anticholinergic and in males.

2. **Serotonergic agents:** Effects similar to tricyclic antidepresants but fewer side effects.

3. **Theophyllines:** Benefits to sleep apnea in terms of reduced AHI diluted by adverse effect on sleep quality.

4. **Sex steroids (medroxyprogesterone):** Act principally by central respiratory stimulation but unlikely to benefit sleep apnea unless there is associated hypoventilation.

5. **Anti-hypertensives:** Treat an important complication or comorbidity but may also directly benefit the patient's sleep apnea.

6. **Wake promoting agents (modafinil):** May benefit selected cases in which hypersomnolence is a major factor not adequately controlled by measures to treat the sleep apnea.

activation by CO_2 is sufficient to overcome airway collapse in SA. Needless to say, there are methodological problems associated with stabilizing the CO_2 level throughout the night, which severely may hamper the applicability of this treatment modality.

OTHER PHARMACOLOGICAL APPROACHES

A number of other pharmacological approaches have been attempted in SA. A slight reduction of SA was found after application of nicotine as a chewing gum (38) or via a transdermal delivery system (39). However, nicotine also disturbs sleep and may induce gastrointestinal side effects, which limits its usefulness. In a small study of 10 SA patients (40), the benzodiazepine antagonist flumazenil had no significant effects on SA and sleep structure. A putative glutamate antagonist sabeluzole (41) reduced hypoxemic events in a plasma concentration dependent manner in a double blind controlled trial of SA patients, but the subjective effects were relatively modest. Modafinil, a vigilance promoter, improved alertness and reduced complaints of sleepiness in a double blind controlled study of SA patients, but it failed to influence any of the respiratory parameters studied (42).

Indirect approaches to influence SA frequency include pharmacological treatment of nasal congestion. Although vasoconstricting and anti-inflammatory agents are likely to be widely used for this purpose, there are no objective data actually evaluating their usefulness in SA. Similarly, the increasingly effective anti-obesity agents are likely to represent a new and indirect method to treat SA pharmacologically. To date, however, there have been no well designed studies of the impact of controlled weight reduction after these agents in SA.

TREATMENT OF SLEEP APNEA IN ENDOCRINE DISORDERS

The prevalence of SA is increased in acromegaly and hypothyroidism. In acromegaly, treatment with the somatostatin analog octreotide reduces central SA, and to a less extent, obstructive SA. This effect is not directly related to the degree of growth hormone suppression (43). There is controversy regarding the effect of thyroxine on SA frequency in patients with hypothyroidism, particularly in the presence of coexisting obesity. (44–46). The degree of myxedematous involvement in the upper airway (47) may also influence treatment.

> **⌐ Key points box 10.3**
>
> **Effectiveness of pharmacological agents**
>
> 1. Pharmacological agents currently available are less effective than nasal CPAP in managing SA and are limited by side effects.
> 2. However, several agents have been shown to produce significant objective benefits and may be indicated in selected cases, particularly when nasal CPAP is poorly tolerated.
> 3. Since different pharmacological agents produce their effects by different mechanisms, combination therapy may be more effective, although few studies have addressed this question.

CENTRAL SLEEP APNEA (CSA)

ACETAZOLAMIDE

The well-documented beneficial effects of acetazolamide on CSA likely result from the induction of metabolic acidosis, which in turn stimulates respiratory drive. The frequency of CSA was reduced by approximately 70% and was accompanied by an improvement of daytime symptoms after 1 week of therapy (48). In more recent studies this effect on CSA was demonstrated to remain after 1 month of therapy, but there was no effect on obstructed breathing events (49). An additional long-term study demonstrated a surprising persistent effect on CSA up to 6 months after discontinuation of therapy. This finding has led to the suggestion that acetazolamide induces a long-lasting resetting of the CO_2 response threshold (50). Despite these promising results, the clinical use of acetazolamide is limited owing to potential side effects, such as electrolyte changes, precipitation of calcium phosphate salts in alkaline urine, and paresthesias.

THEOPHYLLINE

Recent data suggest a favorable effect of theophylline in CSA associated with congestive heart failure (Cheyne-Stokes breathing). In a small placebo controlled trial of patients with compensated heart failure, CSA apnea index (AI) was reduced by approximately 60% after theophylline administration, compared with approximately 20% after placebo (51). The degree of intermittent hypoxia was reduced along with these changes, whereas the right and left ventricular ejection fractions remained unchanged. Plasma concentrations of theophylline obtained were well within the range recommended in the treatment of for example, bronchial asthma. Interestingly, cardiac output has been described to increase after theophylline, and it remains to be clarified whether the main effect on CSA is explained by the respiratory stimulant properties or the positive inotropic effect of the drug. At present there are not sufficient data to support general recommendations of theophylline treatment in this type of breathing disorder. Further studies focusing on the effect of theophylline on mortality and quality of life would be useful in these patients.

⟳ Key points box 10.4

Central sleep apnea

- Acetazolamide has both short-term and long-term effects but is its use limited by adverse effects.
- Theophylline may be beneficial, particularly where there is associated heart failure
- CSA related to heart failure may benefit from oxygen therapy, and benzodiazepines may be helpful in selected cases by reducing an elevated respiratory drive.

OTHER TREATMENTS

There have been attempts to treat CSA associated with cardiac failure with supplemental oxygen and CPAP therapy (52). The value of CPAP treatment on cardiac function in these patients is strongly supported by studies from one group (54) and larger multi-center trials have been initiated. A final, somewhat different treatment approach includes the use of short-acting benzodiazepines, which may have a beneficial effect by suppressing the degree of respiratory drive that contributes to the Cheyne-Stokes pattern of CSA (53).

CONCLUSIONS

No highly effective pharmacological treatment of SA has yet been described. However, a wealth of data suggest that SA frequency and severity, as well as the associated daytime symptoms, may be favorably modified by pharmacological agents. Although no single drug has been shown to reduce SA by more than 50% in controlled studies, it should be pointed out that a 50% level of efficacy may compare favorably with other treatment modalities. CPAP and surgery are hampered by limited compliance (CPAP) or incomplete long-term effectiveness (surgery). For these reasons, the present lack of highly effective therapeutic modalities is likely to induce a future intense search for possible candidate drugs.

Interestingly, the drugs used to date appear to have unique properties in the sense that they affect different aspects and forms of SA, such as predominantly obstructive or central apneas or apneas appearing during NREM or REM sleep. This finding suggests that improved disease classification and thereby better selection of treatment candidates or possibly different forms of pharmacological combination therapy may represent future avenues of development. The lack of adequate animal models of SA has restricted the possibilities for rational drug development. Therefore, it is possible that future identification of SA drug therapy may result from by chance observations from drug therapy of other medical disorders.

There is a great lack of outcome data from drug therapy studies in SA. In fact, a consensus on optimal outcome variables to be used in therapy trials in SA patients has not been reached. Should this be related to subjective well-being, reduction of an elevated cardiovascular risk, reduction of SA, or simply polysomnographically assessed sleep? Clarification of these issues will not only increase the possibility of identifying an effective pharmacological treatment but also appropriately define its role in the management of SA.

REFERENCES

1. Phillipson EA. Sleep apnea—a major public health problem. N Engl J Med 1993; 328:1271–1273.

2. Schmidt HS, Clark RW, Hyman PR. Protriptyline: an effective agent in the treatment of the narcolepsy-cataplexy syndrome and hypersomnia. Am J Psychiatry 1977; 134(2):183–185.

3. Brownell LG, West P, Sweatman P, et al. Protriptyline in obstructive sleep apnea. A double-blind trial. N Engl J Med 1982; 307:1037–1042.

4. Clark RW, Schmidt HS, Schaal SF, et al. Sleep apnea: treatment with protriptyline. Neurology 1979; 29:1287–1292.

5. Smith PL, Haponik EF, Allen RP, et al. The effects of protriptyline in sleep-disordered breathing. Am Rev Respir Dis 1983; 127:8–13.

6. Nykamp K, Rosenthal L, Folkerts M, et al. The effects of REM sleep deprivation on the level of sleepiness/alertness. Sleep 1998; 21(6):609–614.

7. Rubin AH, Alroy GG, Peled R, et al. Preliminary clinical experience with imipramine HCl in the treatment of sleep apnea syndrome. Eur Neurol 1986; 25:81–85.

8. Meyer-Madaus H, Haug HJ, Kessler C. [Imipramine in sleep apnea syndrome] Imipramin bei Schlafhypopnoesyndrom. Dtsch Med Wschr 1991; 116(45):1734–1735.

9. Schmidt HS. L-tryptophan in the treatment of impaired respiration in sleep. Bull Eur Physiopathol Respir 1983; 19:625–629.

10. Hanzel DA, Proia NG, Hudgel DW. Response of obstructive sleep apnea to fluoxetine and protriptyline. Chest 1991; 100:416–421.

11. Kraiczi H, Hedner J, Dahlof P, et al. Effect of serotonin uptake inhibition on breathing during sleep and daytime symptoms in obstructive sleep apnea. Sleep 1999 22(1):61–67.

12. Rose D, Khater-Boidin J, Toussaint P, et al. Central effects of 5-HT on respiratory and hypoglossal activities in the adult cat. Respir Physiol 1995; 101(1):59–69.

13. Veasey SC, Panckeri KA, Hoffman EA, et al. The effects of serotonin antagonists in an animal model of sleep-disordered breathing. Am J Respir Crit Care Med 1996; 153(2):776–786.

14. Popovic RM, White DP. Upper airway muscle activity in normal women: influence of hormonal status. J Appl Physiol 1998; 84(3):1055–1062.

15. Cistulli PA, Barnes DJ, Grunstein RR, et al. Effect of short-term hormone replacement in the treatment of obstructive sleep apnoea in postmenopausal women. Thorax 1994; 49(7):699–702.

16. Stewart DA, Grunstein RR, Berthon-Jones M, et al. Androgen blockade does not affect sleep-disordered breathing or chemosensitivity in men with obstructive sleep apnea. Am Rev Respir Dis 1992; 146:1389–1393.

17. Cook WR, Benich JJ, Wooten SA. Indices of severity of obstructive sleep apnea syndrome do not change during medroxyprogesterone acetate therapy. Chest 1989; 96:262–266.

18. Rajagopal KR, Abbrecht PH, Jabbari B. Effects of medroxyprogesterone acetate in obstructive sleep apnea. Chest 1986; 90:815–821.

19. Sutton FD Jr, Zwillich CW, Creagh CE, et al. Progesterone for outpatient treatment of Pickwickian syndrome. Ann Intern Med 1975; 83:476–479.

20. Saaresranta T, Irjala K, Polo-Kantola P, et al. Hormonal alterations related to progestin-induced sustained improvement of nocturnal ventilation in postmenopausal women. Proceedings, 'Diagnosis and treatment of sleep related breathing disorders,' Grenoble, December 1988; 1999; 78.

21. Bayliss DA, Millhorn DE, Gallman EA, et al. Progesterone stimulates respiration through a central nervous system steroid receptor-mediated mechanism in cat. Proc Natl Acad Sci USA 1987; 84(21):7788–7792.

22. Hannhart B, Pickett CK, Moore LG. Effects of estrogen and progesterone on carotid body neural output responsiveness to hypoxia. J Appl Physiol 1990; 68(5):1909–1916.

23. Grieger E, Schneider H, Weichler U, et al. Therapy control of theophylline evening dosage in patients with sleep-related respiratory disorders—follow-up study. Pneumologie 1993; 47(Suppl 1):166–169.

24. Kempf P, Mossinger B, Muller B, et al. Comparative studies on the effect of nasal CPAP, theophylline and oxygen in patients with sleep apnea syndrome. Pneumologie 1991; 45 (Suppl 1):279–282.

25. Guilleminault C, Hayes B. Naloxone, theophylline, bromocriptine, and obstructive sleep apnea. Negative results. Bull Eur Physiopathol Respir 1983; 19:632–634.

26. Espinoza H, Antic R, Thornton AT, et al. The effects of aminophylline on sleep and sleep-disordered breathing in patients with obstructive sleep apnea syndrome. Am Rev Respir Dis 1987; 136:80–84.

27. Mulloy E, McNicholas WT. Theophylline in obstructive sleep apnea. A double-blind evaluation. Chest 1992; 101(3):753–757.

28. Roehrs T, Merlotti L, Halpin D, et al. Effects of theophylline on nocturnal sleep and daytime sleepiness/alertness. Chest 1995; 108(2):382–387.

29. Schwartz AR, Rowley JA, O'Donnell C, et al. Effect of hypertension on upper airway function and sleep. J Sleep Res 1995; 4(Suppl 1):83–88.

30. Wilson CR, Manchanda S, Crabtree D, et al. An induced blood pressure rise does not alter upper airway resistance in sleeping humans. J Appl Physiol 1998; 84(1):269–276.

31. Carley DW, Trbovic SM, Radulovacki M. Hydralazine reduces elevated sleep apnea index in spontaneously hypertensive (SHR) rats to equivalence with normotensive Wistar-Kyoto rats. Sleep 1996; 19(5):363–366.

32. Weichler U, Herres-Mayer B, Mayer J, et al. Influence of antihypertensive drug therapy on sleep pattern and sleep apnea activity. Cardiology 1991; 78:124–130.

33. Issa FG. Effect of clonidine in obstructive sleep apnea. Am Rev Respir Dis 1992; 145:435–439.

34. Kantola I, Rauhala E, Erkinjuntti M, et al. Sleep disturbances in hypertension: a double-blind study between isradipine and metoprolol. J Cardiovasc Pharmacol 1991; 18 (Suppl 3): S41–S45.

35. Heitmann J, Grote L, Knaack L, et al. Cardiovascular effects of mibefradil in hypertensive patients with obstructive sleep apnea. Eur J Clin Pharmacol 1998; 54(9–10):691–696.

36. Gold AR, Schwartz AR, Bleecker ER, et al. The effect of chronic nocturnal oxygen administration upon sleep apnea. Am Rev Respir Dis 1986; 134:925–929.

37. Hudgel DW, Hendricks C, Dadley A. Alteration in obstructive apnea pattern induced by changes in oxygen-and carbon-dioxide–inspired concentrations. Am Rev Respir Dis 1988; 138:16–19.

38. Gothe B, Strohl KP, Levin S, et al. Nicotine: a different approach to treatment of obstructive sleep apnea. Chest 1985; 87:11–17.

39. Davila DG, Hurt RD, Offord KP, et al. Acute effects of transdermal nicotine on sleep architecture, snoring, and sleep-disordered breathing in nonsmokers. Am J Respir Crit Care Med 1994; 150(2):469–474.

40. Schönhofer B, Köhler D. Benzodiazepine receptor antagonist (flumazenil) does not affect sleep-related breathing disorders. Eur Respir J 1996; 9:1816–1820.

41. Hedner J, Grunstein R, Eriksson B, et al. A double-blind, randomized trial of sabeluzole—a putative glutamate antagonist—in obstructive sleep apnea. Sleep 1996; 19(4):287–289.

42. Heitmann J, Cassel W, Grote L, et al. Does short-term treatment with modafinil affect blood pressure in patients with obstructive sleep apnea? Clin Pharmacol Ther 1999; 65(3):328–335.

43. Grunstein RR, Ho KK, Sullivan CE. Effect of octreotide, a somatostatin analog, on sleep apnea in patients with acromegaly. Ann Intern Med 1994; 121:478–483.

44. Rajagopal KR, Abbrecht PH, Derderian SS, et al. Obstructive sleep apnea in hypothyroidism. Ann Intern Med 1984; 101:491–494.

45. Kapur VK, Koepsell TD, deMaube J, et al. Association of hypothyroidism and obstructive sleep apnea. Am J Respir Crit Care Med 1998; 158(5 Pt 1):1379–1383.

46. Grunstein RR, Sullivan CE. Sleep apnea and hypothyroidism: mechanisms and management. Am J Med 1988; 85: 775–779.

47. Orr WC, Males JI, Imes NK. Myxedema and obstructive sleep apnea. Am J Med 1981; 70:1061–1066.

48. White DP, Zwillich CW, Pickett CK, et al. Central sleep apnea. Improvement with acetazolamide therapy. Arch Intern Med 1982; 142:1816–1819.

49. Debacker WA, Verbraecken J, Willemen M, et al. Central apnea index decreases after prolonged treatment with acetazolamide. Am J Respir Crit Care Med 1995; 151:87–91.

50. Verbraecken J, Willemen M, De Cock W, et al. Central sleep apnea after interrupting longterm acetazolamide therapy. Respir Physiol 1998; 112(1):59–70.

51. Javaheri S, Parker TJ, Wexler L, et al. Effect of theophylline on sleep-disordered breathing in heart failure. N Engl J Med 1996; 335(8):562–567.

52. Naughton MT, Bradley TD. Sleep apnea in congestive heart failure. Clin Chest Med 1998; 19(1):99–113.

53. Bonnet MH, Dexter JR, Arand DL. The effect of triazolam on arousal and respiration in central sleep apnea patients. Sleep 1990; 13:31–41.

54. Bradley TD, Holloway RM, McLaughlin PR, Ross BL, Walters J, Liu PP. Cardiac output response to continuous positive airway pressure in congestive heart failure. Am Rev Resp Dis 1992; 145:377–382.

11 ORAL APPLIANCES FOR SNORING AND OBSTRUCTIVE SLEEP APNEA SYNDROME

John A Fleetham

INTRODUCTION

Oral appliances (OA) have been used for many years to correct upper airway obstruction (1). More recently OA have been developed as an alternative approach to nasal continuous positive airway pressure (CPAP) therapy in the management of snoring and obstructive sleep apnoea syndrome (OSAS) (2–5). This chapter reviews the different types of OA and the currently available data concerning their mechanism of action, efficacy and side effects, and treatment guidelines.

APPLIANCE TYPE

OA advance either the mandible or the tongue. There are other minor design differences in the many OA currently available that may also affect their success and treatment compliance. Mandibular advancement OA utilize traditional dental techniques to attach the appliance to one or both dental arches (6–9). Construction usually requires dental impressions, bite registration, and fabrication by a dental laboratory. Some appliances are available in a prefabricated form (Fig 11.1A) that can be molded to the patient's teeth in an office setting (10). Some appliances restrict mouth opening by means of clasps, whereas others allow relatively unhindered movement. Lateral and vertical jaw movement may reduce the risk of temporomandibular joint discomfort and facilitate oral breathing in patients who have nasal obstruction. OA sometimes include tubes or openings for oral breathing or pressure relief. Several appliances feature a posterior extension of the maxillary component to modify the position of the soft palate or tongue. Recent advances in dental materials have improved the flexibility and strength of thermosensitive acrylic resin materials used in the construction of OA, which appear to be associated with better oral retention.

More recently OA with an adjustable hinge have been developed (Fig 11.1B,C) that allow progressive advancement of the mandible after initial construction until the optimal mandibular position is achieved. The amount of anterior posterior mandibular movement and the speed which with this can be changed varies considerably among patients. There is some preliminary experience with overnight titration of mandibular advancement in the sleep laboratory, which should help reduce the time involved in determining the optimal degree of mandibular advancement. Some of the original adjustable OA had a lingually located hinge mechanism that encroached on tongue space and decreased rather than increased upper airway size. This problem does not exist with the more recent adjustable mandibular advancement OA. Mandibular advancement OA require at least 10 teeth in each of the maxillary and mandibular arches. Furthermore, the patient should be able to advance his or her mandible by at least 5 mm without discomfort.

The other major type of OA available is the tongue retainer, which keeps the tongue in an anterior position during sleep by means of negative pressure in a soft plastic bulb. It fits over both the mandibular and maxillary arches and

---

⊶ Key points box 11.1

Appliance type

1. Oral appliances (OA) advance either the mandible or tongue.
2. Mandibular advancement appliances usually require individual fabrication, and the more recently developed more OA allow progressive advancement of the mandible.
3. Tongue retention appliances are suitable for edentulous patients.

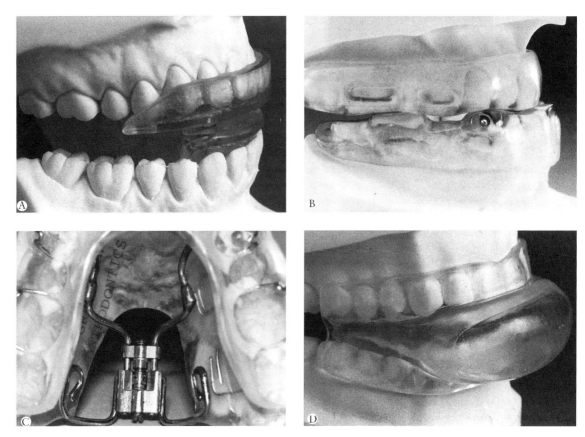

Fig 11.1 *Lateral views of a prefabricated nonadjustable (A) and a fabricated adjustable (B) mandibular advancement OA and prefabricated tongue retaining device (D). C shows the screw mechanism from the adjustable OA that connects the mandibular and maxillary components and enables gradual advancement of the mandible.*

has a flange that fits between the lips and teeth, keeping the appliance anterior in the mouth (Fig. 11.1D). This appliance was one of the first to be developed and is available in both a fabricated and prefabricated form (11–13). It can be used in edentulous patients and is the OA of choice for patients with no teeth, limited anterior posterior mandibular movement, or large tongues.

MECHANISM OF ACTION

The majority of OA are designed to maintain the mandible or tongue (or both) in a protruded posture during sleep, thereby preventing upper airway occlusion. Proposed mechanisms of action of OA include increased upper airway size, decreased upper airway compliance,

activation of upper airway dilator muscles, and stabilization of mandibular posture. A variety of upper airway imaging techniques have been used to assess changes in upper airway size and function with OA in patients with OSAS. These imaging techniques include cephalometry, computed tomography (CT), magnetic resonance (MR) imaging, and videoendoscopy (14). Voluntary mandibular and tongue protrusion has been shown to increase upper airway size and alter upper airway shape (15). Several studies have demonstrated an increase in the anteroposterior diameter of the upper airway after OA insertion (7, 10, 16–18) (Fig. 11.2). This increase was predominantly in the oropharynx and hypopharynx, but some studies have also suggested an effect on the velopharynx (7, 16). In patients with mild to moderate

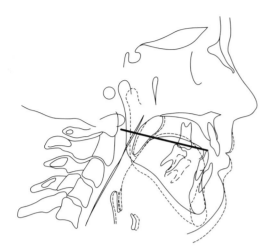

Fig 11.2 *Lateral cephalometry with (broken line) and without (solid line) a mandibular repositioning appliance in a patient with OSAS. The horizontal line represents the narrowest cross-section of the oropharynx (From Lowe AA, Fleetham JA, Ryan CF, et al. Effects of a mandibular repositioning appliance used in the treatment of obstructive sleep apnoea on tongue muscle activity. Prog Clin Biol Res 1990; 345:395–405. Copyright 1990, reprinted by permission of Wiley-Liss, a division of John Wiley and Sons, Inc.)*

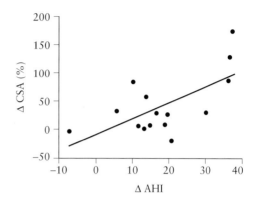

Fig 11.3 *The relationship between change in AHI (Δ AHI) and the proportional change in cross-sectional area (Δ CSA) of the velopharynx with mandibular advancement OA implacement. (From Ryan CF, Lowe LL, Peat D, et al. Mandibular advancement oral appliance therapy for obstructive sleep apnea: effect on awake calibre of the velopharynx. Thorax 1999; 54: 972–7, printed by permission.)*

OSAS, treated with a mandibular advancement OA, upper airway cross-sectional area has been shown to increase by a mean 18% in the hypopharynx and 25% in the velopharynx, and without a significant increase in the oropharynx (19). The lateral diameter of the velopharynx increased to a greater extent than the anterior posterior diameter. The reduction in apnea-hypopnea index (AHI) with the OA was related to the increase in the velopharynx cross-sectional area (Fig. 11.3). All of these upper airway imaging studies have been performed during wakefulness, and it is unknown whether the same changes occur during sleep.

EFFICACY AND SIDE EFFECTS

Some of the currently available OA have obtained Federal Drug Administration (FDA) marketing approval for snoring and OSAS, which does not require proof of clinical efficacy but does provide some safety review. The majority of the data concerning the efficacy and side effects of OA

in the treatment of snoring and OSAS are from uncontrolled case series studies, which are subject to study design problems such as regression to the mean and selection and reporting bias. In a 1995 review of 19 case series involving 304 patients (3) 70% of patients with snoring or OSAS treated with OA had a greater than 50% reduction in AHI, and AHI was reduced to 10 events/hour or less in 51% of patients (6–13, 16, 18, 20–24). At least three additional case series have been published since that review with similar results (25–27). More recently the quality of OA clinical research has become more rigorous, with the completion of at least four prospective randomized clinical trials comparing the efficacy and side effects of several OA and nasal CPAP. In a 2 week crossover study comparing a nonadjustable mandibular OA with nasal CPAP in 21 patients with OSAS, subjective sleepiness was improved equally with both treatments (28). The OA advanced the mandible by approximately 65% maximal protrusion and reduced AHI by 39%, compared to a 60% reduction with nasal CPAP. Fifty-one patients with mild to moderate OSAS treated with either a non adjustable or an adjustable mandibular advancement OA were compared with those treated with nasal CPAP in a 4 month crossover study (29, 30). Treatment success was defined as a reduction in AHI to < 10/hour and relief of symptoms, treatment failure as failure to reduce AHI to < 10/hour with or without failure to relieve symptoms, and compliance failure as inability or unwillingness to use the treatment. Of the patients treated with the non adjustable OA 48% were treatment successes, compared to 61% for the adjustable OA and 66% for CPAP (Table 11.1). Both OA and CPAP were effective in reducing symptoms, but OA was less effective in improving sleep oxygenation. The long-term preference was overwhelmingly in favor of OA therapy. Fourteen patients had treatment success with both treatments: 12 of these patients preferred OA and 2 preferred CPAP as a long-term treatment. A recent randomized prospective parallel multicenter study compared the efficacy and side effects of an adjustable mandibular advancement OA versus CPAP in 101 patients with OSAS (31). Efficacy was assessed by symptom and quality of life questionnaire, a subjective and objective measurement of daytime vigilance, and polysomnography. This study demonstrated that patients were less willing or able to tolerate long-term treatment with an OA than with nasal CPAP. OA and nasal CPAP both improved daytime symptoms, quality of life, AHI, sleep fragmentation, and arterial oxygen desaturation. However, nasal CPAP was more effective at improving AHI and sleep fragmentation than OA.

A variety of reports have attempted to identify which patients are most likely to obtain a successful response to OA therapy (32). Patients with OSAS that occurs predominantly in the supine position appear more likely to have a successful response with a mandibular advancement OA (33). It has been proposed that treatment success is inversely related to pretreatment AHI, but this relationship may just be a function of the definition of treatment success (16, 23). Several upper airway skeletal and soft tissue measurements made from pretreatment lateral cephalometry have been shown to be associated with treatment success, but there is considerable overlap between good and poor treatment response (16, 34). Upper airway fluoroscopy has also been proposed as a technique to guide successful OA therapy (35). The utility of any treatment guidelines based on OSAS severity or upper airway anatomy now requires prospective evaluation. Although OA design has been proposed as an important determinant of treatment success, to date there have been very few prospective comparative studies evaluating different OA designs (36).

Only patient-reported compliance data are available on OA therapy. In recent randomized clinical trials, 96% patients reported using OA for > 75% nights and 80% patients used OA > 75% of each night, compared to 67% and 67% respectively, for nasal CPAP (29). However, previous experience with nasal CPAP suggests that patient reports tend to overestimate actual use. Attempts to develop a covert OA compliance monitor have been fraught with technological difficulties, and at present no data on covert OA appliances are available.

Minor side effects are common in the first month of OA therapy but usually resolve with time. These side effects include excessive salivation, mouth dryness, and sore teeth or jaw. Limited data are available on long-term complications of OA therapy. Temporomandibular joint dysfunction appears uncommon, but tooth movement can occur, causing change in dental occlusion. Side effects can be decreased by adjustment of the appliance to reduce pressure on the anterior teeth and avoidance of excessive mandibular advancement. The cost of OA therapy varies depending on the OA used and the extent and expertise of the dental supervision. Costs can equal or exceed those associated with nasal CPAP therapy. OA usually remain

Table 11.1 Treatment outcome

	Nonadjustable OA	Adjustable OA	Nasal CPAP
Treatment success[a]	48%	61%	66%
Treatment failure[b]	28%	35%	0%
Compliance failure[c]	24%	4%	34%

[a] Resolution of symptoms and reduction in AHI < 10/hour.
[b] Ongoing clinical symptoms or AHI > 10/hour.
[c] Inability or unwillingness of patient to continue to use the treatment.

effective for at least 5 years, but they can break and require either repair or replacement.

TREATMENT GUIDELINES

Nasal CPAP remains the primary treatment for symptomatic patients with OSAS who do not respond to conservative measures. The most recent randomized clinical trials data indicate that nasal CPAP is more effective at improving apnea severity and sleep fragmentation than OA. Furthermore, it takes longer to obtain optimal treatment with an OA than with nasal CPAP, which can be a significant issue in patients with excessive daytime sleepiness. However, there can be substantial problems with patient acceptance and long-term compliance with nasal CPAP (37). OA have been clearly shown to improve symptoms, quality of life, apnea severity, sleep fragmentation, and arterial oxygen desaturation and should be considered in symptomatic patients with OSAS who are unwilling or unable to comply with nasal CPAP therapy. OA therapy may also be indicated as an adjuvant to nasal CPAP when the patient is away from home or does not have access to electrical power. OA have also been used as combination therapy in patients who have had an unsuccessful response to uvulopalatopharyngoplasty (UPPP) (38). OA should only be prescribed by a sleep disorder specialist in collaboration with a dentist or orthodontist with a major interest in OA therapy. Both the American Sleep Disorders Association (39) and the Sleep Disorder Dental Society have developed practice guidelines for OA therapy. These guidelines emphasize the importance of combined medical and dental evaluation prior to OA treatment. Patients should not have major periodontal disease, and all dental restorations should be complete prior to OA therapy. It is important to reassess all patients after OA therapy. Some patients feel subjectively better despite no objective change in OSAS severity. OA can decrease rather than increase upper airway size in some patients by causing downward rotation of the mandible (30). This highlights the importance of repeat sleep monitoring in all patients with moderate to severe OSAS treated with OA.

A recent survey of dentists revealed that only 18% of patients underwent sleep monitoring after OA treatment (40). Patients treated with OA also require long-term dental follow-up evaluation to ensure adequate OA retention and comfort. OA may require adjustment after any new dental restorations.

CONCLUSIONS

The treatment of snoring and OSAS should be individualized for each patient based on age, severity of symptoms, magnitude of clinical complications, and cause of upper airway obstruction. OA are an effective treatment for both snoring and OSAS in selected patients. In general, OA should be reserved for symptomatic patients who are unwilling or unable to comply with nasal CPAP. OA therapy should be supervised by both medical and dental specialists with a major interest in the management of sleep-disordered breathing.

REFERENCES

1. Robin P. Glossoptosis due to atresia hypotrophy of the mandible. Am J Dis Child 1934; 48:541–547.

2. Lowe AA. Dental appliances for the treatment of snoring and obstructive sleep apnea. In Kryger MH, Roth T, Dement WC eds. Principles and practice of sleep medicine, 2nd edn. Philadelphia: WB Saunders; 1994:722–735.

3. Schmidt Nowara W, Lowe A, Wiegand L, et al. Oral appliances for the treatment of snoring and obstructive sleep apnea: a review. Sleep 1995; 18:501–510.

4. Millman RP, Rosenberg CL, Kramer NR. Oral appliances in the treatment of snoring and sleep apnea. Clin Chest Medicine 1998; 19:69–75.

5. Bennett LS, Davies RJ, Stradling JR. Oral appliances for the management of snoring and obstructive sleep apnea. Thorax 1998; 53(Suppl 2):58–64.

6. Bernstein AK, Reidy RM. The effects of mandibular repositioning on obstructive sleep apnea. Cranio 1988; 6:179–181.

7. Bonham PE, Currier GF, Orr WC, et al. The effect of a modified functional appliance on obstructive sleep apnea. Am J Orthod Dentofacial Orthop 1988; 94:384–392.

8. Clark GT, Arand D, Chung E, et al. Effect of anterior mandibular positioning on obstructive sleep apnea. Am Rev Respir Dis 1993; 147:624–629.

9. George PT. A modified functional appliance for treatment of obstructive sleep apnea. J Clin Orthod 1987; 21:171–175.

10. Schmidt Nowara WW, Meade TE, Hays MB. Treatment of snoring and obstructive sleep apnea with a dental orthosis. Chest 1991; 99:1378–1385.

11. Cartwright RD, Samelson CF. The effects of a nonsurgical treatment for obstructive sleep apnea. The tongue-retaining device. JAMA 1982; 248:705–709.

12. Cartwright RD. Predicting response to the tongue retaining device for sleep apnea syndrome. Arch Otolaryngol 1985; 111:385–388.

13. Cartwright R, Stefoski D, Caldarelli D, et al. Toward a treatment logic for sleep apnea: the place of the tongue retaining device. Behav Res Ther 1988; 26:121–126.

14. Fleetham JA. Upper airway imaging in relation to obstructive sleep apnea. In Clin Chest Med 1992; 13:399–416.

15. Ferguson KA, Love LL, Ryan CF. Effect of mandibular and tongue protrusion on upper airway size during wakefulness. Am Rev Crit Care Med 1997: 155:1748–1754.

16. Eveloff SE, Rosenberg CL, Carlisle CC, et al. Efficacy of a Herbst mandibular advancement device in obstructive sleep apnea. Am J Respir Crit Care Med 1994; 149:905–909.

17. Johnson LM, Arnett GW, Tamborello JA, et al. Airway changes in relationship to mandibular posturing. Otolaryngol Head Neck Surg 1992; 106:143–148.

18. Lowe A, Fleetham J, Ryan F, et al. Effects of a mandibular repositioning appliance used in the treatment of obstructive sleep apnea on tongue muscle activity. In: Issa FG, Suratt PM, Remmers JE, eds. Sleep and respiration. New York: Wiley Liss; 1990:395–405.

19. Ryan CF, Lowe LL, Peat D, et al. Mandibular advancement oral appliance therapy for obstructive sleep apnea: effect on awake calibre of the velopharynx. Thorax 1999; 54:972–7.

20. Ichioka M, Tojo N, Yoshizawa M, et al. A dental device for the treatment of obstructive sleep apnea: a preliminary study. Otolaryngol Head Neck Surg 1991; 104:555–558.

21. Knudson RC, Meyer JB Jr, Montalvo R. Sleep apnea prosthesis for dentate patients. J Prosthet Dent 1992; 68:109–111.

22. Meier-Ewert K, Brosig B. Treatment of sleep apnea by prosthetic mandibular advancement. In: Peter JH, Podszus T, von Wichert P, eds. Sleep-related disorders and internal disease. Munich: Springer Verlag; 1987:341–346.

23. O'Sullivan RA, Hillman DR, Mateljan R, et al. Mandibular advancement splint: an appliance to treat snoring and obstructive sleep apnea. Am J Respir Crit Care Med 1995; 151:194–198.

24. Nakazawa Y, Sakamoto T, Yasutake R, et al. Treatment of sleep apnea with prosthetic mandibular advancement (PMA). Sleep 1992; 15:499–504.

25. Menn SJ, Loube DI, Morgan TD, et al. The mandibular repositioning device: role in the treatment of obstructive sleep apnea. Sleep 1996; 19:794–800.

26. Marklund M, Franklin KA, Sahlin C, et al. The effect of a mandibular advancement device on apneas and sleep in patients with obstructive sleep apnea. Chest 1998; 113:707–713.

27. Stradling JR, Negus TW, Smith D, et al. Mandibular advancement devices for the control of snoring. Eur Respir J 1998; 11:447–450.

28. Clark GT, Blumenfeld I, Yoffe N, et al. A crossover study comparing the efficacy of continuous positive airway pressure with anterior mandibular positioning devices on patients with obstructive sleep apnoea. Chest 1996; 109: 1477–1483.

29. Ferguson KA, Ono T, Lowe AA, et al. A randomized crossover study of an oral appliance vs. nasal-continuous positive airway pressure in the treatment of mild-moderate obstructive sleep apnea. Chest 1996; 109:1269–1275.

30. Ferguson KA, Ono T, Lowe AA, et al. A short-term controlled trial of an adjustable oral appliance for the treatment of mild to moderate obstructive sleep apnoea. Thorax 1997; 52:362–368.

31. Fleetham JA, Lowe A, Vazquez JC, et al. A long term randomized parallel multicentre study of an oral appliance vs. nCPAP in the treatment of obstructive sleep apnea. Am Rev Crit Care Med 1998; 157:A285.

32. Lowe AA. Can we predict the success of dental appliance therapy for the treatment of OSA based on anatomical considerations? Sleep 1993; 16:593–595.

33. Marklund M, Persson M, Franklin KA. Treatment success with a mandibular advancement device is related to supine-dependent sleep apnea. Chest 1998; 114: 1630–1635.

34. Mayer G, Meier-Ewert K. Cephalometric predictors for orthopaedic mandibular advancement in obstructive sleep apnoea. Eur J Orthod 1995; 17:35–43.

35. L'Estrange PR, Battagel JM, Harkness B, et al. A method of studying adaptive changes of the oropharynx to variation in mandibular position in patients with obstructive sleep apnoea. J Oral Rehabil 1996; 23:699–711.

36. Hans MG, Nelson S, Luks VG, et al. Comparison of two dental devices for treatment of obstructive sleep apnea syndrome (OSAS). Am J Orthod Dentofacial Orthop 1997; 111:562–570.

37. Engleman HM, Martin SE, Douglas NJ. Compliance with CPAP therapy in patients with the sleep apnoea/hypopnoea syndrome. Thorax 1994; 49:263–266.

38. Millman RP, Rosenberg CL, Carlisle CC, et al. The efficacy of oral appliances in the treatment of persistent sleep apnea after uvulopalatopharyngoplasty. Chest 1998; 113: 992–996.

39. ASDA Standards of Practice Committee. Practice parameters for the treatment of snoring and obstructive sleep apnea with oral appliances. Sleep 1995; 18:511–513.

40. Loube DI, Strauss AM. Survey of oral appliance practice among dentists treating obstructive sleep apnea patients. Chest 1997; 111:382–386.

CLINICAL SIGNIFICANCE AND MANAGEMENT OF SNORING WITHOUT OBSTRUCTIVE SLEEP APNEA SYNDROME

Victor Hoffstein

INTRODUCTION

Snoring has always been a nuisance for the listener who is wanting to fall asleep but unable to do so because of disturbing noise. Kleitman, in his first authoritative textbook on sleep disorders first published over 40 years ago (1), commented that 'snoring is harmless to the sleeper, but can be very annoying to others who may be awake at the time, . . . '. There are many anecdotes in the popular press describing persons whose snoring was so loud that it disturbed people in other rooms or even on other houses on the street. The remedies to cope with this disturbing, objectionable noise ranged from the passive, such as wearing earplugs, to extremely active, such as homicide.

Discovery that snoring may be more than a mere nuisance, driving the frustrated bed partner out of the bedroom, must be credited to the recognition of the obstructive sleep apnea syndrome (OSAS) in the 1970s (2,3). It was quickly learned that snoring is the most common symptom of OSAS, sharing with it several pathophysiological features, and being the main reason for bringing patients with OSAS to medical attention. It is therefore not surprising that soon after adverse medical consequences of OSAS were recognized, a question arose as to whether the same consequences occur in nonapneic snorers.

Lugaresi and colleagues (2,4) were the first ones to raise the possibility that snoring by itself may be pathological. They pointed out that heavy habitual snoring may be a precursor to obstructive sleep apnea, which they termed 'heavy snorers disease.' They described patients with habitual snoring and daytime sleepiness, but no significant apneas, thus raising a possibility that snoring and daytime sleepiness may be linked. In addition, during their studies of blood pressure fluctuations during sleep in patients with sleep apnea, these authors noticed elevations in the arterial blood pressure during non-apneic snoring.

It is these pioneering observations that lie at the origin of many subsequent studies in the 1980s and 1990s, whose aim was to determine whether snoring is an independent risk factor for daytime dysfunction and for vascular disease—a task as yet not fully completed. In fact, it became clear that snoring itself cannot be regarded as a homogeneous symptom with similar consequences in all snorers. At one end of the spectrum are completely asymptomatic, nonobese, and otherwise healthy snorers whose only reason for seeking medical attention is to comfort their bed partners. These patients are generally referred to as simple snorers ('simple' in this context indicates lack of any other medical signs or symptoms). At the other end of the spectrum are obese, somnolent snorers with medical problems (vascular disease, endocrine abnormalities) whose daytime function is significantly compromised, and whose nocturnal polysomnography not surprisingly reveals sleep apnea. These are apneic snorers. In the middle of the spectrum are patients who have mild daytime dysfunction (sleepiness, tiredness), who snore habitually (usually nightly or almost nightly), who are generally overweight, and whose sleep study confirms the presence of snoring but does not indicate significant sleep apnea. It is this group of patients, sometimes referred to as habitual snorers, complex snorers, primary snorers, or patients with upper airway resistance syndrome (5) that is currently receiving most attention directed toward establishing whether snoring causes their daytime symptoms.

For the sake of clarity, adherence to the conventional use, and consistency, in this chapter we will use exclusively the terms 'apneic' and 'nonapneic' snorers, on whether the respiratory disturbance index (RDI) is greater or lower than 10. All of the discussion in this chapter will refer to nonapneic snorers.

The purpose of this chapter is twofold. Our main aim is to present a synthesis of the available information regarding clinical significance of snoring without sleep apnea. Our second aim is to review the management of snoring. Both areas are under active investigation at present with much progress made in the last decade. Most of the advances in our understanding of snoring and its consequences occurred due to close linkage between snoring and sleep apnea.

Prior to late 1970s or early 1980s there were no studies in peer-reviewed medical literature dealing with treatment of snoring. Only anecdotal reports describing various gadgets or home remedies were available. One notable exception is the work by Robin (6), who summarized, with great perception and foresight, various aspects of snoring, including both medical and surgical treatment. During the past 20 years many articles have appeared dealing with treatment of snoring, using a diversity of techniques, including lifestyle modification, drug therapy, use of various appliances designed to increase the patency of the upper airway, and surgery. We review the advances achieved in treatment of snoring, evaluate and synthesize the available information, and present an integrated approach to management of nonapneic snoring.

Before concentrating on these principal goals, as reflected in the title of this chapter, we briefly review the epidemiology and pathogenesis of snoring.

EPIDEMIOLOGY, PATHOGENESIS, AND MEASUREMENT OF SNORING

EPIDEMIOLOGY

Snoring is common, but exactly how common is still a matter of debate. Review of 16 studies published between 1980 and 1998, comprising more than 32,000 subjects, reveals very wide variability in the prevalence of snoring. Rates range from 5–86% in men and from 2–57% in women with a mean prevalence of 32% in men and 21% in women.

It is too simplistic to conclude from these results that snoring varies widely among different countries and different populations. It undoubtedly does, but population differences are only one of the factors contributing to the variability in the prevalence of snoring. Most of the variability is inherent in the methodology employed to gather the data. Snoring is an unusual symptom; it is not complained about by the patient, but by the patient's bed partner.

The importance of having a bed partner to assess snoring is illustrated in the study of Stradling and Crosby (7); when spouses were present during interviews, the prevalence of snoring more than doubled. Remission of snoring with age over 55 or 65 years, found in some studies (8, 9), may be related to the absence of a bed partner. Even if the snoring history is obtained in the presence of a bed partner, there is still a great deal of subjectivity, since perception of sound differs between different persons (10).

Several authors emphasized that the importance of using similar and validated questionnaires for assessment of snoring (11–13). Gislason et al. (11) looked at several large studies, each one reporting different prevalence of snoring (ranging from 9–44%), and noted marked differences in the type of questions being asked to assess snoring, speculating that the differences are methodological rather than factual. When Janson et al. (12) studied random samples of men and women of similar ages in Sweden, Iceland, and Belgium, using identical questionnaire (translated and back-translated to verify the accuracy and meaning) and identical scale to asses snoring, almost identical results were obtained. Finally, overrepresentation of patients with sleep apnea in the population sample will result in increased prevalence of snoring.

Studies originating in the United States, including the widely quoted Wisconsin Sleep Cohort Study (14), consistently indicate that snoring occurs in 35–45% of and in 15–28% women.

PATHOGENESIS OF SNORING

Snoring is a sound produced by the vibrations of upper airway walls, which lack cartilaginous support. These vibrations can occur at any part of the upper airway, from the soft palate superiorly almost to the larynx inferiorly. Quinn et al. (15) performed sleep nasendoscopy in 50 nonapneic snorers. They observed isolated vibrations of the soft palate most frequently. However, 30% of their patients had vibrations at other sites, such as the epiglottis, base of the tongue, and tonsils, confirming that the entire upper airway, rather than a single isolated segment, may be responsible for the generation of snoring sounds. It is these vibrations that generate the low frequency sound usually perceived as snoring.

Theoretical models have been developed to examine the mechanism of snoring (16–18). These models predict that when inspiratory flow exceeds a certain critical value, the airway becomes unstable and may either close and stay closed (as in apnea) or repetitively open and close (as in snoring). This repetitive collapse and reopening of the airway, with vibratory motion of the airway walls, generates the sound of snoring. The critical value of the inspiratory flow that leads to airway closure is determined by airway geometry, its compliance, and resistance. Although the physics of the model is quite complex, involving principles of flow dynamics through collapsible tubes, the models make several predictions regarding factors that promote airway closure and therefore will influence snoring.

Some of these predictions have been verified experimentally. For example, reduction in the rigidity of airway walls will worsen snoring, whereas breathing lighter gas mixture (e.g., helium-oxygen mixture) will reduce it. Dynamic closure of the airway walls in patients with sleep apnea during conditions of inspiratory flow limitation was observed directly by Isono et al. (19). Focal neurogenic lesions in the upper airway muscle fibers, consistent with what may be expected as a result of vibration-induced injury, have been observed in snorers (20).

Identification of the site of vibrations during snoring may have important positive and negative implications for surgical treatment. Existing observations of diffuse airway involvement already explain why surgery of the palate and uvula is not uniformly successful. Although sleep nasendoscopy is theoretically an attractive method of preoperative assessment, its invasive nature, discomfort, and uncertainties in interpreting the results preclude its routine use in clinical practice.

MEASUREMENT OF SNORING

It is disappointing that we do not have an objective and standard measurement of snoring. Unlike the case of sleep apnea, in which relatively standard measurement techniques are available, snoring is not measured routinely in all sleep laboratories. Even when it is measured, the methodologies of measurement and analysis are sufficiently diverse as to preclude quantitative comparisons among different studies. These diversities include microphone placement, acoustic definition of snores, and methods of analyzing the sound signal. Several different techniques for measuring snoring, used by various investigators, are described in a recent comprehensive review (18).

Nonapneic patients referred because of snoring are frustrated when, after spending a night in the sleep laboratory, all they are told is that they do not have sleep apnea, whereas what they expect is a comment about their snoring. The sleep physician generally relies on the impression of a sleep technologist to determine whether the patient snored or not. Considering that snoring may lead to important surgical decisions, it is unsatisfactory that we cannot quantitate it properly for use in diagnosis and follow-up evaluation of interventions.

The argument for not measuring snoring during nocturnal polysomnography is that the test is done to rule out sleep apnea, not to diagnose snoring. Quality of sound, and particularly its disturbing character, is a subjective perception on the part of the listener. Snoring is variable from night to night, and a frequently presented argument is that the results of a one night laboratory investigation should not influence treatment decisions. Since we have no standards for measuring snoring, we do not know much about its night-to-night variability and the factors influencing this variability.

However, being able to measure snoring has important implications. First, it would help to eliminate some of the subjectivity present in the studies of the health outcomes of snoring; undoubtedly, examination of the relationship between snoring and health outcomes would become more robust and probably less variable, if we could relate objective health outcomes to objective measure of snoring. Second, measurement of snoring could be combined with other respiratory monitoring (e.g., measurements of airflow) to develop a useful ambulatory (i.e., in-home) screening test for sleep apnea. Lastly, it would add an objective measurement when assessing treatment outcomes.

Understanding the pathophysiology of snoring and having a standard and validated method for measuring snoring may open an opportunity for mathematical modeling of the airway to determine the site (or sites) of vibrations. We recall from previous discussion that snoring occurs only when critical relationships between airway area, compliance of the airway wall, and flow rate are satisfied; this implies that snoring sound may be generated at any site within the upper airway. Depending on the particular situation, some sites may be more susceptible to vibrations than others; they may be referred to as primary sites of snoring. It is also possible that critical conditions are satisfied at multiple sites within the airway. Direct observations of the airway in sleeping apneic and nonapneic snorers (15, 21, 22) suggest that multiple sites of partial collapse are in fact more common than single sites.

Nevertheless, being able to assess objectively the severity of snoring and determine the primary site of vibrations would help to make a more informed decision regarding surgery, maximize the success rate, and objectively determine the outcome.

Several laboratories measure and analyze sound as a part of full nocturnal polysomnography. One popular analytic technique is spectral analysis and digital processing of snoring sounds. This approach is attractive for several reasons. First, examination of the power spectrum may enable us to define and quantitate snoring. Generally it is a low frequency sound with most energy contained between 0 and 6000 Hz. Results obtained to date indicate that power spectrum of snoring sound is variable and depends on airway anatomy, body position, route of breathing, and similar factors. Second, it may be possible to use the measured power spectrum of snoring to reconstruct airway geometry and identify the position of the 'snoring generator.' There are patients whose power spectrum shows only a single well-defined narrow peak, suggesting that there is a single anatomical site within the airway where snoring is generated. Most patients exhibit peaks at different frequencies, implying the existence of several sites along the airway, which vibrate producing the sound. This is confirmed by pressure measurements at several sites within the airway (21, 22). It would appear that in most patients snoring is a result of diffuse, rather than local, abnormality of the upper airway. This is why surgical correction, which focuses only on a narrow segment of the airway, may not fully resolve snoring; after surgery a different segment of the airway may begin to vibrate, producing snoring sound.

No matter what method is used to measure snoring, the important point is to validate the measuring system, so that sound measured during sleep represents snoring rather than other nocturnal noise. It is this 'biological' validation of the correspondence between measured sound and subjective perception of this sound as snoring that is the biggest obstacle in the objective quantification of snoring.

CLINICAL SIGNIFICANCE OF SNORING

MARKER OF SLEEP APNEA

Snoring is the most common symptom of sleep apnea. It is frequently the sole reason for referring the patient to a sleep laboratory. Performing a sleep study on every snorer would be expensive and time-consuming. Consequently, the ability to predict high and very low likelihood of sleep apnea in specific patients would be very useful by allowing patients to be prioritized for polysomnography.

Several models incorporating snoring together with other symptoms (or signs) of sleep apnea have been described. Analytical methods included 1) linear regression analysis to determine contributions of snoring and other variables to variability of apnea-hypopnea index (AHI), 2) logistic regression to determine the odds for demonstrating sleep apnea in snorers with or without other symptoms or signs of OSAS, and 3) calculations of sensitivity, specificity, positive and negative predictive values, and diagnostic accuracy of snoring, alone or in combination with other features of sleep apnea. The methods employed in different studies vary significantly by type of population (general versus clinic), wording of questions about snoring, number of subjects, whether polysomnography was performed consistently and what type, and methods of analysis. It is therefore not surprising that the results also vary considerably. For example, in snorers referred to an otolaryngologist for treatment and evaluation of possible sleep apnea, prevalence of sleep apnea is over 70% (23). In a population of patients referred to a medical sleep disorders center to rule out sleep apnea, in which some, but not all, are habitual snorers, the prevalence of OSAS is about 50% (24). In the general population the prevalence of OSAS is less than 10% (14). Another example of the crucial importance of the type of population and the wording of questions on the final results is the study of Crocker et al. (25), who found that snoring was not a significant determinant of AHI. Kump et al. (26) and Bliwise et al. (27) found that subjects who snore severely have more that 20 times greater odds for sleep apnea than subjects who never snore.

Most of the studies to date identify snoring as an independent and significant predictor of sleep apnea. Other significant predictors of apnea, in addition to snoring, were bed partner's observations of cessation of breathing, excessive daytime sleepiness, choking or gasping for breath, male sex, age, neck circumference, hypertension, and alcohol intake.

For a clinician working in a sleep disorder center, who wants to know the likelihood that a particular patient has OSAS, the following guidelines may be offered.

Asymptomatic patients referred with a chief complaint of snoring have approximately a 20–30% of having sleep apnea. Patients who snore and have other symptoms or signs of sleep apnea (important signs being obesity, hypertension, increased neck circumference) have a 50–70% chance of having sleep apnea.

RELATIONSHIP TO VASCULAR DISEASE

Early observations by Lugaresi et al. (2) demonstrated that snoring is associated with elevations in systemic blood pressure during sleep. These observations raised a possibility that nocturnal fluctuations of blood pressure may lead to sustained daytime hypertension. Subsequent epidemiological investigations, carried out mainly in Scandinavian countries, found that snoring is an independent risk factor for vascular disease, such as hypertension, coronary artery disease, and cerebrovascular disease. Although many of these studies implied that snoring is an independent risk factor for vascular disease, review of the data up to 1995 (28, 29) indicates that the association is not independent and is probably due to confounding factors, mainly unsuspected sleep apnea, obesity, and lifestyle factors (smoking, alcohol, lack of exercise). Let us examine whether more recent investigations alter this conclusion.

Several large studies addressing snoring and hypertension are available. There are two lines of evidence. First, data from an epidemiological study carried out in Sweden involving over 2500 randomly selected subjects are available (30). These subjects were followed for 10 years, and the relationship between snoring and appearance of hypertension was examined. The authors found that only subjects aged 30–49 years who reported habitual snoring at the beginning of the study and at follow-up evaluation 10 years later had odds ratio of 2.6 for development of hypertension. No polysomnography was performed, snoring and hypertension were self-reported, confidence intervals for the odds ratio were wide (1.5–4.5), and no association between snoring and hypertension was found in subjects 50 years old and older. Furthermore, no significant increase in cardiovascular mortality associated with snoring was found over 10 years of follow-up study (31). Even snorers with excessive daytime sleepiness did not demonstrate a significant increase in the relative risk of cardiovascular mortality.

The second line of evidence is based on the data reported in subjects from the Wisconsin Sleep Cohort Study (14, 32, 33). Over 1000 subjects had full polysomnography and careful measurements of evening and morning blood pressure. Odds ratio for hypertension for subjects with AHI < 15 (versus AHI = 0) was 1.8. Measured blood pressures, without adjustment for obesity, age, and other factors, were 123/81 mm Hg for those with AHI < 2 versus 130/85 mm Hg for those with AHI between 5 and 15. After adjustment for the confounding factors, a regression model obtained using the cohort data predicted only 0.12 mm Hg increase in diastolic blood pressure for each additional apnea or hypopnea. This implies that a nonapneic snorer with AHI = 10 has a diastolic blood pressure only 1.2 mm Hg higher than a person with AHI = 0.

The above results indicate that there is a dose-response relationship between sleep-disordered breathing and blood pressure, with nonapneic snoring representing the very beginning of this relationship. However, these data do not allow us to conclude that the association between snoring and hypertension is of clinical significance. Finally, it should be remembered that an association, even if it exists, does not imply causality. There are no long-term data at all to determine the possibility of a causal relationship between snoring and hypertension.

SNORING AND DAYTIME DYSFUNCTION— UPPER AIRWAY RESISTANCE SYNDROME (UARS)

If, in addition to snoring, a person complains of daytime tiredness and fatigue, sleep apnea is suspected (34), and such a patient is frequently referred to a sleep disorders center. However, in many such patients nocturnal polysomnography does not demonstrate sleep apnea (AHI < 10). This is not surprising since these symptoms are very nonspecific and are commonly present in the community population. It was therefore always assumed that nonapneic tired and sleepy snorers are like that for reasons other than breathing abnormalities during sleep.

In 1991 Guilleminault et al. (35) advanced a hypothesis that nonapneic snoring may by itself lead to daytime sleepiness, even in the absence of sleep apnea. They studied 15 habitual snorers who exhibited episodes of increased respiratory effort (i.e., more negative esophageal pressure) during snoring, without significant changes in airflow to classify these episodes as hypopneas, indicative of increased upper airway resistance. These episodes were accompanied by short electroencephalographic (EEG) arousals. The authors postulated that arousals fragmented sleep resulting in daytime sleepiness, which can be reversed by treatment with continuous positive airway pressure (CPAP). Two years later, in 1993, the same authors introduced a new term, – 'upper airway resistance syndrome' (UARS), to describe sleepy nonapneic patients, not necessarily habitual snorers, who have cyclical increases in upper airway resistance during breathing (36). These increases are usually accompanied by mild reduction in airflow, not enough to define them as hypopneas. Most importantly, these episodes of increased upper airway resistance are terminated by arousals that fragment sleep and may lead to daytime symptoms. This term gained tremendous popularity, to some extent owing to the fact that sleep specialists suddenly found themselves in a position to attach a specific diagnosis, that of UARS, to a large group of their patients (nonapneic snorers with nonspecific daytime symptoms) and recommend various trials of treatment.

Much work is currently going on to elucidate the pathophysiology, definition, diagnosis, and the very existence of this syndrome, particularly because in many epidemiological studies snoring continues to emerge as an independent correlate of daytime dysfunction (37–40). Irrespectively of the final outcome, one major contribution of this pioneering work is already clear—the importance of nocturnal arousals (some of them very short, lasting less than 3 s) and sleep fragmentation in causing daytime neuropsychological deficits (41). Until now these symptoms were thought to be present only in patients with significant sleep apnea and were considered to be related to hypoxemia and arousals, which occur at termination of apneas and hypopneas. We now know that these symptoms are present in patients with very mild disorder, less than 15 respiratory events per hour of sleep (42), who do not have significant nocturnal hypoxemia. Moreover, these symptoms are improved after reduction of nocturnal elevations in upper airway resistance with nasal CPAP. The attention is now shifted away from apneas, hypopneas, and hypoxemia as being primary determinants of daytime function, to arousals and increases in sympathetic activity due to elevations in upper airway resistance, with or without snoring. These arousals may influence not only daytime function but also the autonomic activity, causing transient increases in blood pressure during sleep (43), perhaps leading to hypertension (44).

This emphasis on arousals led to a reassessment of the definition of arousals and sleep fragmentation. Increases in EEG frequency shorter than 3 s are now accepted as an arousal. There is evidence that sleep may be fragmented by episodic increases in sympathetic activity manifesting as changes in heart rate and respiration, even without conventional EEG changes. Since normal asymptomatic individuals exhibit EEG arousals during sleep, it is necessary to determine the normal range of arousal index. Some results indicate that depending on age, normal asymptomatic persons may have 14–30 arousals per hour of sleep (45).

At this time it is still too premature to accept fully the existence of the UARS as a new disease causing daytime sleepiness, tiredness, memory deficits, inability to concentrate, reduction in work performance, and hypertension. Very few measurements, aside from the pioneering work of Guillemnault et al. referred to earlier, exist with simultaneous monitoring of upper airway resistance and sleep architecture, coupled with full assessment of daytime function. There are no long-term follow-up studies documenting improvement in daytime function, reduction in sleep fragmentation, and normalization in airway resistance with treatment.

Until such information becomes available, it is appropriate to diagnose UARS, as defined by Guilleminault et al. (44), in 'patients with or without regular heavy snoring and increased respiratory efforts during sleep associated with brief decreases (within one to three breaths of the arousal) in tidal volume, leading to transient EEG arousals and a complaint of daytime tiredness or sleepiness.' Unequivocal diagnosis of UARS requires monitoring of upper airway pressure (ideally esophageal and pharyngeal pressure at several sites) and airflow. This is not done routinely. In the absence of esophageal pressure monitoring, frequent arousals during sleep in a nonapneic patient with daytime sleepiness should raise a suspicion of UARS. Snoring, if present, indicates increases in upper airway resistance during sleep and strengthens the diagnosis, but the absence of snoring does not negate it.

HEARING LOSS

Another possible result of chronic exposure to episodic nocturnal noise may be hearing loss. It is well known that hearing loss accompanies the aging process (termed presbycusis or presbyacusis), but the precise reason for it is unknown. A commonly postulated cause of presbycusis is cumulative exposure to environmental noise. Consequently, it is an attractive and plausible hypothesis that snoring, probably the most common, most frequent, and most persistent noise affecting many persons, results in progressive loss of hearing acuity. This possibility was first raised by Prazic (46), but it was never tested in a large group of patients Only one study exists in which audiograms, sleep, and snoring were measured in 219 patients (47). The results indicate no significant relationship between snoring and hearing loss, rendering unlikely the hypothesis that snoring leads to presbycusis.

○┓ Key points box 12.1

Snoring

■ Snoring is very common in the general population, but precise prevalence figures are difficult to determine because of the subjective nature of the complaint and the absence of objective, standardized techniques to quantitate the degree of snoring.

■ Habitual, heavy snoring is clinically important because of its relationship to OSAS and to UARS.

MANAGEMENT

Should nonapneic snoring be treated at all? I believe it should, for two reasons. First, it is a symptom that is troublesome to patients' families and bed partners. Many snorers grow to be self-conscious and ashamed of their snoring, which leads to compromised social interactions; they frequently fear sharing a room, not simply a bed, with another person. They suffer marital discord, are unwilling to travel when shared sleeping accommodations may be required, and frequently are afraid of being ridiculed. Second, according to the discussion presented above, the health effects of snoring are still not fully known, and as long as there is a possibility that snoring may be associated with adverse consequences, it should be treated.

Treatment of nonapneic snoring is conceptually similar to treatment of sleep apnea. The methods are largely the same, but the emphasis on which particular method to employ differs depending on whether the patient has sleep apnea. Many of these methods are reviewed in sections dealing with treatment of sleep apnea. In this section we concentrate only on the effectiveness of various methods

for treatment of nonapneic snoring. We discuss treatment of snoring under two general headings—medical and surgical.

MEDICAL TREATMENT

Medical management of snoring can be grouped into several categories, as given in Table 12.1.

Lifestyle Modifications

This means removal of risk factors associated with snoring. They are, in order of importance; obesity, alcohol ingestion, drugs (sedatives, hypnotics, muscle relaxants), and smoking.

■ **Weight Loss.** Being overweight (25 < body mass index (BMI) < 30) or obese (BMI > 30) is probably the most common and most important risk factor predisposing to snoring. Patients frequently give a history of increase in snoring concomitant with weight gain. Surveys of sleep clinic populations invariably indicate high prevalence of obesity in snorers referred for detection of possible sleep apnea; regression analysis with AHI as a dependent variable always demonstrates strong correlation with indices of obesity (generally BMI). Surveys of general populations identify obesity as being one of the most important determinants of snoring (48).

There are good theoretical arguments as well as experimental evidence pointing to the abnormalities in upper airway mechanics as favoring appearance of snoring in obese persons. Studies of pharyngeal function in snorers show fat deposits around lateral airway walls, as well as infiltration of muscle tissue by adipose cells. These factors result in reduced airway area and increased compliance of pharyngeal walls—conditions that predispose to the appearance of snoring and, in some persons, to sleep apnea.

Table 12.1 Medical treatments of nonapneic snoring

1. Lifestyle modification: dealing with the risk factors (weight loss, alcohol, muscle relaxants and sedatives, smoking)
2. Positional training
3. Medications
4. Nasal dilators
5. CPAP
6. Oral appliances

Influence of weight loss on snoring has been addressed almost exclusively in the context of investigations dealing with sleep apnea (49), almost never in the context of treatment of nonapneic snoring (50). These investigations demonstrate significant reduction in AHI and either disappearance or marked improvement in snoring. Although it is not possible to predict the amount of weight loss required to abolish snoring in each individual patient, it is clear that achievement of ideal body weight (based on BMI < 25) is not necessary in the majority of patients. In many of them, snoring will improve after a loss of only a few kilograms.

Treatment of obesity is complex, requires a team effort, and needs to be individualized and closely supervised. This topic is beyond the scope of this review, but such treatment is comprehensively described in a recent summary statement (51).

- **Alcohol Ingestion.** Alcohol use constitutes another common risk factor for snoring and apnea. Many, although not all, epidemiological studies of snoring and prevalence of other apnea symptoms in the general population show a positive correlation between snoring and alcohol ingestion. It is a common observation that nocturnal ingestion of alcohol will convert a nonsnorer into a snorer and a nonapneic snorer into an apneic snorer (52). The effect of alcohol is dose-related, may be evident even after a single drink, is most pronounced within the first hour postingestion, and, depending on the dose ingested, may last for several hours. It is prudent to recommend that snorers abstain from ingestion of any alcohol in the evening. The mechanisms by which alcohol worsens snoring and sleep apnea include increase in inspiratory resistance, greater inspiratory effort, loss of pharyngeal muscle tone, and impaired arousal responses. No studies examining changes in snoring with withdrawal of alcohol exist.

- **Sedatives, Hypnotics, and Muscle Relaxants.** Another common advice given to snorers is to avoid the sedatives, hypnotic drugs, and muscle relaxants, which may increase snoring by the same mechanism as alcohol. This advice originates from the earlier literature, some of them case reports, describing increases in the number of apneas after ingestion of benzodiazepines. More recent studies do not demonstrate any significant worsening of snoring or apnea in patients with milder forms of this disorder treated with brotizolam, flurazepam, triazolam, flunitrazepam, or zopiclone. This does not mean that the use of these generally overprescribed medications in nonapneic snorers should be condoned. However, when required for a specific indication, such medications may be prescribed, provided that the patient is aware of the possibility that snoring may be worsened or sleep apnea may appear, and that appropriate follow-up evaluation is arranged.

- **Smoking.** Probably the weakest correlate of snoring is smoking. The only evidence for its role in snoring comes from epidemiological studies (53) showing positive correlation between smoking and snoring. There are no studies examining the effect of smoking cessation on snoring (i.e., a causal relationship has not been demonstrated). Theoretical arguments in favor of the pathological role of smoking involve detrimental changes in airway physiology secondary to airway inflammation.

Positional Training

Many bed partners disturbed by their mate's loud snoring will testify to the fact that snoring is reduced or completely eliminated after the snorer moves from the back to the side. This common observation led to many early devices designed to prevent the snorer from lying on the back; tennis balls sewn into the pajama top is one of the better known remedies.

Studies of the airway properties during sleep demonstrate that in patients with sleep apnea the upper airway becomes more unstable when supine than in the lateral position or at 30 degrees of elevation. Neck flexion and extension affect upper airway properties, and this led to the development of special pillows designed to keep the neck extended and head to the side. However, there are no data showing that this manipulation abolishes snoring.

Most studies dealing with positional effects address sleep apnea rather than nonapneic snoring. Very few studies deal specifically with snoring. Braver et al. (50, 54) studied asymptomatic snorers with mild sleep apnea but were unable to find any difference in the number of snores between sleeping on the side and sleeping on the back. This does not necessarily imply lack of improvement in the perception of snoring, which may not correlate with objective measurement. However, it is also true that many patients referred because of snoring will generally snore in any position; this is why they were referred to the clinic in the first place.

Although, as mentioned previously, rigorous scientific data showing beneficial effect of body or head position on snoring are lacking, this treatment is so benign and inexpensive that patients whose bed partners report positional snoring should be advised to try sleeping on the side or with the head elevated to 45 degree angle.

Medications

No medications are available to cure snoring. However, since nasal obstruction is a risk factor for snoring (55), several medications have been used to relieve it in the hope that snoring will be ameliorated. Nasal decongestants and corticosteroids are the ones employed most commonly. There is a marked paucity of scientific data to determine if these medications are useful. They should not be used indiscriminately in all snorers, but patients with nonanatomical nasal obstruction should be given a trial of these nasal sprays. Other medications used to treat snoring include protriptyline (in the hope that it will increase pharyngeal muscle tone and reduce compliance) and intranasal lubricants (which may reduce the turbulence in the upper airways). However, there are too few data to recommend the use of these agents at this time for treatment of snoring.

Nasal Dilators

Mechanical nasal dilators, first introduced at the turn of the 20th century, achieved considerable popularity in the late 1980s and 1990s, with the realization that nasal obstruction, particularly in the region of the nasal valve, is associated with sleep-disordered breathing. The two most popular nasal dilators, that received most attention in the literature, are Nozovent (56) and Breathe Right (57). The former is a reusable internal dilator that fits into the nostrils, dilating the region of the nasal valve; the latter is a disposable, one-time only external dilator with adhesive backing that fits over the ridge of the nose. Both types of dilators reduce measured nasal resistance and increase flow in awake individuals. Their effect on snoring is variable. Subjective results indicate improvement in snoring in up to 50% of patients. Objective results, obtained during polysomnographic monitoring of snoring sounds with and without nasal dilators, indicate no change in snoring index (58, 59).

Both dilators are well tolerated, are inexpensive, and have no side effects. Since they may improve snoring in some patients, it is reasonable to offer these devices for 2 weeks as a therapeutic trial.

Nasal CPAP

Nasal CPAP is the mainstay of treatment of sleep apnea and is described in greater detail elsewhere in this chapter. It is well known that application of positive pressure will relieve snoring as well as sleep apnea. There are no systematic long-term studies regarding acceptance of nasal CPAP as treatment for nonapneic snoring. Most nonapneic snorers regard nasal CPAP as an 'overkill' and are reluctant to accept this treatment. There is some objective information regarding CPAP compliance in nonapneic snorers, obtained usually as a part of other investigations (42). Only a minority of nonapneic snorers (about 20%) accept nasal CPAP, using it less than 3 hours/night.

Poor compliance with CPAP clearly presents a problem in recommending it as treatment of choice to nonapneic snorers with UARS. Patient education and an opportunity of gradual acclimatization with CPAP help to improve the tolerance. It is important to have properly trained personnel (usually a respiratory technologist) who can deal with patients' questions and complaints. This may improve compliance enough to ensure that the patient accepts CPAP for at least 1 month as a therapeutic trial; if a definite subjective benefit is perceived by the patient at the end of the trial period, the compliance issue will become less important. If there is no subjective benefit, other therapeutic options must be considered.

The relationship between the pressure that abolishes snoring and that which resolves sleep apnea has not been well studied. Although intuitively it might seem that the former is lower than the latter, this is frequently not the case. There are many apneic persons on CPAP set to resolve sleep apnea (as determined during a titration study) whose bed partners continue to complain about snoring. It is not unusual that during CPAP titration study snoring is noted to disappear, but apneas persist. Consequently, disappearance of snoring is unreliable as a method for determining the optimum CPAP and cannot replace a proper CPAP titration study.

Oral Appliances

These appliances are currently considered to be the treatment of choice, in preference to CPAP, for nonapneic snoring. They are not new. Some of the earlier appliances, designed to keep the mouth closed and to force breathing through the nose, were first patented in the nineteenth century. However, their rise in popularity dates only to the last 20 years, undoubtedly due to the recognition of the sleep apnea syndrome and relatively limited alternatives available for successful treatment of this condition and its most common symptom—snoring.

Currently close to two dozen oral appliances are available on the market. They all fall into two categories: tongue-retaining devices (TRD) and mandibular advancement appliances (MAA). The latter can be either fixed or adjustable (i.e., allowing variable amounts of mandibular protrusion). Variable MAA are now the most commonly used oral appliances. They are custom-fitted to the patient's mouth, and the amount of mandibular protrusion is adjusted to achieve a compromise between patient's comfort and disappearance of snoring.

The efficacy of oral appliances as treatment of nonapneic snoring is not easy to assess. Most of the studies concentrated on sleep apnea; a review of 22 studies published between 1986 and 1998 describing the effects of MMA in 364 patients indicate a success rate (defined as reduction in AHI from greater than 10 to less than 10) of approximately 55%. In only some of these studies were questions included about snoring in the assessment protocol, and only in two studies (60,61) was snoring measured objectively. Both of these studies demonstrated subjective and objective reduction in snoring in all patients, suggesting a 100% response rate. However, both studies had a number of design limitations (highly selected group of patients, not all patients available for follow-up evaluation), which precludes accepting this perfect response rate as a norm for oral appliances. Other studies, of which one by Ferguson et al. (62) had the most rigorous design, indicate response rates of 55–100%.

Many technical advances have occurred in recent years with regard to the design and manufacturing of these appliances. The materials are soft, are nonirritating, and can be custom-fit for each individual patient. The design of some appliances allows the mandible to protrude by more than 15 mm without removing the appliance from the mouth. We still do not know about the long-term efficacy and side effects of these appliances, particularly whether they cause any changes in maxillomandibular alignment. They need to be fit individually for each patient, and proper follow-up evaluation to deal with possible patient discomfort must be assured. It is important that the appliance be constructed by a dentist who has a working knowledge of this field.

Considering the reported efficacy of these appliances, and given the technological advances that make these devices easily adjustable, more comfortable, and better accepted by the patients, they should be receiving increasing attention for treatment of nonapneic snoring.

SURGICAL TREATMENT

Surgery has traditionally been regarded as a very attractive approach to deal with snoring, as indicated by the fact that snorers are frequently referred to ear, nose, and throat surgeons for treatment of their snoring.

As a result, much has been published regarding the efficacy of surgical treatment of snoring. However, there are many shortcomings inherent in almost all of the studies. This not only makes the comparison and pooling of the results difficult but also inhibits interpretation of the results and inhibits giving a definitive answer regarding the efficacy of surgical treatment. These problems and differences in experimental design affect the final outcome and must be kept in mind when interpreting the results. They are summarized in Table 12.2.

Table 12.2 Factors affecting surgical results

1. Follow up time: snoring changes with length of time following surgery (short, unknown, variable)
2. Sleep studies: apneic subjects may respond differently than nonapneic subjects (not done at all, done only preoperatively or postoperatively, done only in selected patients)
3. Retrospective analysis: bias toward patients for whom follow-up data exist
4. Influence of confounding factors: weight, alcohol, drugs
5. Assessment of snoring: is it really improved? (objective measurement of sound; subjective assessment: self [discrete answers, analogue scales], bed partner; telephone versus face-to-face interview; improvement versus complete disappearance)
6. Surgical technique: is one surgeon (or procedure) better than another?

Surgery for snoring can be generally divided into nasal and pharyngeal. Let us first consider nasal surgery.

Nasal Surgery

Many snorers complain of nasal obstruction. Inability to breathe through the nose forces a more resistive route of breathing, resulting in a more negative intrathoracic pressure and turbulent flow through the upper airway. This facilitates vibrations of pharyngeal walls, leading to snoring. In theory, relief of nasal obstruction may promote nasal breathing in some patients, thus reducing snoring. In practice, however, the success of nasal surgery in abolishing snoring is far from perfect. Almost all of the published reports deal only with short-term results, which are generally very good, with up to 95% of patients reporting improvement or sometimes even complete relief of snoring. Nevertheless, with a few exceptions, there are virtually no studies that examined whether this beneficial effect persists beyond the first year postoperatively. In fact, anecdotal evidence suggests that it seldom does.

It is not possible to predict preoperatively which patients will respond to nasal surgery; neither static measurements of nasal structure (radiographic imaging) nor dynamic measurements of nasal function (rhinometry) serve as sufficiently reliable indicators of postoperative success. Consequently, it is prudent to adopt a conservative approach and reserve surgery only for snorers with anatomical nasal obstruction (deviated septum, nasal polyps, and similar problems).

Pharyngeal Surgery (nonlaser)

This is the most common surgical approach to treatment of snoring. The initial procedure described by Ikematsu (63) involved partial resection of the uvula, the soft palate, and mucosa of the posterior tonsilar pillars; the author of the study reported approximately 80% success rate . Fujita et al. (64) modified this procedure, which they termed uvulopalatopharyngoplasty (UPPP), applied it to snorers with sleep apnea, and reported that snoring was abolished in almost all patients. This initial report started almost an avalanche of UPPP investigations, most of them very descriptive and subjective, and generally favorable. Many modifications of the original technique have been described and used in small numbers of patients. The discussion below summarizes the combined results of pharyngeal surgery.

A sampling of 44 UPPP reports between 1981 and 1999, describing a total of 3730 snorers, indicates an average success rate of .84% (range, 18–100%) for improvement in snoring, This result must be interpreted with caution, in the context of all the caveats summarized above. High initial success rate may be more than halved (e.g., from 80% to less than 40%) with one additional year of follow-up evaluation. Although 90% of patients may report 'improvement.' only fewer than 20% of them will admit complete disappearance of snoring. Depending on the type of questions asked and whether a bed partner is present during the interview, there may be a substantive disagreement between the snorer and the bed partner regarding 'improvement.' Up to 10% of nonapneic snorers may develop sleep apnea (with or without snoring), which may go unnoticed if appropriate postoperative follow-up evaluation is not done (65).

There are no definite preoperative criteria to ensure success of UPPP for treatment of snoring. Various techniques are used for airway assessment during wakefulness and sleep, employed mainly for investigation of sleep apnea rather than nonapneic snoring. They include static imaging (e.g., cephalometry), dynamic imaging (e.g., fast computed tomography, ultrafast magnetic resonance imaging), and clinical assessment (e.g., Müller maneuver, simulated snoring). They are generally used only during wakefulness. Techniques of airway assessment used during sleep include nasendoscopy, pressure measurements along the airway to identify the site of significant narrowing or collapse, and ultrafast imaging. Based on the very limited information regarding their usefulness, none of them can be recommended for routine preoperative assessment, although individual clinics may have their own protocol utilizing these techniques.

Probably the most useful preoperative test is a sleep study, simply because it can identify snorers with sleep apnea who can therefore be offered a more successful treatment. Accumulated clinical experience suggests that pharyngeal surgery is most successful in patients with obvious anatomical abnormality (e.g., large tonsils) or in nonobese, young persons with idiopathic snoring and without other major health problems.

Immediate postoperative side effects of UPPP include pain, dysphagia, nasal reflux, hypernasal speech, and, rarely, significant bleeding. Most of them are self-limited and resolve within several weeks. Long-term side effects, mainly nasal speech and nasal regurgitation, are rare. Overall, the procedure is safe. The reluctance to offer it to patients as a treatment of choice stems from the uncertainty about its efficacy rather than fear of complications.

Pharyngeal Surgery (Laser)

In laser assisted uvulopalatoplasty (LAUP), modified resection of the uvula and soft palate is performed using laser rather than a scalpel, as in conventional UPPP. Two incisions are made vertically at the base of the soft palate along each side of the uvula; the tip of the uvula is vaporized. The palate incisions heal, causing contractions of the soft tissues, stiffening of the palate, and presumably reduction in vibrations.

Unlike the case in UPPP, there is generally no resection of pharyngeal or tonsilar tissue. The surgery is performed in an office setting with local anesthesia. It is done sequentially, during several office visits in 2–3 week intervals. The patient is given time for the incisions to heal and an opportunity to determine the effect of surgery on snoring. If snoring persists, further vaporization of the uvula and incisions of the palate are performed. The end point is reached either when the patient is satisfied with the result or technically when no further uvular or palatine surgery can be performed—whichever comes first.

This procedure, described initially by Kamami (66), gained tremendous popularity in North America in the early 1990s, because it offered an alternative to UPPP that did not require hospitalization, could be done without general anesthetic, was technically less complex than UPPP, was thought to be less painful and have fewer side effects, and was actively promoted by the laser industry. It became the procedure of choice for nonapneic snoring.

However, as North American experience with LAUP accumulated, a different picture began to emerge. First, it became clear that the procedure is not as pain-free as was initially thought; the pain may be quite severe, although self-limited and lasting only during the immediate postoperative period, no more than a few weeks. Second, the procedure is associated with similar complications as the conventional UPPP, although probably less frequently; Walker and Gopalsami (67) reported 3.5% overall complications rate in 754 LAUP procedures involving 541 patients. Lastly, and most importantly, the success rate of LAUP for treatment of nonapneic snoring is similar to that of conventional UPPP: a review of 26 studies published between 1990 and 1999 and involving almost 3000 patients indicates an improvement rate of 81–87%. The

only advantage of LAUP over conventional UPPP is the convenience of an office procedure and absence of general anesthesia.

The Standards of Practice Committee of the American Sleep Disorders Association, having reviewed the early literature on LAUP did not recommend the use of this procedure for treatment of sleep apnea but recommended it only for nonapneic snoring (68). It is possible that after the procedure a nonapneic snorer may develop sleep apnea without significant snoring. Since 20–65% of snorers may have sleep apnea, all candidates for LAUP should have a preoperative sleep study to rule out sleep apnea. They should also have regular postoperative follow-up evaluations with at least one postoperative polysomnogram within the first 6 months.

Other Surgical Procedures

Surgical procedures involving repositioning of the mandible are used for treatment of sleep apnea, but these are almost never considered for treatment of snoring. Consequently, we shall not discuss them here.

---

o—ₘ   Key points box 12.2

Management of snoring

- Habitual snoring warrants treatment because of its disruptive social effects and potential adverse health consequences.

- The management of snoring should include weight reduction in obese individuals and avoidance of alcohol intake.

- Several mechanical devices are available to reduce snoring, including nasal dilators and oral appliances. The efficacy of such devices is highly variable.

- Nasal continuous positive airway pressure during sleep is effective in abolishing snoring, but it is generally not acceptable to otherwise asymptomatic snorers.

- Pharyngeal surgery can be very effective in the treatment of snoring, but rates of success are highly variable and cannot be predicted in advance.

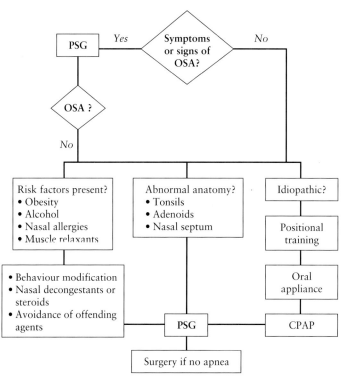

Fig 12.1 Investigation and treatment of habitual snorers. PSG, polysomnography; CPAP, continuous positive airway pressure.

Another recently described procedure is somnoplasty or ablation of the palatal tissue using radiofrequency (RF) waves. This simple, repeatable office procedure reduces the volume of the palate and presumably leads to palatal stiffening and reduction in snoring. There is only one peer-reviewed study describing this procedure in 22 snorers (69). Preliminary short-term results are favorable; the procedure appears to be safe and relatively effective. It reduced subjective snoring score by 77% in the patients studied. Obviously, at this stage it is too early to properly evaluate the usefulness of this procedure for treatment of snoring.

CONCLUSIONS

Snoring has traditionally been regarded only as a social nuisance. However, it is also a sign of a health hazard, being one of the most common symptoms of sleep apnea. It may share with OSAS some of its adverse health consequences, such as daytime dysfunction and possibly vascular disease. Definitive demonstration of the direct causal link between snoring and these health outcomes must await further studies. In the interim, habitual snorers referred to sleep clinic must be assessed to rule out sleep apnea, and investigated or treated according to the protocol summarized in Figure 12.1. If there is a surgically correctable anatomical lesion, baseline polysomnography should be performed followed by surgery. In the absence of surgically correctable lesion, and if non-invasive approaches are unsuccessful, polysomnography should be performed to rule out sleep apnea, and surgical approach discussed with patient.

REFERENCES

1. Kleitman N. Sleep and wakefulness. Chicago: University of Chicago Press, 1963.
2. Lugaresi E, Coccagna G, Farneti P, et al. Snoring. Electroenceph Clin Neurophysiol 1975; 39:59–64.
3. Guilleminault C, Tilkian A, Dement WC. The sleep apnea syndromes. Ann Rev Med 1976; 27:465–484.
4. Lugaresi E. Mondini S, Zucconi M, et al. Staging of heavy snorers disease: a proposal. Bull Eur Physiopathol Resp 1983; 19:590–594.

5. Guilleminault C, Stoohs R, Clerk A, et al. A cause of excessive daytime sleepiness: the upper airway resistance syndrome. Chest 1993; 104:781–787.

6. Robin IG. Snoring. Proc R Soc Med 1968; 61:575–582.

7. Stradling JR, Crosby JH. Relation between systemic hypertension and sleep hypoxemia and snoring: analysis in 748 men drawn from general practice. Br Med J 1990; 300:75–78.

8. Honsberg AE, Dodge RR, Cline MG, et al. Incidence and remission of habitual snoring over a 5- to 6-year period. Chest 1995; 108:604–609.

9. Lindberg E, Taube A, Janson C, et al. A 10-year follow up of snoring in men. Chest 1998; 114:1048–1055.

10. Hoffstein V, Mateika S, Anderson D. Snoring: Is it in the ear of the beholder ? Sleep 1994; 17:522–526.

11. Gislason T, Janson C, Tomasson K. Epidemiological aspects of snoring and hypertension. J Sleep Res 1995; 4: (Suppl 1):145–149.

12. Janson C, Gislason T, De Backer W, et al. Daytime sleepiness, snoring, and gastrooesophageal reflux amongst adults in three European countries. J Intern Med 1995; 237:277–285.

13. Young TB. Some methodological and practical issues of reported snoring validity. Chest 1991; 99:531–532.

14. Young T, Palta M, Dempsey J, et al. The occurrence of sleep-disordered breathing among middle-aged adults. N Engl J Med 1993; 328:1230–1235.

15. Quinn SJ, Daly N, Ellis PDM. Observation of the mechanism of snoring using sleep nasendoscopy. Clin Otolaryngol 1995; 20:360–364.

16. Gavriely N, Jensen O. Theory and measurement of snores. J Appl Physiol 1993; 74:2828–2837.

17. Huang L. Mechanical modeling of palatal snoring. J Acoust Soc Am 1995; 97:3642–3648.

18. Dalmasso F, Prota R. Snoring: analysis, measurement, clinical implications, and applications. Eur Respir J 1996; 9:146–159.

19. Isono S, Feroah TR, Hajduk EA, et al. Interaction of cross-sectional area, driving pressure, and airflow of passive velopharynx. J Appl Physiol 1997; 83:851–859.

20. Friberg D, Ansved T, Borg K, et al. Histological implications of a progressive snorers disease in an upper airway muscle. Am J Respit Crit Care Med 1998; 157: 586–593.

21. Skatvedt O. Continuous pressure measurements during sleep to localize obstructions in the upper airways in heavy snorers and patients with obstructive sleep apnea syndrome. Eur Arch Otorhinolaryngol 1995; 252:11–14.

22. Boudewyns AN, Van de Heyning PH, De Backer WA. Site of upper airway obstruction in obstructive apnea and influence of sleep stage. Eur Respir J 1997; 10:2566–2572.

23. Tami TA, Duncan HJ, Pfleger M. Identification of obstructive sleep apnea in patients who snore. Laryngoscope 1998; 108:508–513.

24. Deegan PC, McNicholas WT. Predictive value of clinical features for the obstructive sleep apnea syndrome. Eur J Respir Dis 1996; 9:117–124.

25. Crocker BD, Olson LG, Saunders NA, et al. Estimation of the probability of disturbed breathing during sleep before a sleep study. Am Rev Respir Dis 1990; 142:14–18.

26. Kump K, Whalen C, Tishler PV, et al. Assessment of the validity and utility of a sleep-symptom questionnaire. Am J Respir Crit Care Med 1994; 150:735–741.

27. Bliwise DL, Nekich JC, Dement WC. Relative valididty of self-reported snoring as a symptom of sleep apnea in sleep clinic population. Chest 1991; 99:600–608.

28. Waller PC, Bhopal RS. Is snoring a cause of vascular disease? An epidemiological review. Lancet 1989; 1:143–146.

29. Hoffstein V. Is snoring dangerous to your health? Sleep 1996; 19:506–516.

30. Lindberg E, Janson C, Gislason T, et al. Snoring and hypertension: a 10 year follow-up. Eur Respir J 1998; 11:884–889.

31. Lindberg E, Janson C, Svärdsudd K, et al. Increased mortality among sleepy snorers: a prospective population-based study. Thorax 1998; 53:631–637.

32. Young T, Finn L, Hla KM, et al. Snoring as a part of dose-response relationship between sleep-disordered breathing and blood pressure. Sleep 1996; 19:S202–S205.

33. Young T, Peppard P, Palta M, et al. Population-based study of sleep-disordered breathing as a risk factor for hypertension. Arch Intern Med 1997; 157:1746–1752.

34. Snoring and sleepiness. Editorial. Lancet 1985; 1:925–926.

35. Guilleminault C, Stoohs R, Duncan S. Snoring (I). Daytime sleepiness in regular heavy snorers. Chest 1991; 99:40–48.

36. Guilleminault C, Stoohs R, Clerk A, et al. A cause of excessive daytime sleepiness: the upper airway resistance syndrome. Chest 1993; 104:781–787.

37. Jennum P, Sjøl A. Self-assessed cognitive function in snorers and sleep apneics. An epidemiological study of 1,504 females and males aged 30–60 years: the Dan-MONICA II study. Eur Neurol 1994; 34:204–208.

38. Ulfberg J, Carter N, Talbäck M, et al. Excessive daytime sleepiness at work and subjective work performance in the general population and among heavy snorers and patients with obstructive sleep apnea. Chest 1996; 110:659–663.

39. Kim HC, Young T, Matthews CG, et al. Sleep-disordered breathing and neuropsychological deficits: a population-based study. Am J Respir Crit Care Med 1997; 156:1813–1819.

40. Whitney CW, Enright PL, Newman AB, et al. Correlates of daytime sleepiness in 4578 elderly persons: the cardiovascular health study. Sleep 1998; 21:27–36.

41. Martin SE, Engleman HM, Deary IJ, et al. The effect of sleep fragmentation on daytime function. Am J Respir Crit Care Med 1996; 153:1328–1332.

42. Engleman HE, Kingshott RN, Wraith PK, et al. Randomized placebo-controlled crossover trial of continuous positive airway pressure for mild sleep apnea/hypopnea syndrome. Am J Respir Crit Care Med 1999; 159:461–467.

43. Lofaso F, Goldenberg F, d'Ortho MP, et al. Arterial blood pressure response to transient arousals from NREM sleep in non-apneic snorers with sleep fragmentation. Chest 1998; 113:985–991.

44. Guilleminault C, Stoohs R, Shiomi T, et al. Upper airway resistance syndrome, nocturnal blood pressure monitoring, and borderline hypertension. Chest 1996; 109:901–908.

45. Boselli M, Parrino L, Smerieri A, et al. Effect of age on EEG arousals in normal sleep. Sleep 1998; 21:351–357.

46. Prazic M. Snoring and presbyacusis. Acta Otolaryngol 1973; 75:216–219.

47. Hoffstein V, Haight J, Cole P, et al. Does snoring contribute to presbycusis? Am J Respir Crit Care Med 1999; 159:1351–1354.

48. Bloom JW, Kaltenborn WT, Quan SF. Risk factors in general population for snoring: importance of cigarette smoking and obesity. Chest 1988; 93:678–683.

49. Strobel RJ, Rosen RC. Obesity and weight loss in obstructive sleep apnea: a critical review. Sleep 1996; 19:104–115.

50. Braver HM, Block AJ, Perri MG. Treatment for snoring: combined weight loss, sleeping on the side, and nasal spray. Chest 1995; 107:1283–1288.

51. Executive summary of the clinical guidelines on the identification, evaluation, and treatment of overweight and obesity in adults. Arch Intern Med 1998; 158:1855–1867.

52. Issa FG, Sullivan CE. Alcohol, snoring, and sleep apnea. J Neurol Neurosurg Psychiatry 1982; 45:353–359.

53. Wetter DW, Young TB, Bidwell TR, et al. Smoking as a risk factor for sleep-disordered breathing. Arch Intern Med 1994; 154;2219–2224.

54. Braver HM, Block AJ. Effect of nasal spray, positional therapy, and combination thereof in the asymptomatic snorer. Sleep 1994; 17:516–521.

55. Young T, Finn L, Kim H. Nasal obstruction as a risk factor for sleep-disordered breathing. J Allergy Clin Immunol 1997; 99:S757–S762.

56. Petruson, B. Snoring can be reduced when nasal airflow is increased by the nasal dilator Nozovent. Arch Otolaryngol Head Neck Surg 1990; 116:462–464.

57. Ulfberg J, Fenton G. Effect of Breathe Right nasal strip on snoring. Rhinology 1997; 35:50–52.

58. Hoffstein V, Mateika S, Metes A. Effect of nasal dilation on snoring and apneas during different stages of sleep. Sleep 1993; 16:360–365.

59. Liistro G, Rombaux P, Dury M, et al. Effect of Breathe Right on Snoring: a polysomnographic study. Respir Med 1998; 92:1076–1078.

60. O'Sullivan RA, Hillman DR, Mateljan R, et al. Mandibular advancement splint: an appliance to treat snoring and obstructive sleep apnea. Am J Respir Crit Care Med 1995; 151:194–198.

61. Stradling JR, Negus TW, Smith D, et al. Mandibular advancement devices for the control of snoring. Eur Respir J 1998; 11:447–450.

62. Ferguson KA, Ono T, Lowe A, et al. A randomized cross-over trial of an oral appliance vs. nasal-continuous positive airway pressure in the treatment of mild-moderate obstructive sleep apnea. Chest 1996; 109:1269–1275.

63. Ikematsu T. Study of snoring. Ther J Jpn Otorhinolaryngol 1964; 64:434–435.

64. Fujita S, Conway W, Zorick F, et al. Surgical correction of anatomic abnormalities in obstructive sleep apnea syndrome: uvulopalatopharyngoplasty. Otolaryngol Head Neck Surg 1981; 89:923–934.

65. Friberg D, Carlsson Nordlander B, Larsson H, et al. UPPP for habitual snoring: a 5-year follow up with respiratory sleep recordings. Laryngoscope 1995; 105:519–522.

66. Kamami YV. Laser CO_2 for snoring—preliminary results. Acta Otorhinolaryngol Belg 1990; 44:451–456.

67. Walker RP, Gopalsami C. Laser-assisted uvulopalatoplasty: postoperative complications. Laryngoscope 1996; 106:834–838.

68. Standards of Practice Committee of the American Sleep Disorders Association. Practice parameters for the use of laser-assisted uvulopalatoplasty. Sleep 1994; 17:744–748.

69. Powell NB, Riley RW, Troell RJ, et al. Radiofrequency volumetric tissue reduction of the palate in subjects with sleep-disordered breathing. Chest 1998; 113:163–174.

PART FOUR
COMPLICATIONS

13

NEUROPSYCHIATRIC AND BEHAVIORAL COMPLICATIONS OF OBSTRUCTIVE SLEEP APNEA SYNDROME

Christian Guilleminault and Luciana Palombini

INTRODUCTION: DYSFUNCTIONAL BREATHING DURING SLEEP

Many different factors can contribute to partial or complete occlusion of the upper airway during sleep. The presence of familial aggregates of subjects with this abnormal occlusion during sleep indicates that genetic as well as environmental risk factors are involved (1, 2). An abnormal degree of occlusion of the upper airway during sleep implies that the normal coordination between inspiratory and upper airway dilator muscles during sleep is inappropriate, with a dysfunction of the careful balance that normally exists in nonaffected subjects. The factors that lead to this dysfunction are still poorly understood and rarely investigated. This dysfunction may exist very early in life. Infants 3 to 6 weeks old have been shown to have obstructive sleep apnea syndrome (OSAS) and hypopnea and abnormal inspiratory efforts during sleep (3, 4). The fact that this dysfunction is seen during a specific state of alertness (i.e., sleep) indicates that a specific neuronal condition is necessary for the phenomenon to occur. The interaction between the neuronal status and the development of the dysfunction, however, is mostly observational. Despite its vagueness, terminology such as 'instability of the controlling neurological network' has been used when considering apneas at sleep onset.

SLEEP STAGES AND AROUSALS

There are some established facts: in nonobese subjects, apneas and hypopneas are more commonly seen during stage I and II non–rapid eye movement (NREM) sleep, but are much less frequently noticed during stage 4 NREM sleep (5). In subjects with an abnormal increase in respiratory efforts ('upper airway resistance syndrome' or UARS), greater inspiratory effort is seen in stages 3–4 NREM sleep without alpha electroencephalographic (EEG) arousal than during stages 1 and 2 NREM sleep, indicating that the arousal threshold is different depending on the NREM sleep stage. It also appears that there is a lesser occurrence of classic apneas and hypopneas during slow wave sleep than during stages 1–2 NREM sleep. These observations have led to speculation that the stimuli associated with dysfunctional breathing during sleep will be more likely to induce a cortical EEG arousal in the so-called 'light sleep' stages (1–2 NREM sleep) than in slow wave sleep. It is only very recently, with the use of spectrum analysis of the EEG, that this speculation has received some support (see below).

In some normal weight subjects, apneas and hyponeas are observed only during NREM sleep and not during REM sleep (6). The absence of occlusion phenomenon during REM sleep in these subjects has been attributed to 1) REM sleep–related muscle atonia, which causes the action of the inspiratory accessory muscles to cease and leads to a decrease in the 'sucking' pressure applied on the upper airway dilators; and 2) a different control of ventilation during REM sleep.

Why such 'improvement' is not seen in overweight subjects has also been speculated to be related to the muscle atonia of REM sleep, with a greater chance for the fatty pads to express lateral pressure on the upper airway. This pressure is due to the disappearance of tone in the muscles that make up the lateral walls and leads to a further mechanical narrowing of the airway. Muscle atonia would also affect the intercostal muscles and the abdominal muscles, which have been shown to contract during expiration in the NREM sleep of obese OSAS subjects. During REM sleep, abdominal obesity leads to a flattening of the diaphragm in a supine subject and a further reduction in tidal volume with an increased perfusion-ventilation mismatch. These hypotheses have received some support from studies considering breathing during

REM sleep in normal and obese subjects (which have demonstrated a mild reduction of tidal volume and a slight increase in breathing frequency during REM sleep in normal subjects), and from investigations of abdominal muscle activity during NREM and REM sleep. But once again, little work has been done here.

○┐ Key points box 13.1

Sleep and breathing

- Sleep-disordered breathing is always associated with abnormal respiratory efforts during sleep, which have an impact on the sleeping EEG.
- REM sleep is associated with a different neuronal firing pattern than NREM sleep. Therefore, sleep-disordered breathing that is present in NREM sleep may be absent in REM sleep or indicated only by an increase in breathing frequency.

VICIOUS CYCLES

The dysfunction during sleep may also be related to progressive impairment of specific reflexes during sleep. The appearance of a full-blown syndrome may involve progressive blunting of specific neuronal responses, leading to a 'vicious cycle' (7). Experiments have demonstrated that sleep deprivation blunts arousal responses and worsens OSAS, increasing the duration and the frequency of abnormal breathing events. Alcohol and central nervous system depressant drugs have been shown to induce similar changes (8–11). Alcohol seems to act by affecting the timing of the reflex contractions of the upper airway dilators. Normally, the upper airway dilators must begin their contraction at least one synaptic time (i.e., 500 ms) before the beginning of the contraction of the diaphragm. This coordinated reflex will prevent an abrupt application of a negative intrathoracic (and transpharyngeal) pressure on an unprepared pharyngeal region. This coordination is impaired by alcohol (and possibly by central nervous system depressant drugs). Impaired coordination of this reflex has also been induced experimentally in subjects treated with diaphragmatic pacing or with poncho or currasse negative pressure ventilators (12,13). In these last cases, the inspiration is artificially triggered at the periphery, without involvement of the subcortical structures

responsible for an integrated respiratory response, and, as with alcohol, the abrupt application of a negative intrathoracic pressure on the unprepared pharynx leads to an obstructive sleep hypopnea and, sometimes, to a complete apnea.

The Stockholm group recently reported on a series of investigations demonstrating the existence of another vicious cycle (14–16). Systematic investigations of the pharyngeal region have shown that OSAS patients have abnormal palatal sensory responses, particularly to thermic stimuli, and show histological evidence of peripheral neuropathy in the tissues obtained after uvulopalato pharyngoplatsy (UPPP). The hypothesis is that snoring (a vibratory phenomenon), the 'sucking' of the tissues related to the abnormally high negative transpharyngeal pressure, and the ensuing local but repetitive edema are responsible for the neurological lesions and neurophysiological consequences.

These last findings may support the hypothesis of a progressive worsening of poor respiratory coordination on an abnormal anatomical terrain. The progressive worsening would be related to development of a dysfunction of the neuronal control of an integrated reflex responsible for maintaining the patency of the upper airway during sleep, further worsened by development of a local peripheral neuropathy. The initial mechanism, however, has not been explained.

EARLY RECOGNITION OF RISK FACTORS FOR SLEEP-DISORDERED BREATHING

Studies in infants with obstructive sleep apnea have identified at least three risk factors: 1) a morphotype (the dolichocephalic child), which may be related to developmental and, possibly, genetic factors; 2) low or absent hypoxic and hypercapnic responses, which have been shown to be associated with 'obstructive ventilation during sleep'; these reflex responses have been shown to be both genetically determined and environmentally induced (or at least significantly worsened) in older children and adults; and 3) the presence very early in life of environmental factors (most frequently upper airway allergies and infection) leading to abnormal nasal resistance.

The role of abnormal nasal resistance early in life has been extensively studied in the infant rhesus monkey. As can be seen, some of these risk factors involve the neuronal control of ventilation during sleep.

Risk factors for sleep-disordered-breathing
- Environmental factors can aggravate sleep-disordered breathing.
- Snoring may result in the development of an upper airway neuropathy.
- Risk factors for sleep-disordered breathing are both genetic and environmental and are often identifiable in early childhood.

NEUROBEHAVIORAL CHANGES AND ABNORMAL BREATHING DURING SLEEP

Many more investigations have been performed on subjects with a known occlusive breathing disorder during sleep to assess the impact of their abnormal respiratory pattern. One of the immediate problems of these studies is that, as seen above, there may be a progressive evolution of the dysfunction with the presence of a vicious cycle. The consequences observed may thus be placed on a continuum. Some of these consequences have been observed only in subjects with comorbid factors, such as obesity, which has its own complications, including hypoventilation during REM sleep or severe repetitive hypoxemia. To reconcile the different reports in the literature, it is necessary to clearly understand the notion that the dysfunction leading to the occlusive breathing during sleep may be an independent factor (as shown by regression analysis) in the occurrence of the studied symptoms, but the 'weight' of this factor in the constellation of problems presented by the studied subjects may not be very great. Unfortunately, many of the studies that have been performed investigated only a small number of subjects, or the stepwise and multiple regression analyses necessary to determine the strength of the reported findings were not available.

DAYTIME SLEEPINESS AND NOCTURNAL SLEEP

Daytime sleepiness is a landmark symptom of any occlusive sleep disorder and was emphasized in the initial descriptions of OSAS and UARS. Daytime sleepiness was the symptom that initiated the first efforts to understand abnormal breathing during sleep, in an attempt to identi-

fy the different types of patients encomposed by the term 'pickwickian syndrome' (17, 18). Many studies have indicated the difficulty of subjectively recognizing and objectively quantifying sleepiness. Patients will often use terms such as 'fatigue' and 'tiredness' to describe the consequences of sleepiness. Physicians may also have difficulty recognizing daytime sleepiness. In one study, many women with a sleep-related breathing disorder were found to have been classified by previous physicians as having 'chronic fatigue syndrome' or 'depression' instead of sleepiness (19).

Subjective Scales to Evaluate Sleepiness

The most commonly used scale for the evaluation of sleepiness is the Epworth Sleepiness Scale (ESS). It was initially studied on a small group of OSAS subjects. Some of the instructions in the ESS, however, raise questions about its value; for example, it asks subjects who do not regularly perform one of the studied activities (such as driving) to imagine the activity and its consequences. Studies by other groups have been unable to clearly determine what this scale really measures. The scale, however, is widely used, probably because it is easy to administer. Considering this widespread use, it would be worth doing a larger population study to see its distribution. Other scales, such as the Stanford Sleepiness Scale (SSS), are harder to administer, requiring the collection of many data points during one day. The Karolinska Sleepiness Scale (KSS) does not require as much effort, but, like the SSS, it investigates one specific day, whereas the ESS has a more general goal: it considers an overall behavior pattern which, by comparison, is vague in terms of daily variability.

Objective Tests to Evaluate Sleepiness

The objective tests used to evaluate sleepiness are said to reflect the artificial conditions under which they are administered. The most commonly used, the Multiple Sleep Latency Test (MSLT), investigates 'physiological sleepiness' during the day (20). The Maintenance of Wakefulness Test (MWT) tries to assess the ability to stay alert in a monotonous and sleep-inducing situation (21). These two test have been widely used, but their specificity and sensitivity have never been determined on a large population, despite many studies done on small subject groups. In the clinical field, these tests are criticized as being time consuming and effort intensive. Uncertainty of the limits of pathology and uncertainty about the changes associated with normal aging are more serious problems associated with the tests. Attempts have been made to develop more sensitive scoring methods for these tests and to develop shorter tests derived from the same premises (22–24).

Tests that investigate reaction time and lapses have also been used to study sleepiness. The use of the simple reaction time test led to the development of two commercially available computer-based portable systems (25). Once again, however, there have been few publications on their use in the study of occlusive sleep disorders. The underlying assumption is that impaired alertness results from sleep disruption, which is the consequence of the abnormal breathing during sleep. Many different factors can contribute to impaired alertness, however. Sleep disruption should be viewed as a 'risk factor' for impaired alertness, a factor that may become major if the fragmentation of sleep is chronic. Normal subjects who were submitted to experimentally induced sleep fragmentation at a rate of approximately one fragmentation per minute had abnormal scores on MSLTs and reaction time tests (26, 27). There is no information, however, on the effect of experimentally induced sleep fragmentation if the fragmentation is only intermittent during the night or involves longer intervals between stimuli.

Investigations of OSAS patients with chronic sleep fragmentation have shown disconcerting results when the investigation of nocturnal sleep was compared to MSLT results. No significant relationship was found between the number of abnormal breathing events (respiratory disturbance index RDI) and the results of the MSLT (28, 29). In one study, 25% of subjects with severe OSAS had very abnormal daytime results, with the abnormal presence of two or more sleep-onset REM periods during the five 15

min naps taken during the day (29). In these studies, however, the abnormal sleep during the daytime tests was significantly related to the amount of stage 1 NREM sleep during the night, not to the scored sleep fragmentation.

NOCTURNAL SLEEP SCORING AND SLEEP-DISORDERED BREATHING

One issue in the understanding of dysfunctional breathing during sleep is related to the current methods for scoring sleep records. Sleep was initially scored using a very reductionist technique, based on an atlas developed to study normal subjects (30). Over time, it became apparent that such an approach was inappropriate, and efforts were made to remedy these historical developments. The original scoring method required a minimum of 16 s of alpha EEG to define an 'arousal.' The current international definition requires a minimum of 3 s of alpha EEG in the central leads of the 10–20 international electrode placement system to define an arousal (31). Visual recognition of a 3 s EEG arousal is more difficult, however, and interscorer reliability has been poorer than with the previously defined scoring system.

Another issue is the improved definition of an 'occlusive breathing event.' Use of better monitoring technology (esophageal pressure, nasal canula) has refined the previously used definition, despite the fact that no consensus statement has been published. The notion that respiratory efforts may vary during sleep is obvious. The limit of an 'abnormal effort' during sleep, however, is difficult to define and may be sleep stage dependent if the EEG is the considered outcome variable, as noted above (32–34). Abnormal respiratory effort seems to be the consequence of oronasal flow limitation and its causes, but the recognition of the abnormality will depend on the technique used to recognize the flow limitation (32–34). Once again, some research has been done, but normative data are lacking.

POWER SPECTRUM ANALYSIS AND SLEEP-DISORDERED BREATHING

Instead of relying on visual analysis of the EEG to define sleep, several other techniques may be used. The most common and oldest techniques involve the use of spectral analysis of the EEG and period-amplitude analysis, or a combination of the two. As with any analytic technique, these approaches have their limitations and pitfalls, but they can give information on the disturbances of sleep

---

> **⊶ Key points box 13.3**
>
> Scales to evaluate sleepiness
> - Self-administered scales are often unreliable in evaluating daytime sleepiness.
> - The most commonly used scale (the Epworth Sleepiness Scale) has not been fully validated.
> - Objective tests of sleepiness must be interpreted on the basis of what the tests measure.

associated with occlusive breathing disorders during sleep. In a study performed by the Stanford group, a comparison was performed on age, sex, and BMI matched OSAS, UARS and normal subjects (35). Subjects were monitored with nocturnal polysomnography under the same conditions, with the same equipment and for the same sleep duration. The analysis was based on the EEG monitored in the central leads (C3 and C4). In this analysis, the total power in each frequency band was calculated to give a within-band window comparison over time. This method was used to evaluate the magnitude of the potential change within a specific frequency band over 30 s, in order to compare the change of activity to that of other frequency bands. This approach gives an evaluation of the change of the relative power over time with each frequency band.

Figure 13.1 is a graphic representation of $8\frac{1}{2}$ hours of recording of one matched subject in each of the groups. As can be seen, all the subjects with occlusive disorders during sleep, regardless of type, had significantly different results from controls (analyses of variance [ANOVA] p < 0.01). They had a significantly lower relative power density in the 'sleep spindle' band (12–14 Hz). The 'sleep hypopnea syndrome' patients (74), and the UARS patients had a significantly higher relative power density in the alpha EEG bands from 8 to 10 Hz and in the theta bands (6 and 7 Hz). The UARS patients had a greater power density in the 7 to 9 Hz bands than any other group (ANOVA p < 0.05). The authors hypothesized that respiratory efforts, when very intense, lead to alpha EEG arousals in the UARS subjects. Patients with OSAS slept during the apneic events, had more 'awakenings' (EEG arousals ≥ 30 s in duration) but fewer very short 'arousals,' and had a combined decrease in oxygen saturation and increase in respiratory efforts during the apneic events. Despite the small sample size, the analysis confirmed that subjects with different sleep-disordered breathing syndromes all suffer serious disturbances of nocturnal sleep, even though the nature of the disturbance differs with each syndrome.

POWER SPECTRAL ANALYSIS IN UARS— EEG SLEEP DISTURBANCES, ALPHA EEG, AND VISUAL SCORING

Another study, also performed by the Stanford group, focused only on subjects with UARS (36). A respiratory pattern, referred to by the authors as a 'crescendo,' had previously been defined based on esophageal pressure (Pes) monitoring during sleep. This pattern is particularly seen in stages 1 and 2 NREM sleep. It is characterized by a progressively more negative end inspiratory esophageal pressure with each successive breath (a 'crescendo' requires a minimum of three successive breaths but usually consists of more) (37). The first breaths in the 'crescendo' are not associated with an abnormal flow limitation, simultaneously monitored with the help of a face mask and a pneumotachograph. Abnormal airway resistance and flow limitation usually occur in the one or two breaths preceding a visually scored alpha EEG arousal (32, 37). This EEG change is associated with a decrease in respiratory effort, as seen on the esophageal pressure curve. This change has been called 'Pes reversal.' In the study, all 'crescendos' in stage 2 NREM sleep in the different recordings were identified. The related sleep EEG was carefully scored, and the 30 s before and after the Pes reversal were visually identified for study (36). The visual scoring revealed that not all crescendos were terminated by a visually scored alpha EEG arousal. Crescendos either 1) terminated in an arousal; 2) terminated without an arousal but with an associated increase in chin muscle tone; or 3) terminated without such changes. Spectral analysis of the central leads of the EEG performed on the 30 s prior to and after the Pes reversal indicated some common features. At 30 s before the Pes reversal, the EEG showed normal stage 2 NREM sleep and stayed that way for two or sometimes three breaths. There was thereafter a decrease of the relative power of the 12 to 14 Hz band (sleep spindles). An increase in the relative power in the delta (0.5 to 2.5 Hz) band occurred as a next step and peaked at the time of the Pes reversal. This was a significant change seen in all subjects.

The analysis also revealed differences is relationship to the visual scoring at the time of and after the Pes reversal. A significant increase in the relative power of the alpha and beta bands was seen in the events that led to an EEG arousal and in events that were associated with a small burst of chin electromyographic (EMG) waves. Alpha and beta EEG changes were greater in events ending in EEG arousal, and the changes involved more breaths after the Pes reversal. No significant increase in the relative power of the alpha and beta bands was noted in events that terminated without an

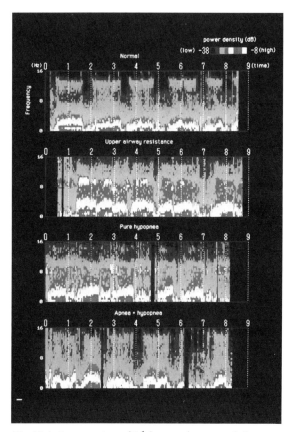

Fig 13.1 *Presentation of $8\frac{1}{2}$ hours of nocturnal sleep recording in four age, sex, and BMI matched subjects (three different sleep-disordered breathing conditions and one normal control). Long 'awakenings' and body movement – related EEG artifacts were deleted visually prior to performing fast Fourier transformation (FFT) analysis. A Hamming window was applied. The power within each 5 s window was normalized to the total power of all windows during a 30 s epoch for the respective bands. Frequencies in Hertz are presented on the ordinate (y) axis; time in hours is presented on the abscissa (x) axis. The 0.1 to 0.5 Hz range was not investigated due to the possibility of artifacts. The color scale is indicative of the relative power of the different frequency bands studied, from 0.5 to 16 Hz (see text). (From Guilleminault C, Kim YD, Horita M, et al. Power spectral deep EEG findings in patients with obstructive sleep apnea and upper airway resistance syndrome. Clin Neurophysiol 1999; Suppl. 50:118.)*

arousal or an associated increase in chin EMG waves, despite a Pes reversal. The increase in the relative power of the delta band, however, was significantly greater even after the Pes reversal (36).

There was also an interaction between the type of the EEG change that was noted at the time of the Pes reversal and in the following breaths. Despite the fact that a Pes reversal occurred in all three conditions, there was a significantly smaller decrease in esophageal pressure (i.e., persistence of a higher respiratory effort) when only the relative power of the delta band increased. In these instances, a new crescendo started immediately.

In summary, a greater reduction of respiratory effort occurred when the relative power of the alpha band significantly increased at Pes reversal, and normal breathing persisted for a significantly longer period when this pattern was noted. The study, thus, indicated that an increase in the relative power of alpha band may occur without a visually scored alpha EEG arousal, and that an increase in the relative power of the delta band and a disappearance of the sleep spindle band occur earlier and may be an indication of much earlier sleep disturbance not visually seen.

OVERALL EEG CHANGES AND RELATIONSHIP TO GOOD SLEEP

The presence of sleep spindles has been associated with a decrease in body movements (38) and with the blocking of externally applied sleep disturbing noises (39). The presence of sleep spindles has been considered an index of a good quality sleep. Increased respiratory efforts eliminate this pattern and probably leave the cortex more vulnerable to stimulation. The question of what the increase in relative power in the delta bands means is unsolved. It has been considered to be an expression of the cortical stimulation response to the subcortical structures to avoid arousal. It seems to be an unadapted response as far as breathing effort is concerned, as abnormal breathing immediately reoccurs. All of these responses are associated with an increase in heart rate in subjects without autonomic nervous system lesions (40). This suggests that the use of heart rate to dissociate these complex responses is inadequate. But further studies are required, as investigation of EEG components may also reveal more visually scored computer analyzed R-R intervals.

Future of EEG Analysis

Currently, most EEG investigations involve linear analysis techniques. Even though studies considering interhemispheric correlation and EEG coherence have not been performed on subjects with occlusive breathing disorders during sleep, these linear analysis techniques will have limitations. To bring further information on brain functioning, we may apply spatiotemporal pattern analysis. The neuronal network is modified differently depending on the condition during sleep. This activity is always in some state of disequilibrium. Biological signals, such as the EEG, are unlikely to remain stationary over long intervals. Nonlinear analysis (i.e., looking for chaotic attractors) is probably a better approach to understanding not only the sleep disturbance related to breathing during sleep but also the reported impaired responses to cognitive tests. The absence of a time series long enough to remain stationary over a sufficient period of time is a difficulty that has to be resolved before having a very appropriate way of investigating a 'change of state' (increased respiratory effort, for example). New tools have been proposed, however, to investigate the global structures of attractor, reconstructed from very short time series. Linear mode complexity is an example of these tools. Such new approaches have the best chance of bringing information on the changes occurring in the cortical neurological network, using the EEG as an index of these changes (41, 42).

Cognitive Tests and Abnormal Breathing During Sleep

The literature investigating the impact of occlusive disorders during sleep has one major problem: often no clear dissociation was made between normoweight and obese patients. This is unfortunate, as obesity has its own impact, including oxygen desaturation. Neuropsychological tests are not without problems themselves, as learning effect is common and as circadian timing of the test administration has an impact on results. Neuropsychological testing usually includes a battery of tests to investigate different subsets of the cognitive process. However, certain tests that look at broad categories of cognition, such as attention, memory, and executive functions, may not be sensitive enough if a defect, induced by specific environmental factors (sleep-disordered breathing), leads to a disruption of a subcategory of a specific cognitive function. This means that if the right test is not performed, a specific impairment may be missed.

Several studies have looked at patients with repetitive obstructive sleep apnea as monitored by polygraphic recording during sleep, but commonly without having discremenated between OSAS patients and obese patients with an obstructive sleep apnea pattern. Most studies have explored attention, long and short memory spans, learning abilities, verbal fluency, planning and programming abilities, and categorizing abilities, among others (43–54). As pointed out by Naegele et al. (53), many of the neuropsychometric tests indicating abnormal results compared to age, sex and, sometimes, BMI matched controls involved mental processes supposedly associated with frontal neuronal networks. Patients made more errors on tests indicative of verbal and visual learning disability and reduced memory span, particularly short-term memory. They were also reported to have a decreased ability to initiate new mental processes and to inhibit

---

> ⚲ **Key points box 13.4**
>
> **Sleep EEG analysis**
>
> - Spectrum analysis of the nocturnal sleep EEG indicates that subjects with sleep-disordered breathing syndromes all suffer from sleep disturbances, but the nature of the EEG disturbance differs with each syndrome.
> - Visual scoring of sleep recordings often fails to recognize alpha EEG arousals.
> - A sleep disturbance may be indicated only by bursts of increased delta frequency.
> - The impact on breathing of changes in brain activity, indicated by EEG analysis, depends on whether alpha or delta bursts occur with the abnormal breathing effort.
> - The use of nonlinear EEG analysis will make it possible to determine dynamic changes in cortical networks resulting from sleep-disordered breathing; an approach that will be useful in assessing daytime sleepiness and cognitive impairment.

automatic ones, showing a trend toward perseveration and a decrease in planning abilities and in manual dexterity. Impairment of the ability to perform on certain simple tests, such as reaction time tests, leads some researchers to use these simple computer administered tests to appreciate the gross level of daytime impairment in sleep-disordered patients.

REACTION TIME AND EVOKED RESPONSES

The psychovigilance test (PVT), for example, in which subjects push a button to eliminate a rectangle that appears randomly, about 10 times over a 10 min period, on the top of a handheld microprocessor, has been widely used, including as an outcome measure of treatment (25). Other clinical neurophysiological tests have been administered, either on their own or in association with psychometric testing. Auditory event–related potentials, particularly changes in P 300 wave, have also been explored (55). PVT results in subjects with dysfunctional breathing during sleep have indicated the presence of lapses, slow response time, and an increased variability of response time, similar to what is seen in subjects who have been subjected to experimental sleep deprivation or alcohol intake above the legally defined limit for drunkenness. P 300 amplitude was observed to be significantly decreased while its latency was increased.

COGNITIVE DEFECTS AND THE ROLE OF COMORBIDITY

Different statistical manipulations suggested that sleep fragmentation and repetitive oxyhemoglobin desaturation were related to the observed cognitive defects, but this is a controversial issue. Some studies have emphasized the return to completely normal functioning with treatment with nasal CPAP; others, particularly those of Bedard et al. (48, 50) and Naegele et al. (54), have emphasized the persistence of cognitive dysfunction. When persistent dysfunction was noted, it involved short-term memory or planning abilities and manual dexterity. Unfortunately, the studies reporting persistence of cognitive impairment may have been flawed. Depending on the study, there was no objective evaluation of compliance with the prescribed treatment, nor was there any evaluation of the persistence of microarousals and the persistence of abnormal breathing efforts during sleep.

Finally, and most importantly, the subjects with residual problems were obese. Obesity has its own set of compli-

cations, and it is possible that the metabolic changes associated with obesity (particularly those linked to glucose and insulin metabolism) (56, 57) may have their own deleterious effect on brain functioning. Treatment with nasal CPAP would have no impact on the complications due to the comorbid associations. The attribution of the persistence of cognitive dysfunction, despite appropriate treatment, to the direct action of the occlusive sleep phenomenon needs further investigation. Strokes have also been seen in persons with sleep-disordered breathing, and occlusive sleep disorders are a risk factor for stroke. However, the cognitive dysfunctions reported here are not linked to a specific vascular territory, and the evaluation of the studied patients does not support the concept of microstroke as responsible for the reported persistent dysfunction.

Oπ Key points box 13.5

Sleep disordered breathing and cognitive functions

- Patients with sleep-disordered breathing may demonstrate abnormalities in tests of simple reaction time and in auditory evoked responses.
- The cognitive dysfunction that occurs in patients with sleep-disordered breathing usually improves with treatment; failure to do so may indicate the presence of comorbid factors.

MOOD AND OSAS

Depression was listed as one of the common findings in the initial description of OSAS (58). Since then, several studies have looked at the relationship between mood, OSAS, and effect of treatment with nasal CPAP (59–63). The reports have shown discrepancies in results. Some of these discrepancies may have been related to the instruments used to evaluate the mood disorder. Reynolds et al. (59), using DMS-3 (Diagnostic and statistical manual of mental disorders – 3rd edition) and investigating 25 men with polysomnographically defined OSAS, found that 40% of the subjects met the diagnostic criteria for an affective disorder. Interestingly, these authors indicated that 61% of the variance in depression rating could be explained by four variables: age, REM activity, REM sleep latency, and presence or absence of antihypertensive medication. Presence of this last factor could suggest a participation or the existence of a comorbity or a specific role of antihypertensive drugs in the presence of depression in OSAS. Millman et al. (61) had 55 patients with polysomnographically defined OSAS who completed the Zung Self Rating Depression Scale (SDS). These authors found that 25 subjects (45%) had SDS scores ≥ 50, which is consistent with depression. In contrast to the study of Reynolds et al. (59), however, the scores did not correlate with antihypertensive medications. Millman et al. did not correlate either with age, RDI, or oxygen saturation nadir. When subjects were divided into two groups, however, with an SDS score of 50 taken as a cut-off point, the group with SDS scores > 50 had a significantly higher RDI. The authors also indicated that after treatment with nasal CPAP, the group with SDS scores that were initially over 50 had significantly lower SDS scores. This last result was criticized due to absence of a control group or placebo CPAP.

Engleman et al. (51) had a prospective parallel group study with subjects randomly treated either conservatively or with nasal CPAP. Mood was again assessed with scales, and depression was a clear finding. Compared to conservatively treated and noncompliant CPAP subjects, the 14 subjects who complied with nasal CPAP treatment significantly improved their depression scores. Two or more recent studies enlarged the scope of the investigation, adding anxiety to depression. Borak et al. (62) investigated 20 OSAS subjects at baseline and again at 3 and 12 months. It is unclear how compliance to treatment was evaluated, and no control group was available. Once again, these authors found abnormal anxiety and depression scale scores in the majority of their OSAS subjects, with a significant and clinically relevant correlation between anxiety scores and the RDI. They could not, however, show a relationship between nasal CPAP use and improvement of anxiety and depression scores, although they did show improvement in cognitive test results.

The largest group study was reported by Pillar and Lavie (63). The evaluation of anxiety and depression was performed using the SCL-90 (symptom self-report inventory) questionnaire on 2271 patients (1977 men and 294 woman) with OSAS recognized by clinical evaluation and polysomnography. To deal with the great discrepancy in the number of men and woman, the study group was stratified into subgroups according to sex, age, and RDI. Anxiety and depression scores were found elevated in the two sexes, but there were no

BMI, RDI, or age related differences in anxiety, depression, or any of the other SCL-90 dimensions in men. The results were very different in women. Depression and anxiety scores were significantly higher in women than in men for all age groups and all levels of RDI. This sex difference is common in many illnesses, but the depression scores were higher in women with a high RDI than in women with a low RDI. The authors concluded that, in men, the existence of depression or anxiety was not correlated with the presence of OSAS, but that, in women, there was an association between higher anxiety and depression scores and the presence of severe OSAS.

These different studies support the concept that OSAS is associated with depression and anxiety, particularly in woman, with a relationship in this sex between severity of the psychiatric symptoms and severity of the breathing disorder (with RDI taken as an index of severity). In men, there is probably a relationship between the presence of depressive symptoms and sleep-disordered breathing in a subgroup of OSAS patients. The current investigations did not make it possible to define clearly the group of men with OSAS developing these depressive symptoms. There are preliminary indications that the symptoms of depression and anxiety may be relieved with appropriate treatment with nasal CPAP; however, these preliminary indications need to be confirmed by a well-constructed, placebo-controlled study.

PREVALENCE OF BEHAVIORAL PROBLEMS ASSOCIATED WITH SLEEP-DISORDERED BREATHING

Prevalence studies in the general population are few. Two teams (Gislason et al. [64, 65] and Ohayon et al. [66]) have performed general population studies. Another team (67) has performed a large cohort study and extrapolated the findings to the general population. But only the Ohayon et al. team (68, 69) has investigated the prevalence of abnormal behavior during sleep and the various associations with occlusive breathing disorders during sleep. These authors have studied the prevalence of night terrors, sleep walking, sleep paralysis and hypnagogic hallucinations on representative samples of the general population (15 years of age and older) of western European countries, and have determined their relationship to sleep-disordered breathing. Sleep paralysis was reported by 6.2% of the combined population of Germany and Italy; and 15% of this subgroup (0.93% of the general population) suffered some form of sleep-disordered breathing (69). The prevalence of night terrors, sleep walking, and confusional arousals was determined on a representative sample of the general population of the United Kingdom aged 15 years or older. Night terrors were reported by 2.2% of the sample, sleep walking by 2%, and confusional arousals by 4.2%. Night terrors, sleep walking, and confusional arousals associated with sleep-disordered breathing were reported by 0.2%, 0.08%, and 0.15% of the general population, respectively (68). Once mental disorders were eliminated, sleep-disordered breathing was the most common disorder associated with these parasomnias. The notion that sleep-disordered breathing should be looked for when these parasomnias are reported, however, is not common knowledge.

A last issue that has received little attention is the risk of violence from sleep. No population studies have been done on the prevalence of sleep-related nocturnal violence. Self-inflicted injuries or injuries to others are seen in association with night terrors, sleep walking, confusional arousals, and REM behavior disorder. Studies have indicated that being male and having a seizure disorder during sleep are two risk factors for sleep-related violence (70, 71). Sleep-disordered breathing can lead to

anoxic seizure (72), however, and the question has been raised as to the role of the added hypoxia in the occurrence of confusional status, which may lead to the injury of self or others. Any medicolegal evaluation for sleep-related abnormal behavior, including violence, must include monitoring for occlusive breathing disorders during sleep.

CONCLUSIONS

It was in 1975 that OSAS was first outlined, clearly indicating the presence of an entity affecting many subjects that did not fit the 'pickwickian syndrome' description. In 1977, a review of 25 patients with OSAS indicated that daytime tiredness, fatigue, and sleepiness were complaints in all subjects and that other behavioral problems were noted (58). Since that time, much progress has been made in our understanding of occlusive upper airway problems during sleep and EEG changes leading to and associated with these breathing abnormalities. Some of the other behavioral changes associated with sleep-disordered breathing have been confirmed, but more investigation is needed to understand the prevalence of these compliants and the mechanisms behind them.

REFERENCES

1. Redline S, Tosteson T, Tishler PV, et al. Studies in the genetics of obstructive sleep apnea: familial aggregation of symptoms associated with sleep-related breathing disorders. Am Rev Respir Dis 1992; 145:440–444.

2. Guilleminault C, Partinen M, Hollman K, et al. Familial aggregates in obstructive sleep apnea syndrome. Chest 1995; 107:1545–1551.

3. Guilleminault C, Ariagno R, Korobkin R, et al. Mixed and obstructive sleep apnea and near miss for SIDS: 2. 'near miss' and normal control infants: comparison over age. Pediatrics 1979; 64:882–891.

4. Guilleminault C, Stoohs R. From 'apnea of infancy' to obstructive sleep apnea syndrome in the young child. Chest 1992; 102:1065–1071.

5. Kraizci H, Hedner J, Dahlof P, et al. Effect of serotonin uptake inhibition on breathing during sleep and daytime symptoms in obstructive sleep apnea. Sleep 1999; 22:61–67.

6. Tilkian AG, Guilleminault C, Schroeder JS, et al. Hemodynamics in sleep induced apnea: studies during wakefulness and sleep. Ann Intern Med 1976; 85:714–719.

> **⊶ Key points box 13.6**
>
> **Moods in OSAS**
> - Sleep-disordered breathing is associated with depression and anxiety, particularly in women; but an etiological link has yet to be established.
> - The prevalence of neurobehavioral disturbances in sleep-disordered breathing is unknown, because of the lack of appropriate population studies.
> - After mental disorders, sleep-disordered breathing is the most common disorder associated with night terrors, sleep-walking, and confusional arousal. These parasomnias can be associated with violent behavior.

7. Guilleminault C. Diagnosis, pathogenesis and treatment of the obstructive sleep apnea syndromes. Adv Intern Med Pediatr 1985; 52:2–57.

8. Guilleminault C. Sleep apnea syndromes: impact of sleep and sleep states. Sleep 1980; 3:227–246.

9. Issa FG, et al. Alcohol, snoring and sleep apnea. J Neurol Neurosurg Psychiatry 1982; 45:353–359.

10. Bonora et al. Selective depression by ethanol of upper airway respiratory motor activity in cats. Am Rev Respir Dis 1984; 130:156–161.

11. Mendelsson WB, et al. Flurazepam induced sleep apnea syndrome in a patient with insomnia and mild sleep-related respiratory changes. J Nerv Ment Dis 1981; 169: 261–264.

12. Quera-Salva MA, Guilleminault C. Post-traumatic central sleep apnea in a child. J Pediatr 1987; 110:906–909.

13. McNicholas WT, Coffey M, Boyle T. Effects of nasal airflow on breathing during sleep in normal humans. Am Rev Respir Dis 1993; 147:620–623.

14. Friberg D, Ansved T, Borg K, et al. Histological indications of a progressive snorers disease in upper airway muscle. Am J Respir Crit Care Med 1998; 157:586–893.

15. Friberg D, Gazelius B, Hokfelt T, et al. Abnormal afferent nerve endings in the soft palatal mucosa of sleep apneoics. Regul Pept 1997; 71:29–36.

16. Friberg D, Gazelius B, Lindblad LE, et al. Habitual snorers and sleep apneoics have abnormal vascular reactions of the soft palatal mucoso on afferent nerve stimulation. Laryngoscope 1998; 108:431–436.

17. Gastaut H, Tassinari CA, Duron B. Etude polygraphique des manifestations épisodiques (hypniques et respiratoires) diurnes et nocturnes du syndrome du Pickwick. Rev Neurol (Paris) 1966; 2:167–186.

18. Gastaut H, Tassinari CA, Duron B. Polygraphic study of the episodic diurnal and nocturnal manifestations of the Pickwickian syndrome. Brain Res 1966; 2:167–186.

19. Guilleminault C, Stoohs R, Kim Y, et al. Sleep-related upper airway disordered breathing in women. Ann Intern Med 1995; 122:493–501.

20. Carskadon MA, Dement WC. The multiple sleep latency test: what does it measure? Sleep 1982; 5:S67–S72.

21. Mitler MM, Gujavarty KS, Browman C. Maintenance of wakefulness test: a polygraphic technique for evaluation of treatment efficacy in patients with excessive somnolence. Electroencephalogr Clin Neurophysiol 1982; 53:658–661.

22. Roth B, Nevsiloma S, Sonka K, et al. An alternative to the multiple sleep latency test for determining sleepiness in narcolepsy and hypersomnia: a polygraphic score of sleepiness. Sleep 1986; 9:243–245.

23. Roth B, Nevsiloma S, Sonka K, et al. A quantitative polygraphic study of daytime somnolence and sleep in patients with excessive diurnal sleepiness. Arch Suisse Neurol Neuropsychiatry 1984; 135:265–272.

24. Philip P, Ghorayeb I, Leger D, et al. Objective measurement of sleepiness in summer vacation long-distance drivers. Electroencephalogr Clin Neurophysiol 1997; 102:383–389.

25. Dinges DF, Powell JW. Microcomputer analyses of performance on a portable simple visual RT task during sustained operations. Beh Res Meth Instr Comp 1985; 17:652–655.

26. Bonnet MH. Effect of sleep disruption on sleep performance and mood. Sleep 1985; 8:11–19.

27. Philip P, Stoohs R, Guilleminault C. Sleep fragmentation in normals. Sleep 17:242–247.

28. Roth T, Hartse KM, Zorik F, et al. Multiple naps and the evaluation of daytime sleepiness in patients with upper airway sleep apnea. Sleep 1980; 3:425–440.

29. Guilleminault C, Partinen M, Quera-Salva MA, et al. Determinants of daytime sleepiness in obstructive sleep apnea. Chest 1988; 94:32–37.

30. Rechtschaffen A, Kales A. A manual of standardized terminology, techniques and scoring system for sleep stages of human subjects. Washington DC: US Public Health Service, US Government Printing Office, 1968.

31. American Sleep Disorders Association. Atlas task force: scoring of the EEG arousals—rules and examples. Sleep 1993; 15:173–184.

32. Guilleminault C, Stoohs R, Clerk A, et al. A cause of excessive daytime sleepiness: the upper airway resistance syndrome. Chest 1993; 104:781–787.

33. Hosselet JJ, Norman RG, Ayappa I, et al. Detection of flow limitation with a nasal canula/pressure transducer system. Am J Respir Crit Care Med 1998; 157:1461–1467.

34. Clark SA, Wilson CR, Satoh M, et al. Assessment of inspiratory flow limitation invasively and non-invasively during sleep. Am J Respir Crit Care Med 1998; 158:713–722.

35. Guilleminault C, Kim YD, Horita M, et al. Power spectral sleep EEG findings in patients with obstructive sleep apnea and upper airway resistance syndrome. Clin Neurophysiol 1999 (in press).

36. Guilleminault C, Beck J, Carillo O. EEG arousal and upper airway resistance syndrome. Electroencephalogr Clin Neurophysiol 1997; 103:501.

37. Guilleminault C, Kim YD, Stoohs R. Upper airway resistance syndrome. Oromaxillofac Surg Clin North Am 1995; 7:243–256.

38. Gaillard JM, Auber C. Specificity of benzodiazepine action on human sleep confirmed. Another contribution of automatic analysis of polygraphic recordings. Biol Psychiatry 1975; 10:185–197.

39. Yamadori H. Role of the spindles in the onset of sleep. Kobe J Med Sci 1971; 17:97–111.

40. Guilleminault C, Connolly S, Winkle R, et al. Cyclical variation of the heart in sleep apnea syndrome: mechanisms and usefulness of 24-hour electrocardiography as a screening technique. Lancet 1984; i:126–131.

41. Broomhead DB, King GP. Extracting qualitative dynamics from experimental data. Physica D 1986; 20:217–236.

42. Sirovich L. Chaotic dynamics of coherent structure. Physica D 1989; 37:126–145.

43. Berry DTR, Mebb WB, Block AJ, et al. Nocturnal hypoxia and neuropsychological variables. J Clin Exp Neuropsychol 1986; 8:229–238.

44. Findley L, Barth JT, Powers DC, et al. Cognitive impairment in patients with obstructive sleep apnea and association hypoxemia. Chest 1986; 90:686–690.

45. Greenberg GD, Watson RK, Deptula D. Neuropsychological dysfunction in sleep apnea. Sleep 1987; 10:254–262.

46. Telakivi T, Kajaste S, Pertinem M, et al. Cognitive function in middle-aged snorers and controls: role of excessive daytime somnolence and sleep related hypoxic events. Sleep 1988; 11:454–462.

47. Dederian SS, Bridenbaugh RH, Rajogopal KR. Neuropsychological symptoms in obstructive sleep apnea improve after treatment with nasal CPAP. Chest 1988; 94:1023–1027.

48. Bedard MA, Montplaisir J, Richer F, et al. Obstructive sleep apnea syndrome: pathogenesis of neuropsychological deficits. Clin Exp Neuropsychol 1991; 13:950–964.

49. Montplaisir J, Bedard MA, Richer F, et al. Neurobehavioral manifestation in obstructive sleep apnea syndrome before and after treatment with continuous positive airway pressure. Sleep 1992; 15 (Suppl):S17–S19.

50. Bedard MA, Montplaisir J, Malo J, et al. Persistent neuropsychological deficits and vigilance impairment in sleep apnea syndrome after treatment with continuous positive airway pressure. J Clin Exp Neuropsychol 1993; 15:330–341.

51. Engleman HM, Cheshire KE, Deary IJ, et al. Daytime sleepiness, cognitive performance and mood after continuous positive airway pressure for the sleep apnea-hypopnea syndrome. Thorax 1993; 48:911–914.

52. Jennum P, Sjol A. Self assessed cognitive function in snorers and sleep apneics. An epidemiological study of 1504 females and males aged 30 to 60 years: the Dan-MONICA II study. Eur Neurol 1994; 34:204–208.

53. Naegele B, Thouvard V, Pepin JL, et al. Deficits of cognitive executive functions in patients with sleep apnea syndrome. Sleep 1995; 18:43–52.

54. Naegele B, Pepin JL, Levy P, et al. Cognitive executive dysfunction in patients with obstructive sleep apnea syndrome after CPAP treatment. Sleep 1998; 21:392–397.

55. Rumbach L, Krieger J, Kurtz D. Auditory event-related potentials in obstructive sleep apnea: effects of treatment with nasal continuous positive airway pressure. Electroencephalogr Clin Neurophysiol 1991; 80:454–457.

56. Strohl KP, Novak RD, Singer W, et al. Insulin level, blood pressure and sleep apnea. Sleep 1994; 17:614–618.

57. Stoohs R, Facchini F, Guilleminault C. Insulin resistance and sleep-disordered breathing in healthy humans. Am J Respir Crit Care Med 1996; 154:170–174.

58. Guilleminault C, Tilkian A, Eldridge FL, et al. Sleep apnea syndrome due to upper airway obstruction: a review of 25 cases. Arch Intern Med 1977; 137:296–300.

59. Reynolds CF 3rd, Kupfer DJ, McEachran AB, et al. Depressive psychopathology in male sleep apneics. J Clin Psychiatry 1984; 45:287–290.

60. Bliwise DL, Yesavage JA, Sink J, et al. Depressive symptoms and impaired respiration in sleep. J Consult Clin Psychol 1986; 54:734–735.

61. Millman RP, Fogel BS, McNamara ME, et al. Depression as a manifestation of obstructive sleep apnea: reversal with nasal continuous positive airway pressure. J Clin Psychiatry 1989; 50:348–351.

62. Borak J, Cieslicki JK, Koziej M, et al. Effects of CPAP treatment on psychological status in patients with severe obstructive sleep apnoea. J Sleep Res 1996; 5:123–127.

63. Pillar G, Lavie P. Psychiatric symptoms in sleep apnea syndrome: effects of gender and respiratory disturbance index. Chest 1998; 114:697–703.

64. Gislason T, Revnisditir H, Kristbjarnarson H, et al. Sleep habits and sleep disturbances among the elderly: an epidemiologic survey. J Intern Med 1993; 234:31–39.

65. Gislason T, Almquist M, Eriksson G, et al. Prevalence of sleep apnea syndrome among Swedish men—an epidemiologic study. J Clin Epidemiol 1988; 41:571–576.

66. Ohayon MM, Guilleminault C, Priest RG, et al. Snoring and breathing pauses: results in the general population of the United Kingdom. Br Med J 1997; 314:860–863.

67. Young T, Palla M, Dempsey JA, et al. The occurrence of sleep-disordered breathing among middle age adults. N Engl J Med 1993; 328:1230–1235.

68. Ohayon M, Guilleminault C, Priest RG. How frequent are night terrors, sleep walking and confusional arousals in the general population? Their relationship to other sleep and mental disorders. J Clin Psychiatry 1999, (in press).

69. Ohayon M, Zulley Z, Guilleminault C, et al. Prevalence and pathological associations of sleep paralysis in the general population. Neurology 1999 (in press).

70. Guilleminault C, Moscovitch A, Leger D. Forensic sleep medicine, nocturnal wandering and violence. Sleep 1995; 18:740–748.

71. Guilleminault C, Leger D, Philip P, et al. Nocturnal wandering and violence: review of a sleep clinic population. J Forensic Med 1998; 43:158–163.

72. Cirignota F, Zucconi M, Mondini S, et al. Cerebral anoxic attacks in sleep apnea syndrome. Sleep 1989; 12: 400–404.

73. Guilleminault C, Eldridge F, Simmons FB, et al. Sleep apnea syndrome: can it induce hemodynamic changes? West J Med 1975; 123:7–16.

74. Gould GA, Whyte KE, Airlie M, et al. The sleep hypopnea syndrome. Am Rev Resp Dis 1988; 137: 895–898.

14

CARDIOVASCULAR COMPLICATIONS OF OBSTRUCTIVE SLEEP APNEA SYNDROME

John R Stradling and Robert J O Davies

INTRODUCTION

The interactions between irregular breathing at night and the cardiovascular system are fascinating examples of human physiology in action. Unraveling both the acute effects of apneas and the longer-term effects has kept many minds occupied and provided the basis for a large amount of research over the years. The fascination lies in the short-term changes in blood pressure (BP) and cardio-vascular perturbation with each apnea (Fig. 14.1) as well as the possibility of longer-term effects that might con-tribute to a person's risk of myocardial infarction or stroke. Whereas much is known about the acute cardio-vascular changes, many of the proposed longer-term effects remain largely hypothetical and unproven. This chapter reviews what is, and is not, known and tries to synthesize a view that will inform the practicing clinician. This will have some relevance to looking after current patients with sleep apnea, but more importantly will allow the clinician to assess any future studies claiming

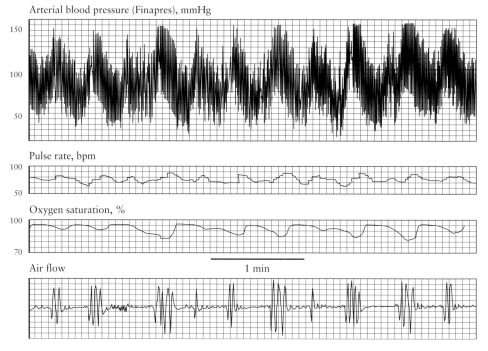

Fig 14.1 *Five minute tracing of beat-to-beat arterial BP during about 9 cycles of OSAS. Note the large rises in BP coincident with the return of breathing and the period of hypoxemia (from a finger oximeter). Note also the simultaneous oscillations in heart rate.*

that sleep apnea is the occult contributor to much unexplained cardiovascular disease.

Any future proof of such a relationship could have profound effects on the management to sleep apnea, which at present is treated largely because of the disabling hypersomnolence brought about by sleep fragmentation. At present the treatment of OSAS with continuous positive airway pressure (CPAP) would probably not be accepted by many asymptomatic patients in order to reduce some small future risk of stroke. However, once a simpler and less unpleasant treatment is available, this will become an issue, similar to the treatment of asymptomatic hypertension with drugs.

ACUTE SYSTEMIC CARDIOVASCULAR CHANGES IN OSAS

Obstruction to airflow occurs as 'awake' muscle tone is withdrawn from pharyngeal dilator muscles and improves when this wakefulness-related muscle tone returns. Thus, fluctuating central nervous system activity during sleep is an integral part of the syndrome and has important effects on the cardiovascular control centres. In addition, in most patients with OSAS, there is a reflex increase in inspiratory effort during the obstructed periods, producing larger swings in pleural pressure than are normally present. These larger swings in pleural pressure influence the pressures in and around the heart and great vessels. Finally, the later consequences of a period of obstructed breathing, hypoxia and hypercapnia, will reflexly influence cardiovascular control mechanisms. Disentangling the relative effects of these changes on heart rate, blood pressure, and cardiac output during obstructive apneas has been difficult.

INSPIRATORY EFFORT

During the course of an obstructive apnea there is usually gradually increasing inspiratory effort. This results probably from three mechanisms. First there will be an immediate increase in inspiratory muscle firing from muscle spindle feedback, then an almost immediate effect resulting from a reduced inflation reflex, and finally a slow increase due to stimulation of the chemoreceptors by the evolving hypercapnia and hypoxia. Each frustrated inspiratory effort is like a short-lived Müller maneuver with a recovery period in between, during expiration. The length of the inspiration is too short for much in the way

of immediate reflex compensatory mechanisms to respond. This means that each fall in intrathoracic pressure is transmitted almost fully to the peripheral arterial system (1). Because the heart is in the chest, any falls in intrathoracic pressure similarly lower intracardiac pressures relative to extrathoracic structures. Hence, an inspiratory effort of 40 mm Hg will lower arterial pressure by about 40 mm Hg. This means there will be less arterial perfusion pressure available, and the left ventricle (LV) will not empty itself as well; thus, the ejection fraction will fall. This produces an increase in both the afterload and preload to the LV as well as a demonstrable increase in its volume (2, 3). Because the expiratory phase removes this subatmospheric pleural pressure and allows recovery, the effects on LV function are not as great as during a held Müller maneuver.

The intermittent subatmospheric pressures may also increase venous return into the thorax by 'aspirating' blood from the venae cavae. The extent to which this happens is debated and may depend on the initial pressure in the venae cavae. If the venous filling pressure is high enough to prevent the development of a subatmospheric pressure within the venae cavae at their point of entry into the thorax, more blood will be aspirated. There is some evidence for this with leftward displacement of the interventricular septum from an enlarging right ventricle during an apnea (4). However, if the intrathoracic vena caval pressure falls to below atmospheric during an obstructed inspiration, a 'choke point' will develop due to collapse of the vessel at the point of entry into the thorax, limiting any extra inflow (5, 6). With LV outflow reduced, and right ventricle (RV) inflow increased (assuming incomplete recovery during the expiratory phase), there will tend to be an increase in the total thoracic blood volume, providing an increase in preload to the LV at the end of each apnea.

HYPOXIA AND AROUSAL FROM SLEEP

In addition, during the apnea the average BP and heart rate tend to fall overall. Part of this must be associated with the return to sleep, which normally lowers BP via a drop in cardiac output, with a change in baroreceptor set point (7). Additionally, part of the explanation will be the transmission of increasingly subatmospheric pleural inspiratory pressures through to the arterial system (mentioned above). Part of the bradycardia is probably vagally induced and is likely to be due to the 'diving reflex' (8). This is most obvious in diving mammals and acts to preserve brain oxygenation (9). In the presence of apnea (no pulmonary infla-tion) and trigeminal nerve stimulation, hypoxia produces a bradycardia and sympathetically induced vasoconstriction, mainly in the muscles. Trigeminal nerve stimulation occurs during diving in response to facial stimulation by cold water and in OSAS may result from excessive pharyngeal stimulation (10). This reflex muscular vasoconstriction reduces oxygen delivery to nonessential organs during a breathhold dive, and the bradycardia prevents too high a rise in BP as a consequence. This increase in sympathetic tone to the muscles can be clearly demonstrated (Fig. 14.2)

and drops out quickly once the apnea is terminated (11). Coincident with apnea termination is a rise in BP of well over 15 mm Hg (Fig. 14.1), sometimes over 50 mm Hg, a rise in heart rate, but a fall in cardiac output for 2 or 3 beats (with a rise thereafter). This rise in BP is probably conse-quent upon the arousal-related increase in sympathetic out-put (12) to other vascular beds (e.g., the skin), a hangover of vasoconstriction in muscular beds despite the cessation of sympathetic flow to them, and a rise in heart rate (Fig. 14.3). The extra LV preload from blood retained in the thorax during the apneic period may allow the heart to increase cardiac output later on in the arousal.

Exactly how much of this BP rise is due to the attendant hypoxia is debated. To the extent that the hypoxia prob-ably contributes to the vasoconstriction during the apnea (13), which may then persist into the early postapneic phase, hypoxia may play a part. However, in patients with OSAS, abolition of the hypoxia during the apnea hardly blunts the BP rise at all (14). In addition, the BP rise, but not the cardiac output changes, can be mimicked by noise-induced arousals (12, 15). Awake studies have sug-

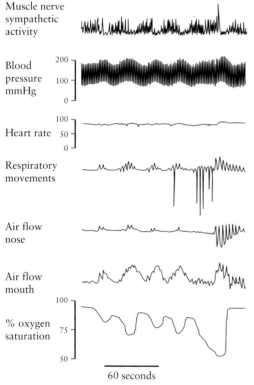

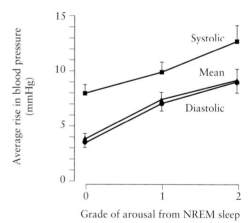

Fig 14.2 *Two minute tracing of sympathetic nerve activity (to a leg muscle) during about 5 cycles of OSAS. Note that the highest nerve activity is during the latter part of the apneas with an abrupt fall at the resumption of breathing when blood pressure is still rising. (From Hedner J, Ejnell H, Sellgren J, et al. Is high and fluctuating muscle nerve sympathetic activity in the sleep apnoea syndrome of pathogenetic importance for the development of hypertension? J Hypertens 1988; 6[Suppl]: S529–S531.)*

Fig 14.3 *The average rise in the blood pressure over 10 s in normal subjects during sleep in response to a noise. A grade 0 arousal is when the noise had apparently produced no discernible increase in EEG frequency. A grade 1 arousal is an increase electromyogram (EMG) or cortical EEG high frequency for > 1 and < 10 s, and a grade 2 for > 10 s. (From Davies RJO, Belt PJ, Robert SJ, et al. Arterial blood pressure responses to graded transient arousal from sleep in normal humans. J Appl Physiol 1993; 74: 1123–1130.)*

gested that perhaps even minor asphyxia might be important in generating a BP rise (16,17), although it is likely that responses during sleep differ from those whole awake.

Thus, the three main components of OSA—frustrated increases in inspiratory effort, hypoxemia (or asphyxia), and arousal—probably all contribute to the dramatic changes in heart rate and BP seen acutely with each apnea.

After the institution of CPAP, the acute changes in BP and heart rate are abolished (Fig. 14.4). However, the average BP does not fall immediately (14). The cause of this short-term persistence is not clear, but it may be due to release of circulating catecholamines during the apneic periods (18, 19) and persisting high sympathetic tone (20, 21). In the presence of preexisting ischemic heart disease, these rises in circulating catecholamines, accompanied by the hypoxemia, may be responsible for some of the malignant arrhythmias and episodes of angina occurring in some OSAS patients (22, 23) actually during apneic periods (Fig. 14.5). The severe bradycardias sometimes seen are vagally induced and not thought to be dangerous in their own right.

○▬ **Key points box 14.1**
Acute cardiovascular changes during apneas (systemic circulation)
■ During apneas: Muscle bed vasoconstriction Bradycardia (diving reflex) Falls in pleural pressure with each inspiration Falls in BP with each inspiratory effort These impede left ventricular emptying
■ 25% fall in cardiac output, pooling of blood in thorax
■ Large rises in BP at the end of every apnea and hypopnea
■ These rises mainly due to arousal and increased sympathetic tone
■ Initial further fall in cardiac output, followed by a rise

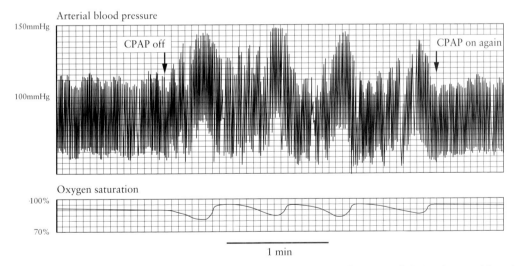

Fig 14.4 *Five minute tracing of beat-to-beat arterial BP in an asleep patient during nasal CPAP therapy. After about 1 min the pressure at the mask is lowered and the OSA returns, with a resumption of BP surges due to arousal, and inspiratory pressure falls during the obstructed inspiratory efforts. After 3 min the CPAP pressure is returned to a therapeutic level with abolition of the large BP changes. Note that respiratory oscillations of about 5 mm Hg are still present due to the pleural pressure swings during normal breathing.*

Apnea during sleep

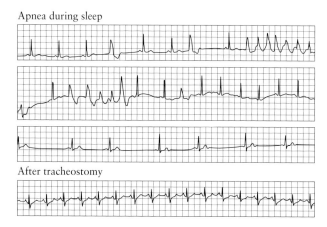

After tracheostomy

Fig 14.5 *Electrocardiographic (ECG) tracing during sleep in a patient with severe OSAS. Note the bradycardia with short bursts of ventricular tachycardia. Regular rate and rhythm are restored after tracheostomy removes the OSAS. (From Tilkian AG, Motte J, Guilleminault C. Cardiac arrhythmias in sleep apnea. In: Guilleminault C, Dement WC, eds. Sleep apnea syndromes. New York: Alan R. Liss; 1978: 197–210.)*

ACUTE CHANGES IN THE PULMONARY CIRCULATION

Direct measurements of pulmonary artery pressure (PAP) during OSAS do of course have the respiratory pleural pressure swings superimposed (Fig. 14.6). If transmural pressures are looked at, referenced to esophageal pressure, there appears to be a rise in PAP during the apnea with a further brief rise at apnea termination. In addition, there seems to be a more gradual rise in PAP over many cycles of apnea (24, 25). This of course might be expected, given that hypoxia constricts the pulmonary arterioles directly. In humans, administration of oxygen, however, does not seem to abolish the within-apnea changes, similar to the systemic circulation, although such maneuvers do allow $PaCO_2$ to rise a little, which in the pulmonary circulation is also vasoconstrictive. In anesthetised animals, added oxygen diminishes the pulmonary artery pressure rise during simulated OSAS and allows PAP to fall (26) (Fig. 14.7). Far more severe hypoxia was used in these experiments compared to that usually seen in patients with OSA, and of course there is no central nervous system arousal at the end of each apnea. An alternative explanation for the PAP rise seen in humans, already discussed above, is that increased venous return engendered by increasingly subatmospheric pleural pressures may provide an added preload to the right ventricle and thus increase right-sided cardiac output against a constant or slightly higher pulmonary vascular resistance. In addition, the higher pulmonary venous pressure due to reduced LV ejection fraction, also discussed previously, will contribute to higher pulmonary vascular pressures.

At present the most likely situation seems to be that any within-apnea changes in PAP are due to increased venous return, the postapneic rise to arousal, with the longer-term rises within a night due to hypoxemia.

⚬━ Key points box 14.2

Acute cardiovascular changes during apneas (pulmonary circulation)

- Small rise in pulmonary artery pressure during apnea
- Bigger rise at apnea end
- In humans, neither of these are prevented by maintaining normoxia
- Progressive rise in baseline pulmonary artery pressure over the night, prevented by normoxia

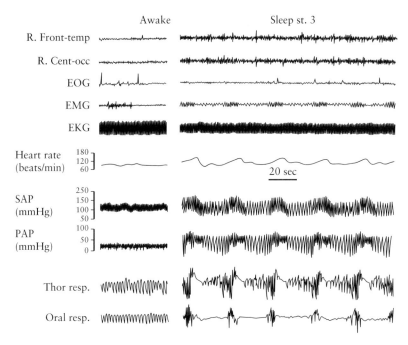

Fig 14.6 Three minute tracing of (PAP) and systemic arterial pressures (SAP) during about 5 cycles of OSAS, compared to a short section of awake recording. Note the rise in PAP (enlarged scale compared to systemic trace) at apnea end, with pleural pressure swings superimposed, indicating that the pressures have been referenced to atmospheric, rather than intrathoracic (esophageal), and are not therefore transmural. (From Coccagna G, Mantovani M, Brignani F, et al. Continuous recording of the pulmonary and systemic arterial pressure during sleep in syndromes of hypersomnia with periodic breathing. Bull Eur Pathophysiol Respir 1972; 8: 1159–1172.)

CHRONIC SYSTEMIC CARDIOVASCULAR CHANGES IN OSAS

HYPERTENSION

Given the considerable acute changes in the systemic circulation during obstructive apneas, it is not unreasonable to suppose there might be significant adverse consequences in the long term. The main debate in this area has been over effects on diurnal (awake) BP and therefore on the possible risk of cerebrovascular events or myocardial infarction. It is often assumed that cardiac or cerebrovascular events might occur more commonly as a result of the raised diurnal blood pressure; however, there is no reason why these outcomes might not result directly from the surges in BP occurring during the apneas. Although much effort has been put into establishing or failing to establish a link between OSAS and diurnal hypertension, what really matters is whether there is real long-term morbidity. In theory, therefore, the ideal studies to prove any association would simply involve the collection of an OSAS group along with a non-OSAS control group, matched for all the known cardiovascular risk factors, such as age, sex, obesity (particularly upper body obesity), tobacco consumption, alcohol consumption, exercise levels, and blood levels of substances such as cholesterol and uric acid. Unfortunately, OSAS itself, and of course snoring, appears to be directly related to some of these factors. This makes disentangling confounding variables and establishing OSAS as a true independent predictor of cardiovascular events extremely difficult. Another problem is that some of these 'known' risk factors for cardiovascular events were established before there was a proper understanding of OSAS. Thus,

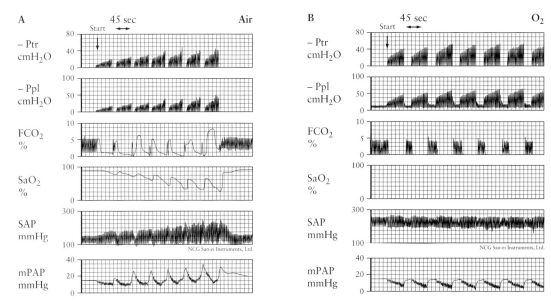

Fig 14.7 *Simulated OSAS in dogs that have been anesthetized, which removes any influence of central nervous system arousals. Panel A is without added oxygen, which results in falls of oxygen saturation to 25% or so. In association with this fall, the transmural PAP (mPAP) rises with each apnea. In panel B hypoxemia has been prevented with the addition of added oxygen. In the absence of hypoxemia there are falls in PAP which the authors argue may be due to a reduced venous return resulting from venous collapse during the large inspiratory efforts. Note that in this anesthetized animal preparation, without central nervous system arousals, relief of hypoxia also blunts the systemic rises in BP (SAP), unlike in sleeping humans with OSAS. (From Iwase N, Kikuchi Y, Hida W, et al. Effects of repetitive airway obstruction on O_2 saturation and systemic and pulmonary artery pressure in anesthetized dogs. Am Rev Respir Dis 1992; 146: 1401–1410.)*

for example, part of the apparent relationship between obesity and BP might in fact be due to OSAS. Hence, allowing for obesity first in studies assessing the independent contribution of OSAS to BP might make the investigator come to the erroneous conclusion that there was none. A further complication in such studies is that OSAS varies considerably from night to night (27). However, if there is a contribution to cardiovascular morbidity then we assume it will have been the average amount of OSAS over some years that will be important. Hence measuring OSAS during a one night study in a strange environment, and quantifying it as apnea-hypopnea index (AHI), is unlikely to be a good measure of the true 'load' (Fig. 14.8) and certainly less precise than a one-off measurement of body weight to quantify obesity, for example.

A number of other approaches to this problem exist, and their contributions to the debate are discussed here.

There have been many recent and extensive reviews of this area (28–32).

POPULATION STUDIES

When early case series of patients with OSAS were published (33, 34), many patients were found to have hypertension. It was assumed that the OSAS played a part in this until careful studies were performed controlling for obesity and other confounding variables (35–37). The better the degree of controlling, the less the OSAS appeared to be an independent predictor of hypertension, except perhaps for early morning BP (38, 39). However, as mentioned earlier, it may be an error to allow for obesity and only use the results from one sleep study. In addition, after years of suffering from OSAS it may be that the patent's compensatory measures developed to a varying extent, which limit the hypertension or even reverse it.

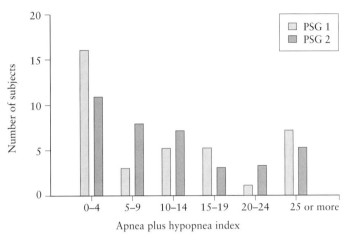

Fig 14.8 *Variability in AHI between two polysomnographic studies on patients being investigated for OSAS. Note the differing number of persons in each level of AHI activity between the two studies, with no particular overall shift to more or less severe OSAS in the second study. (From Chediak AD, Acevedo Crespo JC, Seiden DJ, et al. Nightly variability in the indices of sleep-disordered breathing in men being evaluated for impotence with consecutive night polysomnograms. Sleep 1996; 19: 589–592.)*

Other approaches have been to assess the prevalence of OSAS in patients first diagnosed as having hypertension. Again, early on, uncontrolled studies suggested a high prevalence of OSAS in hypertensive objects (40), but closer controlling largely removed any association in most studies (41).

Early epidemiological studies in community populations on the association between sleep-disordered breathing and hypertension found habitual snoring (or other markers of OSAS) to be predictive of hypertension (42, 43). Again, allowing for confounding variables largely abolished this association (44–46). Three more recently published large epidemiological surveys of OSAS and BP have again come to different conclusions. The large Wisconsin study (47, 48) suggested an effect of OSAS (measured as apneas and hypopneas) on BP even in a 'normal' community population. Interestingly, even small amounts of OSAS (AHI 5–15) seemed to be an independent risk factor, with more severe OSAS (AHI > 15) being no worse (Fig. 14.9). Although general obesity was allowed for, upper body obesity was not. An Australian study (49), using simpler definitions of OSAS, failed to find a significant independent relationship with daytime BP. The MONICA II study from Denmark (50) found a significant association between OSAS (or reported snoring) and sex, BMI, alcohol, and tobacco. An apparent association between OSAS and daytime BP disappeared

when these factors were allowed for first in a multiple regression analysis.

IMPACT OF NASAL CPAP ON BLOOD PRESSURE

Attempts have been made to assess the effects of nasal CPAP on the BP in patients with OSAS. Such an approach clearly needs some form of a control, which most studies have not had. An untreated group of OSAS patients is essential, and the alternative of using poor CPAP compliers is not as good, since noncompliers will be different in other ways other than CPAP usage. Uncontrolled studies have given conflicting results with some groups finding falls in BP (51) after CPAP (Fig. 14.10) and others not (52) despite a fall in peripheral muscle sympathetic nerve activity. Selecting hypertensive OSAS patients (on the grounds they will be the ones who can have BP falls) will always produce a fall in BP when measured for a second time, owing to regression to the mean. In incompletely controlled studies from our unit, there appears to be a small effect of CPAP after a month's treatment compared to placebo, of the order of 2 mm Hg. Acute nasal CPAP withdrawal leads to a small increase in BP in some patients (53). The other control group that would be advisable is hypertensive patients without OSAS given CPAP, since the changes in

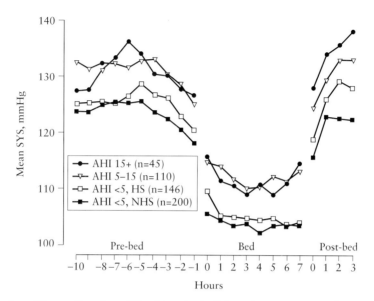

Fig 14.9 *Twenty-four hour BP recordings from 501 subjects in the Wisconsin community study. Note that the mean BP is highest in the subjects found to have either 5–15 or > 15 apneas or hypopneas hour of sleep. Those with an AHI of < 5 are subdivided into those with (HS) and without (NHS) a history of snoring. The most suggestive evidence of a 'dose-response' relationship between obstructive upper airway problems and BP comes from the immediately postsleep period at the far right of the graph, but these data are not corrected for obesity. (From Young T, Finn L, Hla KM, et al. Snoring as part of a dose-response relationship between sleep-disordered breathing and blood pressure. Sleep 1996; 19: S202–S205.)*

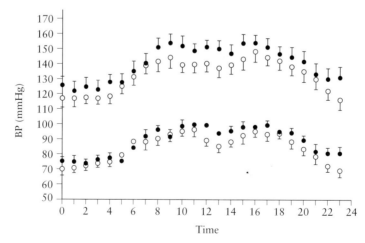

Fig 14.10 *Twenty-four hour BP recordings before (closed circles) and after (open circles) nasal CPAP therapy for OSAS. Note that these patients with OSAS were significantly hypertensive prior to CPAP, and that during the day there was about a 10 mm Hg fall in systolic pressures after therapy. (From Wilcox I, Grunstein RR, Hedner JA, et al. Effect of nasal continuous positive airway pressure during sleep on 24-hour blood pressure in obstructive sleep apnea. Sleep 1993; 16: 539–544.)*

intrathoracic pressure alone could conceivably influence fluid balance and BP, independent of an effect on OSAS. Any failure of the BP to fall significantly after the introduction of nasal CPAP could be because the baroreceptor resetting associated with the hypertension might now be irreversible.

Some recent studies have tried to circumvent these limitations but have introduced other uncertainties. Brooks et al. (54, 55) have set up an extraordinary model of OSAS in dogs. Chronically tracheotomized dogs have valves at the entrance to the tracheotomy controlled remotely by a computer that can also process the electroencephalographic (EEG) signals transmitted remotely from implanted electrodes. The computer can be programmed to close off the tracheotomy whenever the dog falls asleep and to open it again when it awakens. Thus, OSA in this model can be turned on and off at will. After the sudden onset of OSA, continued nightly for up to 3 months, there is a sustained rise in daytime BP of about 15 mm Hg as well as the expected episodic rises with each apnea during sleep (Fig. 14.11). After cessation of the OSA the daytime BP falls again, over the course of a week also. Simulation of the acute BP rises at night, using noise to repeatedly awaken the dogs rather than OSA, did not produce an associated rise in daytime BP. This suggests that, although it is the arousal that causes the acute rises in BP, something else causes the sustained daytime rise: candidates might be the hypoxemia, the hypercapnia, the increased swings in pleural pressure, or combinations of these two stimuli. The limitations of this dog model are the species difference, the sudden onset of the OSA (rather than the usual slow progression seen in humans), and the relatively short exposure. These last two factors may not allow for compensatory measures to develop. However, this model provides some of the most powerful evidence for an effect of OSAS on the awake BP.

MYOCARDIAL INFARCTION AND CEREBROVASCULAR DISEASE

Using myocardial infarction or cerebrovascular disease as an end point, and examining a relationship with prior symptoms of snoring and OSAS, has also produced conflicting results (56–60). Most studies lose any association with OSAS when other factors, especially upper body obesity, are adequately allowed for (61). Studying patients after their

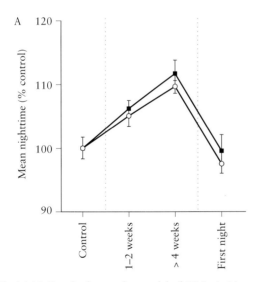
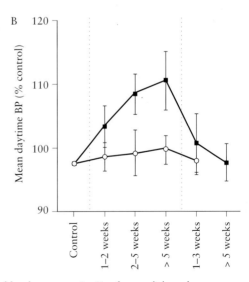

Fig 14.11 *Results from a dog model of OSA. A, Mean overnight blood pressures (as % of control) have been measured in response to OSA (black squares) and intermittent noise (open circles) 'administered' between the dotted lines during sleep periods. Note that the rise in BP is fairly similar. B, The daytime BP are displayed. Note that the dogs subjected to over a month of OSA (black squares) have elevated mean pressures but the dogs exposed to noise during sleep (open circles) do not have elevated awake pressures. (From Brooks D, Horner RL, Kozar LF, et al. Obstructive sleep apnea as a cause of systemic hypertension. Evidence from a canine model. J Clin Invest 1997; 99: 106–109.)*

acute events presents problems, since both stroke and heart failure can cause sleep-disordered breathing (62–65).

Although many textbooks and introductions to papers on cardiovascular complications of OSAS assume a causal relationship has been robustly established, this is not true. Until certain studies have appeared, clinicians will have to keep an open mind. The studies required are 1) a randomized placebo-controlled trial of nasal CPAP versus placebo on 24 hour BP profiles, although the time interval necessary to show or exclude an effect is unclear, 2) case-controlled studies with control individuals perfectly matched to the OSAS patients for upper body obesity, smoking, alcohol consumption, and similar factors, perhaps looking at surrogate markers of damage such as LV failure, renal impairment, subtle cerebrovascular disease, or blood markers of myocardial and endothelial damage, as well as 24 hour BP profiles. It is unlikely that placebo-controlled trials of therapy will be performed with end points such as myocardial infarction or stroke until a very much more palatable form of therapy than nasal CPAP becomes available that could be used extensively by asymptomatic patients.

O→ **Key points box 14.3**

Chronic changes in OSAS (systemic circulation)

- Increased catecholamine levels and sympathetic tone when awake
- Increased diurnal BP in OSAS mainly due to confounding variables:

Obesity	Upper body obesity
Alcohol	Smoking
Exercise	

- Small independent effect of OSAS on morning blood pressure
- Nasal CPAP may reduce blood pressure a small amount on average
- No robust evidence to implicate OSAS in stroke or myocardial infarction
- There are still major areas of uncertainty

CHRONIC PULMONARY CIRCULATION CHANGES IN OSAS

As with the systemic circulation, it was originally assumed that sustained rises in the PAP would occur with OSAS.

However, evidence implies that this usually only occurs when there is daytime hypoxemia as well (66). This is usually related to the presence of one or more additional factors, such as small airways obstruction (67–69), neuromuscular disease, or extreme obesity (Fig. 14.12). It appears that, rather like erythropoietin release (70), more prolonged hypoxia is necessary to raise PAP chronically; the transient falls of oxygen levels with complete recovery in between do not seem to be enough on their own. However, in other series of OSAS patients without lung disease who had noninvasive PAP measurements, some had raised levels in association with OSA alone (71), but the pulmonary hypertension seen under these circumstances was very modest and unlikely to be of any clinical significance.

O→ **Key points box 14.4**

Chronic changes in OSAS (pulmonary circulation)

- Pulmonary artery pressure (PAP) is rarely raised without diurnal hypoxemia
- Diurnal hypoxemia usually due to associated small airways obstruction
- Rises in PAP are modest and unlikely to be clinically significant

CONCLUSIONS

There is no doubt that obstructive sleep apneas induce profound changes in the cardiovascular system, with large rises in BP associated with each arousal. Although the rises are dramatic, there is not yet any evidence that these surges damage target organs. Little robust evidence exists that OSAS produces a sustained rise in awake BP, although the evidence for this is increasing, particularly early morning pressures. Again, whether these sustained pressures produce secondary damage is not clear, but by analogy with other causes of hypertension, they might do so. At present there is insufficient evidence to justify the prescription of nasal CPAP for cardiovascular reasons (except in the small subgroup with ischemic heart disease and nocturnal angina or malignant arrhythmias). When a simpler and more acceptable treatment for OSAS is available, placebo-controlled trials will be possible, just as occurred when acceptable oral hypotensive agents became available. Then we will be in a position to advise our patients whether their asymptomatic sleep apnea should be treated to lower future cardiovascular risk.

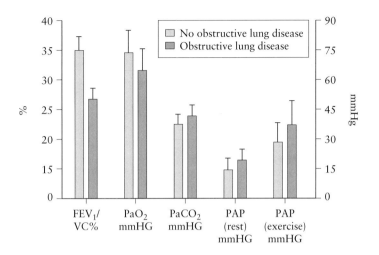

Fig 14.12 *Effect of obstructive lung disease in patients with OSAS on resting blood gases and invasively measured PAP, at rest and during exercise. Note that the presence of obstructive lung disease and mild extra hypoxemia is associated with modestly higher PAP, which are unlikely to be of clinical significance. (From Weitzenblum E, Krieger J, Oswald M, et al. Chronic obstructive pulmonary disease and sleep apnea syndrome. Sleep 1992; 15: S33–S35.)*

⊶ Key points box 14.5

Conclusions

- Clear evidence exists that OSAS causes nocturnal hypertension.
- There is limited evidence that OSAS causes diurnal hypertension.
- The evidence is that poor OSAS causes cardiovascular morbidity (strokes and myocardial infarction).
- There is no evidence that OSAS causes harmful pulmonary hypertension.
- Further properly controlled studies are badly needed.
- Currently there is no justification for treating OSAS with nasal CPAP for cardiovascular reasons alone.
- Treating asymptomatic OSAS will become an issue when there is simpler treatment.

REFERENCES

1. Lea S, Ali NJ, Goldman M, et al. Systolic blood pressure swings reflect inspiratory effort during simulated obstructive sleep apnoea. In Horne J, ed. Sleep 90. Bochum: Pontenagel Press, 1990; 178–181.

2. Karam M, Wise RA, Natarajan TK, et al. Mechanism of decreased left ventricular stroke volume during inspiration in man. Circulation 1984; 69:866–873.

3. Lugaresi E, Cirignotta F, Coccogna G, et al. Clinical significance of snoring. In: Saunders NA, Sullivan CE, eds. Sleep and breathing. New York, Marcel Dekker, 1984:283–298.

4. Shiomi T, Guilleminault C, Stoohs R, et al. Leftward shift of the interventricular septum and pulsus paradoxus in obstructive sleep apnea syndrome. Chest 1991; 100:894–902.

5. Gardner AMN, Fox RH. The return of blood to the heart. London, John Libbey; 1989:70–75.

6. Condos WRJ, Latham RD, Hoadley SD, et al. Hemodynamics of the Mueller maneuver in man: right and left heart micromanometry and Doppler echocardiography. Circulation 1987; 76:1020–1028.

7. Bristow JD, Honour AG, Pickering TG, et al. Cardiovascular and respiratory changes during sleep in normal and hypertensive subjects. Cardiovas Res 1969; 3:476–485.

8. Zwillich C, Devlin T, White D, et al. Bradycardia during sleep apnea: characteristics and mechanism. J Clin Invest 1982; 69:1286–1292.

9. Angell-James JE, DeBurgh-Daly M. Cardiovascular responses in apnoeic asphyxia: role of arterial chemoreceptors and the modification of their effects by a pulmonary inflation reflex. J Physiol Lond 1969; 201: 87–104.

10. Andreas S, Hajak G, von Breska B, et al. Changes in heart rate during obstructive sleep apnoea. Eur Respir J 1992; 5:853–857.

11. Hedner J, Ejnell H, Sellgren J, et al. Is high and fluctuating muscle nerve sympathetic activity in the sleep apnoea syndrome of pathogenetic importance for the development of hypertension? J Hypertens S 1988; 6 (Suppl):S529–S531.

12. Davies RJO, Belt PJ, Robert SJ, et al. Arterial blood pressure responses to graded transient arousal from sleep in normal humans. J Appl Physiol 1993; 74:1123–1130.

13. Leuenberger U, Jacob E, Sweer L, et al. Surges of muscle sympathetic nerve activity during obstructive apnea are linked to hypoxemia. J Appl Physiol 1995; 79:581–588.

14. Ali NJ, Davies RJO, Fleetham JA, et al. The acute effects of continuous positive airway pressure and oxygen administration on blood pressure during obstructive sleep apnea. Chest 1992; 101:1526–1532.

15. Ringler J, Basner RC, Shannon R, et al. Hypoxemia alone does not explain blood pressure elevations after obstructive apneas. J Appl Physiol 1990; 69:2143–2148.

16. van den Aardweg JG, Karemaker JM. Repetitive apneas induce periodic hypertension in normal subjects through hypoxia. J Appl Physiol 1992; 72: 821–827.

17. Morgan BJ, Denahan T, Ebert TJ. Neurocirculatory consequences of negative intrathoracic pressure vs. asphyxia during voluntary apnea. J Appl Physiol 1993; 74:2969–2975.

18. Fletcher EC, Miller J, Schaaf JW, et al. Urinary catecholamines before and after tracheostomy in patients with obstructive sleep apnea and hypertension. Sleep 1987; 10:35–44.

19. Dimsdale JE, Coy T, Ziegler MG, et al. The effect of sleep apnea on plasma and urinary catecholamines. Sleep 1995; 18:377–381.

20. Carlson JT, Hedner J, Elam M, et al. Augmented resting sympathetic activity in awake patients with obstructive sleep apnea. Chest 1993; 103:1763–1768.

21. Morgan BJ, Crabtree DC, Palta M, et al. Combined hypoxia and hypercapnia evokes long-lasting sympathetic activation in humans. J Appl Physiol 1995; 79:205–213.

22. Tilkian AG, Motta J, Guilleminault C. Cardiac arrhythmias in sleep apnea. In: Guilleminault C, Dement WC, eds. Sleep apnea syndromes. New York, Alan R. Liss; 1978:197–210.

23. Franklin KA, Nilsson JB, Sahlin C, et al. Sleep apnoea and nocturnal angina. Lancet 1995; 345:1085–1087.

24. Marrone O, Bellia V, Pieri D, et al. Acute effects of oxygen administration on transmural pulmonary artery pressure in obstructive sleep apnea. Chest 1992; 101:1023–1027.

25. Marrone O, Bonsignore MR, Romano S, et al. Slow and fast changes in transmural pulmonary artery pressure in obstructive sleep apnoea. Eur Respir J 1994; 7:2192–2198.

26. Iwase N, Kikuchi Y, Hida W, et al. Effects of repetitive airway obstruction on O_2 saturation and systemic and pulmonary artery pressure in anesthetized dogs. Am Rev Respir Dis 1992; 146:1402–1410.

27. Chediak AD, Acevedo Crespo JC, et al. Nightly variability in the indices of sleep-disordered breathing in men being evaluated for impotence with consecutive night polysomnograms. Sleep 1996; 19:589–592.

28. Waller PC, Bhopal RS. Is snoring a cause of vascular disease? An epidemiological review. Lancet 1989; 1:143–146.

29. Stradling JR. Sleep apnoea and systemic hypertension. Thorax 1989; 44:984–989.

30. Working group on OSA and hypertension, Carlson J, Davies R, et al. Obstructive sleep apnea and blood pressure elevation. What is the relationship? Blood Pressure 1993; 2:166–182.

31. Fletcher EC. The relationship between systemic hypertension and obstructive sleep apnea: facts and theory. Am J Med 1995; 98:118–128.

32. Silverberg DS, Oksenberg A. Essential hypertension and abnormal upper airway resistance during sleep. Sleep 1997; 20:794–805.

33. Guilleminault C, Tilkian A, Dement WC. The sleep apnea syndromes. Ann Rev Med 1976; 27:465–484.

34. Guilleminault C, Simmons FB, Motta J, et al. Obstructive sleep apnea syndrome and tracheostomy. Arch Intern Med 1981; 141:985–988.

35. Millman RP, Redline S, Carlisle CC, et al. Daytime hypertension in obstructive sleep apnea. Prevalence and contributing risk factors. Chest 1991; 99:861–866.

36. Davies RJO, Crosby J, Prothero A, et al. Ambulatory blood pressure and left ventricular hypertrophy in untreated obstructive sleep apnoea and snoring, compared to matched controls, and their response to treatment. Clin Sci 1994; 86:417–424.

37. Hoffstein V. Blood pressure, snoring, obesity, and nocturnal hypoxaemia. Lancet 1994; 344:643–645.

38. Grunstein R, Wilcox I, Yang TS, et al. Snoring and sleep apnoea in men: association with central obesity and hypertension. Int J Obes Relat Metab Disord 1993; 17:533–540.

39. Hoffstein V, Mateika J. Evening-to-morning blood pressure variations in snoring patients with and without obstructive sleep apnea. Chest 1992; 101:379–384.

40. Kales A, Bixler ED, Cadieux RJ, et al. Sleep apnoea in a hypertensive population. Lancet 1984; 2:1005–1008.

41. Warley AR, Mitchell JH, Stradling JR. Prevalence of nocturnal hypoxaemia amongst men with mild to moderate hypertension. Q J Med 1988; 68:637–644.

42. Koskenvuo M, Kaprio J, Partinen M, et al. Snoring as a risk factor for hypertension and angina pectoris. Lancet 1985; 1:893–896.

43. Lugaresi E, Cirignotta F, Coccagna G, et al. Some epidemiological data on snoring in cardiocirculatory disturbances. Sleep 1980; 3:221–224.

44. Schmidt-Nowara WW, Coultas DB, Wiggins C, et al. Snoring in a Hispanic-American population. Risk factors and association with hypertension and other morbidity. Arch Intern Med 1990; 150:597–601.

45. Gislason T, Aberg H, Taube A. Snoring and systemic hypertension — an epidemiological study. Acta Med Scand 1987; 222:415–421.

46. Stradling JR, Crosby JH. Relation between systemic hypertension and sleep hypoxaemia or snoring: analysis in 748 men drawn from general practice. Br Med J 1990; 300:75–78.

47. Hla KM, Young TB, Bidwell T, et al. Sleep apnea and hypertension. Ann Intern Med 1994; 120:382–388.

48. Young T, Finn L, Hla KM, et al. Snoring as part of a dose-response relationship between sleep-disordered breathing and blood pressure. Sleep 1996; 19:S202–S205.

49. Olson LG, King MT, Hensley MJ, et al. A community study of snoring and sleep-disordered breathing. Health outcomes. Am J Respir Crit Care Med 1995; 152:717–720.

50. Jennum P, Sjol A. Snoring, sleep apnoea and cardiovascular risk factors: the MONICA II Study. Int J Epidemiol 1993; 22:439–444.

51. Wilcox I, Grunstein RR, Hedner JA, et al. Effect of nasal continuous positive airway pressure during sleep on 24-hour blood pressure in obstructive sleep apnea. Sleep 1993; 16:539–544.

52. Hedner J, Darpo B, Ejnell H, et al. Reduction in sympathetic activity after long-term CPAP treatment in sleep apnoea: cardiovascular implications. Eur Respir J 1995; 8:222–229.

53. Stradling JR, Partlett J, Davies RJO, et al. Effect of short-term graded withdrawal of nasal continuous positive airway pressure on systemic blood pressure in patients with obstructive sleep apnoea. Blood Pressure 1996; 5:234–240.

54. Brooks D, Horner RL, Kozar LF, et al. Obstructive sleep apnea as a cause of systemic hypertension. Evidence from a canine model. J Clin Invest 1997; 99:106–109.

55. Brooks D, Horner RL, Kimoff RJ, et al. Effect of obstructive sleep apnea versus sleep fragmentation on responses to airway occlusion. Am J Respir Crit Care Med 1997; 155:1609–1617.

56. Koskenvuo M, Kaprio J, Telakivi T, et al. Snoring as a risk factor for ischaemic heart disease and stroke in men. Br Med J 1987; 294:16–19.

57. Spriggs DA, French JM, Murdy JM, et al. Historical risk factors for stroke: a case control study. Age Ageing 1990; 19:280–287.

58. Spriggs DA, French JM, Murdy JM, et al. Snoring increases the risk of stroke and adversely affects prognosis. Q J Med 1992; 83:555–562.

59. Bassetti C, Aldrich MS, Chervin RD, et al. Sleep apnea in patients with transient ischemic attack and stroke: a prospective study of 59 patients. Neurology 1996; 47:1167–1173.

60. Hung J, Whitford EG, Parsons RW, et al. Association of sleep apnoea with myocardial infarction in men. Lancet 1990; 336:261–264.

61. Lavie P, Herer P, Peled R, et al. Mortality in sleep apnea patients: a multivariate analysis of risk factors. Sleep 1995; 18:149–157.

62. Bassetti C, Aldrich MS, Quint D. Sleep-disordered breathing in patients with acute supra-and infratentorial strokes. A prospective study of 39 patients. Stroke 1997; 28: 1765–1772.

63. Good DC, Henkle JQ, Gelber D, et al. Sleep-disordered breathing and poor functional outcome after stroke. Stroke 1996; 27:252–259.

64. Alex CG, Onal E, Lopata M. Upper airway occlusion during sleep in patients with Cheyne-Stokes respiration. Am Rev Respir Dis 1986; 133:42–45.

65. Kryger MH, Hanly PJ. Cheyne-Stokes respiration in cardiac failure. Prog Clin Biol Res 1990; 345:215–224.

66. Bradley TD, Rutherford R, Grossman RF, et al. Role of daytime hypoxemia in the pathogenesis of right heart failure in the obstructive sleep apnea syndrome. Am Rev Respir Dis 1985; 131:835–839.

67. Weitzenblum E, Krieger J, Apprill M, et al. Daytime pulmonary hypertension in patients with obstructive sleep apnea syndrome. Am Rev Respir Dis 1988; 138:345–349.

68. Bradley TD, Rutherford R, Lue F, et al. Role of diffuse airway obstruction in the hypercapnia of obstructive sleep apnea. Am Rev Respir Dis 1986; 134:920–924.

69. Weitzenblum E, Krieger J, Oswald M, et al. Chronic obstructive pulmonary disease and sleep apnea syndrome. Sleep 1992; 15:S33–S35.

70. Goldman JM, Ireland RM, Berthon-Jones M, et al. Erythropoietin concentrations in obstructive sleep apnoea. Thorax 1991; 46:25–27.

71. Sajkov D, Cowie RJ, Thornton AT, et al. Pulmonary hypertension and hypoxemia in obstructive sleep apnea syndrome. Am J Respir Crit Care Med 1994; 149:416–422.

72. Coccagna G, Mantovani M, Brignani F, et al. Continuous recording of the pulmonary and systemic arterial pressure during sleep in syndromes of hypersomnia with periodic breathing. Bull Eur Physiopathol Respir 1972; 8:1159–1172.

73. Weitzenblum E, Krieger J, Oswald M, et al. Chronic obstructive pulmonary disease and sleep apnea syndrome. Sleep 1992; 15:S33–S35.

15 HORMONAL AND METABOLIC DISTURBANCES IN SLEEP APNEA

Ronald R Grunstein

INTRODUCTION

Human neuroendocrine and metabolic physiology is often influenced by behavioral states of sleep and wakefulness. Plasma levels of pituitary and other hormones also spontaneously fluctuate across the 24 hour period. These endocrine rhythms have often been labeled either sleep related (when the predominant change in fluctuation is nocturnal) or circadian (when the rhythm appears to be regulated by an internal clock rather than periodic changes in the external environment). The predominant influences are intrinsic circadian rhythmicity and sleep, which interact to varying degrees to produce the characteristic 24 hour rhythm of each hormone. Other factors such as meals and exercise may also cause some changes in hormone level (1).

The recognition of breathing disorders in sleep has paralleled the advances in understanding of neuroendocrine biology. However, despite the existence of sleep apnea as a unique mix of sleep fragmentation and hypoxic exposure, little is known about the interrelationships between endocrine and metabolic pathophysiology and sleep apnea. There are a number of areas of common interest. Epidemiological features of sleep apnea include marked male preponderance and an association with obesity and advancing age (2, 3). Sleep apnea has also been linked to impaired life quality, sexual dysfunction in adults, poor growth in children, and endocrine conditions such as acromegaly, hypothyroidism, and Cushing disease. Some hormonal treatments such as progesterone have been used therapeutically in sleep apnea, whereas other treatments, such as growth hormone or testosterone, may worsen sleep-disordered breathing. Upper body obesity is characteristic in sleep apnea patients and this type of adiposity is associated with a wide range of metabolic abnormalities that promote morbidity and mortality (4).

Sleep apnea may interact with endocrine rhythms via a number of mechanisms. First, repetitive apneas will cause sleep fragmentation and disorganization of sleep stages and cycles. Second, hypoxia may have direct central effects on neurotransmitters (5), which in turn will affect hypothalamic-pituitary hormone production. Third, sudden arousal from sleep may produce a central 'stress' response leading to hormonal changes (6). Fourth, daytime sleep episodes may interact with daytime hormone rhythms. Finally, all of the above factors may interact and lead to changes in the central control of sleep and endocrine rhythms.

SLEEP APNEA AND NEUROENDOCRINE CHANGES— CONFOUNDING BY OTHER VARIABLES

Assessment of the influence of sleep apnea on endocrine function requires close consideration of confounding factors, such as age, obesity, and other associated diseases, such as chronic lung disease. Confounding can be controlled for with multivariate analysis or by treatments that eliminate the disease process (e.g., weight reduction for obesity or continuous positive airway pressure [CPAP] for sleep apnea). However, in analyzing the confounding effect of obesity in sleep apnea, weight reduction may not answer the question, as both sleep apnea and obesity could resolve in parallel.

ENDOCRINE FUNCTION IN SLEEP APNEA—EFFECT OF TREATMENT

GROWTH HORMONE (GH)

GH secretion is closely linked with sleep (7, 8). GH may act directly on tissues, but in most body organs GH acts through an intermediate mediator, somatomedin C, now known as insulin-like growth factor-1 (IGF-1), which is synthesized in the liver and other organs in response to GH (7). As GH is secreted in a pulsatile fashion and has a relatively short serum half-life (22 min), a single random GH level provides little information on the 24 hour GH production of an individual person. However, a single IGF-1 level has a high level of correlation with 24 hour mean plasma GH and can be used clinically as an index of GH status (9).

GH secretion is pulsatile and episodic, but unlike many other hormones, it does not have a dominant independent circadian rhythm. The first studies measuring GH during polysomonographically monitored sleep indicated that there was a consistent relationship between GH secretion and slow wave sleep (SWS). Although subsequent investigators have challenged this observation, recent studies, using more frequent sampling to better characterize GH secretory bursts, have found a close association between GH and SWS (7, 8). The presence of SWS is not obligatory for GH secretion, but Van Cauter et al. (8) observed that 70% of GH pulses occuring during sleep were associated with SWS.

In obesity, GH production is decreased in both 24 hour mean levels and in response to stimuli (7, 10). This reduction in GH output is related to increased fat mass rather than weight. Most studies suggest that the reduced GH output in obesity is reversed with weight loss (7, 10). Furthermore, IGF-1 levels are reduced in obesity (11).

GROWTH HORMONE AND SLEEP APNEA

In a cross-sectional study of 225 men undergoing sleep studies (11), IGF-1 levels were reduced in men with sleep apnea (Fig. 15.1), and this was related to the severity of the apnea (both desaturations per hour and minimum oxygen saturation in sleep). The decreased IGF-1 levels were also related to aging and coexisting obesity but also independently to sleep apnea. The role of sleep apnea in these cross-sectional results was confirmed by the reversal of these reduced IGF-1 levels with 3 months of nasal CPAP treatment without any significant accompanying weight change (11) (Fig. 15.2). As circulating IGF-1 levels are dependent on GH secretion, these data suggested that the lower plasma IGF-1 levels reflected reduced GH secretion.

There are a number of possible reasons why GH secretion may be reduced in sleep apnea. Sleep is fragmented

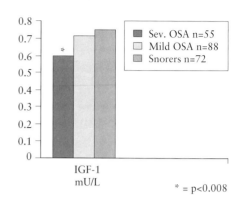

Fig 15.1 *Insulin-like growth factor-1 levels in patients with severe OSAS (Sev. OSA), mild OSAS (Mild OSA) and snorers. Patients with severe OSAS have significantly reduced IGF-1 levels (p < .008).*

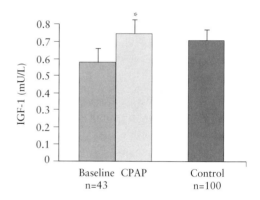

Fig 15.2 *Insulin-like growth factor 1 (IGF-1) levels in 43 men with sleep apnea before (gray bar) and after (open bar) 3 months of nasal CPAP. These results are contrasted with those of 100 men of similar age (solid bar) to establish normative values for IGF-1.*

and SWS is markedly reduced or absent in sleep apnea (12), and this may cause a reduction in sleep-entrained GH secretion. Growth hormone concentrations are virtually absent in severe sleep apnea (11). However, as discussed previously, reduced GH secretion in sleep apnea may be explained by coexisting central obesity. The best evidence supporting a role for sleep apnea in reducing GH secretion in sleep is provided by studies measuring GH concentrations before and after elimination of sleep apnea without change in confounding variables. Early case studies suggested that both CPAP and tracheostomy led to an increase in GH levels. Other studies measuring GH during sleep before and after CPAP provide further evidence of an increase in sleep-related GH secretion with correction of the sleep-breathing abnormality only (13–16).

Recently, we compared GH concentrations at baseline, after 1 week of an oral anti-androgen drug, flutamide, for sleep apnea and again after CPAP (13, 17). There was no difference in sleep, breathing, or hormonal variables between the two baseline studies and flutamide. On CPAP treatment, apneic breathing and shifts between sleep stages were markedly reduced, and the average length of SWS epochs was increased. Compared with the baseline studies, there were significant increases in GH concentrations and pulse frequency on CPAP treatment. After CPAP treatment, GH pulses were 11 times more likely to be preceded by an epoch of SWS compared with the baseline. There was no weight change in the patient explaining these results.

These findings suggested that pulsatile GH secretion is facilitated by periods of uninterrupted SWS on CPAP treatment. Fragmentation of SWS by apnea-induced arousals may reduce both the frequency and magnitude of the pulse of GH associated with SWS. Support for this hypothesis is provided by experimental data in healthy volunteers. GH secretion in response to growth hormone releasing hormone (GHRH) infusion is enhanced at night, particularly in SWS as opposed to rapid eye movement (REM) sleep, when the response to GHRH is similar to wakefulness (8). Arousals following GHRH infusion interrupt the normal GH response, which is restored after resumption of sleep (8). As the pulsatile secretion of GH results from the interaction of GHRH and somatostatin at the level of the somatotrope, it is certainly possible that repetitive arousals in sleep apnea may impair the GH response to endogenous bursts of GHRH into the pituitary portal circulation. Interestingly, patients with fibromyalgia characteristically have intrusions of alpha-electroencephalographic (EEG) (awake) activity fragmenting SWS, and low GH concentrations have been reported in this condition (18).

The biological significance of reduced GH and IGF-1 levels in sleep apnea is unclear. Severe sleep apnea in the pediatric population is characterized by failure to thrive, short stature, and other growth disturbances that can be corrected by elimination of the upper airway obstruction (19). It is possible that impaired GH secretion may play a role in these observations. Detailed studies of GH secretion in otherwise healthy children with sleep apnea are lacking. Waters et al. (16) examined GH secretion in sleep in patients comparent with 19 subjects with achondroplasia with a mean age of 11 years. Five subjects were restudied after treatment for obstructive sleep apnea syndrome (OSAS). In this group of five subjects, improved respiratory distress index (RDI) and reduced sleep state transitions were not associated with significant changes in GH secretion rate by sleep stage. However, GH secretion peak during the first 2 hours of SWS was initially absent, appearing only after treatment of OSAS. Other workers have speculated on other mechanisms for poor growth, including increased energy expenditure (20). The potential effects of reduced GH concentrations in adults with severe sleep apnea are speculative and are discussed later.

In conclusion, sleep apnea is associated with reduced GH concentrations, possibly due to less SWS, although an additional effect of intermittent hypoxia cannot be fully excluded. GH concentrations rise after nasal CPAP treatment. Further research is required to assess the relationship between this rise in GH concentrations and health outcomes.

⊶ Key points box 15.1

Growth hormone and acromegaly

1. Growth hormone (GH) secretion closely relates to slow wave sleep (SWS).

2. GH secretion is reduced in obesity and improves with weight loss.

3. GH secretion is also low in sleep apnea, probably due to loss of SWS and increases with nasal CPAP therapy.

4. Both central sleep apnea (CSA) and obstructive sleep apnea syndrome (OSAS) are common in acromegaly.

5. CSA in acromegaly likely relates to disordered central respiratory control. The mechanism of OSAS is unclear and does not appear to simply relate to narrowing of the upper airway.

6. The impact of treating acromegaly on sleep apnea is variable.

ACROMEGALY AND SLEEP APNEA

INTRODUCTION

Acromegaly is a condition of GH excess in adults characterized by the insidious development of coarsening of facial features, bone proliferation, and soft tissue swelling (9). It is usually secondary to a GH producing pituitary adenoma, which may be either a microadenoma or macroadenoma. Rarely the GH excess commences prior to puberty and closure of the epiphyses, and then the condition is termed gigantism. It occurs with equal frequency in both sexes with a prevalence of 50–70 cases per million. The clinical features may be due to the local effects of an expanding pituitary mass in addition to the effects of excess GH secretion, which include disordered somatic cell growth and insulin resistance. The mortality of untreated or partially treated acromegaly is about double the expected rate in healthy subjects matched for age (21). Acromegaly was first described as a clinical entity by Marie in 1886. Ten years later, Roxburgh and Collis (22) described daytime sleepiness and Chappell and Booth (23) observed upper airway obstruction as features of acromegaly, but the association between sleep apnea and acromegaly was only described 80 years later (24).

PREVALENCE OF SLEEP APNEA IN ACROMEGALY

Sleep-disordered breathing is extremely common in acromegaly. We had previously estimated that about 60% of our unselected patients with acromegaly have sleep apnea (25). Almost all of our patients were noted to have heavy snoring. In a Finnish study, using the static charged bed respiratory screening device, 10 of 11 patients had sleep apnea (91%), compared with 29.4% of the general population (26). In the only other large study of sleep apnea prevalence, Rosenow et al. (27) studied 54 patients with treated acromegaly from a larger sample of 100 patients. They excluded patients with previously known sleep apnea. Despite these exclusion criteria, 39% of the remaining 54 patients had sleep apnea. Treatment of acromegaly and the limited monitoring techniques used in the study may also have reduced prevalence. Sleep apnea was associated with increasing age and tended to be more common in men and women over the age of 50 year. Obesity does not appear to be a predisposing factor to sleep apnea in acromegaly. Increases in body mass index (BMI) in

acromegaly may be due to increased muscle mass rather than the increased body fat typically seen in obesity (9).

ETIOLOGY OF CENTRAL AND OBSTRUCTIVE SLEEP APNEA IN ACROMEGALY

The first reports of the association of sleep apnea with acromegaly suggested that macroglossia was an important etiological factor in producing sleep apnea as the large tongue narrowed the hypopharynx and collapsed backwards in sleep. However, endoscopy during apneic periods (28) revealed no posterior movement of the tongue, suggesting that macroglossia was not the primary factor in upper airway obstruction. In this report, primary pharyngeal collapse into the laryngeal vestibule was observed. Attempted treatment with a nasopharyngeal airway past the tongue did not prevent apnea. More recently, Pelttari et al. (25) observed no dynamic narrowing behind the tongue on nasopharyngoscopy.

We have observed a high rate of central apnea in patients with acromegaly (25) (34% of the total group of patients with sleep apnea). Other investigators (29), using full sleep studies, reported that two of their three patients with sleep apnea and acromegaly had predominantly or exclusively central apnea. A waxing and waning central apnea pattern of breathing on static charge sensitive bed studies has also been reported as more common in acromegaly than in typical upper airway obstruction (25).

The high prevalence of central apnea in acromegaly suggests that abnormalities of central respiratory control are involved. This has been supported by our finding that patients with central sleep apnea had significantly lower awake arterial carbon dioxide levels than those with obstructive apnea (25, 30), and increased ventilatory responsiveness was observed in the central apnea group (30). Central apnea occurs in association with a wide range of disorders, and many potential mechanisms have been described, including disordered central respiratory control. The precise cause in acromegaly is unclear, but there are a number of possible hypotheses, including alterations in central somatostatin pathways disinhibiting respiratory control (30). Other mechanisms include an effect of GH on central respiratory control, either directly or by altering metabolic rate. This is supported by the correlation between GH hypersecretion and prevalence of central apnea (30). Interestingly, apparent central apneas have been observed in beagles exposed to medroxyprogesterone, which causes GH increases and an acromegaly-like condition.

DISEASE ACTIVITY IN ACROMEGALY AND SLEEP APNEA

In view of the morbidity and mortality of acromegaly, it is important to define active and inactive (cured) disease. High circulating IGF-1 and GH levels reflect increased GH production and therefore disease activity. Studies describing 'cure' after pituitary surgery often use inadequate criteria of disease inactivity (9). True cure involves observing a physiological 24 hour GH secretion, normal IGF-1 levels, and normal GH responses to glucose. Even in patients with acromegaly and normal IGF-1 and GH profiles, GH secretory patterns are still different from those in normal subjects.

Most studies have observed persisting sleep apnea despite treatment of acromegaly by pituitary surgery. We have found no correlation between disease activity and sleep apnea severity (25). No significant differences were observed in mean GH and IGF-1 levels in patients with and without sleep apnea. In this study, 23 patients had detailed 24 hour GH secretory profiles, among whom 16 had sleep apnea (two predominantly CSA and 14 predominantly OSAS). In this subgroup with more extensive GH measurements, no significant differences in mean GH and GH pulsatility were found between patients with and without sleep apnea. In contrast, Rosenow et al. (27) reported lower GH levels in patients with milder sleep apnea. Studies using octreotide, a somatostatin analogue, have shown powerful GH reduction with parallel decrease in apnea severity (31). However, even in this study, a relationship was seen between the decrease in apnea and decrease in GH levels (31).

At present it is not known what proportion of patients with both sleep apnea and acromegaly will have complete resolution of their sleep apnea after cure of acromegaly. This will require careful prospective studies with accurate monitoring of true cure of acromegaly. However, it is clear that sleep apnea does occur in cured acromegaly. The combination of inactive acromegaly and sleep apnea may occur for a number of reasons. First, sleep apnea is a common disorder and may be coincident to acromegaly in patients with other risk factors for sleep apnea. Second, it may take a long time after normalization of GH secretion for effects of acromegaly to resolve, or there may be permanent effects on upper airway function or sleep-breathing regulation.

Although there appears to be no relationship between disease activity and severity of sleep apnea, patients with CSA have a much higher IGF-1 and fasting GH levels than patients with OSAS (25, 30) (Fig. 15.3).

MORBIDITY AND MORTALITY OF ACROMEGALY AND SLEEP APNEA

The adverse health risks of both acromegaly and sleep apnea are well established. Both disorders are associated with an increased risk of hypertension (9). In acromegaly

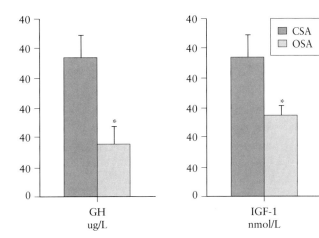

Fig 15.3 Random GH and IGF-1 levels in patients with CSA (n = 14, solid bars, CSA) and OSAS (n = 29, open bars, OSA). CSA patients have higher levels of biochemical activity.

the blood pressure level is sometimes reduced by successful transsphenoidal surgery. One postulated mechanism for hypertension in acromegaly is sodium and water retention secondary to GH overproduction (9).

We have found strong links between hypertension and sleep apnea in our patients with acromegaly, suggesting that sleep apnea may be another important mechanism causing hypertension (25). Over 50% of our patients with both acromegaly and sleep apnea had hypertension. All patients without sleep apnea were normotensive. Patients who were hypertensive had significantly higher respiratory disturbance indices and greater degrees of sleep hypoxemia than those who were normotensive. Mean 24 hour GH and IGF-1 levels and degree of obesity were not significantly different in those with hypertension compared to those without hypertension. Using multiple regression, both RDI and age were found to be independent predictors of hypertension (25).

Somnolence has long been recognized as part of the clinical spectrum of acromegaly. Although sleep apnea is the most likely cause, a direct effect of increased GH in promoting sleep and sleepiness has been suggested. Alternatively, sleepiness in the absence of sleep apnea may be due to effects of radiotherapy (32). Wright et al. (21) reviewed the causes of death in patients with acromegaly at four London hospitals and found an excess of deaths due to cardiovascular and respiratory causes. They commented 'The excess of deaths due to respiratory disease was an unexpected finding for which there was no obvious explanation.' There is no apparent excess of chronic lung disease in acromegaly. Lung function is usually normal or supernormal. With our new understanding of the high prevalence of sleep apnea in acromegaly, it is likely that this is the mechanism of deaths at that time attributed to respiratory disease. Another potential link is sleep apnea and upper airway obstruction complicating anesthesia in these patients. One recent Swedish report of deaths in acromegaly found five postoperative deaths in 62 total consecutive deaths in patients with acromegaly (33).

Sex Hormones and Sleep Apnea

Male Hormonal Disorders

Several case reports in the early 1980s described development of sleep apnea after testosterone therapy (34–36). Other investigation (37) reported the development of sleep apnea in a 54 year old woman with renal failure after androgen administration. The sleep apnea resolved on withdrawal of the medication and recurred when the drug was reintroduced. These author also observed an increase in supraglottic resistance after androgen administration. More recently, sleep apnea associated with an endogenous benign testosterone-producing ovarian tumor has been described (38). The OSAS resolved after tumor removal. These cases certainly suggest that testosterone may be important in the regulation of breathing during sleep and in the pathogenesis of sleep apnea. Testosterone also was reported to exacerbate sleep apnea in a 13 year old boy associated with an increase in upper airway collapsibility during sleep (39).

Two studies have systematically examined the sleep-breathing effects of exogenous testosterone on hypogonadal patients. Matsumoto et al. (40) studied five patients and observed development of sleep apnea in one patient and worsening of preexisting sleep apnea in another. There was no effect in the other three patients. Schneider et al. (41) investigated 11 hypogonadal men before and after testosterone replacement. There was a significant increase in apneas in the group as a whole, but clinically significant increases occurred in only three patients. The two studies show that testosterone-induced or testosterone-exacerbated sleep apnea is not a consistent finding in hypogonadal patients. The clinical message from these studies is that patients commencing on androgen replacement therapy should be questioned closely for sleep apnea symptoms and monitored during the course of their therapy to check if such symptoms develop. The possibility of more extensive use of testosterone therapy in eugonadal men for contraception or for 'andropause' will likely bring testosterone-induced apnea into clinical practice.

Low testosterone levels have been reported in men with sleep apnea (11, 42). In the largest study (11), hormone level suppression by sleep apnea was independent of age, degree of obesity, and presence of awake hypoxemia and hypercapnia. Testosterone levels increase with treatment of sleep apnea using nasal CPAP or even successful uvulopalatopharyngoplasty (UPPP) (11, 42). These androgen abnormalities in sleep apnea (decreased sex hormone – binding globulin [SHBG] and free and total testosterone) are qualitatively as well as quantitatively distinct from those reported in aging (increased SHBG, decreased free and total testosterone) and obesity (decreased SHBG and total testosterone, normal free testosterone). Importantly, despite the fall in plasma free and total testosterone levels, there was no increase in basal plasma gonadotropin (luteinizing hormone [LH], follicle-stimulating hormone [FSH]) levels. These findings, together with the retention of pituitary sensitivity to exogenous gonadotrophin releasing hormone (GnRH) in sleep apnea (43), point to a hypothalamic abnormality as the cause of the fall in testosterone levels. This explanation would be similar to the postulated level of the dysfunction of the GH – IGF-1 axis in sleep apnea. The lack of change in plasma LH levels does not imply that LH secretion is entirely normal in men with sleep apnea, since LH is secreted in an intermittent fashion (44). It is certainly possible that pulsatile LH secretion is abnormal in sleep apnea, but no published data are available.

The potential causes of this hypothalamic abnormality are essentially similar to those involved in reduced GH secretion. Testosterone levels are significantly reduced by sleep deprivation and fragmentation (45). Therefore, sleep fragmentation in sleep apnea may lead to disruption of sleep-entrained rhythms in LH and testosterone. Hypoxemia in sleep apnea may be involved as, unlike GH, there are several reports of low sex steroid levels in chronic airflow limitation in studies with small patient numbers (46). In other, larger studies (11), the apparent effects of awake hypoxemia and impaired lung function were entirely accounted for by sleep hypoxemia. It is possible that the sexual dysfunction reported in sleep apnea may be mediated by the sex hormone changes seen in sleep-disordered breathing. The low testosterone levels may also interact with low IGF-1 levels and impair anabolism. Androgens may exacerbate sleep apnea, and it is possible that the fall in androgen levels may be part of an adaptive homeostatic mechanism to reduce sleep-disordered breathing. However, androgen lowering therapy with the nonsteroidal androgen antagonist flutamide did not alter sleep-disordered breathing or awake ventilatory drive (17).

FEMALE SEX HORMONES AND SLEEP

The low prevalence of sleep apnea in premenopausal women compared to women after the menopause and the increase in prevalence of sleep-disordered breathing among postmenopausal women have led to studies examining the therapeutic role of progestational hormones in sleep apnea (47). The level of awake genioglossus electromyogram (EMGgg) is highest in the luteal phase, second highest in the follicular phase, and lowest in postmenopausal women (48). Importantly, EMGgg increases after hormone therapy. Progesterone levels fall after the menopause and progestogins have been shown to

stimulate ventilation during the luteal phase of the menstrual cycle, in pregnancy, in normal male subjects, and in conditions of alveolar hypoventilation (49).

In general, the therapeutic results for progestogins have been disappointing. Recent reports, including a double blind study at high doses (47), have revealed no improvement in indices of sleep apnea severity. Block et al. (49) were unable to demonstrate a protective effect of progesterone upon postmenopausal females with sleep apnea syndrome. The apparent 'protection' of premenopausal status against sleep apnea has provoked some interest in hormone replacement as a therapy for sleep apnea in women. Pickett et al. (50) used combined therapy with both progestogen and an estrogen in women who had had a surgical menopause. They demonstrated improvement, but the pretreatment apnea was very mild. Estrogen alone or in combination with progesterone in sleep-disordered breathing had no effect on sleep apnea in 15 postmenopausal women with moderate OSAS despite a doubling of serum estrogen level (51). It is still possible that longer term or higher dose treatment may provide more positive results.

It is important to recognize that menopause is associated with increased central obesity. Whether this is a specific menopausal effect or simply reflects aging is unclear (44).

However, this increasing central obesity may explain the association between menopause and sleep apnea prevalence. Some female hormonal disorders are associated with obesity and in this way possibly may be linked to sleep apnea. Obesity occurs in approximately 50% of hyperandrogenic anovulatory women, some of whom also have non–insulin-dependent diabetes mellitus (NIDDM). One example of this is the polycystic ovary syndrome (45).

⊶ Key points box 15.2

Sex hormones

1. Testosterone may predispose to sleep apnea, although testosterone levels are low in patients with established disease (possibly as an adaptive mechanism).

2. Although there are theoretical and experimental reasons to believe that progestational hormones might benefit sleep apnea, clinical trials of these agents in sleep apnea have been disappointing.

HYPOTHYROIDISM AND SLEEP APNEA

Apneic breathing in myxedema was noted by Massumi and Winnacker (53), and the presence of sleep apnea was later confirmed by other investigators (54). Though myxedema coma is now rare, in retrospect many cases were probably due to severe sleepiness and obtundation secondary to severe sleep apnea, coupled with the hypercapnic respiratory failure of sleep apnea. Several mechanisms have been suggested to explain the association between sleep apnea and hypothyroidism. These include reduced upper airway patency due to myxedematous infiltration of tissues, impaired function of upper airway muscles, and reduced central drive to upper airway muscles (55).

Several recent studies have questioned the strength of the association between sleep apnea and hypothyroidism. Lin et al. (56) studied 20 hypothyroid patients. All reported snoring but only two patients had moderate to severe OSAS and three had mild OSAS. Pelttari et al. (57) compared 26 patients with hypothyrodism to 188 euthyroid controls. Half (50%) of the hypothyroid patients and 29.3% of the control subjects had at least some episodes of partial or complete upper airway obstruction. Severe obstruction with episodes of repetitive apnea were present in 7.7% of the patients and in 1.5% of the controls. However, this association was largely explained by coexisting obesity and male sex. It has also been claimed that routine thyroid function testing in sleep apnea is not cost effective (58) except in certain high-risk groups, such as elderly women. Two large sleep cohort studies have been completed with conflicting conclusions regarding the strength of the association between sleep apnea and hypothyroidism (59, 60). It is likely that the prevalence of the association in sleep apnea cohorts is too low, and further case control studies in larger cohorts of sleep apnea patients are needed. In contrast, there are no prospectively collected data from large groups of hypothyroid patients. It has been asserted that the prevalence of sleep apnea in this group is high (61).

The effect of adequate thyroid hormone replacement on sleep apnea in hypothyroidism has been variable. Orr et al. (62) described three obese patients with myxedema and sleep apnea and reported cure of sleep apnea when the patients became euthyroid. Other case reports (50) describe similar cures. Rajagopal et al. (61) noted a significant reduc-

tion in apnea index for both obese and nonobese patients. Mean apnea index (AI) fell from 99.5 to < 20 in the six obese patients without weight change, and in all patients there was an associated decrease in apnea duration. The three nonobese patients had reduced AI of < 5 after achieving euthyroid status. In contrast, in another study of 10 patients (55), only two had a complete resolution of their sleep apnea when they became euthyroid. Five patients had moderate improvement in sleep apnea although they continued to require nasal CPAP, whereas three patients had worsening in their apnea frequency.

The failure of sleep apnea to resolve after thyroxine treatment supports the view of a chance rather than causal association. An alternative explanation may be that hypothyroidism induces long term changes in upper airway mechanics (63) or breathing control that do not resolve immediately after a euthyroid state is achieved. However, in two sleep apnea case-control studies, past hypothyroidism did not appear to be a risk factor for sleep apnea (53, 59).

A number of studies have suggested a link between sleep apnea and cardiovascular complications in the initial stages of thyroid hormone replacement therapy. It is well recognized that rapid restoration of the euthyroid state in hypothyroid patients may entail significant cardiovascular morbidity and mortality (55). This is particularly so in the elderly or in those with preexisting cardiovascular disease. We observed one male patient with extremely long apneas lasting over 2 min, yet his oxyhemoglobin desaturation fell to only 64% (55). Undoubtedly his low metabolic rate and oxygen consumption (reduced to 50% of normal) contributed to his ability to maintain such saturation despite long apneas. After commencing thyroxine treatment an increase in basal metabolic rate and oxygen consumption may occur more rapidly than clearance of abnormal myxedematous mucoprotein from the upper airway and normalization of depressed ventilatory responses. Long apneas may then be associated with a lower oxyhemoglobin saturation as the oxygen consumption rate increased, therefore posing a potential risk of dangerous hypoxemia for a patient with compromised coronary blood supply. We have also observed two female patients who had cardiac complications after commencing thyroxine treatment prior to a sleep study and to the use of nasal CPAP therapy. One had a myocardial infarction with residual nocturnal angina after her thyroxine dosage was increased. Her nocturnal angina resolved after nasal CPAP was commenced. Another had nocturnal ventricular arrythmias and unstable angina noted after thyroxine therapy was commenced. Both complications resolved with CPAP therapy. We are also aware of an elderly obtunded patient with myxedema (and had witnessed long apneas) who died in her sleep 24 hours after commencing a minimal dose of 25 μg of thyroxine. No sleep study had been performed and no CPAP treatment commenced. Abouganem et al. (64) reported extreme bradycardia and hypotension complicating sleep apnea in a patient with myxedema successfully managed with nasal CPAP prior to commencing thyroxine treatment. Orr et al. (62) described a myxedematous patient with OSAS and cardiac arrythmias who underwent a tracheostomy, resolving both the OSAS and arrythmias. It would seem appropriate to institute thyroid hormone replacement cautiously in patients with hypothyroidism, sleep apnea, and probable cardiovascular disease.

⊙━ Key points box 15.3

Hypothyroidism
Studies on the association of hypothyroidism with sleep apnea have produced conflicting conclusions, and thyroid replacement therapy in hypothyroid patients with sleep apnea has shown inconsistent benefits.

DISORDERED CORTICOSTEROID SECRETION AND SLEEP APNEA

Patients with corticosteroid excess secondary to Cushing disease characteristically have truncal obesity, hypertension, and depression. In the only published data, about one third of patients appear to have sleep apnea (63). Patients with Cushing disease who do not have sleep apnea exhibit poorer sleep continuity, shortened REM latency, and increased first REM period density compared to normal subjects (65, 66).

DIABETES AND OBESITY

DIABETES AND CENTRAL OBESITY
Sleep apnea is common in diabetic persons (67) and even more common in diabetic patients with autonomic neur-

opathy (68). The fundamental link between diabetes and sleep disorders is sleep apnea, through a co-association with obesity (4, 69).

Central obesity is often a more crucial determinant of morbidity and mortality than total adiposity (69). Centrally obese individuals have increased risk of cardiovascular and cerebrovascular disease, diabetes, hypertension, hyperlipidemia, hyperuricemia, and insulin resistance relative to peripherally obese individuals. Central obesity is the commonest metabolic abnormality in sleep apnea. In sleep apnea, the predominant pattern of obesity is central (4). The health risks of obesity and sleep apnea are similar, and data are complicated by mutually confounding variables (4). Attempts at separating out the two disorders have suggested that they are additive in the pathogenesis of obesity-related morbidity (70).

Central obesity is a powerful epidemiological predictor of sleep apnea (4, 70), and weight reduction may lead to marked improvement in sleep apnea severity. However, there are certainly fewer data addressing the reverse possibility – that sleep apnea may promote the development of obesity. Unfortunately, no long-term longitudinal studies examining the developmental relationship between upper airway obstruction and obesity exist. It is tempting to think that chronic intermittent hypoxia and sleep fragmentation over years in sleep apnea can lead to changes in central control of energy regulation, appetite control, feeding, and metabolism that would promote weight gain and thus worsen sleep apnea further. Moreover, if this is the case, could this vicious cycle be broken by successful CPAP therapy? Or, are there clear interindividual differences in underlying hypothalamic function leading to divergent responses in energy balance in patients with sleep apnea?

During sleep, energy expenditure (EE) typically falls relative to the awake basal state (71). In severe sleep apnea, sleep EE appears to increase during apneic sleep and falls with CPAP therapy (71). This would seem to be paradoxical; such EE changes would favor weight loss prior to CPAP and weight gain after CPAP. However, the 24 hour EE may be different in untreated sleep apnea with reduced spontaneous physical activity (SPA—such as routine physical activities) due to fatigue and sleepiness producing a net decrease in EE, despite increased EE in sleep due to respiratory effort and sleep fragmentation. Other intriguing data suggest that patients with sleep apnea may have altered serotonergic sensitivity in the hypothalamus. Hudgel et al. (72) observed that the cortisol response to L-5-HTP, a serotonin precursor, was elevated relative to that in control nonapneic subjects and was not readily explained by changes in weight. Subsequent data have shown that treatment with nasal CPAP reverses the elevated cortisol response to serotonergic stimulation (73). These latter investigators have speculated that the exaggerated cortisol responses in sleep apnea indicate supersensitivity of post synaptic serotonergic receptors in the hypothalamus caused by a serotonergic 'deficient' state induced by sleep apnea. Certainly short periods of sleep deprivation in humans and animals produce evidence of increased serotonin turnover (74), but whether chronic sleep fragmentation and hypoxemia in sleep apnea produce serotonin depletion in the hypothalamus and other regions is entirely speculative.

Interestingly, there are parallel findings of a serotonin-deficient state in central obesity (75). Bjorntorp (75) has described a cluster of disorders associated with central obesity, including abnormalities of the hypothalamic–pituitary–end organ axes (low growth hormone and testosterone, high cortisol), a 'defeat' reaction to stress with psychosocial disability and carbohydrate craving promoted by a low serotonergic state. Specific serotonergic agonists have been used as treatments in central obesity. The observed low testosterone and GH in sleep apnea also occurs in central obesity. In central obesity, recombinant GH appears to reduce central body fat (76). Perhaps restoration of GH secretion during sleep with nasal CPAP in sleep apnea may have similar effects. A recent report suggests that nasal CPAP will reduce visceral fat deposits even without a change in BMI in patients with sleep apnea (77).

Another area of common ground is insulin sensitivity. Central obesity is associated with hyperinsulinemia and insulin resistance (78). Certainly some data also point to increased insulin levels in sleep apnea independent of weight and central obesity (78) (Fig. 15.4). Nasal CPAP also improves insulin sensitivity in NIDDM (67). However, in community cohorts, any relationship between sleep apnea and insulin resistance appears to be mediated by obesity (79).

Recently, Vgontzas et al. (80) have argued that daytime sleepiness is a frequent complaint of obese patients even among those who do not have sleep apnea (80). They investigated 73 obese patients without sleep apnea who were consecutively referred for treatment of their

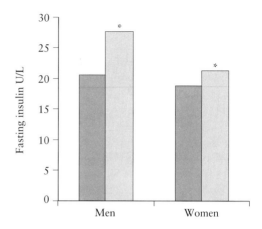

Fig 15.4 *Fasting insulin levels are higher in severely obese men and women with a high likelihood of sleep apnea (black bars, n = 338 men and 155 women) versus those with low likelihood sleep apnea (white bars, n = 216 men and 481 women). Adapted from ref. 78.*

obesity and 45 controls matched for age. In comparison to controls, obese patients were sleepier on objective testing during the day, and their nighttime sleep was more disturbed. Although this is intriguing, it would be important to confirm these findings using rigorous measurement of upper airway resistance and arousals. If proven, they may indicate that somnogeneic cytokines, (such as tumor necrosis factor alpha and interleukins) produced by central fat masses (81, 82) can cause daytime sleepiness, which is distinct from the arousals and sleep fragmentation produced by upper airway obstruction.

⚬┅ Key points box 15.4

Diabetes

1. Sleep apnea is common in diabetes, probably through a coassociation with obesity.
2. Central obesity is a powerful predictor of sleep apnea and has been associated with similar hormonal abnormalities as in OSAS, such as insulin resistance and low growth hormone and testosterone levels.

REFERENCES

1. Van Cauter E, Refetoff S. Multifactorial control of the 24 hour secretory profiles of pituitary hormones. J Endocrinol Invest 1985; 8:381–391.

2. Young T, Palta M, Dempsey J, et al. Occurrence of sleep-disordered breathing among middle-aged adults. N Engl J Med 1993; 328:1230–1235.

3. Bearpark H, Elliott L, Grunstein R, et al. Snoring and sleep apnea: a population study in Australian men. Am J Respir Crit Care Med 1995; 151:1459–1465.

4. Grunstein RR, Wilcox I, Yang TS, et al. Snoring and sleep apnoea in men: association with central obesity and hypertension. Int J Obesity 1993; 17:533–540.

5. Pastuszko A, Wilson DF, Ericinsk M. Neurotransmitter metabolism in rat brain synaptosomes: effect of anoxia and pH. J Neurochem 1982; 38:1657–1667.

6. Grunstein RR, Stewart DA, Lloyd H, et al. Acute withdrawal of nasal CPAP in obstructive sleep apnea does not cause a rise in stress hormones. Sleep 1996; 19:774–782.

7. Veldhuis JD, Iranmanesh A. Physiological regulation of the human growth hormone (GH)–insulin-like growth factor type I (IGF-I) axis: predominant impact of age, obesity, gonadal function, and sleep. Sleep 1996; 19(10 Suppl):S221–S224.

8. Van Cauter E, Caufriez A, Kerkofs M, et al. Sleep, awakenings, and insulin-like growth factor 1 modulate the growth hormone (GH) secretory response to GH-releasing hormone. J Clin Endocrinol Metab 1992; 74:1451–1459.

9. Melmed S, Acromegaly. N Engl J Med 1990; 322:966–977.

10. Iranmanesh A, Veldhuis JD. Clinical pathophysiology of the somatotropic (GH) axis in adults. Endocrinol Metab Clin North Am 1992; 21:783–817.

11. Grunstein RR, Handelsman DJ, Lawrence S, et al. Neuroendocrine dysfunction in sleep apnea: reversal by nasal continuous positive airway pressure. J Clin Endocrinol Metab 1989; 68:352–358.

12. Issa FG, Sullivan CE. The immediate effects of nasal continuous positive airway pressure treatment on sleep pattern in patients with obstructive sleep apnoea syndrome. Electroencephalogr Clin Neurophysiol 1986; 136: 755–761.

13. Grunstein RR. Metabolic aspects of sleep apnea. Sleep 1996; 19(10 Suppl):S218–S220.

14. Goldstein SJ, Wu RHK, Thorpy MJ, et al. Reversibility of deficient sleep entrained growth hormone secretion in a boy with achondroplasia and obstructive sleep apnoea. Acta Endocrinol (Copenh) 1987; 16:95–97.

15. Cooper BG, White JES, Ashworth L, et al. Hormonal and metabolic profiles in subjects with obstructive sleep apnoea syndrome and the acute effects of nasal continuous positive airway pressure treatment. Sleep 1995; 18:172–179.

16. Waters KA, Kirjavainen T, Jimenez M, et al. Overnight growth hormone secretion in achondroplasia: deconvolution analysis, correlation with sleep state, and changes after treatment of obstructive sleep apnea. Pediatr Res 1996; 39(3):547–553.

17. Stewart DA, Grunstein RR, Berthon-Jones M, et al. Androgen blockade does not affect sleep-disordered breathing or chemosensitivity in men with obstructive sleep apnea. Am Rev Respir Dis 1992; 146(6):1389–1393.

18. Bennett RM, Clark SR, Campbell SM, et al. Low levels of somatomedin C in patients with the fibromyalgia syndrome. Arthritis Rheum 1992; 35:1113–1116.

19. Stradling JR, Thomas G, Williams P, et al. Effect of adeno-tonsillectomy on nocturnal hypoxemia, sleep disturbance and symptoms in snoring children. Lancet 1990; 335:249–253.

20. Marcus CL, Carroll JI, Koerner CB, et al. Determinants of growth in children with OSA syndrome. J Paediatr 1994; 125:556–562.

21. Wright AD, Hill DM, Lowy C, Mortality in acromegaly. Q J Med 1970; 39:1–16.

22. Roxburgh F, Collis AJ. Notes on a case of acromegaly. Br Med J 1896; 2:63–65.

23. Chappell WF, Booth JA. A case of acromegaly with laryngeal symptoms and pharyngeal symptoms. J Laryng Otol 1896; 0:142–150.

24. Laroche C, Festal G, Poenaru S, et al. Une observation de respiration periodique chez une acromegalie. Ann Med Intern 1976; 127:381–385.

25. Grunstein RR, Ho KY, Sullivan CE. Acromegaly and sleep apnea. Ann Intern Med 1991; 115:527–532.

26. Pelttari L, Polo O, Rauhala E, et al. Nocturnal breathing abnormalities in acromegaly after adenomectomy. J Clin Endocrinol (Oxf) 1995; 43(2):175–182.

27. Rosenow F, Reuter S, Deuss U, et al. Sleep apnoea in treated acromegaly: relative frequency and predisposing factors. Clin Endocrinology 1996; 45:563–9.

28. Cadieux RJ, Kales A, Santen RJ, et al. Endoscopic findings in sleep apnea associated with acromegaly. J Clin Endocrinol Metab 1982; 55:18–22.

29. Perks WH, Horrocks PM, Cooper RA, et al. Sleep apnea in acromegaly. Br Med J 1980; 280;894.

30. Grunstein RR, Ho KY, Berthon-Jones M, et al. Central sleep apnea is associated with increased ventilatory response to carbon dioxide and hypersecretion of growth hormone in patients with acromegaly. Am J Respir Crit Care Med 1994; 150(2):496–502.

31. Grunstein RR, Ho KY, Sullivan CE. Effect of octreotide, a somatostatin analog, on sleep apnea in patients with acromegaly. Ann Intern Med. 1994; 121(7):478–483.

32. Faithfull S. Patients' experiences following cranial radiotherapy: a study of the somnolence syndrome. J Adv Nurs 1991; 16(8):939–946.

33. Bengtsson B-A, Eden S, Ernst I, et al. Epidemiology and long term survival in acromegaly. Acta Med Scand 1988; 223:327–335.

34. Sandblom RE, Matsumoto AM, Schoene RB, et al. Obstructive sleep apnea induced by testosterone administration. N Engl J Med 1983; 308:506–510.

35. Strumpf IJ, Reynolds SF, Vash P, et al. A possible relationship between testosterone, central control of ventilation, and the Pickwickian syndrome (abstract). Am Rev Respir Dis 1978; 117:A183.

36. Harman E, Wynne JW, Block AJ. The effect of weight loss on sleep-disordered breathing and oxygen desaturation in morbidly obese men. Chest 1982; 82:291–293.

37. Johnson MW, Arch AM, Remmers JE. Induction of the obstructive sleep apnea syndrome in a woman by exogenous androgen administration. Am Rev Respir Dis 1984; 129:1023.

38. Dexter DD, Dovre EJ. Obstructive sleep apnea due to endogenous testosterone production in a woman. Mayo Clin Proc 1998; 73(3):246–248.

39. Cistulli PA, Grunstein RR, Sullivan CE. Effect of testosterone administration on upper airway collapsibility during sleep. Am J Respir Crit Care Med 1994; 149:530–532.

40. Matsumoto AM, Sandblom RE, Schoene RB, et al. Testosterone replacement in hypogonadal males: effects on obstructive sleep apnea, respiratory drives and sleep. Clin Endocrinol (Oxf) 1985; 22:713–717.

41. Schneider BK, Pickett CK, Zwillich CW, et al. Influence of testosterone on breathing during sleep. J Appl Physiol 1986; 61:618–624.

42. Santamaria JD, Prior JC, Fleetham JA. Reversible reproductive dysfunction in men with obstructive sleep apnea. Clin Endocrinol 1988; 28:461–470.

43. Stewart DA, Grunstein RR, Sullivan CE, et al. Neuroendocrine changes in sleep apnea are not related to a pituitary defect. Sleep Res 1989; 18:308.

44. Pincus SM, Mulligan T, Iranmanesh A, et al. Older males secrete luteinizing hormone and testosterone more irregularly, and jointly more asynchronously, than younger males. Proc Natl Acad Sci USA 1996; 93(24):14100–14105.

45. Akerstedt T, Palmblad J, de la Torre B, et al. Adrenocortical and gonadal steroids during sleep deprivation. Sleep 1980; 3:23–30.

46. d'A Semple P, Beastall GH, Brown TM, et al. Sex hormone suppression and sexual impotence in hypoxic pulmonary fibrosis. Thorax 1984; 39:46.

47. Cook WR, Benich JJ, Wooten SA. Indices of severity of obstructive sleep apnea syndrome do not change during medroxyprogesterone acetate therapy. Chest 1989; 96:262–266.

48. Popovic RM, White DP. Upper airway muscle activity in normal women: influence of hormonal status. J Appl Physiol 1998; 84(3):1055–1062.

49. Block AJ, Wynne JW, Boysen PG, et al. Menopause, medroxyprogesterone and breathing during sleep. Am J Med 1980; 70:506–510.

50. Pickett CK, Regensteiner JG, Woodard WD, et al. Progestigin and estrogen reduce sleep-disordered breathing in postmenopausal women. J Appl Physiol 1989; 66:1656–1661.

51. Cistulli PA, Barnes DJ, Grunstein RR, et al. Effect of short-term hormone replacement in the treatment of obstructive sleep apnoea in postmenopausal women. Thorax 1994; 49(7):699–702.

52. Goudas VT, Dumesic DA. Polycystic ovary syndrome. Endocrinol Metab Clin North Am 1997; 26(4):893–912.

53. Massumi RA, Winnaker JL. Severe depression of the respiratory center in myxedema. Am J Med 1964; 36:876–882.

54. Duron B, Quinchard J, Fullana N. Nouvelles recherches sur le mechanisme des apneés du syndrome de pickwick. Bull Physiopathol Respir 1972; 8: 1277–1288.

55. Grunstein RR, Sullivan CE. Hypothyroidism and sleep apnea. Mechanisms and management. Am J Med 1988; 85:775–779.

56. Lin CC, Tsan KW, Chen PJ. The relationship between sleep apnea syndrome and hypothyroidism. Chest 1992; 102(6):1663–1667.

57. Pelttari L, Rauhala E, Polo O, et al. Upper airway obstruction in hypothyroidism. J Intern Med 1994; 236: 177–181.

58. Winkelman JW, Goldman H, Piscatelli N, et al. Are thyroid function tests necessary in patients with suspected sleep apnea? Sleep 1996; 19:790–793.

59. Kapur VK, Koepsell TD, de Mawbe J, et al. Association of hypothyroidism and sleep apnea. Am J Respir Crit Care Med 1998; 158: 1379–1383.

60. Sjokdt NM, Aktar R, Easton PA. Screening for hypothyroidism in sleep apnea. Am Rev Respir Crit Care Med 1999; 160:732–735.

61. Rajagopal KR, Abbrecht PH, Derderian SS, et al. Obstructive sleep apnea in hypothyroidism. Ann Intern Med 1984; 101:471–474.

62. Orr WC, Males JL, Imes NK. Myxedema and obstructive sleep apnoea. Am J Med 1981; 70:1061–1066.

63. Petrof BJ, Kelly AM, Rubinstein NA, et al. Effect of hypothyroidism on myosin heavy chain expression in rat pharyngeal dilator muscles. J Appl Physiol 1992; 73: 179–187.

64. Abouganem D, Taylor AL, Donna E, et al. Extreme bradycardia during sleep apnea caused by myxedema. Arch Intern Med 1987; 147:1497–1499.

65. Shipley JE, Schteingart DE, Tandon R, et al. Sleep architecture and sleep apnea in patients with Cushing's disease. Sleep 1992; 15(6):514–518.

66. Shipley JE, Schteingart DE, Tandon R, et al. EEG sleep in Cushing's disease and Cushing's syndrome: comparison with

patients with major depressive disorder. Biol Psychiatry 1992; 15; 32(2): 146–155.

67. Brooks B, Cistulli PA, Borkman M et al. Effect of nasal continuous positive airway pressure treatment on insulin sensitivity in patients with Type II diabetes and obstructive sleep apnea. J Clin Endocrinol Metab 1994; 79: 1681–1685.

68. Ficker JH, Dertinger SH, Siegfried W, et al. Obstructive sleep apnoea and diabetes mellitus: the role of cardiovascular autonomic neuropathy. Eur Respir J 1998; 11(1): 14–19.

69. Bjorntorp P. Obesity. Lancet 1997; 350(9075):423–426.

70. Grunstein RR, Stenlof K, Hedner J, et al. Impact of self reported sleep apnea symptoms on psycho-social performance in the Swedish Obese Subjects (SOS) Study. Sleep 1995; 18: 635–643.

71. Stenlof K, Grunstein RR, Hedner J, et al. Energy expenditure in obstructive sleep apnea: effects of treatment with continuous positive airway pressure. Am J Physiol 1996; 271: E1036–1043.

72. Hudgel DW, Gordon EA, Meltzer HY. Abnormal serotonergic stimulation of cortisol production in obstructive sleep apnea. Am J Respir Crit Care Med 1995; 152: 186–192.

73. Hudgel DW, Gordon EA. Serotonin-induced cortisol release in CPAP-treated obstructive sleep apnea patients. Chest 1997; 111(3):632–638.

74. Heiser P, Dickhaus B, Opper C, et al. Platelet serotonin and interleukin-1 beta after sleep deprivation and recovery sleep in humans. J Neural Transm 1997; 104(10): 1049–1058.

75. Bjorntorp P. Neuroendocrine abnormalities in human obesity. Metabolism 1995; 44(2 Suppl 2): 38–41.

76. Johannsson G, Marin P, Lonn L, et al. Growth hormone treatment of abdominally obese men reduces abdominal fat mass, improves glucose and lipoprotein metabolism, and reduces diastolic blood pressure. J Clin Endocrinol Metab 1997; 82(3): 727–734.

77. Chin K, Shimizu K, Nakamura T. et al. Changes in intrabdominal visceral fat and serm leptin levels in patients with obstructive sleep apnea following nasal continuous positive airway pressure. Circulation 1999; 100: 706–712.

78. Grunstein RR, Stenlof K, Hedner J, et al. Impact of obstructive sleep apnea and sleepiness on metabolic and cardiovascular risk factors in the Swedish Obese Subjects (SOS) Study. Int J Obesity 1995; 151:410–418.

79. Stoohs RA, Facchini F, Guilleminault C. Insulin resistance and sleep-disordered breathing in healthy humans. Am J Respir Crit Care Med 1996; 154(1): 170–174.

80. Vgontzas AN, Bixler EO, Tan TL, et al. Obesity without sleep apnea is associated with daytime sleepiness. Arch Intern Med 1998; 158(12): 1333–1337.

81. Katsuki A, Sumida Y, Murashima S, et al. Serum levels of tumor necrosis factor–alpha are increased in obese patients with noninsulin-dependent diabetes mellitus. J Clin Endocrinol Metab 1998; 83(3): 859–862.

82. Vgontzas AN, Papanicolaou DA, Bixler EO, et al. Elevation of plasma cytokines in disorders of excessive daytime sleepiness: role of sleep disturbance and obesity. J Clin Endocrinol Metab 1997; 82(5): 1313–1316.

Morbidity, Mortality, and Public Health Burden of Sleep Apnea

Susan Redline

INTRODUCTION

Since the late 1960s, the acute pathophysiological effects of obstructive sleep apnea syndrome (OSAS) have been described in increasingly exquisite detail. These effects have been reviewed in the previous chapters. Briefly, the occurrence of sleep-related intermittent upper airway obstruction, manifested as recurrent hypopneas and apneas, results in gas exchange abnormalities, large fluctuations in intrathoracic pressure, and chemoreflex activation (1, 2). These directly or interactively alter sympathetic and parasympathetic nervous system activity and modify the release of neuroendocrine factors. Systemic effects may be widespread may and have an impact on both the cardiovascular system and neurocognitive functions. Cardiovascular consequences are related to alterations in arterial blood pressure, venous blood return, and cardiac afterload with measurable effects on heart rate and rhythm, stroke volume, systemic and pulmonary blood pressures, and, possibly, cerebral perfusion. A range of adverse neurocognitive and behavioral effects also is well described. These have been attributed both to recurrent arousals, causing fragmented sleep and daytime sleepiness, and to the effects of intermittent hypoxemia.

In contrast to the wealth of data that address the acute effects of OSAS, relatively less is known concerning its long-term morbidity. Data from ongoing cohort studies, however, provide growing evidence linking OSAS to chronic health problems. The results of recent randomized control studies that show an amelioration of adverse health effects with treatment of OSAS support a causal role of OSAS in such conditions, underscoring the public health importance of recognizing and treating OSAS in the population.

This chapter reviews data, reported largely between 1995 and 2000, that address chronic morbidities associated with OSAS. Attempts will be made to estimate the overall influence of OSAS-related morbidities on a variety of outcomes, including impact on survival and economic costs (Table 16.1). Finally, the potential effects of intervention on public health are estimated.

OSAS-RELATED MORBIDITIES

BLOOD PRESSURE EFFECTS

Hypertension is perhaps the best-studied outcome of OSAS. Surveys of patients with OSAS or with hypertension have demonstrated that > 50% of patients with one of these conditions also have the other (3–7). Numerous additional studies comparing persons with OSAS or with snoring to subjects without these conditions have demonstrated increased blood pressure levels or a higher prevalence of hypertension in the affected groups (8–10). Many of the studies published prior to 1995, however, suffered from relatively small sample sizes and were criticized because of concern that the observed associations were due to the confounding effects of obesity, a factor strongly associated with both OSAS and hypertension.

Three large population-based studies that have utilized polysomnography now provide clear evidence that an association between OSAS and hypertension is moderately strong and cannot be attributed solely to the effects of obesity or to other measurable, recognized confounders.

The largest and most diverse sample is the Sleep Heart Health Study cohort. This cohort was assembled as part of a multicenter study of 6440 persons recruited from nine diverse geographical locations across the United States. The sample includes subjects with an age range of 40 to 98 years (mean, 64 years) and 23% ethnic minorities (11). Participants were studied with 12 channel in-home polysomnography that provided highly reliable indices of the apnea-hypopnea index (AHI). Prevalence of

Table 16.1 Estimates of potential impact of OSAS on morbidity and mortality

	Magnitude of Effect[a]	Threshold Effect	Dose-Response Relation	Population Variability
Hypertension	+ to ++++	Very low	+	Greater impact in younger and less obese persons
Cardiovascular Disease	+	Low	+ (within range of AHI 1.5–12)	Greater impact in younger persons
Mood or Affect	+ to ++	Intermediate	+	?
Cognition	+ to ++	+	Intermediate to high	Probable, but not defined
Sleepiness	++++	Low	+	?
Mortality	++	?	+	Greater impact in younger persons

[a] + indicates significant effects have been measured in well-designed studies, with odds ratios < 1.5, effect size < 0.25, or % variance explained < 8%.

++ indicate odds ratios > 1.5 but < 3.0, effect sizes .25–.50, or % variance explained 8–15%.

++++ indicates odds ratios > 3.0 or effect sizes ≥ 0.50.

hypertension increased in a linear dose-response fashion with escalating AHI, increasing from 43% among persons with the lowest levels of AHI (AHI < 1.5), to 62% in those with an AHI between 15 and 29, and further to 67% among those with an AHI ≥ 30 (12). As was observed in previous studies, the prevalence of obesity also was strongly associated with OSAS, varying from 16% (among persons within the lowest AHI stratum [AHI < 1.5]) to > 60% (among subjects in the highest AHI stratum [AHI ≥ 30]). Persons with higher AHI levels were also more likely to be male and older. After accounting for the effects of obesity (characterized both by body mass index [BMI] and by indices of body fat distribution), age, sex, race, smoking, and alcohol use, persons with an AHI > 5 significantly were more likely to be hypertensive than similar persons with lower levels of AHI (< 1.5). Specifically, an AHI level of 5–29.9 was estimated to confer a 20–26% excess risk of hypertension, and an AHI ≥ 30 was estimated to confer a 37% excess risk of hypertension.

The Wisconsin Sleep Cohort, a sample of > 1000 state employees aged 30–60 years (mean, 47 years), has provided both cross-sectional and longitudinal estimates of

hypertension risk associated with OSAS. In cross-sectional analyses, significant associations of OSAS with both blood pressure level and prevalence of hypertension were demonstrated (13–15). Using multiple regression analyses, the authors estimated the average expected increase in blood pressure associated with each increment of AHI for persons with a BMI of 30 kg/m^2. These statistical models predicted that each apnea or hypopnea per hour of sleep increased systolic and diastolic blood pressures by 0.24 and 0.12 mm Hg, respectively (or an increase of 3.6 and 1.8 mm Hg, respectively, for an AHI of 15 versus 0). At this same BMI, compared to individuals with an AHI of 0, the relative odds of hypertension (a systolic blood pressure ≥ 140 or diastolic blood pressure ≥ 90 or use of antihypertensive medications) was estimated to be increased threefold (odds ratio 3.07) for persons with an AHI of 30, almost twofold (odds ratio 1.75) for those with an AHI of 15, and by 21% for persons with an AHI of 5. One shortcoming of this (as well as the other cohort studies) was that these cross-sectional analyses did not address the temporal association between OSAS and hypertension or whether OSAS was causally related to the development of hypertension. However, further longitudinal data based on an 8 year follow-up evaluation of the cohort were reported in 2000. These data demonstrated a nearly threefold increased prevalence of (new) hypertension among persons whom at baseline had elevated AHI levels (> 15) (16), strongly suggesting that hypertension may occur in response to OSAS.

A third large cohort (1741 persons) from southern Pennsylvania, consisting of adults ≥ 20 years (mean, 47 years), also has been assembled to examine the relationship between OSAS and hypertension (17). In this cohort, a strong dose-response relationship also was observed between severity of sleep-disordered breathing and hypertension. The relative odds for hypertension for those with an AHI ≥ 15 compared to a group with an AHI of 0 and no snoring, estimated for persons aged 47 years with a BMI of 26.7 kg/m² (the average levels in this cohort) and adjusted for potential confounders, was 6.8. Risk of hypertension also was elevated among persons identified to have milder degrees of sleep-disordered breathing, including snorers with minimal to mild elevations in their AHI (AHI levels > 0 but < 15) (odds ratio 2.3), as well as for snorers with no observed apneas or hypopneas (odds ratio 1.6).

Thus, the three most recently reported large cohort studies are consistent in demonstrating progressive increases in prevalence of hypertension with increasing severity of OSAS. Threshold effects appear measurable even at low levels of AHI, possibly even associated with snoring occurring with minimal apnea activity. Furthermore, these relationships do not appear to be explained solely by obesity of other easily measurable confounders—concerns raised in earlier work. The magnitude of risk appears somewhat debatable, with moderate levels of OSAS associated with odds ratios that may vary about fivefold. However, some of these differences may be explained by heterogeneity of effects among people of varying ages and levels of obesity. Two of the three studies that included a wide range of ages showed stronger relative effects of OSAS in younger than older persons. Two of the studies that examined the modifying influence of obesity on the impact of OSAS on blood pressure also demonstrated much larger effects of OSAS among less obese persons. The relatively greater impact of OSAS on blood pressure level in less obese and younger people could be due to many factors, including population differences in pathophysiological responses to apnea or to genetic factors that modify the expression of OSAS

in different population subsets. Regardless of mechanisms, these observations suggest that younger and nonobese people with OSAS may experience a marked increase in risk of hypertension due to a treatable cause.

The impact of OSAS on blood pressure also has been characterized by studies utilizing 24 hour ambulatory blood pressure recordings. This technology potentially reduces measurement error associated with readings from a single session, allows blood pressure levels to be correlated with sleep-wake states, and identifies abnormalities in relative changes in blood pressure pattern over the day. In relation to OSAS, identification of 'nondippers'—those people whose mean blood pressure does not drop by at least 10% of the wake level—has been of particular interest. Several such studies have demonstrated subjects with OSAS to include a disproportionately large number of 'nondippers' as well as persons with sustained elevations in daytime blood pressure levels (6, 18–20). Most recently, Davies et al. (21) have quantified differences in 24 hour ambulatory blood pressure profiles in 45 patients with OSAS compared to 45 extremely well-matched controls. OSAS patients had significantly higher diastolic blood pressure (by 4.6 mm Hg in the day and 7.2 mm Hg in the night) and higher nocturnal systolic blood pressure (by 9.2 mm Hg). Changes of this magnitude were estimated to potentially increase risk of stroke by 40% and risk of heart disease by 15%.

CARDIOVASCULAR DISEASE (CVD) MORBIDITY

CVD, including coronary artery disease (angina, myocardial infarction) and cerebrovascular disease (stroke and transient ischemic attacks) are reported commonly in persons with OSAS. Increased CVD in people with OSAS could be due to the blood pressure elevations (with effects on the vasculature and heart) commonly observed in this population (as described above). However, the hypoxia or adrenergic responses, or both, that often accompany OSAS also may cause a number of systemic metabolic effects that directly promote atherogenesis, including upregulation of proinflammatory cytokines and prothrombotic processes, and insulin resistance (22, 23). These processes are now recognized as related to a group of 'novel' CVD risk factors that are hypothesized to cause vascular endothelial damage via effects on thrombosis and oxidation of serum and tissue proteins (24).

Most of the evidence relating OSAS and CVD is based on studies of snoring. Both cross-sectional (case-control) and longitudinal studies have reported twofold to four-fold increases in risk of myocardial infarction in snorers compared to non-snorers (25–29). These findings largely persisted even after considering potential confounding with obesity, hypertension, smoking, and alcohol. Snoring also has been associated cross sectionally with reported stroke or transient ischemic attacks (29). Longitudinal data from the Finnish Twin Registry in addition provide evidence that a history of snoring increases risk of combined ischemic heart disease and stroke twofold (28).

Fewer data are available that address CVD in subjects in whom OSAS has been characterized using polysomnography. Retrospective studies of patients studied after a myocardial infarction or after a stroke suggest a marked increase in OSAS in these patient groups (30, 31). However, studies of patients in the immediate postmyocardial or poststroke periods may not provide representative data on breathing patterns that precede the acute CVD events. A major aim of the Sleep Heart Health Study (discussed above) is to provide definitive data regarding the temporal association between OSAS and CVD. Cross-sectional data from this study demonstrate that even modest levels of OSAS (AHI > 12) increase risk of self-reported angina, myocardial infarction, and stroke approximately 30–40% (32). These estimates were adjusted for most major CVD risk factors, including obesity, cholesterol–high density lipoprotein (HDL) level, sex, and smoking. Estimates also were adjusted for blood pressure level, suggesting that the relationship between OSAS and CVD was not mediated solely through the effects of OSAS on hypertension. Interestingly, CVD risk did not increase progressively with increasing levels of AHI above 12. That observation suggested that the effect of OSAS on CVD might be attained at a relatively low level of AHI. The extent to which OSAS is causally related to the development of CVD will be addressed with forthcoming longitudinal analyses.

NEUROCOGNITIVE AND BEHAVIORAL MORBIDITY

A major component of the morbidity of OSAS is thought to relate to short-term and, possibly, long-term neurocognitive deficits caused by exposure to intermittent hypoxemia, hypercapnia, and arousal, acting independently or synergistically (33–35). Deficits have been examined using classic neuropsychological approaches with administration of test batteries that assess a range of functions. These include executive functions (processes involved in planning, initiation, or self-regulation of goal-oriented behavior), attention (including attention span, sustained attention or vigilance, and response times), information processing efficiency, and learning and memory (36).

A wide range of neurocognitive deficits has been reported in patients with OSAS. In general, the largest and broadest range of neuropsychological deficits has been demonstrated in patients with severe OSAS, as evidenced by pathological levels of sleepiness, severe sleep-associated hypoxemia, or with AHIs > 40 (33, 37, 38). Deficits have been reported for general intellectual ability, learning and memory, sustained and focused attention, executive functions, information processing efficiency, and visual and psychomotor performance (33, 39). Some studies have shown an inverse correlation between some of these measures and indices of OSAS (lowest oxygen saturation or total apnea time), suggesting a dose-response relationship between disease severity and neurocognitive deficits (39, 40). Study results suggest that hypoxemia most closely predicts deficits in executive functions and psychomotor skills, whereas sleepiness predicts deficits in attention measures (39, 41).

Interpreting the above study results, however, requires recognition that neurocognitive tests are quite sensitive to noncognitive influences, including age, alcohol consumption, education level, motivation, and baseline intelligence. Many of the preceding studies included subjects representing wide age and apnea ranges, did not include control groups, or included controls that were not well matched to OSAS cases. Thus, some studies may have overestimated deficits attributable to OSAS. Furthermore, these studies provide limited data on the extent to which deficits extend to persons with mild OSAS. Indeed, studies of subjects recruited from the community, or subjects with less severe OSAS, have shown less impairment than studies of severely affected patients seeking help from a specialty clinic. Data from the Wisconsin Sleep Cohort, a population-based study, showed no relationship between the AHI and a 'memory' score based on a word recall test among working middle-aged subjects (40). Weak, but significant, associations were demonstrated between a summary measure of 'psychomotor efficiency' and the AHI, the latter accounting for approximately 4% of the variability in tests dependent on speed. My laboratory has utilized a rigorous neurocognitive testing battery to assess a range of functions in persons carefully screened to be free from confounding medical co-morbidities. We demonstrated small but significant impairments (explaining 4–6% of the test variability) in several domains, including working memory, declarative memory, signal discrimination, and sustained attention (vigilance) (unpublished data). The last-mentioned (vigilance) was the area that was most impaired among persons with mild OSAS (AHI 10–30) (34).

In summary, early studies may have overestimated the effects of OSAS on neurocognitive function. There does, however, appear to be increasing evidence that persons with OSAS, on average, perform more slowly and are less attentive than those without OSAS. The public health impact of these findings is difficult to interpret. For example, the implications of small to moderate impairments in experimentally measured vigilance on performance in daily tasks is unclear. In 'real life' situations, people may differ in their ability to compensate and adapt to vigilance deficits or to deficits in other areas. The extent to which clinically significant effects occur at low levels of OSAS (or whether threshold effects exist, below which function is unimpaired) is, as of yet, also unclear. As described later, additional insight into the public health impact of OSAS rather may be derived from studies of intervention.

It also has been suggested that OSAS may lead to an acceleration of cognitive decline with aging, including increasing risk for dementia (42, 43). The public health impact of OSAS would be even more substantial if the results of prospective studies indicate that OSAS is a cause rather than a consequence of dementia.

SLEEPINESS

Daytime sleepiness is one of the most commonly recognized morbidities of OSAS. Indeed, many definitions of OSAS utilize the dimension 'associated sleepiness' as a necessary element for making this diagnosis or to gauge its severity. The effects of OSAS on daytime sleepiness were discussed in detail in Chapters 2 and 5. Here, it is emphasized that recent data indicate that sleepiness is a concomitant of mild OSAS as well as of more severe conditions. Most recently, the Sleep Heart Health Study reported significant associations of increasing AHI with greater levels of sleepiness, measured by the Epworth Sleepiness Scale (44). This scale provides a score that is constructed from a person's response to an eight item scale

requesting the person to rate his or her likelihood of dozing off in a number of situations. Compared to people with an AHI < 5, the sleepiness scores increased by 8%, 15%, and 29%, respectively, in groups defined by increasing levels of AHI (5 to < 15; 15 to < 30; > 30). Sleepiness, defined on the basis of a score of ≥ 11, was 33% more likely in those with mild OSAS (AHI 15 to < 30) and 67% more likely in those with moderate of greater OSAS (AHI > 30). Furthermore, additional analyses of data from this cohort indicate that snorers, regardless of measurable apnea or hypopnea, also report more sleepiness than nonsnorers.

⊶ Key points box 16.1

OSAS-related morbidities

- Large, population-based studies demonstrate an association between OSAS and hypertension that cannot be attributed to confounders, such as obesity.

- The effects of OSAS on blood pressure appear to be stronger in younger and less obese persons.

- Epidemiological studies suggest that snoring and OSA are risk factors for ischemic heart disease and stroke.

- OSAS may impair neurocognitive function, but the degree of impairment and its impact have not been clearly determined.

- Daytime sleepiness is a common morbidity resulting from OSAS.

IMPACT OF OSAS ON THE INDIVIDUAL PERSON AND SOCIETY

The previously described associations of OSAS with blood pressure, CVD, performance, and behavior may affect public health through a number of ways. In this next section, the influence of OSAS on health is described according to its secondary effects on functional status, accidents, hospitalizations, and mortality.

QUALITY OF LIFE AND FUNCTIONAL STATUS

Quality of life and functional status are related multifaceted concepts. Quality of life refers to 'global well-being,' including physical and psychosocial functions. Functional status specifically refers to the ability to meet needs, fulfill roles, and maintain health and well-being (45, 46). These measures are increasingly used in health services to compare patient subgroups and to assess the impact of different interventions or providers on disease management.

Both quality of life and functional status are increasingly recognized as relevant and important OSAS outcomes (47, 48). Interest in these outcomes stems from recognition that sleepiness, abnormalities in mood or affect (particularly depression, anxiety, and irritability), and physical limitations (occurring secondary to CVD), occur commonly in OSAS and may importantly contribute to impaired quality of life. For example, sleepiness, assessed by the multiple sleep latency test (MSLT), explains a modest but significant amount of the variability in the subscales 'social functioning' and 'energy and fatigue,' and for the summary scores 'functional status' and 'well-being' derived from the Medical Outcomes Survey SF-30, a commonly used generic health-related quality of life instrument (49).

The specific impact of OSAS on quality of life has been assessed by examining the relationship of AHI with quality of life scores. In the Sleep Heart Health Study cohort, participants from the community with AHI levels > 30 were approximately 50% more likely to have low scores on the Medical Outcomes SF-30 subscales of general health, physical functioning, vitality, and social functioning (50). In contrast to the Wisconsin Sleep Cohort, in which poorer scores for several quality of life subscores were observed across the range of OSAS (51), in the Sleep Heart Health Study lower levels of AHI were associated with poorer quality of life only for the vitality subscale. It is not clear whether these study differences relate to differences in the samples (Sleep Heart Health Study cohort is older and more diverse) or analytic approaches. Thus, at this point, it is reasonable to conclude that moderately high levels of AHI negatively affects a broad number of quality of life dimensions. Mildly elevated levels of AHI appear to be associated with reduced vitality, although also may be associated with other dimensions in certain populations.

The psychosocial morbidity associated with OSAS also has been addressed in a large study of obese persons from Sweden (52). Obese people with symptoms of OSAS (snoring, observed apneas, and sleepiness) had significantly increased rates of divorce, impaired work performance, and increased sick leave. Women with OSAS appeared to suffer especially high divorce rates (> seven-fold greater than women without OSAS). On average, subjects with OSAS had five more weeks per year of sick leave than subjects without OSAS. This effect may actually have been underestimated, since it was calculated after adjusting for effects of chronic health conditions, such as hypertension and diabetes, which *per se* may be exacerbated by OSAS. Such excessive rates of sick leave can be anticipated to reduce productivity of the work force and to affect the economy broadly and negatively.

Newer disease-specific quality of life instruments for OSAS are now being used (47, 48). These specifically probe areas of functioning that are likely influenced by mood, energy, and sleep habits (such as social and sexual functions) and ability to perform tasks that require sustained attention. Data from these tools that will be forthcoming over the next few years should further shed light on quality of life in OSAS.

ACCIDENTS

Accidents are the fourth leading cause of death in the United States. Nonfatal accidents also contribute to measurable morbidity by causing permanent injury (affecting > 9 million people/year in the United States) as well as restricted activity days (> 800 million bed days/year) (53). By far the leading type of accidents is motor vehicle accidents. Daytime sleepiness or attentional deficits may be anticipated to increase the risk of accidents in patients with OSAS. Furthermore, vulnerability may be greatest for accidents occurring during long, relatively monotonous tasks, such as driving a motor vehicle.

Several sources of data suggest that persons with OSAS indeed are at considerable risk for vehicular accidents. Anecdotal data and reports from clinics indicate that 30 to 90% of OSAS patients have been involved in accidents, and many of these patients have reported that these accidents were related to sleepiness (53). Findley et al. (54) demonstrated that patients referred to a sleep laboratory and subsequently found to have an AHI > 5 were seven times more likely to have had automobile accidents than referred patients with normal sleep study results. Accident rates for the OSAS group were almost three times greater than the accident rate for all licensed drivers in that state (Virginia). Using a prevalence of OSAS of 1%, they estimated that at least 58,800 of the 2 million accidents per year in the United States would involve persons with

OSAS, an excess of 38,800 accidents per year. In the Wisconsin Sleep Cohort, persons with undiagnosed OSAS but with an AHI > 15 were more than seven times more likely than those with no OSAS to have had multiple automobile accidents in the previous 5 years (55).

Truck drivers, who are predominantly men and often have abnormal sleep-wake schedules, may be an occupational group at particularly high risk for OSAS-related accidents. One study suggested that as many as 78% of long-haul truck drivers have at least mild levels of OSAS, and 10% had evidence of moderate to severe OSAS (56). Another study of long-haul truckers indicated that symptoms of sleep-disordered breathing was an independent predictor of falling asleep at the wheel (57).

These data thus suggest that persons with OSAS are three to seven times more likely to be in car accidents. There are debates, however, over whether a threshold of OSAS exists that increases risk of an accident, and over which characteristics best identify persons with OSAS who are at greatest risk.

MORTALITY

Mortality in OSAS may be increased secondary to CVD or because of fatal vehicular and work-related accidents. Several retrospective studies of patients referred to sleep laboratories and from a few community-based studies provide estimates of the strength of such relationships. As described below, overall effects on mortality appear to be stronger for younger persons.

Two early studies demonstrated increased mortality ratios for patients with severe OSAS treated with conservative therapy or uvulopalatopharyngoplasty (UPPP) (therapeutic efficacy of 50%), as compared to patients treated with tracheostomy or continuous positive airway pressure (CPAP) (58, 59). Both of these studies demonstrated mortality rates of approximately 6% per 5–8 years. Deaths appeared to have been due largely to vascular diseases. Increased mortality was most apparent in subjects < 50 years (i.e, 8 year mortality rate 10% versus 2% for those with more versus less OSAS) (58).

Lavie et al. (60) reported on mortality rates for 1620 OSAS patients (with an apnea index > 10) referred to an Israeli sleep laboratory. Among men < 50 years, all-cause mortality rates were two to four times higher than in the general Israeli population. After adjusting for body mass index (BMI), hypertension, and underlying cardiopulmonary disease, apnea index (AI) predicted all-cause mor-

tality in a dose-dependent fashion. However, mortality due to cardiopulmonary causes was not related to the AI; there was no suggestion of increased mortality with OSAS in older subjects.

Several studies exclusively examined elderly subjects. A nursing home study found that female residents with high levels of OSAS had a greater 10 year mortality rate than female residents with less OSAS; however, OSAS did not predict mortality in men (61). Interestingly, persons with obstructive apnea were more likely to have died in their sleep than subjects without obstructive breathing events. Community-based studies of elderly persons from Australia and California also have examined the relationship of mortality and OSAS (62, 63). Among subjects (mean age of 67 years) followed for up to 10 years, Bliwise et al. (62) demonstrated an almost threefold increase in mortality for subjects with an AHI > 10 as compared to subjects with lower AHIs. This estimate, which was adjusted for age, sex, and BMI, did not reach statistical significance in this sample (n = 198). A smaller effect on mortality was observed among 163 residents of an Australian retirement community followed for only 4 years (63). Both of these studies had limited statistical power to detect any but large effects due to OSAS. It is also possible that older subjects with OSAS may represent a 'survivor' population who are less susceptible to the end-organ effects of the disorder.

The relationship of mortality to symptoms of OSAS also has been examined. In a large, community-based study in Sweden, 3100 respondents to a postal survey were followed for 10 years. Mortality rates in persons < 60 years who reported both snoring and daytime sleepiness were two or three times higher than mortality rates in persons without these symptoms (64). Increased mortality was not found in subjects reporting either snoring or sleepiness, and similar to the Israeli study, increased mortality was not observed among older persons. Excessive death rates were due predominantly to vascular causes, although the number of suicides was also elevated in the symptomatic group. Findings persisted after adjustment for age, obesity, and other medical conditions. In the Honolulu Asian American Aging Study, a study of > 2900 elderly Japanese-American men, a 50% increase in mortality was associated with self-reported sleepiness but not with the symptom 'snoring' (65). The relationship with sleepiness became nonsignificant after adjusting for chronic medical conditions. In a broader age range, a long-term prospective community study conducted as part of National Health and Nutritional Examination Society (NHANES) demonstrated that a history of sleepiness and sleeping > 8 hours increased mortality by 30% (66). These analyses adjusted for multiple potential confounders and were not likely biased by survival or selection biases. The weakness of this study relates to the relative nonspecificity of the symptoms of sleepiness and 'long' sleep to identify people with undiagnosed OSAS.

In summary, many of the studies of mortality have been limited by retrospective data collection, study samples that may represent either 'survivors' (elders) or those who have much comorbidity, relatively small sample sizes or few observed deaths, and lack of appropriate control groups. These limitations make it difficult to assess the overall impact of OSAS and different degrees of OSAS on mortality in unselected subjects. However, the available data do suggest that increased mortality is likely in persons with severe levels of apnea, especially those in whom OSAS first appears in middle life or earlier.

⊙┓ Key points box 16.2

Impact of OSAS

■ Moderate degrees of OSAS have a negative impact on a broad number of quality of life dimensions.

■ OSAS is associated with increased rates of psychosocial morbidity.

■ Persons with OSAS are at increased risk (3–7 times) for motor vehicle accidents.

■ Available data suggest an increased rate of mortality in persons with severe OSAS, particularly when the disorder first appears in midlife or earlier.

ECONOMIC IMPACT OF UNTREATED OSAS

There are a number of sources of economic costs to society due to OSAS. These include costs associated with diagnosing and treating the condition; costs of treating medical conditions that may be precipitated or exacerbated by OSAS (e.g., hypertension and vascular diseases); diminished work productivity due to the direct effects of OSAS (sleepiness and performance deficits) or to complications of associated comorbidities; and the costs of accidents. An emerging, albeit limited, literature suggests that these varied costs are quite substantial. Further, as discussed in the final section of this chapter, some of these costs may be reduced by earlier and more efficient recognition and treatment strategies for OSAS.

HEALTH CARE UTILIZATION COSTS

Two studies from Manitoba, Canada, where there is universal health care and data systems that contain detailed health care costs, indicate that patients with diagnosed OSAS utilize almost twice as many health care resources during their 10 years prior to diagnosis and treatment, compared to age, sex, and neighborhood matched controls followed for a similar time period (67, 68). Increased costs related both to increased overnight hospitalizations (averaging 6.2 versus 3.7 per person over 10 years, for patients and controls, respectively) and for physician claims ($3972 versus $1969) (67).

Kapur et al. (69) also have reported on medical costs of untreated OSAS. In their study, data from a large health maintenance organization in Washington were used to compare costs 1 year prior to diagnosis of patients with OSAS to age and sex-matched controls studied over the same time period. Similar to the Canadian study (67), costs for the OSAS group were about twice as high as for the control group ($2720 versus $1384). Differences in costs persisted after adjusting for differences in chronic diseases between the two groups. Furthermore, among the OSAS cases, a dose-response relationship was observed between increasing AHI and increasing medical care costs. Using these estimates of excessive cost attributable to OSAS and prevalence estimates of moderate OSAS (AHI > 15) in the community (70), these investigators estimated that in the United States untreated OSAS may be responsible for $3.4 billion/year of medical costs.

Costs related to accidents, precipitated or exacerbated by OSAS, constitute a potentially huge economic cost to society. The annual cost of all accidents has been estimated to be at least $143 billion/year in the United States. More than 3% of all accidents are thought to be caused by driver sleepiness (71). The extent to which OSAS contributes to sleepiness in the general population is not precisely known; but even if it is a relatively small cause of sleepiness, OSAS-related accidents can be estimated to contribute to a substantial economic burden.

There are very few data that address the impact of OSAS on loss of work productivity. However, as described above, one population-based Swedish study suggests that obese persons with OSAS take 5 more weeks per year of sick leave than obese persons without OSAS. Additional data are needed to better gauge the potentially broad and diverse ways OSAS may contribute to economic costs to society.

EFFECTS OF TREATMENT ON OSAS-ASSOCIATED MORBIDITIES AND MORTALITY

One of the most important questions concerning OSAS-associated morbidity is whether it can be reduced with early recognition, prevention, or treatment. As reviewed below, an emerging literature suggests that treatment of OSAS may improve sleepiness, quality of life, blood pressure, and at least selective aspects of performance (Table 16.2). These findings suggest the need to develop more focused approaches for efficiently identifying which persons are most likely to benefit from specific therapies, and also for instituting effective programs for OSAS risk reduction.

TREATMENT EFFECTS ON SLEEP QUALITY AND SLEEPINESS

Several studies have demonstrated that symptomatic OSAS patients, usually with moderate to high levels of AHI (> 30), experience improved sleep quality with nasal CPAP therapy. Parameters that have been reported to show the largest improvements are percentage times in stage 1 (66% reduction) and stage 3/4 (fivefold increase) sleep (72), and the arousal index (reduction to one fifth) (73). Daytime sleepiness, assessed by physiological testing (e.g., the multiple sleep latency test [MSLT] or the maintenance of wakefulness test [MWT]) or by subjective reporting (e.g., with the Epworth Sleepiness Scale [ESS]) also has been reported to improve, sometimes dramatically (74–77).

Persons with milder degrees of OSAS also have shown improvements in sleepiness after CPAP therapy. However, in controlled studies of less severely affected persons, improvements in the MSLT or MWT have been small and often nonsignificant (74–76). In contrast, in

Table 16.2 Estimates of effects of OSAS treatment

	Magnitude of Effect[a]
Sympathetic nervous system activity	++
Hypertension	+
Mood or Affect	+/++
Cognition	+
Sleepiness	+++
Mortality	++
Accidents	++
Health care expenditures	++

[a] + indicates significant effects but small have been measured in well-designed studies.

++ indicate 50% or more reduction in rates or costs.

+++ indicate marked improvement in sleepiness (effect size > 0.50).

studies from a variety of settings, consistent improvements in the ESS have been observed across a range of disease severity, with measurable effects in persons with an AHI > 5 and large effects in severely affected persons (74–78). These findings suggest that specific therapy for OSAS can effectively ameliorate the most obviously disabling symptom of the disorder. However, the failure of some studies to show therapy-associated improvements in physiological measurements of sleepiness suggests the need to better understand the bases for persistent physiological sleepiness.

TREATMENT EFFECTS ON HEALTH-RELATED QUALITY OF LIFE

Several well-controlled studies have demonstrated improved health-related quality of life or improved functional status in groups receiving therapeutic levels of CPAP, as compared to groups receiving conservative therapy (weight loss, sleep hygiene), sham CPAP, or an oral placebo (74–79). The domain 'vitality' or 'energy/fatigue' has shown the most consistent improvements across categories of disease severity. Improvements in social functioning or isolation, physical functioning, and general health also have been reported. The importance of these findings is stressed by the increasing recognition that improved well-being and functional status are important outcomes to patients and to health care providers.

It should be emphasized that improved functional status has been demonstrated in subjects with mild levels of OSAS, often without daytime sleepiness. Levels of AHI and daytime sleepiness also have not yet proved to be useful predictors of response to OSAS therapy. Thus, it does not appear to be justifiable to restrict treatment to persons only with moderate or severe disease.

TREATMENT EFFECTS ON MOOD AND COGNITIVE FUNCTION OR PERFORMANCE

Several studies also suggest that treatment of sleep apnea may improve cognition and mood of patients with severe disease (41, 74, 80, 81). Many of the studies reporting positive findings, however, were uncontrolled or enrolled only very severely affected patients. One controlled study of mildly affected patients suggests that both mood (depression) and tasks heavily influenced by attentional abilities may be improved after OSAS treatment (79). Additional work is needed to sort out what cognitive deficits associated with OSAS are due to associated comorbidities, which ones are a direct consequence of the disorder, and which are reversible with therapy.

TREATMENT EFFECTS ON BLOOD PRESSURE

Physiological benefits of CPAP therapy on blood pressure are suggested by the studies demonstrating reductions in sympathetic activity (measured by noradrenaline [norepinephrine] in urine and plasma and by renal and muscle sympathetic activity on nerve recording) after CPAP therapy (18, 82–86). Several small intervention trials have shown that successful treatment of sleep apnea is accompanied by a fall in daytime and nighttime blood pressure readings (18, 82, 87, 88). Using ambulatory blood pressure recording performed on the third night of newly initiated CPAP therapy, Akashiba et al. (18) demonstrated average reductions in daytime systolic and diastolic blood pressure of 3–4 mm Hg and of daytime blood pressure of 6 mm Hg. Furthermore, 68% of the 'nondippers' in this study demonstrated a normal 'dipping' pattern with CPAP therapy. Given the propensity of 'nondippers' to develop stroke and cardiovascular disease complications (89), this finding, if confirmed in randomized controlled studies, may be of especial public health importance.

TREATMENT EFFECTS ON HEALTH CARE UTILIZATION AND ACCIDENTS

Two uncontrolled studies have demonstrated reduced medical encounters after institution of CPAP therapy in OSAS patients as compared to costs prior to therapy (68, 90). In a follow-up investigation to the Manitoba study described above, Bahamanian and colleagues showed a reduction in costs in the 2 years after diagnosis and treatment, as compared to the 5 years prior to diagnosis (68). Reduced physician contacts, consultations, psychotherapy examinations, and hospitalizations were observed. The discrepancy in costs between OSAS patients and controls, initially estimated at $260/year, fell to $174/year after OSAS treatment. The reduction in costs was most evident in persons who adhered to treatment. Findings from Swedish study (90) evaluating hospitalizations 2 years preceding and 2 years after CPAP initiation in 82 patients (54 with cardiopulmonary disease) showed a reduction in hospitalizations from a median of 10 to 0. The authors estimated that the effect could lead to large economic savings.

Krieger et al. (91) reported on self-reported accidents in the one year preceding and one year following CPAP therapy in 547 OSAS patients. They reported a reduction in the number of patients who had had an accident from 60 to 36, with even larger reductions for 'near-miss' accidents (151 to 32). Although these findings were limited because of the use of self-report data and the lack of an untreated control group, they nonetheless suggest very strong and important societal effects of CPAP therapy.

TREATMENT EFFECTS IN SUSCEPTIBLE POPULATIONS

It can be anticipated that the consequences of OSAS, and also the responses to therapy, may differ among subsets of the population with different underlying susceptibilities to sleep fragmentation or hypoxemia. Persons with underlying vascular disease may be especially vulnerable to apnea-associated adrenergic stimulation or hypoxemia exacerbating ischemia. One study that demonstrated a reduction in nocturnal ischemia (measured by reduced ST depression time) in 51 OSAS patients with known ischemic heart disease (92) supports the potential benefit of CPAP therapy in this group of patients. Other studies have demonstrated associations between congestive heart failure and obstructive and central sleep apnea (93–96). Some studies have suggested dramatic improvements in cardiac function with CPAP therapy (94, 96). The extent to which such effects may be due to direct effects on breathing rather than to changes in intrathoracic pressure need to be elucidated.

Alcohol use and sleep deprivation both may exaggerate the effects of OSAS on daytime sleepiness and functioning (97). Persons thus exposed may be especially limited or disabled when also exposed to the effects of OSAS. Many of the studies of neurocognitive functioning in OSAS suggest that persons with similar levels of OSAS may show large variations in neurocognitive performance. These observations imply that there are individual differences in compensatory abilities or vulnerability to the neurocognitive effects of OSAS. Future studies need to address how baseline characteristics (e.g., 'IQ') and other exposures (e.g., head trauma) may influence vulnerability to OSAS.

The elderly, who often have substantial recognized and unrecognized vascular and neurodegenerative diseases, may be particularly vulnerable to the effects of sleep fragmentation and sleep hypoxemia. However, children who are rapidly developing (physically, cognitively, and emotionally) also may be particularly vulnerable to some effects of OSAS. Furthermore, the effects of OSAS could have long-lasting consequences in children.

Future challenges will be to define which patients with OSAS benefit the most from specific therapy aimed at reversing breathing abnormalities during sleep.

Characterization of threshold effects (levels of AHI, sleepiness) that identify those persons who might benefit most from relatively expensive diagnostic (i.e., polysomnography) and therapeutic (i.e., CPAP) interventions will be important for improving the rational utilization of health care resources.

REFERENCES

1. Narkiewicz K, Pesek CA, Kato M, et al. Baroreflex control of sympathetic nerve activity and heart rate in obstructive sleep apnea. Hypertension 1998; 32(6):1039–1043.
2. Somers VK, Dyken ME, Clary MP, et al. Sympathetic neural mechanisms in obstructive sleep apnea. J Clin Invest 1995; 96(4):1897–1904.
3. Fletcher EC, DeBehnke RD, Lovoi BA, et al. Undiagnosed sleep apnea in patients with essential hypertension. Ann Intern Med 1985; 103(2):190–195.
4. Lavie P, Ben-Yosef R, Rubin AE. Prevalence of sleep apnea syndrome among patients with essential hypertension. Am Heart J 1984; 108:373–376.
5. Bartel PR, Loock M, van der Meyden C, et al. Hypertension and sleep apnea in black South Africans. A case control study. Am J Hypertens 1995; 8(12 Pt 1):1200–1205.
6. Portaluppi F, Provini F, Cortelli P, et al. Undiagnosed sleep-disordered breathing among male nondippers with essential hypertension. J Hypertens 1997; 15(11):1227–1233.
7. Carlson JT, Hedner JA, Ejnell H, et al. High prevalence of hypertension in sleep apnea patients independent of obesity. Am J Respir Crit Care Med 1994; 150(1):72–77.
8. Millman RP, Redline S, Carlisle C, et al. Daytime hypertension in obstructive sleep apnea. Chest 1991; 99:861–866.
9. Strohl KP, Novak RD, Singer W, et al. Insulin levels, blood pressure and sleep apnea. Sleep 1994; 17(7):614–618.
10. Grunstein R, Wilcox I, Yang TS, et al. Snoring and sleep apnoea in men: association with central obesity and hypertension. Int J Obes Rel Metab Disord 1993; 17(9):533–540.
11. Quan SF, Howard BV, Iber C, et al. The Sleep Heart Health Study: design, rationale, and methods. Sleep 1997; 20(12):1077–1085.
12. Nieto FJ, Young T, Lind B, et al. Sleep-disordered breathing, sleep apnea, and hypertension: The Sleep Heart Health Study. JAMA 2000; 283:1829–1836.
13. Young T, Peppard P, Palta M, et al. Population-based study of sleep-disordered breathing as a risk factor for hypertension. Arch Intern Med 1997; 157(15):1746–1752.
14. Young T, Finn L, Hla KM, et al. Snoring as part of a dose-response relationship between sleep-disordered breathing and blood pressure. Sleep 1996; 19(10 Suppl): S202–S205.

Key points box 16.3

Treatment effects

- In symptomatic patients with OSAS, treatment with nasal CPAP improves sleep quality and decreases daytime sleepiness.
- Patients with OSAS who are treated with nasal CPAP demonstrate improved quality of life and functional status.
- Several small intervention trials demonstrate that treatment of OSAS is accompanied by decreases in daytime and nighttime blood pressure.
- Treatment of OSAS appears to result in decreased health care utilization costs and decreased rates of automobile accidents.

15. Hla KM, Young TB, Bidwell T, et al. Sleep apnea and hypertension. A population-based study. Ann Intern Med 1994; 120:382–388.

16. Peppard PE, Young T, Palta M, et al. Prospective study of the association between sleep-disorderded breathing and hypertension. N Engl J Med 2000; 342(19):1378–1384.

17. Bixler EO, Vgontzas AN, Lin HM, et al. Association of hypertension and sleep-disordered breathing. Arch Intern Med 2000; 160(15):2289–2295.

18. Akashiba T, Minemura H, Yamamoto H, et al. Nasal continuous positive airway pressure changes blood pressure "non- dippers" to "dippers" in patients with obstructive sleep apnea. Sleep 1999; 22(7):849–853.

19. Pankow W, Nabe B, Lies K, et al. Influence of sleep apnea on 24–hour blood pressure. Chest 1997; 112(5):1253–1258.

20. Wilcox I, Grunstein RR, Hedner JA, et al. Effect of nasal continuous positive airway pressure during sleep on 24-hour blood pressure in obstructive sleep apnea. Sleep 1993; 16(6):539–544.

21. Davies CWH, Crosby JH, Mullins RL, et al. Case-control study of 24 hour ambulatory pressure in patients with obstructive sleep apnoea and normal matched control subjects. Thorax 2000; 55:736–740.

22. Entzian P, Linnemann K, Schlaak M, et al. Obstructive sleep apnea syndrome and circadian rhythms of hormones and cytokines. Am J Respir Crit Care Med 1996; 153(3): 1080–1086.

23. Vgontzas AN, Papanicolaou DA, Bixler EO, et al. Sleep apnea and daytime sleepiness and fatigue: relation to visceral obesity, insulin resistance, and hypercytokinemia. J Clin Endocrinol Metab 2000; 85(3):1151–1158.

24. Kullo IJ, Gau GT, Tajik AJ: Novel risk factors for atherisclerosis. Mayo Clin Proc 2000; 75(4):369–380.

25. Jennum P, Hein HO, Saudicani P, et al. Cardiovascular risk factors in snorers. A cross-sectional study of 3,323 men aged 54 to 74 years: the Copenhagen male study. Chest 1992; 102:1371–1376.

26. Jennum P, Sjol A. Snoring, sleep apnoea and cardiovascular risk factors: the MONICA II Study. Int J Epidemiol 1993; 22(3):439–444.

27. Kaprio J, Koskenvuo M, Partinen M, et al. A twin study of snoring. Sleep Res 1988; 17:365.

28. Koskenvuo M, Kaprio J, Telakivi T, et al. Snoring as a risk factor for ischemic heart disease and stroke in men. Br Med J 1987; 294:16–19.

29. Koskenvuo M, Partinen M, Sarna S, et al. Snoring as a risk factor for hypertension and angina pectoris. Lancet 1985; 1:893–896.

30. Hung J, Whitford EG, Parson RW, et al. Association of sleep apnoea with myocardial infarction in men. Lancet 1990; 336:261–264.

31. Saito T, Yoshikawa T, Sakamoto Y, et al. Sleep apnea in patients with acute myocardial infarction. Crit Care Med 1991; 19(7):938–941.

32. Shahar E, Whitney CW, Boland LL, et al. Sleep-disordered breathing and cardiovascular disease: cross-sectional results of the Sleep Heart Health Study. Am J Respir Crit Care 2000; (In press).

33. Bedard MA, Montplaisir J, Richer F, et al. Obstructive sleep apnea: pathogenesis of neuropsychological deficits. J Clin Exp Neuropyschol 1991; 13:950–964.

34. Redline S, Strauss M, Adams N, et al. Neuropsychological function in mild sleep apnea. Sleep 1997; 20:160–167.

35. Roehrs T, Merrion M, Pedrosi B, et al. Neuropsychological function in obstructive sleep apnea syndrome (OSAS) compared to chronic obstructive pulmonary disease (COPD). Sleep 1995; 18(5):382–388.

36. Lezak MD. Neuropsychological assessment, 3rd edn. New York: Oxford University Press; 1995.

37. Greenberg GD, Watson RK, Deptula D. Neuropsychological dysfunction in sleep apnea. Sleep 1987; 10:254–262.

38. Kales A, Caldwell A, Candieux R, et al. Severe obstructive sleep apnea: II. Associated psychopathology and psychological consequences. J Chron Dis 1985; 38:427–434.

39. Naegele B, Thouvard V, Pepin J, et al. Deficits of cognitive executive functions in patients with sleep apnea syndrome. Sleep 1995; 18:43–52.

40. Kim HC, Young T, Matthews CG, et al. Sleep-disordered breathing and neuropsychological deficits. Am J Respir Crit Care Med 1997; 156:1813–1819.

41. Bedard MA, Montplaisir J, Malo J, et al. Persistent neuropsychological deficits and vigilance impairments in sleep apnea syndrome after treatment with continuous positive airway pressure. J Clin Exp Neuropsychol 1993; 15:330–341.

42. Ancoli-Israel S, Klauber MR, Butlers N, et al. Dementia in institutionalized elderly: relation to sleep apnea. Journal of the American Geriatric Society 1991; 39:258–263.

43. Mant A, Saunders NA, Eyland AE, et al. Sleep-related respiratory disturbance and dementia in elderly females. J Gerontol 1988; 43(5):M140–M144.

44. Gottlieb DJ, Whitney CW, Bonekat WH, et al. Relation of sleepiness to respiratory disturbance index: the Sleep Heart Health Study. Am J Respir Crit Care Med 1999; 159:502–507.

45. Stewart AL, Greenfield S, Hays RD, et al. Functional status and well-being of patients with chronic conditions. Results from the medical outcomes study. JAMA 1989; 262(7):907–913.

46. Patrick DL, Bergner M. Measurement of health status in the 1990s. Ann Rev Publ Health 1990; 11:165–183.

47. Weaver TE, Laizner AM, Evans LK, et al. An instrument to measure functional status outcomes for disorders of excessive sleepiness. Sleep 1997; 20(10):835–843.

48. Flemons WW, Reimer MA. Development of a disease-specific health-related quality of life questionnaire for sleep apnea. Am J Respir Crit Care Med 1998; 158(2):494–503.

49. Briones B, Adams N, Strauss M, et al. Relationship between sleepiness and general health status. Sleep 1996; 19(7):583–588.

50. Baldwin CM, Griffith KA, Nieto FJ, et al. The association of sleep-disordered breathing and sleep symptoms with quality of life in the Sleep Heart Health Study. Sleep 2000; (In press).

51. Finn L, Young T, Palta M, et al. Sleep-disordered breathing and self-reported general health status in Wisconsin Sleep Cohort Study. Sleep 1998; 21:701–706.

52. Grunstein RR, Stenlof K, Hedner JA, et al. Impact of self-reported sleep-breathing distrubances on psychosocial performance in the Swedish obese subjects (SOS) study. Sleep 1995; 18(8):635–643.

53. Leger D. The cost of sleep-related accidents: a report for the National Commission on Sleep Disorders Research. Sleep 1994; 17(1):84–93.

54. Findley LJ, Unverzagt ME, Suratt PM. Automobile accidents involving patients with obstructive sleep apnea. Am Rev Respir Dis 1988; 138(2):337–340.

55. Young T, Blustein J, Finn L, et al. Sleep-disordered breathing and motor vehicle accidents in a population-based cohort. Sleep 1997b; 20(8):608–613.

56. Stoohs RA, Bingham LA, Itoi A, et al. Sleep and sleep-disordered breathing in commercial long-haul truck drivers. Chest 1995; 107(5):1275–1282.

57. McCartt AT, Rohrbaugh JW, Hammer MC, et al. Factors associated with falling asleep at the wheel among long-distance truck drivers. Accid Anal Prev 2000; 32(4):493–504.

58. He J, Kryger MH, Zorick FJ, et al. Mortality and apnea index in obstructive sleep apnea: experience in 385 male patients. Chest 1988; 94(1):9–14.

59. Partinen M, Guilleminault C. Daytime sleepiness and vascular morbidity at seven-year follow-up in obstructive sleep apnea patients. Chest 1990; 97:27–32.

60. Lavie P, PH, Peled R, et al. Mortality in sleep apnea patients: a multivariate analysis of risk factors. Sleep 1995; 18(3):149–157.

61. Ancoli-Israel S, Klauber MR, Kripke DF, et al. Sleep apnea in female patients in a nursing home. Chest 1989; 96:1054–1058.

62. Bliwise DL, Bliwise NG, Partinen M, et al. Sleep apnea and mortality in an aged cohort. Am J Public Health 1988; 78:544–547.

63. Mant A, King M, Saunders NA, et al. Four-year follow-up of mortality and sleep-related respiratory disturbances in non-demented seniors. Sleep 1995; 18(6):433–438.

64. Lindberg E, Janson C, Svardsudd K, et al. Increased mortality among sleepy snorers: a prospective population based study. Thorax 1998; 53(8):631–637.

65. Foley DJ, Monjan AA, Masaki KH, et al. Associations of symptoms of sleep apnea with cardiovascular disease, cognitive impairment, and mortality among older Japanese-American men. J Am Geriatr Soc 1999; 47(5):524–528.

66. Qureshi AI, Giles WH, Croft JB, et al. Habitual sleep patterns and risk for stroke and coronary heart disease: a 10-year follow-up from NHANES I. Neurology 1997; 48:903–911.

67. Ronald J, Delaive K, Roos L, et al. Health care utilization in the 10 years prior to diagnosis in obstructive sleep apnea syndrome patients. Sleep 1999; 22(2):225–229.

68. Bahammam A, Delaive K, Ronald J, et al. Health care utilization in males with obstructive sleep apnea syndrome two years after diagnosis and treatment. Sleep 1999; 22(6):740–747.

69. Kapur V, Blough DK, Sandblom RE, et al. The medical cost of undiagnosed sleep apnea. Sleep 1999; 22(6):749–755.

70. Young T, Palta M, Dempsey J, et al. The occurrence of sleep-disordered breathing in middle-aged adults. N Engl J Med 1993; 328:1230–1235.

71. Lyznicki JM, Doege TC, Davis RM, et al. Sleepiness, driving, and motor vehicle crashes. Council on Scientific Affairs, American Medical Association [see comments]. JAMA 1998; 279(23):1908–1913.

72. Lamphere J, Roehrs T, Wittig R, et al. Recovery of alertness after CPAP therapy. Chest 1989; 96:1364–1367.

73. Loredo JS, Ancoli-Israel S, Dimsdale JE. Effect of continuous positive airway pressure vs placebo continuous positive airway pressure on sleep quality in obstructive sleep apnea. Chest 1999; 116(6):1545–1549.

74. Redline S, Adams N, Strauss ME, et al. Improvement of mild sleep-disordered breathing with CPAP compared with conservative therapy [see comments]. Am J Respir Crit Care Med 1998; 157(3 Pt 1):858–865.

75. Engleman HM, Deary IJ, Douglas NJ. Daytime function after CPAP or placebo in patients with mild sleep apnea/hypopnea syndrome. Am J Resp Crit Care Med 1997; 155:A846.

76. Engleman HM, Martin SE, Dreary IJ, et al. Effect of continuous positive airway pressure treatment on daytime function in sleep apnea hypopnea syndrome. Lancet 1994; 343: 572–575.

77. Hack M, Davies RJ, Mullins R, Choi SJ, et al. Randomised prospective parallel trial of therapeutic versus subtherapeutic nasal continuous positive airway pressure on simulated steering performance in patients with obstructive sleep apnoea. Thorax 2000; 55(3):224–231.

78. Ballester E, Badia JR, Hernandez L, et al. Evidence of the effectiveness of continuous positive airway pressure in the treatment of sleep apnea/hypopnea syndrome. Am J Respir Crit Care Med 1999; 159:495–501.

79. Engleman HM, Kingshott RN, Wraith PK, et al. Randomized placebo-controlled crossover trial of continuous positive air-

way pressure for mild sleep apnea/hypopnea syndrome. Am J Respir Crit Care Med 1999; 159(2):461–467.

80. Engleman HM, Cheshire KE, Deary IJ, et al. Daytime sleepiness, cognitive performance and mood after continuous postiive airway pressure for the sleep apnoea/hypopnoea syndrome. Thorax 1993; 48:911–914.

81. Klonoff H, Fleetham J, Taylor R, et al. Treatment outcome of obstructive sleep apnea: physiological and neuropsychological concomitants. J Nerv Ment Dis 1987; 175:203–212.

82. Minemura H, Akashiba T, Yamamoto H, et al. Acute effects of nasal continuous positive airway pressure on 24-hour blood pressure and catecholamines in patients with obstructive sleep apnea. Intern Med 1998; 37(12): 1009–1013.

83. Hedner J, Ejnell H, Carlson J, et al. Reduction in sympathetic activity after long-term CPAP treatment in sleep apnea: cardiovascular implications. Eur Respir J 1995; 8:222–229.

84. Narkiewicz K, Kato M, Phillips BG, et al. Nocturnal continuous positive airway pressure decreases daytime sympathetic traffic in obstructive sleep apnea. Circulation 1999; 100(23):2332–2335.

85. Saarelainen S, Hasan J, Siitonen S, et al. Effect of nasal CPAP treatment on plasma volume, aldosterone and 24-h blood pressure in obstructive sleep apnoea. J Sleep Res 1996; 5(3):181–185.

86. Bratel T, Wennlund A, Carlstrom K. Pituitary reactivity, androgens and catecholamines in obstructive sleep apnoea. Effects of continuous positive airway pressure treatment (CPAP). Respir Med 1999; 93(1):1–7.

87. Narkiewicz K, Somers VK. The sympathetic nervous system and obstructive sleep apnea: implications for hypertension. J Hypertens 1997; 15(12 Pt2):1613–1619.

88. Voogel AJ, van Steenwijk RP, Karemaker JM, et al. Effects of treatment of obstructive sleep apnea on circadian hemodynamics. J Autonomic Nerv Sys 1999; 77(2–3): 177–183.

89. Verdecchia P, Schillaci G, Guerrieri M. Circadian blood pressure changes and left ventricular hypetrophy in essential hypertension. Circulation 1990; 81:528–536.

90. Peker Y, Hedner J, Johansson A, et al. Reduced hospitalization with cardiovascular and pulmonary diease in obstructive sleep apnea patients on nasal CPAP treatment. Sleep 1997; 20(8):645–653.

91. Krieger J, Meslier N, Lebrun T, et al. Accidents in obstructive sleep apnea patients treated with nasal continuous positive airway pressure: a prospective study. The Working Group ANTADIR, Paris, and CRESGE, Lille, France. Chest 1997; 112:1561–1566.

92. Peled N, Abinader EG, Pillar G, et al. Nocturnal ischemic events in patients with obstructive sleep apnea syndrome and ischemic heart disease: effects of continuous positive air pressure treatment. J Am Coll Cardiol 1999; 34(6):1744–1749.

93. Javaheri S, Parker TJ, Wexler L, et al. Occult sleep-disordered breathing in stable congestive heart failure. Ann Intern Med 1995; 122:487–492.

94. Bradley TD, Holloway RM, McLaughlin PR, et al. Cardiac output response to continuous positive airway pressure in congestive heart failure. Am Rev Respir Dis 1992; 145(Part 1):377–382.

95. Malone S, Liu PP, Holloway R, et al. Obstructive sleep apnoea in patients with dilated cardiomyopathy: effects of continuous positive airway pressure. Lancet 1991; 338:1480–1484.

96. Naughton MT, Liu PP, Bernard DC, et al. A randomized controlled clinical trial of CPAP in patients with heart failure and Cheynes Stokes respiration. Am Rev Respir Dis 1993; 147:A687.

97. Roehrs T, Beare D, Zorick F, et al. Sleepiness and ethanol effects on simulated driving. Alcohol Clin Exp Res 1994; 18:154–158.

PART FIVE

CENTRAL SLEEP APNEA

17

CENTRAL HYPOVENTILATION SYNDROMES AND HYPERCAPNIC CENTRAL SLEEP APNEA

Walter T McNicholas and Eliot A Phillipson

INTRODUCTION

Central hypoventilation syndromes are rare disorders that relate to a defect in central respiratory drive, which results in chronic alveolar hypoventilation, usually without any detectable mechanical ventilatory defects (1, 2). The central hypoventilation may be primary (idiopathic) or secondary to other disorders that cause damage to the brain stem respiratory center. Patients demonstrate both hypoxemia and hypercapnia on arterial blood gas analysis, but they can usually normalize the blood gas values by voluntary hyperventilation (1). These syndromes are sometimes referred to as 'Ondine's curse,' from a character in Greek mythology who was cursed with having to voluntarily control his automatic

body functions, including respiration (2). Patients typically develop recurring episodes of severe respiratory failure, often in association with respiratory infection, since the defective respiratory drive is insufficient to cope with the increased work of breathing associated with respiratory infection (3). Central hypoventilation syndromes must be distinguished from other conditions that can result in chronic hypoventilation, particularly neuromuscular and thoracic cage disorders (Fig. 17.1).

PATHOPHYSIOLOGY

The precise pathophysiological basis of central hypoventilation syndrome is unclear but could relate to abnormalities in

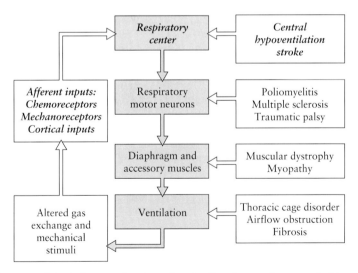

Fig 17.1 *Schematic diagram of the influence of various chronic disorders on the control of breathing at various levels, ranging from the central respiratory center to the lungs. This figure also stresses the feedback system that controls breathing through the chemoreceptors and other afferent inputs. The aspects of respiratory control relevant to central hypoventilation syndromes are highlighted in bold type.*

afferent input from brain stem and peripheral chemorecep-tors, or to defects in the brainstem respiratory center (4), or to both of these. The respiratory center consists of rhythmic respiratory neurons in the medulla and pons, which are located in a dorsal group (nucleus tractus solitarius) and a ventrolateral group (nucleus ambiguus and retroambigu-us). Bilateral damage to these neurons results in failure of automatic respiration. Cases have been reported of the syndrome complicating many neurological disorders; these include encephalitis, cervical cordotomy, bulbar poliomyelitis, brain stem infarction, multiple sclerosis, and Shy-Drager syndrome (5). The hypoventilation in these cases has been shown to be associated with involvement of the brain stem respiratory center in the disease process. Recently, cases of brain stem tegmental necrosis and oli-vary hypoplasia associated with central apnea have been described. Neuropathological findings were localized to the caudal pons and medulla and included tegmental necrosis with involvement of respiratory-related nuclei (6). However, in many cases, there is no detectable underlying neurological abnormality, and the disorder is regarded as primary or idiopathic.

Afferent inputs from chemoreceptors and mechanore-ceptors are important to the maintenance of a normal re-spiratory drive, and defects in these inputs contribute to central hypoventilation. Many pharmacological agents can influence the degree of chemical drive, which may have therapeutic implications. Hypoxic ventilatory depression can be attenuated by aminophylline adminis-tration during wakefulness (7, 8), and CO_2 sensitivity also changes in accordance with the menstrual cycle. There is a significant increase in CO_2 sensitivity between the fol-licular and luteal phases, which is attributed to a stimu-lant effect of progesterone on breathing (9).

Behavioral states (emotive, cognitive, movements, phonation) also influence respiratory drive with consequent effects on respiration. The state of wakeful-ness likewise provides a stimulus to breathing via the reticular activating system, which is obviously lost during sleep.

IMPACT OF SLEEP

During sleep, breathing is predominantly dependent on automatic or metabolic drive from chemoreceptors and mechanoreceptors (10). The effect of sleep stages on the magnitude of chemical drives has been well studied. Ventilatory response to both hypoxia and hypercapnia is reduced in all sleep stages but is most pronounced during rapid eye movement (REM) sleep (11, 12).

Patients with central hypoventilation frequently devel-op severe respiratory insufficiency during sleep (13–15) as a consequence of the reduction in respiratory drive, which is a normal feature of breathing during sleep. Minute ven-tilation falls during sleep, and central sleep apnea (CSA) is a common finding. Severe oxygen desaturation may develop, which partly results from the fact that such patients are likely to be already on the steep part of the oxyhemoglobin dissociation curve. Thus, each unit fall in arterial PO_2 as a result of physiological hypoventilation will be associated with a greater fall in arterial oxygen sat-uration (SaO_2). Furthermore, the changes in rib cage and abdominal contribution to breathing and the changes in functional reserve capacity (FRC) associated with sleep may result in worsening ventilation-to-perfusion relation-ships, which will also aggravate any tendency to hypox-emia.

⟁ Key points box 17.1

Pathophysiology of central hypoventilation

1. Pathophysiology could relate to defective afferent input from chemoreceptors or to defects in the brain stem respiratory center.

2. Defects in the respiratory center could be primary or secondary to a variety of neurological disorders, particularly stroke.

3. Sleep adversely affects ventilation in these disorders by a withdrawal of several important stimulant inputs to ventilation.

4. Patients with central hypoventilation frequently develop prolonged episodes of severe hypoxemia during sleep, and central sleep apnea is common.

CLINICAL PRESENTATION AND DIAGNOSIS

Central hypoventilation syndrome in some patients may go undetected for many years until an episode of acute respira-tory failure develops, usually in association with respiratory infection. Indeed, many patients have a history of recurrent episodes of respiratory failure. The disorder may be discovered in in childhood, but less severe cases may go undetected until adult years. Patients may also manifest unexplained polycythemia or cor pulmonale, which are consequences of chronic hypoxemia. Cases may be familial, and men and women appear to be equally affected. Snoring, morning headaches, and daytime sleepiness are common, but hypertension and dyspnea are not (16).

Patients demonstrate awake hypoxemia and hypercapnia without evidence of muscular weakness or abnormal lung mechanics. Thus, in patients with idiopathic central hypoventilation, pulmonary function test results typically are normal, unless there is coexisting lung disease, and tests of respiratory muscle strength also are normal. A typical finding in these cases is that patients can normalize arterial blood gases by voluntary hyperventilation. In cases in which the central hypoventilation is a consequence of a neurological disorder, such as poliomyelites or brain stem stroke, peripheral muscle weakness may also be found.

Although central hypoventilation syndromes must be distinguished from other causes of hypoventilation, some overlap may occur. For example, some patients with chronic obstructive pulmonary disease (COPD) have a degree of hypoxemia and hypercapnia that appears to be out of proportion to the severity of airflow limitation. These patients, sometimes referred to as 'blue-bloaters,' may have a degree of central respiratory insufficiency in addition to COPD. A further example is the obesity hypoventilation syndrome, in which the increased mechanical ventilatory load caused by gross obesity may unmask an underlying weakness in central respiratory drive, which results in alveolar hypoventilation and blood gas abnormalities that are very similar to those seen in patients with idiopathic central hypoventilation.

SLEEP FINDINGS

The central feature of sleep hypoventilation is an abnormal increase in $PaCO_2$ during sleep, which is usually associated with severe hypoxemia. This hypoxemia may lead to clinical sequelae such as polycythemia, pulmonary hypertension, and cor pulmonale. Hypoxemia is characteristically present to some degree throughout sleep, with oxygen desaturation episodes that occur in addition to, and which are not associated with, distinct apneas and hypopneas. Periods of hypoventilation are usually associated with sustained arterial desaturation lasting up to several minutes. However, this is not a specific finding, since sustained desaturation may also be caused by a change in lung closing volume that can cause a worsening in ventilation perfusion homogeneity. Hypoventilation periods are much more common and severe in rapid eye movement (REM) than in non–rapid eye movement (NREM) sleep.

Apneas and hypopneas may occur in association with hypoventilation; however, sleep hypoventilation should be diagnosed only if the clinical sequelae can be attributed to hypoventilation separate from the apneas and hypopneas. The apneas and hypopneas that occur in association with central hypoventilation syndromes are almost invariably central in origin, and they must be distinguished from other forms of CSA, such as idiopathic central sleep apnea syndrome and Cheyne-Stokes breathing, which are

---

⊶ Key points box 17.2

Clinical features and diagnosis

1. Central hypoventilation syndromes may go undetected for many years, and frequently patients first manifest an episode of acute respiratory failure, usually due to respiratory infection.

2. The chronic hypoxemia that is a feature of this condition predisposes to polycythemia and cor pulmonale.

3. Patients show awake hypoxemia and hypercapnia but can normalize gas exchange by voluntary hyperventilation.

4. Patients with idiopathic central hypoventilation should have normal pulmonary function and normal respiratory muscle strength, but central hypoventilation due to other causes such as stroke may have coexisting features appropriate to the condition.

5. The core finding in central hypoventilation is hypercapnia, which becomes more pronounced during sleep.

6. Central sleep apnea is a common but not essential feature of the disorder, and it differs from other forms of central sleep apnea such as idiopathic and Cheyne-Stokes breathing.

covered in Chapter 18. Patients with these other forms of CSA are generally normocapnic or hypocapnic.

MANAGEMENT

GENERAL PRINCIPLES

Respiratory insufficiency in conditions associated with hypoventilation due to impaired respiratory drive or to impaired neuromechanical coupling will be aggravated by any factor that increases the work of breathing (3), particularly respiratory infection, and such infections in these patients should be treated promptly and vigorously. Clearance of bronchial secretions may also be impaired, and physiotherapy and postural drainage play an important part in management, particularly during acute exacerbations.

OXYGEN THERAPY

The most serious consequence of hypoventilation, particularly during sleep, is hypoxemia. Appropriate oxygen therapy plays an important part in the management of patients with central hypoventilation from any cause. Care must be taken that correction of hypoxemia is not complicated by worsening hypercapnia because of the possibility that correction of hypoxemia may remove an important stimulus to breathing. However, this is less likely in patients with hypoxemia due to central hypoventilation than to other causes of hypercapnic respiratory failure, since most such patients have some defect in the ventilatory responsiveness to hypoxia. Indeed, some reports have suggested that supplemental oxygen may have beneficial effects on ventilation in some patients with central hypoventilation (13), possibly by removal of a depressant effect of hypoxemia on the brain stem respiratory center.

PHARMACOLOGICAL THERAPY

A number of pharmaceutical agents have respiratory stimulant properties that may be helpful in central hypoventilation. Theophylline has effects on respiration in addition to bronchodilation, which may be beneficial in patients with chronic hypoventilation, including central respiratory stimulation (17) and improved diaphragmatic contractility (18). However, the principal limitations of theophyllines in this context are an adverse effect on sleep quality (19) and the relatively high prevalence of gastrointestinal intolerance.

Progesterone, a female hormone, has long been recognized to have respiratory stimulant effects (20, 21), and an illustration of this effect is that women in the later stages of pregnancy tend to become hypocapnic because of the high levels of circulating hormone. The effect appears to be centrally mediated and persists even when peripheral chemoreceptor activity is abolished (22). Progesterone has been used therapeutically in conditions associated with central hypoventilation (23).

Almitrine is not helpful in most patients with central hypoventilation since patients usually have defective carotid body responses to hypoxemia, which is the most important site of action of this drug.

NONINVASIVE ASSISTED VENTILATION

The role of noninvasive assisted ventilation in the management of patients with chronic respiratory failure is discussed in detail in chapter 23, but central hypoventilation syndromes represent one specific indication for this therapy. Noninvasive ventilation is particularly beneficial in patients with respiratory insufficiency due to hypoventilation because of the fact that lung mechanics are usually normal in such patients. Assisted ventilation is usually confined to sleep if possible, for obvious practical reasons, but beneficial effects on gas exchange during wakefulness have been widely reported in patients treated with nocturnal ventilatory support.

Negative Pressure Ventilation

The earliest form of noninvasive ventilation was the 'iron lung' which saved many lives during the poliomyelitis epidemics of the twentieth century. Various forms of noninvasive ventilation have been used over the years, including the rocking bed (24) and the abdominal cuirass (25). Although it is generally effective, negative pressure ventilation can be complicated by the development of upper airway obstruction and obstructive sleep apnea syndrome (OSAS) (26). This complication develops because of the loss of the normal timing relationship between the phasic contraction of the upper airway dilating muscles, which normally contract in association with diaphragmatic contraction to ensure oropharyngeal patency during inspiration (27).

Noninvasive Intermittent Positive Pressure Ventilation (NIPPV)

This technique has now largely replaced other forms of noninvasive ventilation during sleep. NIPPV, which is generally delivered via nasal mask, depends on the patient's maintaining exclusive nasal breathing for efficacy but is helped by the fact that humans are semiobligate nose-breathers, particularly during sleep. However, some patients do breathe through the mouth while on NIPPV, but this problem can usually be overcome by wearing a chinstrap or a full facemask. The mask is usually well tolerated, although some patients with respiratory failure find the nasal mask uncomfortable or claustrophobic, in which case negative pressure ventilation is usually preferred.

Several studies have reported an improvement in daytime blood gas levels and respiratory muscle strength with NIPPV (28–30). The mechanism by which NIPPV produces improvements in daytime blood gas levels likely involves a number of factors, which include resting of the respiratory muscles and a resetting of respiratory drive, particularly at the chemoreceptor level. A reduction in residual volume and in the degree of gas trapping also has been demonstrated with NIPPV, implying a reduction in respiratory load. There have been few reports of NIPPV in the management of central hypoventilation syndromes, perhaps reflecting the rarity of these disorders.

ELECTROPHRENIC PACING

Electrical stimulation of the diaphragm in patients with central respiratory insufficiency has been used in selected cases over the past two decades (31–33). This procedure is highly specialized and involves planting a pacing electrode around the phrenic nerve, either in the cervical or, more commonly, in the high thoracic region. The criteria for successful diaphragm pacing include the need for long-term mechanical ventilatory assistance, a functionally intact phrenic nerve-diaphragm axis, and chest wall stability. The technique has been reported to be effective, particularly in patients with central alveolar hypoventilation (34) and those with a high level quadriplegia (33). Care must be taken to ensure that the phrenic nerve is viable; adequate testing of phrenic nerve function and diaphragmatic contractility should be done in all patients before deciding on this procedure. However, this precaution is more applicable to patients with quadriplegia than to those with central hypoventilation, and the function of the phrenic nerve–diaphragm axis can be tested more easily in patients with central alveolar hypoventilation by recording the response to voluntary hypoventilation. The phrenic nerve is usually tested by means of an external

stimulator applied percutaneously in the neck over the nerve pathway. Diaphragmatic contractility in response to phrenic nerve stimulation can be tested either by recording electromyographic (EMG) activity from surface electrodes or by recording transdiaphragmatic pressure changes with esophageal and gastric balloons (33).

Adults with central alveolar hypoventilation can often be successfully managed with a unilateral phrenic nerve pacemaker, but children generally require bilateral pacemakers because the chest wall is more compliant than in adults and, therefore, a unilateral pacemaker will result in paradoxical movement of the contralateral diaphragm and chest wall with consequent reduction in efficacy.

Approximately 50% of patients develop OSAS as a complication (33), for the same reason as occurs in patients treated with negative pressure ventilation—namely, the loss of the normal timing relationships between upper airway and diaphragmatic contraction, which splints the upper airway open in advance of the onset of inspiration. Such patients may require nasal continuous positive airway pressure (CPAP) or tracheostomy in addition to pacing of the diaphragm. OSAS is more likely in those patients with central alveolar hypoventilation, because these patients have

---

⊙┓ Key points box 17.3

Management

1. Respiratory infections should be treated promptly, since these increase the work of breathing and impair ventilation-to-perfusion matching in the lung.

2. Hypoxemia should be corrected with appropriate oxygen therapy, and in some cases relief of hypoxemia may increase ventilation.

3. Pharmacological agents that stimulate ventilation may help, particularly progesterone and theophylline.

4. Noninvasive assisted ventilation, usually positive pressure via nasal mask, is usually very beneficial in advanced cases.

5. Electrophrenic pacing is also effective, but is often complicated by the development of obstructive sleep apnea.

a reduced upper airway muscle tone and contractility as part of their reduced respiratory drive, whereas patients with high level quadriplegia should have a normal respiratory drive and, therefore, the tone of the upper airway muscles should be higher and thus less likely to be obstructed in response to phrenic nerve stimulation. Attempts have been made to develop pacemakers that synchronize the contractions of upper airway muscles and diaphragm, which would remove the likelihood of upper airway obstruction, but so far these have been without success.

CONCLUSIONS

The impact of sleep on ventilation and gas exchange in patients with chronic respiratory failure due to central alveolar hypoventilation can be dramatic and potentially life-threatening. These effects often go unrecognized, either due to lack of facilities for sleep monitoring or due to a failure by the attending clinician to appreciate the potential impact of sleep on ventilation in these patients. However, appropriate management of the sleep-related deterioration in gas exchange can greatly improve life expectancy, in addition to producing improvements in daytime gas exchange and quality of life. Optimum management requires a careful attention to detail, and such an approach, by optimizing the underlying condition as well as providing appropriate oxygen and drug therapy, can avoid the need for assisted ventilation in many cases. The development of NIPPV by nasal mask has been a major development in this area and has opened up exciting new possibilities for improving the management of patients with central hypoventilation.

REFERENCES

1. Rhoads GG, Brody JS. Idiopathic alveolar hypoventilation: clinical spectrum. Ann Int Med 1969; 71:271–278.

2. Mellins RB, Balfour HH, Turino GM, et al. Failure of automatic control of ventilation (Ondine's curse). Medicine 1970; 49:487–504.

3. Rochester DF, Arora HS. Respiratory muscle failure. Med Clin North Am 1983; 3:573–597.

4. Farmer WC, Glenn WW, Gee JB. Alveolar hypoventilation syndrome. Studies of ventilatory control in patients selected for diaphragmatic pacing. Am J Med 1978; 64:39–49.

5. Udwadia ZF, Athale S, Misra VP, et al. Radiation necrosis causing failure of automatic ventilation during sleep with central sleep apnea. Chest 1897; 92:567–569.

6. Cortez SC, Kinney HC. Brainstem tegmental necrosis and olivary hypoplasia: a lethal entity associated with congenital apnea. J Neuropathol Exp Neurol 1996; 55:841–849.

7. Georgopoulos D, Holtby SG, Berezanski D, et al. Aminophylline effects on ventilatory response to hypoxia and hyperoxia in normal adults. J Appl Physiol 1989; 67:1150–1156.

8. Runold M, Lagercrantz H, Prabhakar NR, et al. Role of adenosine in hypoxic ventilatory depression. J Appl Physiol 1989; 67:541–546.

9. Dutton K, Blanksby BA, Morton AR. CO_2 sensitivity changes during the menstrual cycle. J Appl Physiol 1989; 67:517–522.

10. Feldman JL, Smith JC. Neural control of respiratory pattern in mammals: an overview. In: Dempsey JA, Pack AI, eds. Regulation of breathing. New York: Marcel Dekker; 1995; 39–69.

11. Douglas N, White D, Weil J, et al. Hypercapnic ventilatory response in sleeping adults. Am Rev Respir Dis 1982; 126:758–762.

12. Douglas N, White D, Weil J, et al. Hypoxic ventilatory response decreases during sleep in normal men. Am Rev Respir Dis 1982; 125:286–289.

13. McNicholas WT, Carter JL, Rutherford R, et al. Beneficial effects of oxygen in primary alveolar hypoventilation with central sleep apnea. Am Rev Respir Dis 1982; 125:773–775.

14. Bubis MJ, Anthonisen NR. Primary alveolar hypoventilation treated by nocturnal administration of O_2. Am Rev Respir Dis 1978; 118:947–953.

15. Barlow PB, Bartlett D Jr, Hauri P, et al. Idiopathic hypoventilation syndrome: importance of preventing nocturnal hypoxemia and hypercapnia. Am Rev Respir Dis 1980; 121:141–145.

16. Bradley TD, McNicholas WT, Rutherford R, et al. Clinical and physiologic heterogeneity of the central sleep apnea syndrome. Am Rev Respir Dis 1986; 134:217–221.

17. Eldrige FL, Millhorn DE, Waldrop TG, et al. Mechanism of respiratory effects of methylxanthines. Respir Physiol 1983; 53:239–261.

18. Murciano D, Aubier M, Lecocguic Y, et al. Effects of theophylline on diaphragmatic strength and fatigue in patients with chronic obstructive pulmonary disease. N Engl J Med 1984; 311:349–353.

19. Mulloy E, McNicholas WT. Theophylline improves gas exchange during rest, exercise and sleep in severe chronic obstructive pulmonary disease. Am Rev Respir Dis 1993; 148:1030–1036.

20. Skatrud J, Dempsey J, Kaiser D. Ventilatory response to medroxyprogesterone acetate in normal subjects: time course and mechanisms. J Appl Physiol 1978; 44:939–944.

21. Mikami M, Tatsumi K, Kimura H, et al. Respiration effect of synthetic progestin in small doses in normal men. Chest 1989; 96:1073–1075.

22. Bayliss DA, Millhorn DE, Gallman EA, et al. Progesterone stimulates respiration through a central nervous system steroid receptor mechanism in the cat. Proc Natl Acad Sci USA 1987; 84:7788–7792.

23. Sutton FD, Zwillich CW, Creagh CE, et al. Progesterone for outpatient treatment of Pickwickian syndrome. Ann Intern Med 1975; 83:476–479.

24. Chalmers RM, Howard RS, Wiles CM, et al. Use of the rocking bed in the treatment of neurogenic respiratory insufficiency. Q J Med 1994; 87:423–429.

25. Sawicka EH, Loh L, Branthwaite MA. Domiciliary ventilatory support: an analysis of outcome. Thorax 1988; 43:31–35.

26. Bach JR, Penek J. Obstructive sleep apnea complicating negative-pressure ventilatory support in patients with chronic paralytic/restrictive ventilatory dysfunction. Chest 1991; 99:1386–1393.

27. Strohl KP, Hensley MJ, Hallett M, et al. Activation of upper airway muscles before onset of inspiration in normal humans. J Appl Physiol 1980; 49:638–642.

28. Elliott MW, Mulvey DA, Moxham J, et al. Domiciliary nocturnal nasal intermittent positive pressure ventilation in COPD: mechanisms underlying changes in arterial blood gas tensions. Eur Resp J 1991; 4:1044–1052.

29. Ambrosino N, Nava S, Bertone P, et al. Physiologic evaluation of pressure support ventilation by nasal mask in patients with stable COPD. Chest 1992; 101:385–391.

30. Renston JP, DiMarco AF, Supinski GS. Respiratory muscle rest using nasal BiPAP ventilation in patients with stable severe COPD. Chest 1994; 105:1053–1060.

31. Chervin RD, Guilleminault C. Diaphragm pacing: review and reassessment. Sleep 1994; 17:176–187.

32. Moxham J, Shneerson JM. Diaphragmatic pacing. Am Rev Respir Dis 1993; 148:533–536.

33. Glenn WW, Hogan JF, Phelps ML. Ventilatory support of the quadriplegic patient with respiratory paralysis by diaphragm pacing. Surg Clin North Am 1980; 60:1055–1078.

34. Flageole H, Adolph VR, Davis GM, et al. Diaphragmatic pacing in children with congenital central alveolar hypoventilation syndrome. Surgery 1995; 118:25–28.

18 NONHYPERCAPNIC CENTRAL SLEEP APNEA

T Douglas Bradley

INTRODUCTION

Central sleep apnea (CSA) constitutes a heterogeneous group of disorders whose common feature is a momentary cessation of breathing during sleep due to a transient withdrawal of central respiratory drive to the muscles of respiration. Thus, in contrast to obstructive sleep apnea syndrome (OSAS), in which respiratory drive continues during apnea, in CSA no respiratory efforts or intrathoracic pressure swings are generated. The clinical evaluation and treatment of these disorders is challenging because they are relatively uncommon, can arise from entirely different underlying causes, and have widely varying clinical presentations. In the hypercapnic form of CSA, increases in PCO_2 generally result from reductions in ventilation or outright apneas due to an underlying depression of respiratory drive. In contrast, nonhypercapnic CSA disorders are not associated with either a primary reduction in respiratory drive or respiratory muscle weakness. Instead, these disorders result from respiratory control instability in which increases in respiratory drive frequently play a role. In contrast to hypercapnic CSA, central apneas generally result from episodes of hyperventilation and hypocapnia (1,2).

PATHOGENESIS

Based on theoretical, experimental, and clinical observations, there are a number of mechanisms that could account for transient withdrawal of respiratory drive in subjects whose PCO_2 is either normal or low. These include transient instabilities of respiratory drive, accentuation of respiratory chemoreflexes, and reflex inhibition of respiratory drive by mechanical stimuli.

TRANSIENT INSTABILITY OF RESPIRATORY DRIVE

By definition, patients with nonhypercapnic CSA have either normal or low PCO_2 during both wakefulness and sleep (3). Their CSA is usually associated with classic periodic breathing. Several theoretical and experimental models have been developed to account for fluctuations in respiratory drive that are the hallmark of periodic breathing. Common to all these models is an instability of the respiratory control system in which PCO_2 falls transiently and recurrently below the threshold required to stimulate respiratory output.

Under normal conditions, breathing is regulated by two functionally and anatomically distinct elements, referred to as the metabolic and behavioral respiratory control systems. The function of the metabolic system is to maintain blood gas homeostasis and acid-base balance, which it does through a negative feedback loop. The afferent limb of this loop consists of peripheral and central chemoreceptors that receive sensory information regarding arterial and cerebral PO_2, PCO_2, pH and from the vagus nerves regarding the mechanical ventilatory activity of the airways and lungs. The efferent limb consists of central respiratory motor neurons that stimulate the muscles of respiration to generate an appropriate ventilatory output to maintain blood gas tensions and pH within narrow limits. In contrast, the behavioral control system subserves activities such as phonation that use the ventilatory apparatus for purposes other than gas exchange. Superimposed on these two systems are the stimulatory effects of wakefulness on breathing. This waking neural drive provides a tonic, nonspecific excitation to the respiratory neurons that serves to enhance overall central drive to the respiratory muscles (4). In so doing, it stabilizes breathing and tends to prevent apneas even when the intensity of chemical stimuli falls below the metabolic threshold required to generate ventilation.

During wakefulness, the metabolic and behavioral control systems and the waking neural drive are all operative. However, at the onset of non-rapid eye movement (NREM) sleep, the waking neural drive is abolished and the behavioral control system becomes quiescent (5). As a result, breathing becomes critically dependent on the metabolic control system. Consequently, instabilities of metabolic control are characteristically manifest during NREM sleep.

The respiratory control system is most susceptible to instability at the transition from wakefulness to NREM sleep. During this transition, the instantaneous withdrawal of the waking neural drive results in a simultaneous increase in the threshold PCO_2 required to generate ventilation. The ambient PCO_2 during wakefulness is often below this new threshold level, so that there is a sudden loss of respiratory drive, resulting in a central apnea (4–6) (Fig. 18.1). During apnea, PCO_2 increases at a rate proportional to metabolic CO_2 production, until it reaches

the critical ventilatory threshold level, at which point breathing resumes. If NREM sleep becomes firmly established at this time, stable breathing will resume at a new steady state characterized by a higher PCO_2 set point and at a lower minute ventilation than during wakefulness. Therefore, although the instability of respiratory control that accompanies the normal onset of NREM sleep may cause one or two brief central apneas, it is not sufficient in itself to precipitate periodic breathing with recurrent central apneas. Accordingly, one or more additional sources of respiratory control system instability are required.

One such destabilizing influence is fluctuation in central nervous system (CNS) state. If after the onset of NREM sleep, stable sleep is not established and, instead, CNS state momentarily shifts back to wakefulness, the increased PCO_2 of NREM sleep will be perceived by the control system as relative hypercapnia for wakefulness. A period of hyperpnea will follow, in accordance with the awake ventilatory response to CO_2. If CNS state continues to fluctuate between wakefulness and NREM sleep, waking neural drive and therefore ventilation will also fluctuate. As a result, periodic breathing will ensue during which apneas or hypopneas will alternate with periods of hyperpnea either until sleep becomes firmly established or until there is a prolonged awakening. The magnitude of these ventilatory oscillations during these CNS state transitions will depend on a number of interacting factors, including the ambient PCO_2, the difference between the awake and sleeping PCO_2, the intensity of arousals from sleep, and the magnitude of the awake ventilatory response to CO_2 (1, 5, 6).

Another destabilizing influence is hypocapnia. If ambient PCO_2 is lower and closer to the threshold for apnea than normal during wakefulness, this will predispose to the development of central apnea when the PCO_2 threshold increases at the onset of sleep. If, in addition, PCO_2 does not rise normally at the onset of sleep, there would be a greater tendency for PCO_2 to be below the sleeping threshold and, therefore, for central apnea to occur. A number of studies have shown that patients with nonhypercapnic CSA have a lower PCO_2 during both wakefulness and sleep than do control subjects (2, 7, 8). This lower PCO_2 is probably closer to their apneic threshold than in healthy subjects, since it requires only a 1 to 3 mm Hg decrease in PCO_2 to precipitate a central apnea during NREM sleep in these patients, compared to a reduction of

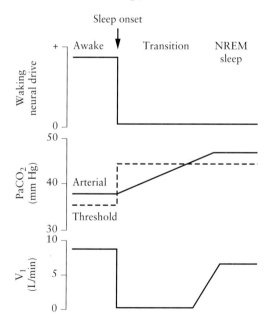

Fig 18.1 The mechanisms underlying central apnea at the onset of sleep. (See text for details.) NREM, Non–rapid eye movement; V_I, minute ventilation. (From Bradley TD, Phillipson EA. Central sleep apnea. Clin Chest Med 1992; 13:493–505.)

3 to 6 mm Hg in a healthy subjects (9–11). Furthermore, whereas the transition from wakefulness to sleep is normally accompanied by a 3 to 4 mm Hg increase in PCO_2, in patients with nonhypercapnic CSA, PCO_2 tends not to increase (12).

Arousals from sleep also interact with hyperventilation to destabilize breathing. They cause augmentation of ventilatory drive over and above that due to a simple shift in CNS state from NREM sleep to wakefulness. As a result, arousals can augment ventilation and drive PCO_2 below the apneic threshold during the following transition to sleep. The more intense the arousal, the greater the augmentation in ventilation, the lower the PCO_2 drops below threshold, and the longer the subsequent central apnea (1). If, on the other hand, arousals are not accompanied by an increase in ventilation, central apneas are unlikely to occur. In the presence of a low background PCO_2, only a small increase in ventilation, such as might occur during a sigh, will be sufficient to drive PCO_2 below the threshold for apnea, even in the absence of arousal. Therefore, arousals from sleep facilitate the development of central

apneas primarily through their effects on ventilation and PCO_2 (Figs. 18.2 and 18.3).

Heightened ventilatory responsiveness to chemical respiratory stimuli during wakefulness can theoretically facilitate respiratory instability for two reasons. First, increased chemoresponsiveness could contribute to the development of chronic hypocapnia (8). Second, the greater the increase in ventilatory responsiveness to chemical stimuli during transitions from NREM sleep to wakefulness, the greater is the potential for augmented ventilation to drive PCO_2 below threshold, triggering a central apnea (5, 6, 13). This phenomenon is known as ventilatory overshoot. Patients with idiopathic CSA have abnormally increased peripheral and central ventilatory responsiveness to CO_2 (8). Persons who develop periodic breathing at high altitude typically have higher ventilatory responsiveness to hypoxia than those who do not develop periodic breathing (14).

According to theoretical models, increased peripheral chemoresponsiveness is more likely to facilitate periodic breathing than is increased central chemoresponsiveness

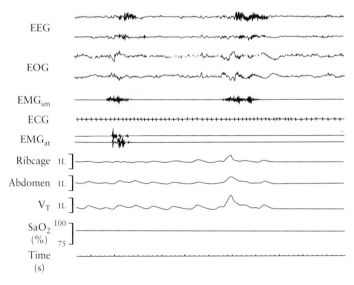

Fig 18.2 Recording from stage 2 sleep demonstrates the transition form stable to periodic breathing in a patient with idiopathic CSA. Two arousals, indicated by increases in EEG and EMGsm activity, are shown. With the first, there is no increase in tidal volume (V_T), and no subsequent apnea. In contrast, the second arousal is accompanied by a large increase in V_T that triggers a central apnea due to a fall in PCO_2 (see Fig. 18.3). EEG, Electroencephalogram; EOG, electrooculogram; EMGsm, submental electromyogram; ECG, electrocardiogram; SaO_2, oxyhemoglobin saturation. (From Xie A, Wong B, Phillipson EA, et al. Interaction of hyperventilation and arousal in the pathogenesis of idiopathic central sleep apnea. Am J Respir Crit Care Med 1994; 150:489–495.)

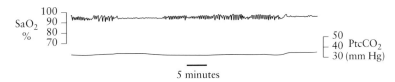

Fig 18.3 *Recordings of nocturnal arterial O_2 saturation (SaO_2) and transcutaneous PCO_2 ($PtcCO_2$) in a patient with idiopathic CSA (same patients as in Fig. 18.2). Recording reads from right to left. Note that the segments containing recurrent central apneas (indicated by oscillations in SaO_2) are preceded by a small decrease in $PtcCO_2$, which corresponds to the second arousal and abrupt increase in tidal volume shown in Figure 18.2. (Modified from Bradley TD, Phillipson EA. Central sleep apnea. Clin Chest Med 1992; 13:493–505.)*

(13). This is because the cycle length of periodic breathing is more in keeping with the shorter circulatory delay between changes in blood gas tensions in the lung and their detection at the carotid bodies than their detection at the central chemoreceptors. Direct evidence in favor of this concept comes from the observation that, in patients with heart failure and CSA, the time delay from a reduction in PCO_2 in the lung until the onset of central apnea is identical to the lung to carotid body circulatory delay (9). Nevertheless, the extent to which increased peripheral versus central chemoreceptor sensitivity contributes to the development of CSA remains to be determined.

Hypoxia could facilitate periodic breathing by stimulating ventilation sufficiently during wakefulness and arousals from sleep to drive arterial and cerebral PCO_2 below the sleeping apneic threshold. This is a mechanism for periodic breathing at high altitude (11). The key role of hypocapnia in the pathogenesis of central apneas in this condition is illustrated by the observation that inhalation of CO_2 under hypoxic conditions abolishes periodic breathing. However, patients with idiopathic CSA and those with heart failure and CSA generally are not hypoxic. Therefore, in these conditions, hypoxia does not play a primary role in the pathogenesis of CSA. Development of hypoxia during central apneas could, however, contribute secondarily to ventilatory overshoot and hypocapnia (13). On theoretical grounds, hypoxia due to pulmonary disease could facilitate the development of CSA, but only if it led to hypocapnia. Hypoxic patients with chronic obstructive airways disease are generally hypercapnic at night and do not have a high prevalence of CSA (15). The prevalence of CSA in hypoxic patients with hypocapnia, such as those with pulmonary fibrotic diseases, has not been determined.

CNS disease leading to hyperventilation could theoretically predispose to the development of CSA. Although early reports suggested a relationship between CNS disease and Cheyne-Stokes respiration with central apneas (CSR-CSA), sleep studies were not performed, and heart failure was not ruled out (16). Cheyne-Stokes respiration is associated with a long periodic breathing cycle length and increased lung-to-chemoreceptor circulation time, both of which are due to a low cardiac output (17). Thus, it is far more likely that the presence of Cheyne-Stokes respiration in patients with cerebrovascular disease is related to concomitant cardiac dysfunction than it is to CNS disease *per se*. Indeed, more recent studies, in which polysomnography was performed, have demonstrated a very high prevalence of OSAS but not of CSA in patients with strokes (18). The prevalence of nonhypercapnic CSA in other types of CNS disease has not been well studied.

Patients with congestive heart failure (CHF) have a high prevalence of CRS-CSA (19,20). One factor that could predispose to CSA in patients with CHF is increased circulation time. This may prolong the delay between changes in arterial blood gas tensions in the lungs and their detection by the peripheral and central chemoreceptors. Thus, at a time when PCO_2 is falling in the lung during hyperpnea, PCO_2 is rising at the peripheral chemoreceptors, further augmenting ventilatory overshoot. This should predispose to ventilatory instability and alternating episodes of hyperpnea and central apnea (13). However, the magnitude of the circulatory delay required to produce periodic breathing in animal experiments far exceeds that observed in CHF (21). Moreover, recent studies in patients with CHF have shown that cardiac output and lung-to-chemoreceptor circulation time do not differ between patients with and without CSA (2,22). These findings do not support a major role for prolonged circulation time in the causation of CSA.

Reflex Inhibition of Central Respiratory Drive

Several reflexes have been described in animals and humans that are capable of triggering transient abolition of central respiratory drive. Perhaps the best known of these is the Hering-Breuer pulmonary inflation reflex (4). However, from a clinical standpoint, inhibitory reflexes arising in the upper airway (pharynx and larynx) are probably more important as potential mechanisms underlying CSA. In sleeping animals, mechanical or chemical stimulation of the larynx can produce a transient inhibition of central respiratory drive (4, 6). In newborn human infants esophageal reflux is thought to be responsible for CSA in some cases. Whether such upper airway reflexes play a role in the pathophysiology of CSA in adult humans has not been established. Patients with idiopathic CSA frequently snore and have increased pharyngeal compliance similar to that seen in patients with OSAS (3, 23, 24). Pharyngeal collapse during central apneas has also been observed in such patients (25). However, it is likely that such collapse is secondary to withdrawal of pharyngeal muscle tone when PCO_2 drops below the apneic threshold during, rather than preceding central apneas. Increased upper airway resistance during snoring could potentially facilitate central apneas by provoking arousals from sleep and triggering hyperventilation and respiratory instability. Although it is possible that each of these mechanisms could cause isolated central apneas, it remains unclear as to whether they could elicit regularly recurring central apneas in association with periodic breathing that would constitute a CSA syndrome.

Key points box 18.1

Pathophysiology of nonhypercapnic CSA

- PCO_2 is low or normal during wakefulness and sleep
- Central apneas are triggered by oscillations in PCO_2 below apnea threshold
- The form of periodic breathing due to respiratory control system instability is characterized by
  - increased peripheral and central ventilatory responsiveness to CO_2
  - PCO_2 chronically close to apnea threshold
  - instability of CNS state at sleep onset
  - apneas occur at transition from wakefulness to NREM sleep or after arousals from sleep
  - apneas commonest in light NREM sleep and less frequent in deep NREM and in REM sleep
  - apnea-related hypoxia usually mild

Clinical and Polysomnographic Features

Nonhypercapnic CSA can be a primary disorder (i.e., idiopathic CSA) or can occur at high altitude or secondary to other medical illnesses, such as acromegaly, CHF, CNS disease, and renal failure. Most research on the clinical and polysomnographic features of CSA has focused on idiopathic CSA and CSA associated with acromegaly and CHF. Conversely, in recent times, little attention has been directed at CSA in the setting of neurological and renal disease. Because of this paucity of literature and the uncertainty as to the clinical significance of nonhypercapnic CSA in association with neurological and renal disease, these disorders are not addressed in this chapter. As well, since periodic breathing with CSA at high altitude is a temporary disorder that arises from normal physiological responses, it is not considered here.

Key points box 18.2

Classification of nonhypercapnic CSA

- Primary
  - Idiopathic CSA
- Secondary
  - Acromegaly
  - Congestive heart failure (Cheyne-Stokes respiration)
  - CNS disease
  - Renal failure
  - High altitude periodic breathing

IDIOPATHIC CENTRAL SLEEP APNEA

Clinical Features

Idiopathic CSA appears to be a very uncommon and probably occurs at less than 5% of the rate of OSAS (26). Recent studies indicate that this form of CSA is associated with the transition from wakefulness to NREM sleep. The key pathophysiological feature of this disorder is a primary tendency to hyperventilate during both wakefulness and sleep in association with increased peripheral and central ventilatory responsiveness to CO_2 (8). The underlying cause of this increased chemosensitivity is unknown. However, the role of hyperventilation in inducing CSA at sleep onset is clear. Specifically, when the waking neural drive to breathing is withdrawn at sleep onset, breathing is not sustained because the decreased PCO_2 resulting from the preceding hyperventilation is below the threshold level required for respiratory rhythm generation during sleep (5, 6). For reasons that are not clear, patients with idiopathic CSA have a prolonged period of transition from wakefulness to established sleep, with the CNS state fluctuating repeatedly between the two states, resulting in recurrent central apneas until sleep becomes firmly established. One possible explanation for this instability in CNS state could be a heightened degree of arousability, which prevents the rapid progression to stable NREM sleep. However, at present, there is no experimental evidence to support such a mechanism.

Patients with idiopathic CSA frequently have clinical features similar to those associated with OSAS. However, patients with CSA tend to be somewhat older (8). There is a striking male preponderance among patients with idiopathic CSA. The reasons for this are not clear but could be related to a tendency to greater sleep fragmentation and a more pronounced augmentation of ventilatory chemoresponsiveness when CNS state shifts from sleep to wakefulness in men than in women (27). These factors could predispose to CNS state instability and could exaggerate the tendency to hyperventilation during arousals (1, 5, 6). Patients with idiopathic CSA are often mildly obese and may complain of excessive daytime sleepiness, restless sleep and snoring, and occasionally of nocturnal choking and nasal obstruction (3). In contrast to patients with OSAS, complaints of insomnia, characterized by difficulty in getting to sleep and frequent nocturnal awakenings, may be prominent (26).

Unlike hypercapnic CSA, idiopathic CSA is not associated with polycythemia or cor pulmonale (3), probably because of the absence of severe hypoxemia during CSA and wakefulness. Arterial O_2 desaturation is relatively mild in this form of CSA because the baseline PaO_2 is usually normal and on the flat upper portion of the oxyhemoglobin dissociation curve. Similarly, cardiac arrhythmias are not a feature of this type of CSA. Thus, patients with idiopathic CSA suffer from a relatively benign form of sleep apnea that is unlikely to lead to serious medical complications.

---

o⟶ Key points box 18.3

Clinical features of idiopathic CSA

- Similarities to obstructive sleep apnea
  - snoring
  - restless sleep
  - nocturnal choking
  - excessive daytime sleepiness
  - marked male predominance
- Differences from obstructive sleep apnea
  - older
  - more frequently suffer insomnia: difficulty in initiating and maintaining sleep
  - apneas more frequent in NREM and less frequent in REM sleep

---

Polysomnographic Features

The characteristic polysomnographic finding in idiopathic CSA is recurrent central apneas occurring at the transition from wakefulness to sleep, alternating with hyperpneas occurring at the time of arousal. Once sleep becomes firmly established, however, the central apneas disappear and breathing becomes regular. Unlike hypercapnic CSA, in idiopathic CSA, apneas and hypopneas are much less frequent in stage 2 and REM sleep and are distinctly uncommon in slow wave sleep (SWS). Furthermore, whereas apnea length in hypercapnic forms of CSA increases from stage 2 to REM sleep, in idiopathic CSA, apnea length remains constant across all sleep stages (3).

Central apneas are typically precipitated either by an abrupt change in CNS state as the patient is drifting off to sleep, or, once sleep has become established, by an abrupt increase in ventilation and decrease in PCO_2 usually associated with arousal (Figs. 18.2 and 18.3). The more intense the arousal, the greater the increase in ventilation, and the longer the subsequent apnea (1) (Fig. 18.4A–D).

The uncommon occurrence of central apneas in SWS is probably due to decreased arousability compared to stages 1 and 2 sleep. The reduced frequency of central apneas in REM compared to stage 2 sleep is probably also partially accounted for by decreased arousability. In

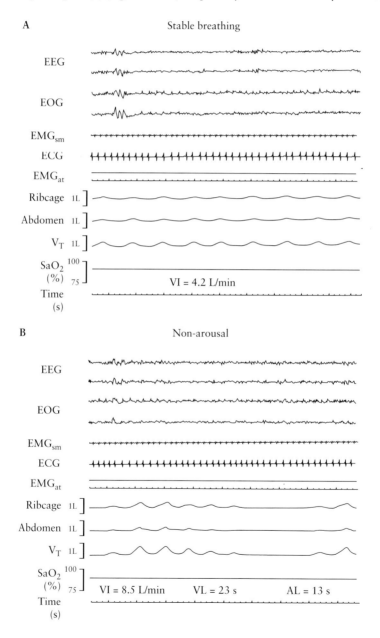

Fig 18.4A,B

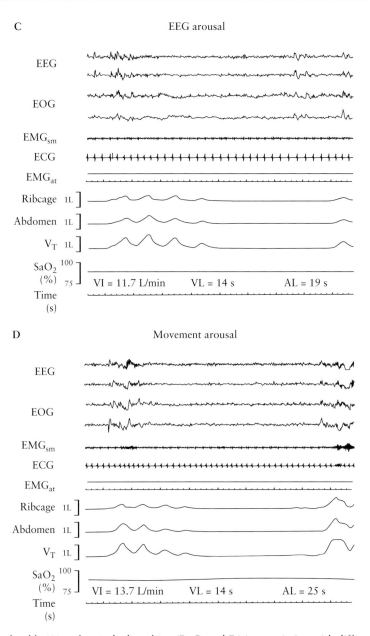

Fig 18.4 *Recording of stable (A) and periodic breathing (B, C, and D) in association with different intensities of arousal during stage 2 sleep in a patient with idiopathic CSA. Arrows indicate the onset of arousal where applicable. With increasing intensity of arousal from nonarousal (B) to EEG arousal (C) to movement arousal (D) there is a progressive increase in minute ventilation (V_I) during the ventilatory phase with a progressive shortening of ventilatory length (VL) and lengthening of the apnea (AL). See text for more complete description. (From Xie A, Wong B, Phillipson EA, et al. Interaction of hyperventilation and arousal in the pathogenesis of idiopathic central sleep apnea. Am J Respir Crit Care Med 1994; 150:489–495.)*

addition, the reduced chemoresponsiveness to chemical stimuli and partial paralysis of respiratory muscles induced by this sleep state increase PCO_2 and prevent the hyperventilation and fall in PCO_2 that typically trigger central apneas.

Because patients with idiopathic CSA generally have no underlying cardiorespiratory disease and normal SaO_2 during wakefulness, their apneas are usually associated with only trivial degrees of arterial O_2 desaturation (3). Similarly, changes in transcutaneous PCO_2 are small but extremely important in perpetuating the disorder. As noted in Fig. 18.3, just before the onset of periodic breathing with CSA, there is a small (2 to 3 mm Hg) decrease in transcutaneous PCO_2 due to an arousal. This small degree of hyperventilation results in recurrent transient loss of central respiratory drive as the state now fluctuates from wakefulness to stage 1 sleep (see previous discussion). This instability in respiratory drive persists until sleep again becomes firmly established, at which point PCO_2 increases and regular breathing ensues (1).

Treatment

Treatment of idiopathic CSA should be considered when a patient complains of symptoms of a sleep apnea syndrome, which could include excessive daytime sleepiness, restless sleep, morning headaches and loud snoring, or insomnia. Because idiopathic CSA is very uncommon, it is not surprising that few studies have specifically addressed its treatment. Furthermore, in the few clinical trials that have been attempted, the type of CSA under consideration was not clearly defined. Nevertheless, guidelines for therapy can be advanced based on pathophysiologic considerations.

Periodic breathing at high altitude can be reversed by the administration of supplemental O_2, which blunts hypoxic responsiveness and allows PCO_2 to rise above the apneic threshold (11). However, as noted earlier, idiopathic CSA is rarely associated with hypoxemia and therefore is usually not responsive to O_2 therapy. Nevertheless, if hypoxemia is present, a trial of supplemental O_2 therapy is appropriate.

Because central apneas are precipitated by fluctuations in PCO_2 below the apnea threshold, raising PCO_2 by inhalation of a CO_2-enriched gas abolishes them (10). Breathing through a face mask with increased deadspace also eliminates CSA. In both cases

an increase of only a 1 to 3 mm Hg in PCO_2 is required to reverse CSA. Unfortunately, administration of a CO_2-enriched gas is not practical and may not be safe in the outpatient setting. A more practical and safer approach may be use of a face mask with increased deadspace. However, by raising PCO_2, both these interventions will increase ventilation and respiratory effort and, therefore, may prove uncomfortable to a patient who is already hyperventilating.

Respiratory stimulants have also been used to treat patients with idiopathic CSA. The rationale for such an approach is that by providing a constant stimulus to breathe, fluctuations in ventilation would be damped irrespective of their effects on PCO_2. The effects of acetazolamide, a carbonic anhydrase inhibitor that stimulates central respiratory drive by causing a metabolic acidosis (28, 29), have been tested in idiopathic CSA. However, these short-term studies were neither randomized nor controlled, and their results were inconsistent. Some investigators reported that acetazolamide reduced the frequency of central apneas and arousals, improved sleep structure, and alleviated symptoms of sleep apnea (28), whereas others failed to find these effects (29). As in the case of CO_2 inhalation, the increased respiratory effort and ventilation arising from use of respiratory stimulants may cause respiratory discomfort. Thus, the efficacy of acetazolamide for idiopathic CSA remains uncertain. The effects of theophylline or medroxyprogesterone on idiopathic CSA are not known.

Because arousal from sleep can precipitate and propagate CSA, sedative medications that blunt arousability and consolidate sleep should theoretically be useful in this disorder. In one study, the effects of a short-acting benzodiazepine, triazolam, was tested during a single night in such patients (30). Although the medication produced a significant reduction in the number of arousals and central apneas, the improvement was modest and may not have been clinically important. The long-term effects of sedatives in idiopathic CSA have not been assessed. In considering the use of sedative medication for CSA, it is critical to establish that the patient has idiopathic CSA rather than hypercapnic CSA. In the latter setting, sedatives are contraindicated because of their potential to aggravate hypercapnia and hypoxia. In addition, the dose of the medication must be selected carefully to avoid a daytime hangover effect. Problems of drug dependency must also be considered. However, further studies on the potential benefits of sedative medications in the treatment of idiopathic CSA appear to be warranted.

Nasal continuous positive airway pressure (CPAP) can also reduce the frequency of central apneas in patients with idiopathic CSA. Because such patients have a highly compliant pharynx (24), the efficacy of CPAP was thought to be due to splinting open of the upper airway, thereby abolishing central apneas arising from reflexes due to pharyngeal collapse (31). Alternatively, upper airway collapse could trigger arousals and hyperventilation, promoting instability of sleep and respiratory control (3). This sequence of events would likewise be interrupted by CPAP. It has also been suggested that CPAP could alleviate CSA by reducing ventilation and increasing PCO_2 above the apnea threshold (32). CPAP can act as an expiratory load and induce a mild degree of CO_2 retention. In addition, CPAP induces an increase in end expiratory lung volume, which would damp oscillations in blood gas tensions and ventilation (33). However, no long-term randomized trials have tested the efficacy of CPAP on symptoms of idiopathic CSA. It also appears that CPAP is not as well tolerated in patients with idiopathic CSA as it is in patients with OSAS. In some patients, idiopathic CSA occurs exclusively in the supine position. This observation suggests a role for upper airway instability in its pathogenesis; hence, avoidance of this sleeping posture might be beneficial (3, 6).

In summary, the treatment of idiopathic CSA presents a problem to the clinician because the disorder is uncommon and there are no well-designed randomized trials to guide therapy. What data are available suggest that a rational approach would involve the use of either CPAP, sedative medications, or acetazolamide. Aggressive therapy is probably not warranted because of the apparent benign nature of the disease.

CENTRAL SLEEP APNEA IN ACROMEGALY
Clinical Features

Recent reports suggest that approximately 30% of patients with acromegaly have CSA (7, 34). Most of these patients have snoring and hypersomnolence, and they have higher levels of growth hormone (GH) and insulin–like growth factor-1 (IGF-1) than acromegalic patients with OSAS or no sleep apnea. Patients with CSA are hypocapnic and have lower awake PCO_2 and higher ventilatory responsiveness to CO_2 than patients with

OSAS or no sleep apnea (7). Slopes of the hypercapnic ventilatory responses were directly related to the levels of GH and IGF-1, suggesting that these substances have effects on breathing control. The severity of CSA was directly related to CO_2 responsiveness and the level of IGF-1. An additional interesting finding was that patients with CSA had a high prevalence of systemic hypertension that was independently related to the presence of CSA. These data suggest that CSA in patients with acromegaly can be manifested as symptoms of a sleep apnea syndrome and that CSA may increase their risk for hypertension. However, there are no reports on either the polysomnographic features or the treatment of CSA in the setting of acromegaly.

CENTRAL SLEEP APNEA AND CHEYNE-STOKES RESPIRATION IN CONGESTIVE HEART FAILURE
Clinical Features

Cheyne-Stokes respiration with CSA (CSR-CSA) is a form of periodic breathing in which apneas and hypopneas alternate with prolonged ventilatory periods characterized by a crescendo-decrescendo pattern of V_T (17, 35, 36). This gradual waxing and waning of V_T, which distinguishes CSR-CSA from other forms of CSA, is a sign of prolonged circulation time and low cardiac output (Fig. 18.5A,B). Unlike OSAS, which probably contributes to the development of CHF, CSR-CSA appears to arise as a result of CHF. Until recently, clinicians have looked upon CSR-CSA as a physiological curiosity. However, this view has changed as it has became apparent that CSR-CSA not only is common in patients with CHF but also has adverse clinical implications.

Epidemiologic studies have consistently reported a high prevalence of CSR-CSA, ranging from 30–40%, in patients with chronic stable CHF (19, 20). This form of breathing is seen more commonly in men than in women, in older than in younger persons, and in association with ischemic rather than idiopathic dilated cardiomyopathy. Atrial fibrillation is frequently associated with CSR-CSA (19). CSA is clearly much more prevalent in patients with CHF than in the otherwise healthy population, suggesting that CHF itself may predispose to its development. The chief risk factor for CSR-CSA, which is shared by idiopathic CSA, is hypocapnia both awake and asleep (1, 12, 35, 37). The cause of hypocapnia in CSR-CSA is probably

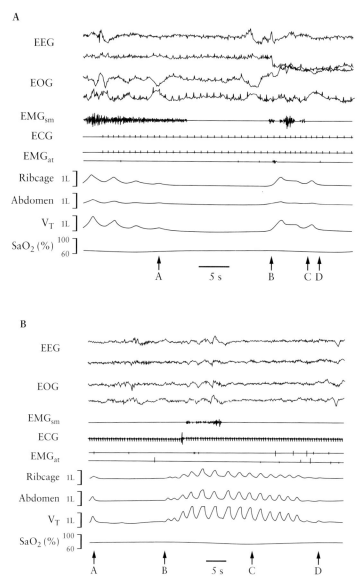

Fig 18.5 *Recordings from a patient with idiopathic CSA **A** and another with heart failure and Cheyne-Stokes respiration with CSA (CSR-CSA) **B** during stage 2 sleep. Compared to the patient with idiopathic CSA, the patient with CSR-CSA has a longer delay from the end of apnea until the nadir of SaO$_2$ (i.e., lung-to-ear circulation time, B-C = 26 s versus 8 s), hyperpnea length (B-D = 46 s versus 7 s) and periodic breathing cycle length (A-D = 65 s versus 25 s), but apnea length is similar (A-B = 21 s versus 18 s). Note also that whereas arousal from sleep occurred at termination of apnea in the patients with idiopathic CSA (indicated by an increase in EMGsm activity), in the patient with CSR-CSA, arousal was delayed until four breaths after apnea termination. See text for more complete description. (From Hall MJ, Xie A, Rutherford R, et al. Cycle length of periodic breathing in patients with and without heart failure. Am J Respir Crit Care Med 1996; 154:376–381.)*

multifactorial. Hypoxia appears not to play an important role because CHF patients with CSR-CSA are generally not hypoxic (2). On the other hand, patients with CHF who have CSR-CSA have higher left ventricular end diastolic volumes and filling pressures than those who do not (12, 22). They are therefore more likely to have pulmonary congestion, which can provoke hyperventilation and hypocapnia by stimulating pulmonary vagal irritant receptors (12, 22, 38). Increased central chemoresponsiveness to CO_2 could also contribute to the development of hypocapnia (39). However, low cardiac output *per se* appears not to be an important factor predisposing to CSR-CSA, since CHF patients with and without CSR-CSA have similar cardiac outputs and ejection fractions (2, 12, 22).

Prospective studies have shown that CHF patients with CSR-CSA have significantly higher death and heart transplantation rates than CHF patients without CSR-CSA matched for age, functional class, and left ventricular ejection fraction (40, 41). Mortality rates are proportional to the frequency of central apneas. The most likely cause of this increased mortality is that patients with CHF and CSR-CSA have higher sympathetic nervous system activity and lower heart rate variability and baroreflex sensitivity than patients without CSR-CSA (41, 42). Increased sympathetic nervous system activity, which probably arises from the combined effects of apnea, apnea-related hypoxia, and arousals from sleep, is a risk factor for mortality in CHF (37, 43). That relationship may be attributable to a number of factors. Increased sympathetic nervous system activity and high circulating catecholamine levels have direct cardiotoxic effects that may contribute to pump failure, elevations in nocturnal blood pressure, and cardiac ischemia (35, 37, 42–44). Patients with CSR-CSA also have increased ventricular ectopy (45). Accordingly, these data suggest that CSR-CSA is part of a viscous cycle whereby CHF leads to CSR-CSA, which provokes greater activation of the sympathetic nervous system that, in turn, aggravates cardiac failure (Fig. 18.6). If true, then alleviation of CSR-CSA could prove beneficial to patients with CHF. On the other hand, it could be that CSR-CSA is simply an outward manifestation of poor cardiac function characterized by left ventricular dilatation and elevated filling pressures (12, 22).

In patients with CSR-CSA, sleep is disrupted by recurrent apneas, hypoxia, and arousals from sleep. These could contribute to symptoms of insomnia, paroxysmal nocturnal dyspnea, and hypersomnolence (46). Symptoms of fatigue normally attributed to low cardiac output could, in some instances, be related to such sleep disruption. However, it is not clear to what extent CSR-CSA leads to symptoms of a sleep apnea syndrome. Although one study (47) showed that patients with CHF and CSR-CSA had a sleep latency significantly shorter than that in CHF patients without this breathing disorder, it appears that many patients with CSR-CSA do not complain of excessive daytime sleepiness (20).

The diagnosis of CSR-CSA is established by polysomnography. However, because no studies have determined symptoms that would predict the presence of CSR-CSA in patients with CHF, indications for polysomnography are not clear. In addition, there is no consensus on whether CSR-CSA should be treated, and if so, by what means. Nevertheless, if the clinician would consider treating CSR-CSA, reasonable indications for polysomnography would be symptoms of a sleep apnea syndrome and symptomatic CHF with left ventricular systolic dysfunction (i.e., ejection fraction < 45%) refractory to medical therapy.

Polysomnographic Features

There are some similarities between the polysomnographic features of CSR-CSA and those of idiopathic CSA. Apneas usually occur either after a change of CNS state from wakefulness to NREM sleep or after an abrupt increase in V_T, often resulting from arousal from sleep (2). The immediate cause of central apneas is a fall in PCO_2 that appears to be sensed at the peripheral, rather than the central, chemoreceptor (9). Apneas and hypopneas occur most frequently in stage 1 sleep and decrease in frequency progressively from stage 2 to stage 3–4 to REM sleep in association with a progressive fall in ventilation and rise in PCO_2 (2).

There are also some important differences in the polysomnographic appearance of CSR-CSA and idiopathic CSA. In contrast to idiopathic CSA, in which apnea is terminated by an abrupt increase in V_T followed by 3 to 5 breaths, in CSR-CSA apnea is terminated by a gradually rising V_T which reaches a peak and then gradually declines until the onset of apnea (Fig. 18.5) (17). There are usually 10 to 14 breaths during hyperpnea, and as a result, the lengths of the hyperpnea and of the periodic breathing cycle are greater than in idiopathic CSA. The

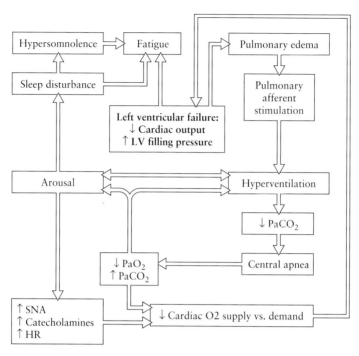

Fig 18.6 *Pathophysiologic scheme of CSR-CSA in association with congestive heart failure. See text for details. SNA, Sympathetic nerve activity; HR, heart rate. (Modified from; Hall MJ, Bradley TD. Cardiovascular disease and sleep apnea. Currt Opin Pulm Med. 1995; 1:512–518.)*

○┓ Key points box 18.4

Clinical significance of Cheyne-Stokes respiration with central sleep apnea in congestive heart failure

- Common: occurs in approximately 30% of patients
- Male predominance
- Risk factors:
  - hypocapnia
  - increased left ventricular filling pressure and end diastolic volume
  - atrial fibrillation
  - older age
- Associated with:
  - increased sympathetic nervous system activity
  - higher prevalence of ventricular ectopy
  - increased risk of death

---

fall in oxyhemoglobin saturation (SaO_2), detected by an oximeter on the ear, does not begin until mid-apnea, and then it declines slowly until reaching its nadir in the middle of hyperpnea. The time from the end of apnea until the nadir of desaturation is reached is the lung to ear circulation time (Fig. 18.5). This measure provides an estimate of the circulation time from the lung to the peripheral chemoreceptors because the ear is adjacent to the carotid body. Lung-to-ear circulation time is directly proportional to hyperpnea and cycle length and inversely proportional to cardiac output. Therefore, the longer hyperpnea and periodic breathing cycle length and the more gradual decline in SaO_2 and rise in V_T after termination of apnea in patients with CHF and CSR-CSA than in patients with idiopathic CSA are due to a lower cardiac output (17). Thus, although low cardiac output and increased circulatory delay are not the cause of central apneas in CSR-CSA, they sculpt the periodic breathing pattern into its characteristic appearance. Hence, while the term 'Cheyne-Stokes respiration' has been used loosely to describe any form of periodic breathing, its use should be reserved for periodic breathing in which the hyperpneic phase is prolonged with a gradual waxing and waning of V_T, as originally described by Cheyne (36).

In CSR-CSA, apnea-related desaturation tends to be mild, and SaO_2 seldom falls below 85% (3). However, more severe desaturation can occur (20, 35, 46). Systemic blood pressure and heart rate oscillate in concert with ventilation during the CSR-CSA cycle, falling during apnea and rising during hyperpnea. The main cause of these oscillations appears to be entrainment by ventilation (48). This respiratory entrainment probably accounts for the very low frequency oscillations in blood pressure and heart rate that have been described in association with CHF (49).

Arousals from sleep frequently occur in association with CSR-CSA. These can lead to fragmentation of sleep, can result in loss of SWS and REM sleep, and may contribute to fatigue and hypersomnolence. Unlike OSAS and idiopathic CSA, arousals frequently, although not always, occur well after the ventilatory phase has begun. Consequently, the functional significance of arousal in CSR-CSA is not clear. Arousals act as a critical protective mechanism that allows airflow to resume after a period of apnea in OSAS (4). This prevents further asphyxiation and may, in some cases, prevent death. As illustrated in Figure 18.5, in CSR-CSA, in which arousal occurs after termination of apnea, it does not serve to initiate airflow, since the ventilatory threshold for chemical stimuli is clearly reached before the arousal threshold. In such circumstances, arousal may serve no useful purpose and, in fact, may potentiate ventilatory drive and propagate CSR-CSA, disrupt sleep, and contribute to paroxysmal nocturnal dyspnea (35, 37). Stimuli provoking arousals probably include asphyxia and physical sensations arising from the act of breathing.

Treatment

There is no consensus on indications for therapy for CSR-CSA in patients with CHF. However, as in the case of idiopathic CSA, it would seem appropriate to consider treatment if there are symptoms of a sleep apnea syndrome or insomnia. In view of the serious nature of the underlying cardiac condition, treatment should also be considered if there are complaints of paroxysmal nocturnal dyspnea, nocturnal angina, nocturnal ventricular arrhythmias associated with apneas, or severe apnea-related hypoxia. There have only been a few trials of therapy for CSR-CSA in patients with CHF. Because of their relatively short duration and the small numbers of patients studied, none can be considered definitive. Therefore, there is no consensus on what constitutes effective therapy for CSR-CSA. Nevertheless, therapeutic guidelines resembling those for idiopathic CSA can be advanced, based on their similar pathophysiologies and the results of these trials. However, an additional consideration in CSR-CSA is the therapy of the underlying cardiac failure.

Because CSR-CSA arises secondary to CHF, appropriate pharmacologic therapy for CHF should be considered the first line of therapy. Only a few small, non-randomized, uncontrolled trials have addressed this issue, however. They described alleviation of CSR-CSA in association with intensification of drug therapy for CHF (50, 51). Neither cardiac function nor symptoms of CSR-CSA were assessed in those studies. There have also been a few case reports describing alleviation of CSR-CSA in patients with CHF after cardiac transplantation (50, 52).

The effects of supplemental O_2 on CSR-CSA in patients with CHF have been studied in several short-term trials. The rationale for using O_2 to treat CSR-CSA in patients with CHF is that correction of apnea-related dips in SaO_2 may suppress peripheral chemoreceptor drive sufficiently to prevent subsequent ventilatory overshoot. Evidence from single night trials of O_2 provide some support for this mechanism. When O_2 was administered at a low flow rate just sufficient to prevent apnea-related dips in SaO_2, neither PCO_2 nor the frequency of central respiratory events changed substantially (9, 44). In contrast, when O_2 was administered at a much higher flow rate, PCO_2 increased and the frequency of central events decreased (53).

Randomized double-blind crossover trials of intranasal O_2 at flow rates of 2 to 4 L/min conducted over longer periods (1 to 4 weeks) in patients with CHF and CSR-CSA demonstrated a modest reduction in the frequency of apneas and hypopneas (54, 55). These were associated with a decrease in nocturnal urinary noradrenaline (norepinephrine) concentration and a slight increase in peak O_2 consumption during exercise testing. However, daytime plasma noradrenaline level did not change, symptoms of CHF did not improve, and cardiac function was not assessed. Nevertheless, these data suggest the potential for O_2 to reduce the severity of CSR-CSA and decrease nocturnal sympathetic nervous system activity.

Balanced against these potential benefits of supplemental O_2, however, are potential detrimental effects that have been described in patients with CHF. These include dose-related increases in systemic vascular resistance, blood pressure, and left ventricular filling pressure and reductions in cardiac output (56). The mechanisms for these adverse effects have not been demonstrated but may involve elaboration of oxygen free radicals that inhibit endothelium dependent vasodilation. Thus, it is not clear that long-term supplemental O_2 would be a safe and effective therapy for CSR-CSA in CHF patients. This issue can only be resolved by longer trials with larger numbers of patients in which the effects of nocturnal O_2 on heart function and prognosis are assessed.

To summarize, although O_2-induced reductions in overnight urinary catecholamine excretion suggests the potential for benefits to the cardiovascular system in some patients with CSR-CSA, it is unlikely to be of benefit when hypoxic dips are minimal. If O_2 is used, it should be administered at a sufficiently low flow rate to avoid hyperoxia and any consequent increase in oxidative stress.

As in the case of idiopathic CSA, raising PCO_2 just 1 to 3 mm Hg, through inhalation of a CO_2 enriched gas mixture, abolishes central apneas and hypopneas in patients with CHF and CSR-CSA (Fig. 18.7A,B) (9). Although inhaled CO_2 or provision of a mask with increased deadspace will alleviate CSR-CSA, neither is liable to be clinically useful because both methods increase minute ventilation and thereby load the inspiratory muscles, which are weak in patients with CHF (57). This could further disrupt sleep because of dyspnea. Raising PCO_2 could also create a potentially dangerous respiratory acidosis. For these reasons, inhalation of CO_2 cannot be recommended for therapy of CSR-CSA at the present time.

Respiratory stimulants could theoretically alleviate CSR-CSA by providing a constant stimulus to breathe even in the presence of low PCO_2. Theophylline increases respiratory drive by a direct stimulatory effect on brain stem respiratory centers. In a small randomized, double-

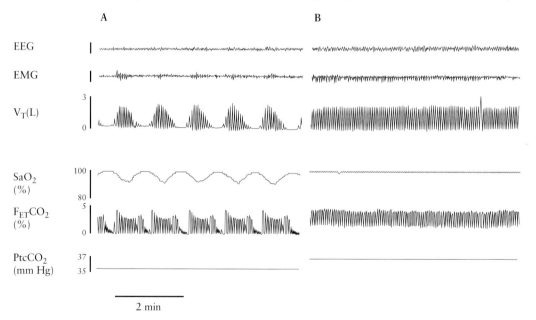

Fig 18.7 *Recordings from a patient during stage 2 sleep while breathing air (A) and CO_2 (B). Central apneas are abolished by CO_2 inhalation in association with an increase in the fraction of end tidal CO_2 ($F_{ET}CO_2$) above the level during hyperpneas preceding apneas, and a 1.6 mm Hg increase in $PtcCO_2$. Abolition of CSR-CSA was also associated with elimination of dips in SaO_2. (From Lorenzi-Filho G, Rankin F, Bies I, et al. Effects of inhaled CO_2 and O_2 on Cheyne-Stokes respiration in patients with heart failure. Am J Respir Crit Care Med 1999; 159:1490–1498.)*

blind, crossover trial lasting 5 days, use of theophylline was associated with a significant reduction in the frequency of central respiratory events, but without any increase in SaO_2, reduction in the frequency of arousals, or improvements in sleep structure. Theophylline did not lead to any improvement in cardiac function (58). However, it could increase cardiac arrhythmias because of its phosphodiesterase inhibitory, sympathoexcitatory, and positive inotropic effects. Other phosphodiesterase inhibitors, such as milrinone, have similar arrhythmogenic effects and have been shown to increase mortality in patients with CHF (59). Another potential problem with theophylline is that it could increase minute ventilation and increase the load on the inspiratory muscles. Therefore, more data are required before theophylline can be recommended as an effective and safe treatment for CSR-CSA in patients with CHF. There are no published reports on the use of acetazolamide or medroxyprogesterone for the treatment of CSR-CSA in patients with CHF. Moreover, the creation of a metabolic acidosis by acetazolamide in such patients might precipitate serious cardiac arrhythmias.

Another potential approach to the treatment of CSR-CSA would be to suppress arousals from sleep and blunt respiratory drive by administering sedative medications. Several benzodiazepines have been tested in patients with CHF and CSR-CSA (60). Although they reduced the number of arousals from sleep, they neither reduced the severity of CSR-CSA nor improved SaO_2. Effects on cardiovascular function were not assessed. Thus, the available evidence does not support the use of sedatives as a treatment for CSR-CSA in patients with CHF.

The most extensively tested therapy for CSR-CSA in patients with CHF is CPAP. CPAP has a number of beneficial acute hemodynamic and autonomic effects when applied to patients with CHF. It increases intrathoracic pressure, which unloads the inspiratory muscles. It also increases the pressure around the heart, which reduces the difference between internal and external left ventricular pressure (i.e., transmural pressure) and thereby decreases both preload and afterload (61, 62). In patients with elevated left ventricular filling pressures, it augments stroke volume and cardiac output (33). Reduced heart rate variability, which is a marker of poor prognosis, is often seen in patients with CHF. CPAP increases heart rate variability in such patients (33). Since CPAP has beneficial effects on cardiac loading conditions, heart rate variability and

cardiac output in CHF patients while awake, it seems reasonable that it could also have longer lasting beneficial effects.

When applied during sleep to patients with CSR-CSA, CPAP generally does not cause an immediate reduction in respiratory events; the reduction occurs only after several weeks. Therefore, the most important goal in initiating nasal CPAP in such patients is not the immediate relief of CSR-CSA, but rather to get the patient accustomed to wearing the apparatus. In general, patients require a 2 to 3 day acclimatization period during which CPAP is slowly raised from 5 cm H_2O to between 10 and 12.5 cm H_2O (37, 46). Since CPAP probably takes several days to weeks to exert its beneficial effects on CSR-CSA, follow-up sleep studies on CPAP should probably be delayed for several weeks after its initiation.

A number of randomized controlled clinical trials of CPAP versus standard pharmacological therapy for CHF have been carried out using this approach in small numbers of patients (fewer than 30). CPAP was applied at pressures of 10–12.5 cm H_2O and was used nightly over 1–3 month periods. CPAP reduced the frequency of central events in association with a significant reduction in ventilation and a significant increase in transcutaneous PCO_2 (32). Since the key determinant of CSR-CSA in patients with CHF is hyperventilation with hypocapnia during sleep, these findings indicated that one mechanism through which CPAP attenuates CSR-CSA is by reducing ventilation and raising PCO_2 above the apneic threshold. The means by which CPAP reduces minute ventilation in CHF patients with CSR-CSA is not clear. The most likely mechanism is alleviation of pulmonary edema by increasing intrathoracic pressure and shifting interstitial lung fluid to the extrathoracic vascular compartment (61). Attenuation of CSR-CSA by CPAP was accompanied by reductions in the frequency of arousals (46). However, in studies in which there was no CPAP acclimatization period and in which CPAP was titrated up over a single night, when the pressure used was less than 10 cm H_2O, or when it was used for less than 1 month, no reductions in the frequencies of central apneas and hypopneas were observed (60, 64).

CPAP has also been shown to improve respiratory muscle function in patients with CHF and CSR-CSA. Patients with CHF frequently suffer from inspiratory muscle weakness, which may play a role in the pathogenesis of their dyspnea. CPAP unloads inspiratory muscles in such patients by reducing the amplitude of inspiratory pleural pressure swings (61). Nightly use of CPAP for 3 months by patients with CHF and CSR-CSA has been shown to improve inspiratory muscle strength and to reduce dyspnea (57). The mechanism for this effect is not well understood, but could involve alleviation of chronic muscle fatigue by inspiratory unloading or improvement in cardiac function with improved muscle perfusion.

Short-term randomized trials have also demonstrated that CPAP has a number of beneficial effects on cardiovascular function. It improves left ventricular ejection fraction and reduces functional mitral regurgitation, indicating improved systolic function and pumping efficiency (46, 65). It reduces both nocturnal urinary and daytime plasma noradrenaline levels, indicating a reduction in sympathetic nervous system activity (42). It also reduces plasma atrial natriuretic peptide levels, indicating a reduction in atrial wall tensions (65). In addition, it reduces the severity of dyspnea and improves quality of life (46). Finally, in a recent randomized trial involving 67 patients with CHF, patients assigned to CPAP experienced a strong trend to reduced rates of death and cardiac transploration over follow up periods of up to five years (66).

The mechanisms by which CPAP leads to these improvements in cardiac and neurohumoral function in patients with CHF and CSR-CSA could include alleviation of apnea-related hypoxic dips and arousals as well as reductions in cardiac filling pressures, diastolic volumes, and left ventricular afterload. However, these improvements cannot be attributed solely to a temporary alteration in loading conditions, since these measurements were made in the daytime several hours after patients had last worn the CPAP apparatus. The mechanism of mechanisms responsible for these carry over effects remain to be determined, but almost certainly favorable chronic alterations in the energetics and biological properties of the myocardium are involved.

In summary, CSR-CSA is common in patients with CHF and is associated with pathological effects on the cardiovascular system. Such effects over time have the potential to cause progression of CHF and to worsen its prognosis (91). As indicated above, specific treatment of CSR-CSA, especially with CPAP or O_2, can have beneficial short-term and medium-term effects on cardiovascular and respiratory function. In the case of treatment with CPAP, the benefits to left ventricular ejection fraction, mitral regurgitation, and atrial natriuretic peptide and nor-adrenaline levels imply the potential to improve survival (42, 46, 65). To date,

however, studies of various interventions for CSR-CSA in patients with CHF have involved too few subjects over too short a duration to provide definitive evidence of long-term benefits. Nevertheless, these studies have provided sufficient evidence of medium-term benefit to warrant larger, longer-term trials of CPAP or supplemental O_2 to evaluate their effects on prognosis in patients with CHF and CSR-CSA.

REFERENCES

1. Xie A, Wong B, Phillipson EA, et al. Interaction of hyperventilation and arousal in the pathogenesis of idiopathic central sleep apnea. Am J Respir Crit Care Med 1994; 150:489–495.

2. Naughton M, Benard D, Tam A, et al. Role of hyperventilation in the pathogenesis of central sleep apnea in patients with congestive heart failure. Am Rev Respir Dis 1993; 148:330–338.

3. Bradley TD, McNicholas WT, Rutherford R, et al. Clinical and physiological heterogeneity of the central sleep apnea syndrome. Am Rev Respir Dis 1986; 134:217–221.

4. Phillipson EA, Bowes G. Control of breathing during sleep. In: Cherniack NS, Widdicombe JG, eds. Handbook of Physiology, vol 2. Control of Breathing. Bethesda, MD: American Physiological Society; 1986:649–849.

5. Trinder J, Whitworth F, Kay A, et al. Respiratory instability at sleep onset. J Appl Physiol 1992; 73:2462–2469.

6. Bradley TD, Phillipson EA. Central sleep apnea. Clin Chest Med 1992; 13:493–505.

7. Grunstein RR, Ho KY, Berthon-Jones M, et al. Central sleep apnea is associated with increased ventilatory response to carbon dioxide and hypersecretion of growth hormone in patients with acromegaly. Am J Respir Crit Care Med 1994; 150:496–502.

8. Xie A, Rutherford R, Rankin F, et al. Hypocapnia and increased ventilatory responsiveness in patients with idiopathic central sleep apnea. Am J Respir Crit Care Med 1995; 152:1950–1955.

9. Lorenzi-Filho G, Rankin F, Bies I, et al. Effects of inhaled CO_2 and O_2 on Cheyne-Stokes respiration in patients with heart failure. Am J Respir Crit Care Med 1999; 159:1490–1498.

10. Xie A, Rankin F, Rutherford R, et al. Effects of inhaled CO_2 and added deadspace on idiopathic central sleep apnea. J Appl Physiol 1997; 82:918–926.

11. Berssenbrugge A, Dempsey J, Iber C, et al. Mechanisms of hypoxia-induced periodic breathing during sleep in humans. J Physiol (London) 1983; 343:507–524.

12. Tkacova R, Hall MJ, Liu PP, et al. Left ventricular volume in patients with heart failure and Cheyne-Stokes respiration during sleep. Am J Respir Crit Care Med 1997; 156:1549–1555.

13. Khoo MC, Kronauer RE, Strohl KP, et al. Factors inducing periodic breathing in humans: a general model. J Appl Physiol 1982; 53:644–659.

14. Lahiri S, Maret K, Sherpa MG. Dependence of high altitue sleep apnea on ventilatory sensitivity to hypoxia. Respir Physiol 1983; 52:281–301.

15. Douglas NJ. Sleep in patients with chronic obstructive pulmonary disease. Clin Chest Med 1998; 19:115–125.

16. Brown HW, Plum F. The neurological basis of Cheyne-Stokes respiration. Am J Med 1961; 30:849–861.

17. Hall MJ, Xie A, Rutherford R, et al. Cycle length of periodic breathing in patients with and without heart failure. Am J Respir Crit Care Med 1996; 154:376–381.

18. Dyken ME, Somers VK, Yamada T, et al. Investigating the relationship between stroke and obstructive sleep apnea. Stroke 1996; 27:401–407.

19. Sin D, Fitzgerald F, Parker JD, et al. Risk factors for central and obstructive sleep apnea in 450 men and women with congestive heart failure. Am J Respir Crit Care Med 1999; 160:1101–1106.

20. Javaheri S, Parker TJ, Liming JD, et al. Sleep apnea in 81 ambulatory male patients with stable heart failure. Types and their prevalence, consequences, and presentations. Circulation 1998; 97:2154–2159.

21. Guyton AC, Crowell JW, Moore JW. Basic oscillating mechanism of Cheyne-Stokes breathing. Am J Physiol 1956; 187:395–398.

22. Solin P, Bergin P, Richardson M, et al. Influence of pulmonary capillary wedge pressure on central sleep apnea in heart failure. Circulation 1999; 99:1574–1579.

23. Brown IG, Bradley TD, Phillipson EA, Zanel N, Hoffstein V. Pharyngeal compliance in snoring subjects with and without obstructive sleep apnea. Am Rev Respir Dis 1985; 132:211–215.

24. Bradley TD, Brown IG, Zamel N, et al. Differences in pharyngeal properties between snorers with predominantly central sleep apnea and those without sleep apnea. Am Rev Respir Dis 1987; 135:387–391.

25. Badr SM, Toiber F, Skatrud JB, et al. Pharyngeal narrowing/occlusion during central sleep apnea. J Appl Physiol 1995; 78:1806–1815.

26. Guilleminault C, Tilkian A, Dement WC. The sleep apnea syndromes. Annu Rev Med 1976; 27:465–484.

27. Hume KI, Van F, Watson A. A field study of age and gender differences in habitual adult sleep. J Sleep Res 1998; 7:85–94.

28. DeBacker WA, Verbraecken J, Willemen M, et al. Central apnea index decreases after prolonged treatment with acetazolamide. Am J Respir Crit Care Med 1995; 151:87–91.

29. Sakamoto T, Nakazawa Y, Hashizume Y, et al. Effects of acetazolamide on the sleep apnea syndrome and its therapeutic mechanism. Psychiatry Clin Neurosci 1995; 49:59–64.

30. Bonnet MH, Dexter JR, Arand DL. The effect of triazolam on arousal and respiration in central sleep apnea. Sleep 1990; 13:31–41.

31. Issa FG, Sullivan CE. Reversal of central sleep apnea using nasal CPAP. Chest 1986; 90:165–171.

32. Naughton MT, Benard DC, Rutherford R, et al. Effect of continuous positive airway pressure on central sleep apnea and nocturnal PCO_2 in heart failure. Am J Respir Crit Care Med 1994; 150:1598–1604

33. Butler GC, Naughton MT, Rahman MA, et al. Continuous positive airway pressure increases heart rate variability in congestive heart failure. J Am Coll Cardiol 1995; 25: 672–679.

34. Grunstein RR, Ho KY, Sullivan CE. Sleep apnea in acromegaly. Ann Intern Med 1991; 115:527–532.

35. Bradley TD. Right and left ventricular functional impairment and sleep apnea. Clin Chest Med 1992; 13:459–479.

36. Cheyne J. A case of apoplexy in which the fleshy part of the heart was converted to fat. Dublin Hospital Rep 1818; 2:216–223.

37. Bradley TD, Floras JS. Pathophysiologic and therapeutic implications of sleep apnea in congestive heart failure. J Card Fail 1996; 2:223–240.

38. Paintal AS. Mechanisms of stimulation of type J pulmonary receptors. J Physiol (Lond) 1969; 203:511–532.

39. Javaheri S. A mechanism of central sleep apnea in patients with heart failure. N Engl J Med 1999; 341:949–954.

40. Hanly PJ, Zuberi-Khokhar NS. Increased mortality associated with Cheyne-Stokes respiration in patients with congestive heart failure. Am J Respir Crit Care Med 1996; 153:272–276.

41. Lanfranchi PA, Braghiroli A, Bosimini E, et al. Prognostic value of nocturnal Cheyne-Stokes respiration in chronic heart failure. Circulation 1999; 99:1435–1440.

42. Naughton MT, Benard DC, Liu PP, et al. Effects of nasal CPAP on sympathetic activity in patients with heart failure and central sleep apnea. Am J Respir Crit Care Med 1995; 152:473–479.

43. Cohn JN, Levine TB, Olivari MT, et al. Plasma norepinephrine as a guide to prognosis in patients with congestive heart failure. N Engl J Med 1984; 311:819–823.

44. Franklin KA, Sandstrom E, Johansson G, et al. Hemodynamics, cerebral circulation, and oxygen saturation in Cheyne-Stokes respiration. J Appl Physiol 1997; 83:1184–1191.

45. Javaheri S, Corbett WS. Association of low $PaCO_2$ with central sleep apnea and ventricular arrhythmias in ambulatory patients with stable heart failure. Ann Intern Med 1998; 128:204–207.

46. Naughton MT, Liu PP, Benard DC, et al. Treatment of congestive heart failure and Cheyne-Stokes respiration during sleep by continuous positive airway pressure. Am J Respir Crit Care Med 1995; 151:92–97.

47. Hanly P, Zuberi-Khokhar N. Daytime sleepiness in patients with congestive heart failure and Cheyne-Stokes respiration. Chest 1995; 107:952–958.

48. Lorenzi-Filho G, Dajani HR, Leung RST, et al. Entrainment of blood pressure and heart rate oscillations by periodic breathing. Am J Respir Crit Care Med 1999; 159:1147–1154.

49. Mortara A, Sleight P, Pinna GD, et al. Abnormal awake respiratory patterns are common in chronic heart failure and may prevent evaluation of autonomic tone by measures of heart rate variability. Circulation 1997; 96:246–252.

50. Dark DS, Pingleton SK, Kerby GR, et al. Breathing pattern abnormalities and arterial oxygen desaturation during sleep in the congestive heart failure syndrome. Improvement following medical therapy. Chest 1987; 91:833–836.

51. Walsh JT, Andrews R, Starling R, et al. Effects of captopril and oxygen on sleep apnoea in patients with mild to moderate congestive heart failure. Heart 1995; 73:237–241.

52. Murdock DK, Lawless CE, Loeb HS, et al. The effect of heart transplantation on Cheyne-Stokes respiration associated with congestive heart failure. J Heart Transplant 1986; 5:336–337.

53. Franklin KA, Eriksson P, Sahlin C, et al. Reversal of central sleep apnea with oxygen. Chest 1997; 111:163–169.

54. Andreas S, Clemens C, Sandholzer H, et al. Improvements in exercise capacity with treatment of Cheyne-Stokes respiration in patients with congestive heart failure. J Am Coll Cardiol 1996; 27:1486–1490.

55. Staniforth AD, Kinnear WJM, Starling R, et al. Effect of oxygen on sleep quality, cognitive function and sympathetic activity in patients with chronic heart failure and Cheyne-Stokes respiration. Eur Heart J 1998; 19.922 928.

56. Haque WA, Boehmer J, Clemson BS, et al. Hemodynamic effects of supplemental oxygen administration in congestive heart failure. J Am Coll Cardiol 1996; 27:353–357.

57. Granton JT, Benard DC, Naughton MT, et al. CPAP improves inspiratory muscle strength in patients with heart failure and central sleep apnea. Am J Respir Crit Care Med 1996; 153:277–282.

58. Javaheri S, Parker TJ, Wexler L, et al. Effect of theophylline on sleep-disordered breathing in heart failure. N Engl J Med 1996; 335:562–567.

59. Packer M, Carver JR, Rodeheffer RJ, et al. Effect of oral milrinone on mortality in severe chronic heart failure. N Engl J Med 1991; 325:1468–1475.

60. Guilleminault CE, Clerk A, Labonowski M, et al. Cardiac failure and benzodiazepines. Sleep 1993; 16:524–528.

61. Naughton MT, Rahman MA, Hara K, et al. Effect of continuous positive airway pressure on intrathoracic and left ventricular transmural pressures in patients with congestive heart failure. Circulation 1995; 91:1725–1731.

62. Lenique F, Habis M, Lofaso F, et al. Ventilatory and hemodynamic effects of continuous positive airway pressure in left heart failure. Am J Respir Crit Care Med 1997; 155:500–505.

63. Bradley TD, Holloway RM, McLaughlin PR, et al. Cardiac output response to continuous positive airway pressure in congestive heart failure. Am Rev Respir Dis 1992; 145:377–382.

64. Davies RJ, Harrington KJ, Ormerod OJ, et al. Nasal continuous positive airway pressure in chronic heart failure with sleep-disordered breathing. Am Rev Respir Dis 1993; 147:630–634.

65. Tkacova R, Liu PP, Naughton MT, et al. Effect of continuous positive airway pressure on mitral regurgitant fraction and atrial natriuretic peptide in patients with heart failure. J Am Coll Cardiol 1997; 30:739–745.

66. Sin DD, Logan AG, Fitzgerald FS, Liu PP, Bradley TD. Effects of continuous positive airway on cardiovascular outcomes in heart failure patients with and without Cheyne-Stokes respiration. Circulation 200; 102:61–66.

PART SIX

SLEEP APNEA IN THE YOUNG AND ELDERLY

19

SLEEP APNEA IN INFANTS AND CHILDREN

Claude Gaultier

INTRODUCTION

Obstructive sleep apnea syndrome (OSAS) was first described specifically in children by Guilleminault et al. (1) as a combination of clinical symptoms and of polysomnography evidence of obstructive apneas. Since this seminal description, criteria for OSAS in children have been refined (2–4). Polysomnographic criteria now include the episodes of partial airway obstruction commonly seen in children with clinical symptoms of OSAS (2, 4). Upper airway resistance syndrome (UARS) is an entity recently described in adults whose diagnosis requires esophageal pressure measurement (5). A recent study by Guilleminault et al. (6) in a large pediatric population found that children with clinical symptoms suggesting OSAS were more likely to have UARS than OSAS. However, most studies of OSAS have used polysomnographic criteria of obstructive apnea-hypopnea or episodes of obstructive hypoventilation (3). This chapter reviews available data on OSAS. It should be borne in mind, however, that UARS probably shares with OSAS the same clinical symptoms, risk of complications, and treatment requirements (6, 7).

EPIDEMIOLOGY

Epidemiological studies of OSAS in children are few and fragmentary in the data they provide. Their results are interesting but provide no conclusions of general validity. Studies of series of patients meeting polysomnographic criteria for OSAS suggest that the peak prevalence is between 2 and 5 years of age (8–10), a finding consistent with the facts that adenotonsillar hypertrophy is the leading cause of OSAS in children and that the facial bones grow more slowly than the lymphoid tissue during childhood (11).

In contrast to the situation in adults, a male bias of OSAS has not been convincingly established in children (12), although it has been suggested by some studies (13, 14).

The frequency of habitual snoring has been evaluated in large pediatric populations (15–19). However, age ranges varied widely (6 months to 6 years [18], 4 to 5 years [17], and 6 to 13 years [15]). The proportion of subjects with habitual snoring varied from 3.2% (18) to 12% (17). Two studies involving use of screening methods in children with habitual snoring estimated the prevalence of OSAS at 0.7% (17) and 3% (18).

The term 'primary snoring' has been used in some studies to designate snoring with a polysomnographic apnea-hypopnea index (AHI) < 1 (20). The natural history of primary snoring has been investigated in two studies with follow-up evaluations of 1–3 years (21, 22).

⊶ Key points box 19.1

Epidemiology and symptoms

1. The prevalence of OSAS in children is in the region of 0.7–3% and peaks between 2–5 years of age.

2. The principal symptoms are snoring and difficulty breathing at night. Daytime sleepiness and obesity are less common in children than in adults.

3. Symptoms of OSAS become worse during upper respiratory infections.

4. Adenotonsillar hypertrophy is the most common pathophysiological factor, but bony abnormalities of the mandible are also frequent.

In one of these studies (21), snoring resolved in 50% of cases, whereas in the other (22) it resolved in only 20% of cases, and two children (10%) developed moderately severe OSAS. However, neither study measured esophageal pressures, leaving open the possibility that some of the children had UARS (23). Finally, a recent study reported data of home overnight cardiorespiratory monitoring in a large population of children 2 to 18 years of age (12). The frequency of OSAS defined by an AHI > 10 was 1.6% (12). The risk for OSAS was estimated to be 3.5 times greater in African-American children than in white children (12).

CLINICAL SYMPTOMS

Detailed analysis of clinical symptoms is the first step toward the diagnosis of OSAS in children. Fairly often, the cause of the symptoms goes unrecognized for some time, occasionally longer than a year. This diagnostic delay explains why even at the present time OSAS is sometimes revealed by severe complications such as acute cardiorespiratory failure (24).

Differences exist between pediatric and adult OSAS in the type and frequency of clinical symptoms (4). Excessive daytime sleepiness, the most prominent clinical symptom of OSAS in adults, is infrequent in children (4). The three main symptoms in infants and children occur at night: snoring, difficulty in breathing with an inward movement of the upper part of the chest during inspiration, and apneas with noisy resumption of breathing (6, 8–10, 25–29). Fairly often, parents report that the child has drenching sweats, restlessness during sleep, and frequent awakenings. Nocturnal enuresis can be at the forefront of the clinical picture in older children (29, 30). Acute upper airway infections are common in younger children (27). The severity of clinical symptoms increases during the infection, then decreases after treatment is initiated. Behavioral disorders (hyperactivity, aggressive behavior) and cognitive impairments have been reported in school children (31–33).

Recent studies have demonstrated reversal of behavioral and learning disorders after appropriate treatment of the OSAS (32, 33). During wakefulness, mouth breathing is common (6, 8–10, 25–29). Failure to thrive is not uncommon in infants and children with OSAS (6, 8–10, 29). OSAS should be looked for routinely during the clinical evaluation of a child with failure to thrive. The mech-

anisms by which growth is stunted remain a matter of debate but include an increase in the work of breathing during sleep, which may be responsible for abnormally high oxygen consumption by the respiratory muscles (34). Disorders in growth hormone secretion due to the disruption in sleep organization have also been implicated (35).

A striking difference from adults is that obesity is not particularly common in children with OSAS (4). However, obese children are at increased risk for OSAS (12), although the magnitude of the increase is not agreed on (36–38). Obese children should be routinely evaluated for clinical symptoms of OSAS, and if any are found investigations during sleep should be performed.

CARDIOVASCULAR COMPLICATIONS

The syndrome combining acute cor pulmonale, pulmonary edema, pulmonary hypertension, and hypoventilation was described in children as early as the 1960s (39). A long diagnostic delay seems to increase the risk of acute cardiorespiratory failure. A trivial upper airway infection is often the precipitating factor. Treatment of the cause of the upper airway obstruction is followed by complete reversal of the hemodynamic disorders (24). The outcome can be fatal in the absence of a prompt diagnosis followed by appropriate treatment (40).

The frequency of heart abnormalities other than acute heart failure has not been accurately determined in pediatric OSAS. Early studies found right ventricular hypertrophy in 3.3% (41) to 55% (42) of cases. Echocardiography is rarely performed on a routine basis, and as a result has not been evaluated in large populations of children with OSAS. Shiomi et al. (43) reported the interesting finding that markedly negative esophageal pressures during sleep are responsible for abnormal motion of the interventricular septum, which is reversible by nasal continuous positive airway pressure (CPAP) (43). Tal et al. (44) reported beneficial effects of tonsillectomy on right ventricular function.

Systemic arterial hypertension is common in adults with OSAS. In an early study of 50 children with severe OSAS, daytime arterial hypertension was found in 10% of patients, who were all older than 10 years of age (8). A recent study of 41 children with a mean age of 5 ± 3 years and moderately severe OSAS (AHI, 10 ± 10) found that diastolic blood pressure was significantly increased during the day and during sleep in comparison to a group of children with snoring but an AHI within the range deemed normal (14).

Heart rhythm disturbances (sinus arrest, second degree atrioventricular block) were reported in a large proportion of cases in early studies (8). Two recent studies (45, 46) produced conflicting results. D'Andrea et al. (45) failed to demonstrate any significant heart rhythm changes in 12 children with partial or complete airway obstruction during sleep. In contrast, using the Poincaré plot analysis to investigate seven children with a mean apnea index of 19.5 ± 5.1, Aljadeff et al. (46) found increased heart rate variability and suggested that investigation of heart rate variability may be a useful screening method for OSAS.

0—■ Key points box 19.2

Cardiovascular complications

1. Acute cardiovascular failure is a rare but potentially fatal complication of childhood OSAS.

2. Right ventricular hypertrophy is common but usually reversible with effective therapy.

3. Systemic hypertension occurs in up to 10% of cases.

DIAGNOSTIC TOOLS

The diagnostic process starts by a careful analysis of the clinical symptoms and an examination of the child to look for mouth-breathing, failure to thrive, obesity, suggestive facial features (long face with retroposition of the mandible and a small chin) (6), and tonsillar hypertrophy (6).

Several groups have sought to determine the sensitivity and specificity of clinical data for identifying OSAS, the goal being to decrease the need for confirmatory polysomnography (6, 25–29, 47). In all the studies but one, the investigators (47) concluded that clinical data had high sensitivity but low specificity. However, polysomnography criteria varied across studies (AHI > 1 [28], > 5 [27, 29], or > 15 [26]), adenotonsillar hypertrophy was a predominant feature in some of the study populations but not in others, and only one study (6) made a distinction between OSAS and UARS. However,

Guilleminault et al. (6) also concluded that clinical symptoms were not sufficiently specific to differentiate OSAS from UARS.

Polysomnography remains the gold standard investigation for the diagnosis of OSAS (48) and even more so for that of UARS (6). The cost of polysomnography is considered high. However, two North American studies have suggested that the cost of polysomnography in children may be offset by the cost of unnecessary tonsillectomies (27, 29).

Polysomnography should ideally be performed overnight. However, polysomnographic evaluation of a daytime nap can be informative, particularly in infants and younger children. A single study has compared overnight versus nap polysomnography in 40 subjects aged 1 month to 16 years (49). Chloral hydrate sedation was used in two thirds of cases. Nap polysomnography was found to have 74% sensitivity and 100% specificity for the diagnosis of OSAS. Thus, an uninformative nap polysomnography study, which is often due to absence of REM sleep, does not rule out OSAS and should be followed by overnight polysomnography. Use of chloral hydrate is inadvisable because it can cause a dramatic exacerbation in the airway obstruction (50, 51). Neither is prior sleep deprivation recommended since it can exaggerate obstructive events (52).

Few normative data on the obstructive apnea index in healthy children have been published. In infants older than 6 weeks, the index of obstructive apneas > 3 s has been reported to be less than 1 (53, 54). Of the three available studies in children older than 1 year and in adolescents (20, 55, 56), two (55, 56) found no obstructive apneas. The third is a more recent study of 50 subjects in whom the mean number of obstructive apneas > 5 s was 0.1 ± 0.5 (range, 0 to 3.1) (20). No normative data have been published on obstructive hypopneas in healthy infants and children. Criteria for OSAS remain poorly defined: whereas some groups (20, 22, 28) consider that an index greater than 1 is significant, others (27, 29) require an index greater than 5 and take into account both obstructive apneas and obstructive hypopneas.

The typical OSAS polysomnography study shows an abnormally high obstructive AHI with predominant occurrence of the obstructive apneas during REM sleep. Outside the periods of apnea, there is a large amount of labored breathing. During periods with ventilation, the chest, which is readily deformable in children (57), moves inward during inspiration. This asynchronous thoracoabdominal motion is particularly marked and prolonged during rapid eye movement (REM) sleep but can occur during non-rapid eye movement (NREM) sleep. Recruitment of accessory respiratory muscles (i.e., the abdominal and intercostal muscles) occurs in some cases (58) but is inhibited during phasic REM sleep (58).

Obstructive hypopnea or periods of obstructive hypoventilation can occur in isolation or in association with obstructive apneas (3). Obstructive hypopnea is defined as an least 50% decrease in the airflow signal accompanied with a decrease in arterial oxygen saturation (SaO_2) (> 3 % [6] or 4 % [48]) with or without arousal (48). Obstructive hypoventilation has been described by Rosen et al. (3) as a decrease in the airflow signal accompanied by a decrease in SaO_2 combined with an increase in the end tidal pressure of CO_2 ($PETCO_2$) and with asynchronous thoracoabdominal motion. $PETCO_2$ or the transcutaneous pressure of CO_2 ($PtcCO_2$), or both, should be measured routinely in children with suspected OSAS (59). Normative data for $PETCO_2$ variations in healthy children have been published (20). In our experience, use of surface electrodes to record diaphragmatic activity helps to determine whether hypopneas or hypoventilation is due to obstruction (58, 60) and can obviate measuring esophageal pressure variations.

Esophageal pressure measurement is still rarely included in polysomnographic studies of infants and children. In addition, very few studies have compared esophageal pressure variations during sleep and wakefulness in healthy children. In two studies of healthy children aged 2 to 14 years (2, 61), the most negative esophageal pressures were in the −8 to −20 cm H_2O range. Lastly, pressure variations seem more reliable than absolute pressure values. Guilleminault et al. (6) compared the reliability of $PETCO_2$ and $PtcCO_2$ to that of esophageal pressure variations for the diagnosis of episodes of increased upper airway resistance. $PtcCO_2$ and $PETCO_2$ identified only 33% and 53% of episodes, respectively (6). Assessment of inspiratory flow limitation using a nasal cannula–pressure transducer system has been reported to be useful in detecting episodes of upper airway resistance during sleep (62). Preliminary data suggest that this method may be useful in children for detecting obstructive apneas and hypopneas. Furthermore, these preliminary data showed that in four children the peak inspiratory esophageal pressure

was more negative during breaths with flow limitations than during normal breaths (63).

Analysis of the arousal response on the polysomnography study is important since it allows us to evaluate the severity of sleep fragmentation. However, arousal response criteria in children are not agreed on. Some groups (6, 64, 65) use only electroencephalographic (EEG) criteria, whereas others (58, 66) also use cardiorespiratory signals. According to the criteria used, the frequency of an arousal response at termination of obstructive apneas or hypopneas varied across studies. In our experience (58) and in that of McNamara et al. (64), an EEG arousal response is uncommon in children with OSAS. In contrast, we share with Mograss et al. (58, 66) the experience that a 'movement-arousal' terminates most obstructive apneas (58, 66).

Sleep organization disturbances were found in an early study (8), whereas in more recent studies (27, 67) sleep organization was found to be normal. These discrepancies are probably ascribable to differences in the severity or duration or both of OSAS. In a small group of infants with OSAS, McNamara et al. (68) found that REM sleep time was decreased, but it returned to normal under nasal CPAP.

Polysomnography is a costly, time-consuming investigation that in France is still rarely performed in children. Evaluation of the diagnostic usefulness of screening methods is important. Nocturnal SaO_2 recording is an inexpensive method, whose results should be analyzed only after artifact elimination (69). Normal values in children have been published (20). Nocturnal SaO_2 recording can assist in the diagnosis since obstructive events can cause a decrease in SaO_2. However, a normal SaO_2 recording does not rule out OSAS (70). SaO_2 recording has been reported to have a better predictive value for OSAS in children who also have a restrictive ventilatory defect than in those who do not (71, 72). SaO_2 determination is of assistance for evaluating the severity of OSAS. Other screening methods include tracheal sound recording (73) and oximetry combined with home video recording (74). None of these methods have been compared to polysomnography at the laboratory in a large group of children with OSAS of varying severity. Jacob et al. (75) evaluated home video and cardiorespiratory recording versus polysomnography at the laboratory in 22 children with OSAS due to adenoid or tonsillar hypertrophy and found no significant differences for the AHI, the number of SaO$_2$ drops, or the number of arousal responses. Although attention is now turning increasingly to home studies, no consensus has been developed as yet regarding the number of signals that are necessary and sufficient for the diagnosis (48). Esophageal pressure recording can be performed only at the laboratory as a second-line investigation if the first-line tests are uninformative (6).

⊶ Key points box 19.3

Diagnosis

1. Clinical features have low specificity for the diagnosis of OSAS in children.
2. The diagnosis of OSAS is often delayed for several years.
3. Polysomnography remains the gold standard, but the AHI threshold for diagnosis is lower than in adults.
4. Limited diagnostic studies in the home will likely become increasingly important in the future, but there have been few comparative studies to date.

PATHOPHYSIOLOGY OF OSAS

The pathophysiology of OSAS in children remains incompletely understood. Many risk factors have been identified and adenotonsillar hypertrophy is the leading cause of OSAS. Other risk factors include malformations of the middle of the face with micrognathia or retrognathia or both (72, 76–79), brain stem abnormalities (71, 80), neuromuscular diseases (81), obesity (36–38), Willi-Prader syndrome (82), sickle cell anemia (83–85), and Marfan syndrome (86). In infants, laryngomalacia can cause severe OSAS (87).

The mechanisms by which adenotonsillar hypertrophy can cause upper airway obstruction during sleep remain unclear. Although the rate of lymphoid tissue growth is normally high between 2 and 6 years of age (11), only 0.7–3% of children develop OSAS (12, 17, 18). The degree of adenotonsillar hypertrophy is not predictive of OSAS (29). However, a high score for adenotonsillar size is common in OSAS patients (25, 29). In a study by Brooks et al. (88), adenotonsillar hypertrophy was cor-

related with the duration but not the number of obstructive apneas.

To explain why some but not all children with adenotonsillar hypertrophy develop OSAS, precipitating factors such as ventilatory control or anatomic abnormalities have been sought. Ventilatory responses to chemical stimuli have been reported to be within the range considered normal both during wakefulness (89) and during sleep (65). However, there is some evidence that subtle abnormalities may occur, particularly toward the end of a night marked by repeated obstructive events responsible for hypercapnia (90). In a study of children with OSAS due to adenotonsillar hypertrophy, Marcus et al. (91) found that the critical upper airway closure pressure was abnormally close to the atmospheric pressure. Neuromuscular control abnormalities associated with an increased propensity for upper airway collapse may promote the development of OSAS. Oropharyngeal size abnormalities have been reported in children with OSAS and adenotonsillar hypertrophy (92, 93). These abnormalities, which are related to the position of the hyoid bone and to the angles estimating the position of the mandible and maxillary bones (93), may increase the risk of OSAS and may be genetically determined (94). However, experiments in monkeys suggest that facial skeleton abnormalities can also occur as a consequence of adenotonsillar hypertrophy (95). In children with OSAS, skeleton abnormalities have been shown to be partly reversible in the medium term after adenotonsillectomy (96, 97).

Adenotonsillar hypertrophy can coexist with other conditions that increase the risk of OSAS because they are characterized by craniofacial malformations (Pierre Robin syndrome, achondroplasia, Crouzon syndrome [72, 76–79]) or neurological abnormalities (myelomeningocele [71, 80]). Sickle cell disease may be a significant risk factor. In a cohort of 55 sickle cell disease patients, Samuels et al. (85) found a high prevalence of obstructive apneas.

TREATMENT

The treatment of adenotonsillar hypertrophy without other abnormalities is discussed first. Polysomnography is recommended before adenotonsillectomy to confirm the existence of OSAS and to evaluate its severity. In practice, adenotonsillectomy is performed based on suggestive clinical symptoms only. The cost of unnecessary adenotonsillectomies should be compared to the cost of routine polysomnography in patients considered for adenotonsillectomy (27, 29). In addition, adenotonsillectomy carries a risk of postoperative complications (bleeding, upper airway obstruction) (98, 99). Two studies (98, 99) have shown that risk factors for postoperative upper airway obstruction include age younger than 3 years and an AHI greater than 10 (98) or 15 (99). Patients with these risk factors should be kept under observation at the hospital for 24 hours after the adenotonsillectomy (98, 99). Nasal CPAP is sometimes indicated before and after the procedure in patients with severe OSAS (13, 100, 101).

Adenotonsillectomy is usually followed by resolution of all clinical symptoms, resumption of growth, and a return to normal of behavior and learning abilities (32, 33). Few studies have evaluated the effect of adenotonsillectomy on respiratory events during sleep (27, 29, 102, 104). Reversal of polysomnography abnormalities is the rule, although some children continue to have clinical symptoms and an abnormal AHI (27, 29, 102). The need for nasal CPAP therapy should be evaluated (13, 101). In two large retrospective studies of the indications of nasal CPAP in children (13, 101), 5% (13) and 17% (101) of patients received nasal CPAP for persistent symptoms after adenotonsillectomy. Nocturnal oxygen therapy has been suggested for patients awaiting adenotonsillectomy for severe OSAS and for those who are unable to tolerate nasal CPAP (105, 106). An editorial by Brouillette and Waters (107) has drawn attention to the risk of alveolar hypoventilation in children given nocturnal oxygen therapy for OSAS. Guilleminault et al. (108) have reported that OSAS can recur several years after adenotonsillectomy, particularly in boys after puberty.

The treatment of the other causes of OSAS raises challenges specific to each cause. In children with OSAS due to craniofacial malformations, neuromuscular disease, or metabolic diseases (Hurler syndrome), fluoroscopic or endoscopic investigations may be useful for identifying the site of obstruction (109–111). Adenotonsillectomy is often the first step of the treatment of these conditions. Inpatient monitoring is mandatory after the procedure since there is a risk of obstructive complications (98,99).

The introduction of nasal CPAP has modified the indications for tracheostomy in infants and children with OSAS due to craniofacial malformations (13, 101, 112). Nasal CPAP is feasible in infants (112). The facemask should be changed as needed as growth proceeds, and the pressure level that is necessary and well tolerated should be determined at regular intervals (13, 101, 112). Full cooperation of the parents is indispensable. Follow-up polysomnography studies should be performed. Compliance is excellent, except occasionally in mentally impaired children (113). Before the feasibility and efficacy of nasal CPAP in infants were demonstrated, treatment by insertion of a nasopharyngeal tube was used successfully in some conditions, such as Pierre Robin syndrome (114).

Nasal CPAP allows one to wait until surgical correction of the craniofacial malformation is performed, usually in adolescence, although some patients have been operated on successfully during childhood (115). Uvulopalatopharyngoplasty (UPPP) has been advocated in children with neurological diseases or Down syndrome and an inability to tolerate nasal CPAP (116).

⊶ Key points box 19.4

Treatment

1. Remove tonsils and adenoids if enlarged, and consider correction of anatomical deformity, if present. Patients need close monitoring in the postoperative period and may require short-term CPAP.

2. Nasal CPAP is usually well tolerated when indicated, even in infants, but involvement of the parents is essential.

3. Nasal CPAP therapy may allow postponement of surgery for anatomical deformities.

FAMILIAL PREDISPOSITION FOR OSAS AND SUDDEN INFANT DEATH SYNDROME

Several recent studies have provided evidence of familial clustering of OSAS (12, 94, 117, 118), possibly due to genetically dependent abnormalities in ventilatory control (117) or skeletal morphology (94, 118). In practice, adults with OSAS should be questioned regarding the presence of clinical symptoms of OSAS in their children, since this can allow an early diagnosis. The frequency of OSAS was found to be equal to 8.4% in a cohort of children recruited as members of families with a member with known OSAS (12).

Tishler et al. (119) have reported clustering in the same families of OSAS and sudden infant death syndrome (SIDS) (119). Some cases of SIDS or apparently life-threatening events in infants may be due to upper airway obstruction (120–122). Guilleminault et al. (120, 121) have described cases of near-miss SIDS infants followed a few years later by OSAS. Nasal CPAP has been used successfully in infants with OSAS or UARS and a history of apparently life-threatening events (68, 112).

CONCLUSIONS

Over two decades after OSAS was first described in children, many questions remain unanswered. Isolated snoring, UARS, and OSAS probably represent a continuum. Polysomnography is the gold standard diagnostic tool. However, in the near future, technological advances will allow the development of highly informative testing methods for use at home. There is a need for consensus on the indications for esophageal pressure measurement and the range of normal variations in this parameter during sleep. Prompt diagnosis is essential to prevent the severe complications of OSAS (acute cardiorespiratory failure, failure to thrive, and impairment of cognitive function). Although adenotonsillar hypertrophy is the leading cause of OSAS, pathophysiological mechanisms remain incompletely understood. Many more uncommon conditions (e.g., craniofacial malformations, neurological diseases) can cause OSAS. Nasal CPAP is feasible in infants and children. To improve our ability to prevent OSAS, further studies of genetic factors and routine examination of children in high-risk families are needed.

REFERENCES

1. Guilleminault C, Eldridge F, Simmons F, et al. Sleep apnea in eight children. Pediatrics 1976; 58:23–31.

2. Guilleminault C, Winkle R, Korobkin R, et al. Children and nocturnal snoring: evaluation of effects of sleep related respiratory resistive load and day time functionning. Eur J Pediatr 1982; 139:165–171.

3. Rosen CL, D'Andrea L, Haddad GG. Adult criteria for obstructive sleep apnea do not identify children with serious obstruction. Am Rev Respir Dis 1992; 146:1231–1234.

4. Carroll JL, Loughlin GM. Diagnosis criteria for obstructive sleep apnea syndrome in children. Pediatr Pulmonol 1992; 14:71–74.

5. Guilleminault C, Stoohs R, Clerk A, et al. A cause of excessive daytime sleepiness: the upper airway resistance syndrome. Chest 1993; 104:781–787.

6. Guilleminault C, Pelayo R, Leger D, et al. Recognition of sleep-disordered breathing in children. Pediatrics 1996; 98:871–882.

7. Downey R, Perkin RM, Macquarrie J. Upper airway resistance syndrome: sick, symptomatic but underrecognized. Sleep 1993; 16:620–623.

8. Guilleminault C, Korobin R, Winkle R. A review of 50 children with obstructive sleep apnea syndrome. Lung 1981; 159:275–287.

9. Brouillette R, Fernbach SK, Hunt CE. Obstructive sleep apnea in infants and children. J Pediatr 1982; 100:31–40.

10. Frank Y, Kravath RE, Pollak CP, et al. Obstructive sleep apnea and its therapy: clinical and polysomnographic manifestations. Pediatrics 1983; 71:742–787.

11. Jeans WD, Fernando DC, Maw AR, et al. A longitudinal study of the growth of the nasopharynx and its contents in normal children. Br J Radiol 1981; 54:117–121.

12. Redline S, Tishler PV, Schluchter M, et al. Risk factors for sleep-disordered breathing in children. Am J Respir Crit Care Med 1999; 159:1527–1532.

13. Waters KA, Everett FM, Bruderer JW, et al. Obstructive sleep apnea: the use of nasal CPAP in 80 children. Am J Respir Crit Care Med 1995; 152:780–785.

14. Marcus CL, Greene MG, Carroll JL. Blood pressure in children with obstructive sleep apnea. Am J Respir Sit Care Med 1998; 157:1098–1103.

15. Corbo GM, Fuciarelli F, Foresi A, et al. Snoring in children: association with respiratory symptoms and passive smoking. Br Med J 1989; 299:1491–1494.

16. Teculescu DB, Caillier I, Perrin P, et al. Snoring in French preschool children. Pediatr Pulmonol 1992; 13:239–244.

17. Ali NJ, Pitson DJ, Stradling JR. Snoring, sleep disturbance, and behaviour in 4–5-year-olds. Arch Dis Child 1993; 68:360–366.

18. Gislason T, Benediktsdottir B. Snoring, apneic episodes, and nocturnal hypoxemia among children 6 months to 6 years old. Chest 1995; 107:963–966.

19. Hultcrantz E, Löfstrand-Tideström B, Ahlquist-Rastad J. The epidemiology of sleep related breathing disorder in children. Int J Pediatr Otolaryngol 1995; 32:563–566.

20. Marcus CL, Omlin K, Basinki DJ, et al. Normal polysomnographic values for children and adolescents. Am Rev Respir Dis 1992; 146:1235–1239.

21. Ali NJ, Pitson D, Stradling JR. Natural history of snoring and related behaviour problems between the ages of 4 and 7 years. Arch Dis Child 1994; 71:74–76.

22. Marcus CL, Hamer A, Loughlin GM. Natural history of primary snoring in children. Pediatr Pulmonol 1998; 26:6–11.

23. Guilleminault C, Pelayo R. And if the polysomnogram was faulty? Pediatr Pulmonol 1998; 26:1–3.

24. Sofer S, Weinhouse E, Tal A, et al. Cor pulmonale due to adenoidal or tonsillar hypertrophy or both in children: non invasive diagnosis and follow-up. Chest 1988; 93:119–122.

25. Leach J, Olson J, Hermann J, et al. Polysomnographic and clinical findings in children with obstructive sleep apnea. Arch Otolaryngol Head Neck Surg 1992; 118:741–744.

26. Goldstein NA, Sculerati N, Walsleben JA, et al. Clinical diagnosis of pediatric obstructive sleep apnea validated by polysomnography. Otolaryngol Head Neck Surg 1994; 111:611–617.

27. Suen JS, Arnold JE, Brooks LJ. Adenotonsillectomy for treatment of obstructive sleep apnea in children. Arch Otolaryngol Head Neck Surg 1995; 121:525–530.

28. Carroll JL, Mc Colley SA, Marcus CL, et al. Inability of clinical history to distinguish primary snoring from obstructive sleep apnea syndrome in children. Chest 1995; 108: 610–618.

29. Wang RC, Elkins TP, Keech D, et al. Accuracy of clinical evaluation in pediatric obstructive sleep apnea. Otolaryngol Head Neck Surg 1998; 118:69–73.

30. Weider DJ, Sateia MJ, West RP. Nocturnal enuresis in children with upper airway obstruction. Otolaryngol Head Neck Surg 1991; 105:427–432.

31. Rhodes SK, Shimoda KC, Wais LR, et al. Neurocognitive deficits in morbidly obese children with obstructive sleep apnea. J Pediatr 1995; 127:741–744.

32. Hansen DE, Vandenberg B. Neuropsychological features and differential diagnosis of sleep apnea syndrome in children. J Clin Child Psychol 1997; 26:304–310.

33. Gozal D. Sleep-disordered breathing and school performance in children. Pediatrics 1998; 102:616–620.

34. Marcus CL, Koerner CB, Pysik Ph, et al. Determinants of growth failure in children with the obstructive sleep apnea syndrome. J Pediatr 1994; 125:556–562.

35. Goldstein SJ, Wu RHK, Thorpy MJ, et al. Reversibility of deficient sleep entrained growth hormone secretion in a boy with achondroplasia and obstructive sleep apnea. Acta Endocrinol 1987; 116:95–101.

36. Mallory GB, Fiser DH, Jackson R. Sleep-associated breathing disorders in morbidly obese children and adolescents. J Pediatr 1989; 115:892–897.

37. Silvestri JM, Weese-Mayer DE, Bass MT, et al. Polysomnography in obese children with a history of sleep-associated breathing disorders. Pediatr Pulmonol 1993; 16:124–129.

38. Marcus CL, Curtis S, Koerner CB, et al. Evaluation of pulmonary function and polysomnography in obese children and adolescents. Pediatr Pulmonol 1996; 21:176–183.

39. Levy AM, Tabakin BS, Hanson JS, et al. Hypertrophied adenoids causing pulmonary hypertension and severe congestive heart failure. N Engl J Med 1967; 397:506–511.

40. Messer J. Mort subite par apnées obstructives chez l'enfant. Arch Fr Pediatr 1984; 41:333–336.

41. Wilkinson AR, McCormick MS, Freeland AP, et al. Electrocardiographic signs of pulmonary hypertension in children who snore. Br Med J 1981; 282:1579–1581.

42. Hunt CE, Brouillette RT. Abnormalities of breathing control and airway maintenance in infants and children as a cause of cor pulmonale. Pediatr Cardiol 1982; 3:429–456.

43. Shiomi T, Guilleminault C, Stoohs R, et al. Obstructed breathing in children during sleep monitored by echocardiography. Acta Paediatr 1993; 82:863–871.

44. Tal A, Leiberman A, Margulis G, et al. Ventricular dysfunction in children with obstructive sleep apnea: radionuclide assessment. Pediatr Pulmonol 1988; 4:139–143.

45. D'Andrea LA, Rosen CL, Haddad GG. Severe hypoxemia in children with upper airway obstruction during sleep does not lead to significant changes in heart rate. Pediatr Pulmonol 1993; 16:362–369.

46. Aljadeff G, Gozal D, Schechtman VL, et al. Heart rate variability in children with obstructive sleep apnea. Sleep 1997; 20:151–157.

47. Brouillette R, Hanson D, David R, et al. A diagnostic approach to children with suspected obstructive sleep apnea. J Pediatr 1984; 105:10–14.

48. American Thoracic Society: Standards and indications for cardiopulmonary sleep studies in children. Am J Respir Crit Care Med 1996; 153:866–878.

49. Marcus CL, Keens TG, Ward SL. Comparison of nap and overnight polysomnography in children. Pediatr Pulmonol 1992; 13:16–21.

50. Hershenson M, Brouillette RT, Olsen E, et al. The effect of chloral hydrate on genioglossus and diaphragmatic activity. Pediatr Res 1984; 18:516–519.

51. Biban P, Baraldi E, Pettenazzo A. The adverse effect of chloral hydrate in children with OSA. Pediatrics 1993; 92: 461–463.

52. Canet E, Gaultier C, D'Allest AM, et al. Effects of sleep deprivation on respiratory events during sleep in healthy infants. J Appl Physiol 1989; 66:1158–1163.

53. Guilleminault C, Ariagno R, Korobkin R, et al. Mixed and obstructive sleep apnea and near miss for sudden infant death syndrome; 2. Comparison of near miss and normal control infants by age. Pediatrics 1979; 64:882.

54. Hoppenbrouwers T, Hodgman JE, Cabal L. Obstructive apnea, associated patterns of movement heart rate, and oxygenation in infants at low and increased risk for SIDS. Pediatr Pulmonol 1993; 15:1–12.

55. Carskadon MA, Harvey K, Dement WC, et al. Respiration during sleep in children. West J Med 1979; 128:477–481.

56. Tabachnick E, Muller NL, Bryan AC, et al. Changes in ventilation and chest wall mechanics during sleep in normal adolescents. J Appl Physiol 1981; 51:557–564.

57. Gaultier C. Cardiorespiratory adaptation during sleep in infants and children. Pediatr Pulmonol 1995; 19:105–117.

58. Praud JP, D'Allest AM, Nedelcoux H, et al. Sleep-related abdominal muscle behavior during partial or complete obstructed breathing in prepubertal children. Pediatr Res 1989; 26:347–350.

59. Morielli A, Desjardins D, Brouillette RT. Transcutaneous and end-tidal carbon dioxide pressures should be measured during pediatric polysomnography. Am Rev Respir Dis 1993; 148:1599–1604.

60. Praud JP, D'Allest AM, Delaperche MF, et al. Diaphragmatic and genioglossus electromyographic activity at the onset and at the end of obstructive apnea in children with obstructive sleep apnea syndrome. Pediatr Res 1988; 23:1–4.

61. Miyazaki S, Itasaka Y, Yamakawa K, et al. Respiratory disturbance during sleep due to adenoid-tonsillar hypertrophy. Am J Otolaryngol 1989; 10:143–149.

62. Hosselet JJ, Norman RG, Ayappa I, et al. Detection of flow limitation with a nasal cannula/pressure transducer system. Am J Respir Crit Care Med 1998; 157:1461–1467.

63. Serebrisky D, Cordero R, Kattan M, et al. Assessment of inspiratory flow limitation in children by nasal cannula/pressure transducer system. Am J Respir Crit Care Med 1999; 159:A485.

64. Mc Namara F, Issa FG, Sullivan CE. Arousal pattern following central and obstructive breathing abnormalities in infants and children. J Appl Physiol 1996; 81:2651–2657.

65. Marcus CL, Lutz J, Carroll JL, et al. Arousal and ventilatory responses during sleep in children with obstructive sleep apnea. J Appl Physiol 1998; 84:1926–1936.

66. Mograss MA, Ducharme FM, Brouillette RT. Movement/arousals. Description, classification and relationship to sleep apnea in children. Am J Respir Crit Care Med 1994; 150:1690–1696.

67. Mc Grath SA, Carroll JL, Mc Colley SA, et al. Normal sleep structure found in children with obstructive sleep apnea. Am Rev Respir Dis 1992; 145:A176.

68. Mc Namara F, Harris MA, Sullivan CE. Effects of nasal continuous positive airway pressure on apnoea index and sleep in infants. J Paediatric Child Health 1995; 31:88–94.

69. Lafontaine VM, Ducharme FM, Brouillette RT. Pulse oximetry: accuracy of methods of interpreting graphic summaries. Pediatr Pulmonol 1996; 21:121–131.

70. Owen GO, Canter RJ. Overnight pulse oximetry in normal children and in children undergoing adenotonsillectomy. Clin Otolaryngol 1996; 21:59–65.

71. Waters KA, Forbes P, Morielli A, et al. Sleep-disordered breathing in children with myelomeningocele. J Pediatr 1998; 132:672–681.

72. Mogayzel PJ, Carroll JL, Loughlin GM, et al. Sleep-disordered breathing in children with achondroplasia. J Pediatr 1998; 131:667–671.

73. Potsic WP. Comparison of polysomnography and sonography for assessing regularity of respiration during sleep in adenotonsillar hypertrophy. Laryngoscope 1987; 97:1430–1437.

74. Stradling JR, Thomas G, Warley AR, et al. Effect of adenotonsillectomy on nocturnal hypoxemia, sleep disturbances, and symptoms in snoring children. Lancet 1990; 335: 249–253.

75. Jacob SV, Morielli A, Mograss MA, et al. Home testing for pediatric obstructive sleep apnea syndrome secondary to adenotonsillar hypertrophy. Pediatr Pulmonol. 1995; 20:241–252.

76. Betancourt D, Beckerman RC. Craniofacial syndromes. In: Beckerman RC, Brouillette RT, Hunt CE, eds. Respiratory control disorders in infants and children Baltimore; Williams & Wilkins: 1992; 294–305.

77. Waters KA, Everett F, Sillence D, et al. Breathing abnormalities in sleep achondroplasia. Arch Dis Child 1993; 69:191–196.

78. Zucconi M, Weber G, Castronovo V, et al. Sleep and upper airway obstruction in children with achondroplasia. J Pediatr 1996; 129:743–749.

79. Marcus CL, Keens TG, Bautista DB, et al. Obstructive sleep apnea in children with Down syndrome. Pediatrics 1991; 88:132–139.

80. Dure LS, Percy AK, Cheek WR, et al. Chiari type I malformation in children. J Pediatr 1989; 115:273–576.

81. Trang TTH, Desguerre I, Goldman M, et al. Sleep-related breathing pattern in young children with neuromuscular disorders. Am Rev Respir Dis 1993; 147:A760.

82. Hertz G, Cataletto M, Feinsilver SH, et al. Sleep and breathing patterns in patients with Prader Willi Syndrome: effects of age and gender. Sleep 1993; 16:366–371.

83. Maddern BR, Ohene-Frempong K, Reed HT, et al. Obstructive sleep apnea syndrome in sickle cell disease. Ann Otol Laryngol 1989; 98:174–178.

84. Davies SC, Stebbens VA, Samuels MP, et al. Upper airways obstruction and cerebrovascular accident in children with sickle cell anaemia. Lancet 1989; 2:283–284.

85. Samuels MP, Stebbens VA, Davies SC, et al. Sleep related upper airway obstruction and hypoxaemia in sickle cell disease. Arch Dis Childh 1992; 67:925–929.

86. Cistulli PA, Sullivan CE. Sleep-disordered breathing in Marfan's syndrome. Am Rev Respir Dis 1993; 147:645–648.

87. Marcus CL, Crockett DM, Davidson-Ward SL. Evaluation of epiglottoplasty as treatment for severe laryngomalacia. J Pediatr 1990; 117:706–710.

88. Brooks LJ, Stephens BM, Bacevice AM. Adenoid size is related to severity but not the number of episodes of obstructive apnea in children. J Pediatr. 1998; 132:682–686.

89. Marcus CL, Gozal D, Arens R, et al. Ventilatory responses during wakefulness in children with obstructive sleep apnea. Am J Respir Crit Care Med 1994; 149:715–721.

90. Gozal D, Arens R, Omlin KJ, et al. Ventilatory responses to consecutive short hypercapnic challenges in children with obstructive sleep apnea. J Appl Physiol 1995; 79: 1608–1614.

91. Marcus CL, Mc Colley SA, Carroll JL, et al. Upper airway collapsibility in children with the obstructive sleep apnea syndrome. J Appl Physiol 1994; 77:918–924.

92. Behlfelt K, Linder-Aronson S, Mc William J, et al. Craniofacial morphology in children with and without enlarged tousils. Eur J Orthodon 1990; 12:233–243.

93. Shintani T, Asakura K, Katauba A. Adenotonsillar hypertrophy and skeletal morphology of children with obstructive sleep apnea syndrome. Acta Otolaryngol 1996; Suppl 523:222–224.

94. Guilleminault C, Partinen M, Hollman K, et al. Familial aggregates in obstructive sleep apnea syndrome. Chest 1995; 107:1545–1551.

95. Vargervik K, Harvold EP. Experiments on the interaction between orofacial function and morphology. Ear Nose Throat J 1987; 66:201–208.

96. Behlfelt K, Linder-Aronson S, Mc William J, et al. Dentition in children with enlarged tonsils compared to control children. Eur J Orthodont 1989; 11:416–429.

97. Hultcrantz E, Larson M, Hellquist R, et al. The influence of tonsillar obstruction and tonsillectomy on facial growth and dental arch morphology. Int J Pediatr Otolaryngol 1991; 22:125–134.

98. McColley SA, April MM, Carroll JL, et al. Respiratory compromise after adenotonsillectomy in children with obstructive sleep apnea. Arch Otolaryngol Head Neck Surg 1992; 118:940–943.

99. Rosen GM, Muckle RP, Mahowald MW, et al. Postoperative respiratory compromise in children with obstructive sleep apnea syndrome: can it be anticipated? Pediatrics 1994; 93:784–788.

100. D'Andrea LA, Traquina DN, Rosen CL. Continuous positive airway pressure (CPAP) for temporary sleep relief of obstructive sleep apnea syndrome (OSAS) in children with adenotonsillar hypertrophy awaiting surgery. Am J Respir Crit Care Med 1994; 149:A886.

101. Marcus CL, Davidson Ward SL, Mallory GB, et al. Use of nasal continuous positive airway pressure as treatment of childhood obstructive sleep apnea. J Pediatr 1995; 127:88–94.

102. Helfaer MA, Mc Colley SA, Pyzik PL, et al. Polysomnography after adenotonsillectomy in mild pediatric obstructive sleep apnea. Crit Care Med 1996; 24:1323–1327.

103. Potsic WP, Pasquariello PS, Corsobaranak C. Relief of upper airway obstruction by adenotonsillectomy. Otolaryngol Head Neck Surg 1986; 94:476–480.

104. Ahlqvist-Rastad J, Hultcrantz E, Svanholm H. Children with tonsillar obstruction: indications for and efficacy of tonsillectomy. Acta Paediatr Scand 1988; 77:831–835.

105. Marcus CL, Carroll JL, Bamford O, et al. Supplemental oxygen during sleep in children with sleep-disordered breathing. Am J Respir Crit Care Med 1995; 152: 1297–1301.

106. Aljadeff G, Gozal D, Bailey-Wahls, et al. Effects of overnight supplemental oxygen in obstructive sleep apnea in children. Am J Respir Crit Care Med 1996; 153:51–55.

107. Brouillette RT, Waters K. Oxygen therapy for pediatric obstructive sleep apnea syndrome: how safe? how effective? Am J Respir Crit Care Med 1996; 153:1–2.

108. Guilleminault C, Partinen M, Praud JP, et al. Morphometric facial changes and obstructive sleep apnea in adolescents. J Pediatr 1989; 114:997–999.

109. Sher AE, Shprinzten RJ, Thorpy MJ. Endoscopic observations of obstructive sleep apnea in children with anomalous upper airways: predictive and therapeutic value. Int J Pediatr Otorhinolaryngol 1989; 17: 1–11.

110. Sher AE. Mechanisms of airway obstruction in Robin sequence: implications for treatment. Cleft Palate Craniofac J 1992; 29:224–231.

111. Gibson SE, Strife JL, Myer CM, et al. Sleep fluoroscopy for localization of upper airway obstruction in children. Ann Otol Rhinol Laryngol 1996; 105:678–683.

112. Guilleminault C, Pelayo R, Clerck A, et al. Home nasal continuous positive airway pressure in infants with sleep-disordered breathing. J Pediatr 1995; 127: 905–912.

113. Guilleminault C, Nino-Murcia G, Heldt G, et al. Alternative treatment to tracheostomy in obstructive sleep apnea syndrome: nasal continuous positive airway pressure in young children. Pediatrics 1986; 78: 797–802.

114. Heaf DP, Helms PJ, Dinwiddie R, et al. Nasopharyngeal airways in Pierre Robin syndrome. J Pediatr 1982; 100:698–703.

115. James D, M L. Mandibular reconstruction in children with obstructive sleep apnea due to micrognathia. Plast Reconstr Surg 1997; 100: 1131–1137.

116. Kosko JR, Derkay CS. Uvulopalatopharyngoplasty: treatment of obstructive sleep apnea in neurologically impaired pediatric patients. Int J Pediatr Otorhinolaryngol 1995; 32: 241–246.

117. Bayadi SE, Millman RP, Tishler PV, et al. A family study of sleep apnea: anatomic and physiologic interactions. Chest 1990; 98:554–559.

118. Redline S, Tosteson T, Tishler PV. Studies of genetics of obstructive sleep apnea: familial aggregation of symptoms associated with sleep-related breathing disturbances. Am Rev Respir Dis 1992; 145: 440–444.

119. Tishler PV, Redline S, Ferrette V, et al. The association of sudden unexpected infant death with obstructive sleep apnea. Am J Respir Crit Care Med 1996; 153:1857–1863.

120. Guilleminault C, Souquet M, Ariagno RL. Five cases of near-miss sudden infant death syndrome and development of obstructive sleep apnea syndrome. Pediatrics 1984; 73:71–78.

121. Guilleminault C, Stoohs R. From apnea of infancy to obstructive sleep apnea syndrome in the young child. Chest 1992; 102:1065–1071.

122. Guilleminault C, Stoohs R, Skrobal A, et al. Upper airway resistance in infants at risk for sudden infant death syndrome. J Pediatr 1993; 122: 881–886.

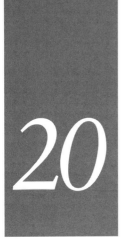

20 SLEEP APNEA IN THE ELDERLY

Jennifer Martin, Carl J Stepnowsky, and
Sonia Ancoli-Israel

INTRODUCTION

Older adults frequently complain of difficulties with sleep. In fact, recent estimates suggest that over 50% of older adults report regular problems with sleep (1). Sleep in older adults may be affected by a number of factors, such as medical illness, psychiatric illness, medication use, circadian rhythm changes, or primary sleep disorders (1). One primary sleep disorder that contributes to the inability of elderly adults to obtain sufficient sleep at night and to subsequent daytime sleepiness is sleep-disordered breathing (SDB). SDB is more common in older adults than in younger adults, and although much controversy exists about the nature of SDB in older adults, it is associated with considerable morbidity and mortality. A number of disorders and characteristics that accompany aging are also signs and symptoms of SDB (see Table 20.1). Since SDB is a treatable disorder regardless of age, it is essential to keep this in mind when evaluating the possibility of SDB in an older person.

Table 20.1 Aging and SDB

Signs Associated with Aging	Signs and Symptoms of SDB
Snoring	Snoring
Fragmented nighttime sleep	Fragmented nighttime sleep
Excessive daytime sleepiness	Excessive daytime sleepiness
Hypertension	Hypertension
Cardiovascular disease	Cardiovascular disease
Cognitive impairment	Cognitive impairment

EPIDEMIOLOGY

Snoring and daytime sleepiness are the most common presenting symptoms of patients with SDB. Older adults are more likely to snore than younger adults (2). Although the prevalence of snoring is greater in younger men than in younger women, the prevalence of snoring is approximately equal in older men and women (3). Data also suggest that elderly adults fall asleep more quickly than younger adults when they are allowed opportunities for sleep throughout the day, indicating that they experience more overall daytime sleepiness (4).

In one of the earliest studies of breathing in sleep, Webb (5) found that 9 of 12 healthy men with an average age of 54 years had periodic pauses in breathing with apneas. Since this initial observation, there have been many studies on the epidemiology of SDB in different age groups. Published studies agree that the prevalence of SDB is higher in the elderly than in middle-aged adults and higher in men than in women, although this sex difference is less dramatic in the elderly than in middle-aged adults (6–8). It also appears that SDB is more common in postmenopausal women than in premenopausal women (9). Studies on menopausal status and SDB generally compare postmenopausal women to age-matched premenopausal women (10). Although such studies have suggested that menopausal status effects the prevalence of SDB, longitudinal studies still need to be conducted to understand the nature of this change in prevalence with the cessation of menses. Additionally, hormone replacement therapy has shown promise in the reduction of SDB in some studies whereas it has shown no effect on SDB in others (11, 12). It is therefore questionable whether estrogen and progesterone are directly protective against the development of SDB or whether other effects of menopause (e.g., changes in lean body mass) indirectly result in an increase in SDB in older women.

In 1989, Ancoli-Israel (7) reviewed epidemiological studies on SDB in healthy elderly subjects and stated that in those studies that reported prevalence rates based on sex, the prevalence rates for elderly women ranged from 19.5 to 60%, whereas the rates for elderly men ranged from 28 to 62%. In those studies reporting combined rates, the prevalence rates ranged from 5.6 to 45%. Many of these studies, however, did not use random sampling, which may account for some of the variability in these prevalence estimates.

In one of the largest studies to date using objective measurement of sleep apnea, Ancoli-Israel et al. (8) found that 24% of randomly selected community-dwelling elderly persons had 5 or more apneas per hour of sleep (apnea index [AI]) and an average AI of 13. An this group, 81% had 5 or more respiratory disturbances per hour of sleep (respiratory disturbance index [RDI]) and an average RDI of 38. For comparison purposes, when more stringent criteria levels were used, the prevalence rates were 10% and 4% for AI greater than or equal to 10 and 20, respectively, and 44% and 24% for RDI levels greater than or equal to 20 and 40, respectively. Enright and colleagues (13) found lower prevalence rates using self-reported snoring with observed apneas. They found that 13% of older men and 4% of older women had these complaints. These results need to be interpreted cautiously as self-report measures of sleep apnea do not correlate highly with objective measures in any age group. These data suggest, however, that there may be a large number of older people living in the community who have SDB but do not report snoring or observed apneas.

Several studies using samples of medically healthy elderly persons have also been reported. Hoch and colleagues (14) studied a group of 105 healthy older adults and found that the median RDI and the prevalence of SDB both increased significantly from 60 to 90 years of age, with 2.9% of those 60–69 years, 33.3% of those 70–79 years, and 39.5% of those 80–89 years having an RDI ≥ 5. Although an RDI ≥ 5 indicates only a mild level of SDB, the difference in prevalence according to the decade of life was striking. In addition to an age effect, significantly more men had an RDI ≥ 10 than did women in the overall sample. Hayward and colleagues (15) studied a random sample of healthy, nondemented retirement village residents and found that 18% had an RDI ≥ 10 and 6% had an RDI ≥ 15. These data suggest that although the prevalence is somewhat lower in

healthy older adults than in random community samples, it is still fairly common.

Bixler et al. (16) recently studied a large group of randomly selected men age 20–100 year. Subjects were randomly selected with 'oversampling' of those with risk factors for SDB (snoring, daytime sleepiness, obesity, hypertension) to be screened in the laboratory. The prevalence of SDB across age groups was examined and was shown to increase with age. This increase in prevalence appeared to be accounted for by an age-related increase in the number of central apneic events. The number of obstructive and mixed apneic events did not appear to increase in a linear fashion relative to age. The prevalence of obstructive sleep apnea syndrome (OSAS) increased up to about age 55 years, after which the prevalence stayed relatively constant. Furthermore, this study reported that SDB in older men is less severe than in younger male patients. Although this study contributed to our understanding of the severity of SDB across the lifespan, it did not address potential differences in this effect between men and women. Additionally, these findings must be interpreted with caution since persons with symptoms were oversampled. The issue of misreporting symptoms in older adults was not addressed in this study. Also, many elderly persons with significant SDB are not obese, which suggests that alternative symptoms (e.g., cognitive difficulties, fragmented sleep) may be as indicative of SDB in the later decades of life as the symptoms used in this study (e.g., obesity, snoring) are in young to middle-aged adults. Nonetheless, these results have implications in the clinical management of men with SDB, which will be discussed later in the chapter.

Data also suggest that nursing home patients are at particularly high risk for development of sleep apnea. Ancoli-Israel et al. (17) studied 233 patients living in nursing homes and found that 70% had RDI ≥ 5. In addition, they reported a strong relationship between mortality and RDI in older women but no relationship between mortality and RDI in older men in their sample, even though SDB was very common in both men and women.

Ancoli-Israel and Coy (18) and Redline and Sanders (19) suggest that the use of varying criteria for defining the presence of SDB accounts for some of the variability in prevalence estimates. No consensus exists on the definition of a hypopnea, with criteria widely varying on minimum amplitude reduction (from any discernible reduction to 50% reduction), associated oxygen desaturation level (from 0% to > 4% desaturation), and associated arousal (required versus not required). There is also no consensus on the definition of an arousal. Furthermore, some studies do not use objectively measured breathing during sleep. For example, Enright et al. (13) used a combination of observed apneas and reported snoring to indicate SDB, yet many persons may not be aware of and therefore not report these symptoms, particularly if they live alone. Some researchers use AI whereas others use RDI. In fact, many studies used an AI criterion of 5, a value thought by many investigators to be too low (18, 19). More work is needed to generate consensus on the criteria that are clinically meaningful for defining the level of SDB that should be used in estimates of prevalence in older adults.

MORBIDITY AND MORTALITY ASSOCIATED WITH SDB

Although they are symptoms of SDB, some physicians may consider snoring and daytime sleepiness a part of 'normal' aging. There is a significant relationship between SDB and its symptoms with morbidity and mortality. Research suggests that persons with SDB are at increased risk for cardiovascular and cognitive consequences. Also, people with SDB are at increased risk for death compared to those without SDB. Unfortunately, the majority of studies have not examined morbidity and mortality exclusively in the elderly to determine whether the risks associated with SDB are comparable to those of younger adults.

SDB AND CARDIOVASCULAR CONSEQUENCES

Sleep apnea has been associated with a number of cardiovascular consequences, including hypertension, cardiac arrhythmias, myocardial infarction, and stroke (see Table 20.2). The specific mechanisms of these effects continue to be examined, but it generally appears that change in blood gases with impairment in respiration and sympathetic nervous system activity contribute significantly to these problems (20). Sleep is normally associated with a reduction in systemic blood pressure; however, persons with SDB often fail to show this decrease in blood pressure during sleep (21). Although the specific mechanisms are still unclear, there is strong evidence linking SDB to nocturnal hypertension, with an increasing body of literature suggesting that SDB is also linked to sustained systemic hypertension (22).

Evidence suggests likewise that snoring may contribute to increased risk for stroke. In a retrospective study of 70 stroke patients, Palomaki et al. (23) found that patients who had a cerebral infarction at night were more likely to report snoring often or always than patients who had a cerebral infarction during the day (68.6% versus 41.2%, respectively). This suggests that the acute effects of snoring/or SDB, or both, may contribute to stroke events during the sleep period, although this does not address the overall increased risk for stroke. Although it is possible that the increase in probability of stroke at night is due entirely to the increase in blood pressure, Koskenvuo et al. (24) found that habitual snoring is an independent risk factor for stroke even after controlling for arterial hypertension. This suggests that SDB may directly increase the risk of stroke, not simply through the effects of SDB on blood pressure. Further examination of the mechanisms underlying this effect are needed.

SDB, COGNITIVE IMPAIRMENT, AND DEMENTIA

SDB at night has been associated with difficulties in concentration, attention, and memory during the day (see Bliwise [25] for a review; see also Table 20.2). Some researchers have demonstrated that the effects of SDB on cognitive functioning are independent of age and other risk factors for cognitive impairment; however, others have failed to show this relationship (15, 26, 27). Studies that have found no relationship often used healthy elderly subjects to eliminate the possibility of effects of other illnesses on cognitive function; however, persons with SDB, especially severe SDB, often have comorbid disease.

Table 20.2 Cardiovascular and cognitive consequences of SDB in the elderly

Cardiovascular Disease
Hypertension
Stroke
Myocardial infarction
Cardiac arrhythmias
Cognitive Functioning
Memory impairments
Attentional difficulties
Difficulty concentrating

In the effort to limit these samples, often those with the most severe SDB (and therefore those most likely to have resultant cognitive impairments) could have been systematically excluded. In addition, it is likely that SDB does not affect all areas of cognitive functioning but only specific cognitive skills. This may also explain the negative findings of some studies that examined only a small number of cognitive tasks. Although there is some controversy about the nature of the relationship between SDB and cognitive functioning, two possible explanations have been suggested. First, cognitive impairment may be due to the transient hypoxia resulting from SDB. In fact, a number of researchers have demonstrated a relationship between oxygen desaturations and cognitive functioning. It is unclear at this time whether the hypoxia from SDB results in irreversible changes in the brain, which may cause nonreversible cognitive impairment. Second, the cognitive impairment may be due to excessive daytime sleepiness resulting from SDB. Persons who are sleep deprived have difficulties on some cognitive tasks, and the effect of SDB on cognitive functioning could simply be an effect of sleep deprivation. At present, there are data to support both hypotheses.

Some studies have shown that SDB is associated with dementia. Dementia describes a group of nonreversible changes that cause impairments in functioning. Ancoli-Israel et al. (28) studied the relationship between SDB and Dementia Rating Scale (DRS) scores in institutionalized elderly and found that higher levels of SDB were significantly associated with decreased overall performance on the DRS and on all of the DRS subscales. The authors suggested that, unlike impairment caused by cortical dementias such as Alzheimer disease (e.g., which involves primarily problems in memory), SDB was associated with widespread impairment including tasks thought to be mediated by subcortical brain areas. In addition, patients who scored in the severe dementia range on the DRS had significantly worse SDB than those who scored in the mild dementia range. It therefore appears that severity of SDB is associated with increased cognitive impairment even in those with both severe SDB and severe cognitive impairment.

Studies on persons with Alzheimer disease, the most common cause of dementia, have indicated that the prevalence of SDB is very high in this population. Hoch et al. (29) compared a group of older adults with Alzheimer disease to a group of older patients with depression and a group of healthy older controls and found that a larger proportion of patients with Alzheimer disease had RDI ≥ 5 and RDI ≥ 10. These data suggest that persons with Alzheimer disease, a specific type of dementing illness, may be at even greater risk for the development of SDB than healthy aged adults. At this point the cause of the increased prevalence in Alzheimer disease patients is unclear. It is possible that, as general brain function deteriorates, respiratory centers are impaired.

In our own laboratory, in an ongoing study on sleep and behavior in institutionalized patients with Alzheimer disease, overnight recordings of sleep-wake and respiration have indicated that SDB was very common, with 80% of patients having an RDI ≥ 10, 47.7% having an RDI ≥ 20, and 51.7% having an AI ≥ 5. Preliminary analyses also indicated that as RDI increased, cognitive functioning decreased. These results suggested that, in patients with Alzheimer disease, RDI may contribute significantly to cognitive functioning even when age, an important predictor of cognitive functioning, was included in the model. We are currently testing whether treatment of SDB in patients with Alzheimer disease may result in some level of improvement in cognitive abilities.

Patients with Parkinson disease, another form of nonreversible dementia, often complain of difficulty with sleep. Parkinson disease, which occurs primarily in older men, involves significant motor disturbances resulting from decreased dopaminergic activity (30). Relatively little work has been done to examine the sleep of Parkinson disease patients. It has been suggested that the significant respiratory difficulties experienced by these patients may cause breathing difficulties at night. Another suggestion has been that the neurological and motor impairments associated with this disorder may cause central sleep apneas, obstructive sleep apneas, or episodes of nocturnal hypoventilation and, in turn, these apneic events may contribute to the sleep fragmentation of which patients often complain (31).

SDB AND MORTALITY

In general, mortality rates from all causes increases 30% during the night, and specifically in those aged 65 and over, between 2:00 A.M. and 8:00 A.M. (32). In addition, persons with SDB are more likely to die at night from any cause than persons without SDB. Data analyzed from the American Cancer Society have shown that those who slept less than 7 hours or more than 8 hours had a higher mortality rate at 6 year follow-up evaluation; 86% of these deaths were in those over the age of 60 years (33). It has been hypothesized that one condition that may have partially accounted for these findings is SDB. Studies of both community dwelling and institutionalized elderly persons have provided some evidence for an association between high AI in the elderly and mortality rates. (17, 34–36)

In a large cohort of sleep apnea patients recruited through a sleep clinic in Israel, Lavie et al. (36) reported that SDB is less predictive of death in individuals over age 70 years than would be expected. In a reanalysis of these data, no significant difference in death rates between those elderly over the age of 70 years and the general population was found (37). Mant et al. (38) found that RDI was not an independent predictor of mortality in a population of nondemented elderly subjects, but that hypertension and other severe illnesses (such as cancer) were predictive.

Ancoli-Israel et al. (39) studied a population-based sample of 426 elderly persons living in the community. Their study showed that those older adults with severe SDB had shorter survival (Fig. 20.1) but that RDI was not an independent predictor of death. Independent predictors of death in this study included cardiovascular disease and pulmonary disease. There is evidence to suggest, though, that these factors may be secondary to or associated with SDB. It is likely that, in older adults, SDB is one of several predisposing factors for cardiovascular and pul-

monary diseases, which, in combination, lead to increased morbidity and mortality.

Recent analyses indicate that having SDB in addition to other diseases may increase mortality risk. In a study of older hospital in-patient men, patients with congestive heart failure (CHF) and SDB had significantly shorter survival than those patients with just CHF, just SDB, or neither. Although SDB alone was not a strong independent predictor of death, in conjunction with congestive heart failure SDB became a serious mortality risk factor. This study also demonstrated that RDI was strongly related to a history of myocardial infarction in these men above and beyond the effects of age, race, income, education, alcohol intake, body mass index, smoking history, and history of hypertension or diabetes (40).

Unfortunately, many of the studies on morbidity and mortality of SDB have involved exclusively or predominantly male patients (16, 35, 41). Additionally, studies that included both men and women often presented only composite data and did not examine sex differences in apnea severity, health consequences, or mortality risk. Since from youth to middle age SDB is less common in women than in men, and since the prevalence is approximately equal in older adults, it is important for future studies to examine the morbidity and mortality risks associated with SDB in older women, especially as these risks may change with menopause and with advancing age.

In summary, a serious consequence of sleep apnea in the elderly seems to be shorter survival time and death during sleep (Table 20.3), particularly if the apnea is associated with heart disease. This finding is consistent with studies on middle-aged adults with sleep apnea (35). Up to the present, there have been no controlled clinical trails or longitudinal studies to determine if treatment of SDB directly decreases morbidity and mortality in elderly adults.

CLINICAL ASSESSMENT AND MANAGEMENT

CLINICAL PRESENTATION AND DIAGNOSIS
Some special considerations must be taken into account in the assessment and management of SDB in the elderly since the cardinal symptoms of sleep apnea—daytime sleepiness and snoring—are particularly common in the elderly. Issues to consider related to clinical presentation of SDB in older adults are summarized in Table 20.4. Nonetheless, as with younger adults, a complete sleep

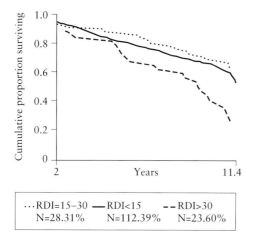

Fig 20.1 Estimated survival for elderly persons with RDI < 15, RDI = 15–30, and RDI ≥ 30 (Mantel-Cox, p = 0.0034). (From Ancoli-Israel S, Kripke DF, Klauber MR, et al. Morbidity, mortality and sleep-disordered breathing in community dwelling elderly. Sleep, 1996; 19:277–282.)

Table 20.3 Mortality and SDB in the elderly

Snoring is associated with increased risk of stroke at night
Patients with SDB are more likely to die at night, during sleep
Patients with SDB are at increased risk of death from cardiovascular or pulmonary disease
Patients with SDB and CHF are at risk for shorter survival

Table 20.4 Clinical presentation of SDB in the elderly

Older Adults with SDB frequently have difficulties in one or more of the following areas:

1. Daytime sleepiness: difficulty sustaining wakefulness during daily activities (e.g., driving, conversation, watching television) or unintentional napping

2. Snoring: patients may be unaware of snoring. Bed partners and/or care giver are valuable resources in assessment of snoring

3. Insomnia: fragmented or restless sleep due to frequent nocturnal awakenings associated with apneic events

4. Nocturnal confusion or daytime cognitive impairment or both: commonly seen as difficulties in concentration, attention, and memory

5. Hypertension

These symptoms should generally not be considered part of normal aging and suggest the need for a thorough diagnostic assessment.

history is critical to accurate assessment. The clinician should not assume that older adults with complaints of daytime sleepiness have SDB simply because of the high base rate, nor should such complaints be discounted as part of 'normal aging.'

As a result of daytime sleepiness, older adults tend to nap more. Although there is some discrepancy in the exact frequency and duration of naps in older adults, it is clear that regular napping is common (42). It is essential to evaluate whether these 'naps' are intentional, planned sleep periods during the day, or whether they are unintentional and due to the inability to sustain wakefulness during the day. It is particularly important in this population to inquire about other medical conditions (e.g., abnormal thyroid function) and medications (e.g., sedative hypnotic medications; antihistamines) that may contribute to daytime sleepiness or may exacerbate breathing difficulties during sleep. Also, as with younger adults, overnight recordings are necessary for the accurate diagnosis of SDB. Self-reported symptoms are insufficient for accurate diagnosis. With

older adults, it may be important to involve the spouse or caregiver in the evaluation and sleep recording process. Older adults may be resistant to spending the night in an unfamiliar environment, such as the sleep laboratory, and they may have difficulties managing the equipment and instructions associated with portable recordings. In addition, older adults may have more difficulty with transportation, less tolerance of tolerating recording equipment, and, in the case of ambulatory recordings, more difficulty removing the recording equipment at the end of the night. All of these factors should be considered in planning the overnight assessment. Considerations in the assessment and diagnosis of older adults are summarized in Table 20.5.

TREATMENT OF SDB IN THE ELDERLY

Age alone should not be the determining factor for deciding whether treatment should be initiated for sleep apnea. Rather, the significance of the patient's symptoms and the severity of the disorder should influence treatment (18). Most patients should initially be started on nasal contin-

Table 20.5 Thorough assessment of SDB in the elderly

1. Obtain complete sleep history
   - symptoms of SDB (unintentional napping, snoring, witnessed apneas)
   - symptoms of other sleep disorders (e.g., leg kicks)
   - sleep-related habits and routines

2. Review medical history and medical records
   - check medication side effects for respiratory impairment, daytime sleepiness, or insomnia
   - look for associated medical illnesses, including hypertension and cardiovascular disease

3. Review or obtain complete psychiatric history
   - ask about current drug and alcohol use
   - ask about current depressive symptoms and past depression
   - evaluate for cognitive impairment or dementia

4. Overnight sleep recording
   - when history is suggestive of SDB, overnight recording is indicated

uous positive airway pressure therapy (CPAP) or bilevel continuous positive airway pressure (BiPAP), which have been shown to effectively manage SDB at night with minimal side effects (43). These devices blow air into the nasal passage and muscular airway, thereby producing positive airway pressure, which acts as a pneumatic splint to keep the airway open during inspiration. Details of treatment with CPAP and BiPAP are summarized elsewhere in this book (Chapter 8).

Whether or not there is a relationship between age and compliance with CPAP therapy remains unresolved. One study, using a desaturation index (oxygen desaturations per hour of sleep) of 20 or greater as a criterion for CPAP therapy, found a slight negative relationship between increasing age and decreased compliance (44). Another study, involving a group of clinic patients, found that older age and more severe RDI were the only significant predictors of compliance (45).

For persons who cannot or will not tolerate positive airway pressure, alternative treatments should be considered (46). For example, oral appliances, although helpful for some persons, require posttreatment evaluation, and older adults with dentures cannot use these devices. Surgical interventions are also sometimes used in the treatment of SDB; however, like oral appliances, surgical interventions require accurate posttreatment assessment. In addition, older adults are at increased risk for complications associated with surgeries.

MEDICATIONS AND ALCOHOL
Sedative and Hypnotic Agents

It is known that elderly persons are prescribed a disproportionately high amount of sedative and hypnotic medications. Persons 60 years old and older receive 66% more prescriptions for sedative or hypnotic medications than those aged 40 to 59 years (47, 48). This is likely due to the fact that older adults complain of and seek treatment for insomnia more often than younger adults. It is also known that most sedative and hypnotic medications are respiratory depressants and may increase the number and duration of apneas in a patient with SDB. In addition to decreased respiration, these medications may also decrease the patient's ability to awaken and terminate an apneic event. It is therefore important to use extreme caution in prescribing these medications for older adults with sleep complaints who may have some SDB.

Alcohol

Although alcohol can exacerbate SDB in any age group, elderly adults metabolize alcohol more slowly than their younger counterparts (49). As a result, the impact of alcohol on SDB may be even greater in older adults. Older adults should therefore be cautioned that even small amounts of alcohol can have a deleterious effect on sleep, and older adults with symptoms of SDB should be encouraged to abstain completely from alcohol.

WHAT IS SDB IN THE ELDERLY?

Despite the growing literature on SDB in older adults, the question of whether SDB in older adults is a distinct condition from that in middle-aged adults remains unanswered. Studies are only beginning to investigate the natural history of SDB in the elderly. Young (50) points out that these studies are challenged by the fact that the natural history of any disease in the elderly is complicated by several factors, including the physiology of aging, comorbid diseases, and differential survival. Young also notes that a distinction needs to be made between those conditions that are age-dependent, in which aging causes pathology, and age-related, in which pathology occurs only during a particular age period. A number of studies have shown that the prevalence of SDB increases steadily, with age suggesting that it is an age-dependent disease (see, for example, Ancoli-Israel et al. [8]). In a study of older men, Bixler et al. (16) suggest that although the prevalence of sleep apnea tends to increase with age, the severity and clinical significance actually decrease with age. This suggests that, although prevalence may be age-dependent, severity and clinical significance may be age-related. Other authors have argued that the morbidity and mortality associated with SDB in the elderly cannot be overlooked, especially in those who are symptomatic (51). As discussed earlier, older adults with SDB appear to be at increased risk for mortality from specific diseases (e.g., cardiovascular diseases), and there is evidence to suggest that older adults with SDB are more likely to die during the sleep period.

At this point, specific conclusions cannot be drawn. The precise nature and significance of SDB in older adults needs to be explored further in longitudinal studies of population and clinic samples.

CONCLUSIONS

Although there is considerable variability in prevalence estimates, it is clear that SDB is common in older adults. It is associated with considerable morbidity and mortality risk. Although snoring and daytime sleepiness, the cardinal symptoms of SDB, are common in older adults, these complaints should be evaluated as potential indicators of SDB, and treatment should be available for older patients as it is for younger patients.

ACKNOWLEDGMENT

Supported by NIA AG02711, NIA AG08415, NHLBI HL44915, the Department of Veterans Affairs VISN-22 Mental Illness Research, Education and Clinical Center (MIRECC), UCSD Cancer Center and the Research Service of the Veterans Affairs San Diego Healthcare System.

REFERENCES

1. Ancoli-Israel S. Sleep problems in older adults: putting myths to bed. Geriatrics 1997; 52:20–30.

2. Norton PG, Dunn EV. Snoring as a risk factor for disease: an epidemiological survey. Br Med J 1985; 291:630–632.

3. Fairbanks DNF. Snoring: an overview with historical perspectives. In: Fairbanks DNF, Fujita S, Ikematsu T, et al. eds. Snoring and obstructive sleep apnea, New York: Raven Press; 1987:1–18.

4. Carskadon MA, Dement WC, Mitler MM, et al. Guidelines for the multiple sleep latency test (MSLT): a standard measure of sleepiness. Sleep 1986; 9:519–524.

5. Webb P. Periodic breathing during sleep. J Appl Physiol 1974; 37:899–903.

6. Young T, Palta M, Dempsey J, et al. The occurrence of sleep-disordered breathing among middle-aged adults. N Engl J Med 1993; 328:1230–1235.

7. Ancoli-Israel S. Epidemiology of sleep disorders. In: Roth T, Roehrs TA, eds. Clinics in geriatric medicine. Philadelphia: WB Saunders; 1989:347–362.

8. Ancoli-Israel S, Kripke DF, Klauber MR, et al. Sleep disordered breathing in community-dwelling elderly. Sleep 1991; 14(6):486–495.

9. Block AJ, Wynne JW, Boysen PG. Sleep-disordered breathing and nocturnal oxygen desaturation in postmenopausal women. Am J Med 1980; 69:75–79.

10. Block AJ, Boysen PG, Wynne JW, et al. Sleep apnea, hypopnea and oxygen desaturation in normal subjects. A strong male predominance. N Engl J Med 1979; 300:513–517.

11. Orr WC, Imes NK, Martin RJ. Progesterone therapy in obese patients with sleep apnea. Arch Intern Med 1979; 139:109–111.

12. Pickett CK, Regensteiner JG, Woodard WD, et al. Progestin and estrogen reduce sleep-disordered breathing in postmenopausal women. J Appl Physiol 1989; 66(4):1656–1661.

13. Enright PL, Newman AB, Wahl PW, et al. Prevalence and correlates of snoring and observed apneas in 5,201 older adults. Sleep 1996; 19:531–538.

14. Hoch CC, Reynolds CFI, Monk TH, et al. Comparison of sleep-disordered breathing among healthy elderly in the seventh, eighth, and ninth decades of life. Sleep 1990; 13(6):502–511.

15. Hayward L, Mant A, Eyland A, et al. Sleep disordered breathing and cognitive function in a retirement village population. Age Ageing 1992; 21(2):121–128.

16. Bixler EO, Vgontzas AN, Ten Have T, et al. Effects of age on sleep apnea in men. Am J Respir Crit Care Med 1998; 157:144–148.

17. Ancoli-Israel S, Klauber MR, Kripke DF, et al. Sleep apnea in female patients in a nursing home: increased risk of mortality. Chest 1989; 96(5):1054–1058.

18. Ancoli-Israel S, Coy TV. Are breathing disturbances in elderly equivalent to sleep apnea syndrome? Sleep 1994; 17:77–83.

19. Redline S, Sanders M. Hypopnea, a floating metric: implications for prevalence, morbidity estimates and case findings. Sleep 1997; 20:1209–1217.

20. Guilleminault C. Clinical features and evaluation of obstructive sleep apnea. In: Kryger MH, Roth T, Dement WC, eds. Principles and practice of sleep medicine, Philadelphia: WB Saunders; 1994:667–677.

21. Shepard JW Jr. Gas exchange and hemodynamics during sleep. Med Clin North Am, 1985; 00:1243–1264.

22. Silverberg DS, Oksenberg A, Iaina A. Sleep-related breathing disorders as a major cause of essential hypertension: fact or fiction? Curr Opin Psychiatry 1998; 7:353–357.

23. Palomaki H, Partinen M, Juvela S, et al. Snoring as a risk factor for sleep-related brain infarction. Stroke 1989; 20:1311–1315.

24. Koskenvuo M, Kaprio J, Heikkila K, et al. Snoring as a risk factor for ischemic heart disease and stroke in men. Br Med J 1987; 294:163–19.

25. Bliwise DL. Review: Sleep in normal aging and dementia. Sleep 1993; 16:40–81.

26. Bliwise DL. Cognitive function and sleep-disordered breathing in aging adults. In: Kuna ST, Remmers JE, Suratt PM, eds. Sleep and respiration in aging adults. New York: Elsevier; 1991:237–244.

27. Findley LJ, Presty SK, Barth JT, et al. Impaired cognition and vigilance in elderly subjects with sleep apnea. In: Kuna ST, Suratt PM, Remmers JE, eds. Sleep and respiration in aging adults. New York: Elsevier, 1991:259–265.

28. Ancoli-Israel S, Klauber MR, Butters N, et al. Dementia in institutionalized elderly: relation to sleep apnea. J Am Geriatr Soc 1991; 39(3):258–263.

29. Hoch CC, Reynolds CFI, Kupfer DJ, et al. Sleep-disordered breathing in normal and pathologic aging. J Clin Psychiatry 1986; 47:499–503.

30. Aldrich MS. Parkinsonism. In: Kryger MH, Roth T, Dement WC, eds. Principles and practice of sleep medicine. Philadelphia: WB Saunders; 1994:783–789.

31. Hardie RJ, Efthimiou J, Stern GM. Respiration and sleep in Parkinson's disease. Neurol Neurosurg Psychiatry 1986; 49:1326.

32. Mitler MM, Hajdukovic RM, Shafor R, et al. When people die. Cause of death versus time of death. Am J Med 1987; 82:266–274.

33. Kripke DF, Simons RN, Garfinkel L, et al. Short and long sleep and sleeping pills: is increased mortality associated? Arch Gen Psychiatry 1979; 36:103–116.

34. Bliwise DL, Bliwise NG, Partinen M, et al. Sleep apnea and mortality in an aged cohort. Am J Public Health 1988; 78:544–547.

35. He J, Kryger MH, Zorick FJ, et al. Mortality and apnea index in obstructive sleep apnea: experience in 385 male patients. Chest 1988; 94:9–14.

36. Lavie P, Herer P, Peled R, et al. Mortality in sleep apnea patients: a multivariate analysis of risk factors. Sleep 1995; 18:149–157.

37. Baltzan M, Suissa S. Mortality in sleep apnea patients: a multivariate analysis of risk factors—a response to Lavie and collaborators. Sleep 1997; 20:377–378.

38. Mant A, King M, Saunders NA, et al. Four-year follow-up of mortality and sleep-related respiratory disturbance in non-demented seniors. Sleep 1995; 18:433–438.

39. Ancoli-Israel S, Kripke DF, Klauber MR, et al. Morbidity, mortality and sleep-disordered breathing in community dwelling elderly. Sleep 1996; 19:277–282.

40. Estline E, Klauber MR, Stepnowsky C, et al. Heart disease and sleep-disordered breathing in older men. J Am Coll Cardiol 1999; submitted

41. Stoohs RA, Gingold J, Cohrs S, et al. Sleep-disordered breathing and systemic hypertension in the older male. J Am Geriatr Soc 1996; 44:1295–1300.

42. Wauquier A, Van Sweden B, Lagaay AM, et al. Ambulatory monitoring of sleep-wakefulness patterns in healthy elderly males and females (> 88 years): the "Senieur" protocol. J Am Geriatr Soc 1992; 40:109–114.

43. American Thoracic Society. Indications and standards for use of nasal continuous positive airway pressure (CPAP) in sleep apnea syndromes. Am J Respir Crit Care Med 1994; 150:1738–1745.

44. Pieters T, Collard P, Aubert G, et al. Acceptance and long-term compliance with nCPAP in patients with obstructive sleep apnoea syndrome. Eur Respir J 1996; 9:939–944.

45. Krieger J, Kurtz D, Petiau C, et al. Long-term compliance with CPAP therapy in obstructive sleep apnea patients and in snorers. Sleep 1996; 19:S136–S143.

46. Lowe AA. Dental appliances for the treatment of snoring and obstructive sleep apnea. In Kryger MH, Roth T, Dement WC, eds. Principles and practice of sleep medicine. Philadelphia: WB. Saunders; 1994:722–735.

47. Prinz PN, Vitiello MV, Raskind MA, et al. Geriatrics: sleep disorders and aging. N Engl J Med 1990; 323(8):520–526.

48. Mellinger GD, Balter MB, Uhlenhuth EH. Insomnia and its treatment. Prevalence and correlates. Arch Gen Psychiatry 1985; 42:225–232.

49. Taasan VC, Block AJ, Boysen PG, et al. Alcohol increases sleep apnea and oxygen desaturation in asymptomatic men. Am J Med 1981; 71:240–245.

50. Young T. Sleep-disordered breathing in older adults: is it a condition distinct from that of middle-aged adults? Sleep 1996; 19:529–530.

51. Fleury B. Sleep apnea syndrome in the elderly. Sleep 1992; 15(6):S39–S41.

PART SEVEN

SLEEP IN OTHER RESPIRATORY DISORDERS

21
NOCTURNAL ASTHMA

Neil J Douglas

INTRODUCTION

Asthma affects at least 5% of the population at least sometime during their lives. Nocturnal cough, wheeze, and breathlessness sometimes represent the first symptoms of asthma, and in some asthmatic persons they are the best marker of deterioration in asthmatic control. Nocturnal asthma is not a different condition from asthma; it is merely one feature of that disease, and a feature that tends to affect mainly those with severe airflow obstruction.

⚬┯ **Key points box 21.1**
Nocturnal asthma
1. Nocturnal asthma symptoms usually reflect inadequate asthma control, and most patients respond to increased preventive therapy.
2. Nocturnal asthma causes significant sleep disturbance, which may result in daytime fatigue and poor cognitive performance.
3. Although severe sleep hypoxemia is rare in nocturnal asthma, a disproportionate number of asthma deaths occur at night.

MECHANISM OF NOCTURNAL ASTHMA

Overnight airway narrowing occurs in normal subjects, but it requires sensitive respiratory function testing for it to be apparent (1). The degree of airway narrowing in normal subjects is small and not enough to give rise to any symptoms. The changes in normal persons are synchronous, suggesting a similar causation. However, the airway narrowing is much more apparent in the asthmatic subject (Fig. 21.1); the mean overnight fall in peak flow rate in normal persons was found in one study to be 8%, and that in asthmatic patients was 50% (2). This exaggeration of a normal response, with airways narrowing in asthmatic persons more marked at night, is similar to their marked responses to a wide variety of other nonspecific factors that may produce trivial airway narrowing in normal persons, such as cold air, methacholine, and histamine.

This 'nocturnal' bronchial narrowing is a circadian feature, the timing of which depends on the timing of the patient's sleep (3, 4), with shift changes producing rapid alterations in the timing of airway narrowing. The critical importance of sleep is underlined by the demonstration that keeping asthmatic persons awake all night markedly reduces the magnitude of overnight fall in peak flow rate (5) (Fig. 21.2). Thus, it appears that sleep time is a central factor in controlling 'nocturnal' airway narrowing.

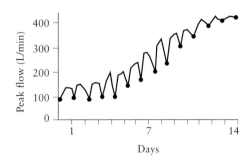

Fig 21.1 *Peak flow rate over a 2 week period in a 62 year old nonallergic asthmatic woman. The flow rate on waking is indicated with a circle. She had marked 'morning dipping'. (From Douglas NJ: Asthma at night. Clin Chest Med 1985; 6: 663–674.)*

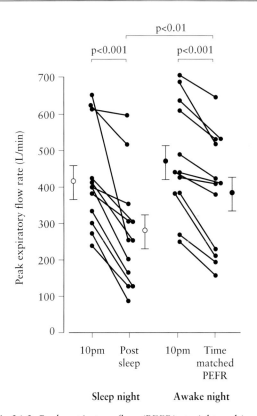

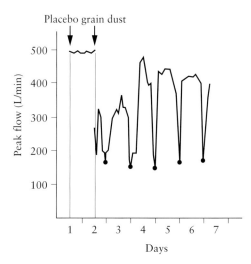

Fig 21.3 Peak flow rates throughout the day after bronchial challenge with placebo and then after challenge with grain dust, initiates nocturnal broncho-constriction. The circles indicate morning flow rates. (Redrawn from Davies RJ, Green M, Schofield NM: Recurrent nocturnal asthma after exposure to grain dust. Am Rev Respir Dis 1976; 114: 1011–1019.)

Fig 21.2 Peak expiratory flow (PEFR) at night and in the morning on both the asleep and the awake nights. All patients developed bronchoconstriction on both nights, but although the 10 P.M. peak flow rates were not significantly different, morning peak flow was higher after the awake night. (From Catterall JR, Rhind GB, Stewart IC, et al: Effect of sleep deprivation on overnight bronchoconstriction in nocturnal asthma. Thorax 1986; 41: 676–680.)

Other factors that have been proposed as possible causes for overnight bronchoconstriction are discussed briefly here.

Cooling of the bronchi due either to a decreased core body temperature during sleep or to the tendency for bedrooms to have a lower temperature at night has been proposed as a mechanism of nocturnal airway narrowing. There is no doubt that airway cooling is a potent cause of airway narrowing in asthmatic persons. However, nocturnal airway narrowing occurs even when the environmental temperatures kept constant throughout the 24 hour cycle (1) so alterations in environmental temperature are not critical factors.

The supine posture has been proposed as a cause for nocturnal asthma. Nevertheless, asthmatic persons left lying supine for 24 hours still exhibit overnight airway narrowing, and lying down does not produce prolonged bronchoconstriction (6).

Allergens in bedding are not the only cause of nocturnal asthma, as nonallergic asthmatic subjects have nocturnal asthma just as frequently (7). However, there is no doubt that exposure to allergens can increase bronchial reactivity in allergic subjects, (8) and this may result in worsening of their nocturnal asthma (9) (Fig. 21.3). Rigorous reduction of house dust mite populations in the bedroom can decrease nocturnal asthma (10). This is likely to be beneficial owing to a reduction in airway reactivity rather than by having a direct effect on allergen-induced bronchoconstriction.

Gastroesophageal reflux has been implicated in nocturnal asthma attacks. However, there is no convincing evidence that this is causally related, and treatment of reflux by either medical or surgical techniques has been found to be of dubious efficacy (11).

A small minority of asthmatic persons who either have the obstructive sleep apnea syndrome (OSAS) or are heavy snorers have coexisting nocturnal asthma. This appears to be as a consequence of their snoring, but the mechanism of this association is unclear (12). I believe that this is a relatively uncommon cause of nocturnal asthma, but one which should be sought as therapy is entirely different.

⊶ Key points box 21.2

Mechanisms of nocturnal asthma

Probable:

1. Circadian factors

2. Sleep state

Possible:

1. Airway cooling

2. Supine posture

3. Allergic factors

4. Gastroesophageal reflux

5. Snoring or sleep apnea

EFFECTOR MECHANISMS RESULTING IN NOCTURNAL AIRWAY NARROWING

Overnight bronchoconstriction is due to circadian variations that are synchronized by sleep time. The possible mechanisms producing bronchoconstriction are described in the following paragraphs.

INCREASED PARASYMPATHETIC AIRWAY TONE

Parasympathetic tone generally increases during sleep (13). Investigations using cholinergic blockade have indicated that some of the overnight bronchial narrowing is due to an overnight increase in parasympathetic tone, but that this does not explain all of the nocturnal bronchoconstriction (14, 15).

DECREASED NONADRENERGIC NONCHOLINERGIC BRONCHODILATING TONE

Creation of the nonadrenergic noncholinergic (NANC) nervous system results in bronchodilatation in man. Activity of the airway NANC system is impaired in the early morning (16), which may contribute to early morning bronchoconstriction.

HORMONAL CHANGES

Circulating levels of both cortisol and catecholamines fall overnight, and it has been proposed that this may explain nocturnal asthma. However, such synchrony does not prove causality, and neither cortisone infusion (17) or catecholamine infusion (18) prevents nocturnal bronchoconstriction. Furthermore, nocturnal asthma often persists despite high dose oral steroid therapy, again suggesting that circadian variation in steroid levels is not an important cause.

AIRWAY INFLAMMATION

There has been considerable speculation that circadian changes in airway inflammatory cell populations may contribute to the development of nocturnal asthma. However, no compelling evidence exists either that consistent changes occur in airway inflammatory cell populations or in mediators or that any causal relationship is present between inflammatory cell populations and nocturnal asthma (19, 20).

⊶ Key points box 21.3

Effector mechanisms of nocturnal bronchoconstriction

Probable

1. Increased parasympathetic nervous system activity

2. Decreased nonadrenergic noncholinergic (NANC) nervous system activity

Possible

1. Hormonal changes

2. Airway inflammation

CONCLUSIONS ON THE EFFECT OF MECHANISMS

Although the precise mechanism by which sleep controls the development of nocturnal asthma is unclear, the most likely candidate is neural control changes effected through increased cholinergic bronchoconstriction and decreased NANC bronchodilatation tone overnight.

EPIDEMIOLOGY

Many asthmatic persons are affected by intermittent nocturnal cough, wheeze, or breathlessness, which is severe enough to disturb their sleep. For many, these are the warning signs of deterioration in asthmatic control, which they use to increase their therapy. Most patients admitted to hospital with attacks of asthma will report recent nocturnal problems, but the frequency is lower in outpatient clinics, family practice asthmatic patients, or population surveys.

CLINICAL FEATURES

The main features of nocturnal asthma are cough, breathlessness, chest tightness, or wheeze, either interfering with sleep or being troublesome first thing in the morning. These may occur every day, or more usually only when the patient's asthma is unstable.

SLEEP

For most asthmatic patients, the major problem is sleep disturbance and feeling tired by day. Polysomnograph provides evidence of sleep disruption with decreased sleep efficiency and increased intervening wakefulness and drowsiness (21–23). This probably results in the impaired cognitive function found in patients with nocturnal asthma compared to age and education matched control subjects (23). Therefore, the resulting sleep problems could have a marked effect on the work and school performance of patients with nocturnal asthma.

During attacks of asthma, patients often have several consecutive nights during which they get little if any sleep because of their nocturnal symptoms. As even one night of sleep deprivation is enough to significantly decrease ventilatory responses to chemostimulation (24), this may be an important factor along with exhaustion and continued airway narrowing in the development of hypoxemia and hypercapnia in some patients with acute severe asthma.

HYPOXEMIA

Severe hypoxemia during sleep is rare in patients with nocturnal asthma, although mild hypoxemia often occurs (21, 22). Desaturation has been observed in some patients before they waken with wheeze (22, 25) but not in all studies (26).

NOCTURNAL ASTHMA ATTACKS

Asthmatic attacks are more common at night than by day with increased presentations both to family physicians and emergency departments (27). This timing is inconvenient to the patient, to their family and friends, and to the medical staff whose assistance is sought.

DEATHS

Asthmatic deaths are fortunately rare, but a disproportionate number of asthmatic deaths occur at night rather than by day (28). These deaths could have many explanations, including the victim being unaware of the development of the attack because he or she was asleep and the inability of hypoxemia, hypercapnia, or increased airflow resistance to rapidly awaken them. Reluctance to seek help during the night could be a factor, but as most ventilatory arrests in already hospitalized asthmatics persons occur at night, the delay in obtaining medical assistance is probably not the only factor (29).

DIFFERENTIAL DIAGNOSIS

Normally the diagnosis is self-evident, but other causes of paroxysmal nocturnal dyspnea may need to be excluded, including (1) pulmonary edema, usually associated with a history of heart disease, chest pain, cardiomegaly, and typical radiographic features and (2) sleep apnea-hypopnea syndrome, which gives rise to brief episodes of choking and in which wheeze is not a feature.

DIAGNOSIS

The patient history in association with evidence of asthma usually suffices for diagnosis. However, it may be necessary to monitor peak expiratory flow rates both for diagnosis and to guide therapy. Peak flow rates should be recorded at a minimum of three times per day, including at first awakening, in the middle of the day, and at bedtime, plus at any additional nocturnal awakenings associated with features of nocturnal asthma. On each occasion, flow rates should be measured in triplicate to assure accuracy. Average overnight falls in peak flow rate of at least

15% in association with a suggestive history is diagnostic of nocturnal asthma.

TREATMENT

The development of nocturnal asthma is a sign of inadequate control of the patient's asthma and should lead to intensification of therapy. This should be directed at improving the patients general asthmatic control and not simply increase the use of bronchodilators at night. Thus, the first step in therapy is to optimize the use of prophylactic agents, usually inhaled steroids, and this is often sufficient (30). Only when either maximum dosage or prophylactic agents have been used or when ideal control of both daytime symptoms and daytime peak flow rates is achieved without preventive nocturnal asthma should therapy be specifically targeted at the nighttime.

Conventional inhaled β_2 agonists bronchodilators only last 4–6 hours. This lack of efficacy late in the night is compounded by the fact that nocturnal airway narrowing tends to be greatest late in the night, even in subjects who have discontinued all bronchodilators. Inhaled atropine-like drugs such as ipratropium last for slightly longer and have the theoretical advantage of directly opposing the increase in parasympathetic tone that is one of the causative factors of nocturnal asthma. Nevertheless, in practice, their role in the management of nocturnal asthma has proved limited and disappointing.

Long-acting inhaled β_2 agonists such as salmeterol and formoterol provide bronchodilation for over 12 hours. Both agents have been shown to decrease symptoms and increase morning peak flow rates in patients with nocturnal asthma (31, 32) (Fig. 21.4). Salmeterol has also been found to improve sleep quality (31) (Fig. 21.5) and quality of life (33). These agents represent a significant advance in the treatment of patients with nocturnal asthma and should be added in all patients whose nocturnal asthma fails to respond to a combination of maximum dose inhaled steroids and inhaled β_2 agonists at bedtime.

Oral sustained release bronchodilators such as theophyllines (34) and β_2 agonists (35, 36) may also improve symptoms and morning peak flow rates. One daily dosage at bedtime may suffice and will minimize daytime side effects (34), but larger doses of theophylline can be given at night than during the day because absorption is slower (37). The effect of theophyllines on sleep quality is

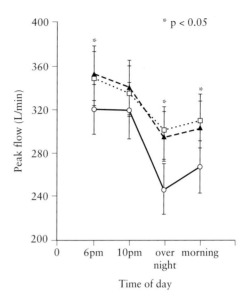

Fig 21.4 *Mean standard error, (SE) peak expiratory flow rate in 18 asthmatic patients receiving placebo (○) or salmeterol 50 μg (□) or 100 μg (▲) twice daily. (Redrawn from Fitzpatrick MF, Mackay TM, Driver H, Douglas NJ: Salmeterol in nocturnal asthma: a double blind, placebo controlled trial of a long acting inhaled β_2 agonist. Br Med J 1990; 301: 1365–1368.)*

disputed. Theophyllines are biochemically related to caffeines, and early studies suggested that they impaired sleep in asthmatic persons (38). However, no sleep disruption was found in normal subjects taking theophyllines (39). Furthermore, there was no difference in sleep quality in patients taking theophyllines in comparison to those on inhaled salmeterol (40). This latter randomized study found no major difference between theophyllines and salmeterol in the management of nocturnal asthma, with only minor benefits in favor of salmeterol, including slightly fewer arousals from sleep, a minor advantage in quality of life, and improved vigilance (40). These differences were minor, which suggests that patient preference and side effects should determine the choice of long-acting bronchodilators. Another randomized trial found that salmeterol was superior to oral sustained release terbutaline in producing nights without awakenings, higher morning peak flow rates, and patient satisfaction (41). Salmeterol 50 μg bd, was similar in efficacy to fluticasone, 250 μg bd, in improving nocturnal asthma (42).

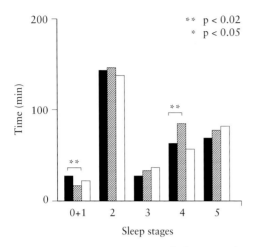

** p < 0.02
* p < 0.05

Fig 21.5 Mean (SE) time spent in each sleep stage by 18 asthmatic patients receiving placebo (solid bar) or salmeterol 50 μg (hatched bar) or 100 μg (open bar) twice daily. (Redrawn from Fitzpatrick MF, Mackay T, Driver H, Douglas NJ: Salmeterol in nocturnal asthma: a double blind, placebo controlled trial of a long acting inhaled β₂ agonist. Br Med J 1990; 301:1365–1368.)

Physicians differ in the rank order of introducing high-dose inhaled steroids or long-acting bronchodilators. With increasing evidence that long-term use of inhaled β_2 agonists does not carry risks, many physicians are now recommending that long-acting inhaled β_2 agonists be used before the dosage of inhaled steroids is increased. Patients who do not respond to the combination of high-dose inhaled steroids plus long-acting bronchodilators may require treatment with oral steroids, either in the short or long term. This usually is sufficient, but not always. When it is not, immunosuppressive therapy with methotrexate may be helpful (43).

In the small number of patients who have both nocturnal asthma and loud snoring or the sleep apnea/hypopnea syndrome, CPAP therapy should be tried (Fig. 21.6) if they do not respond readily to conventional treatment (12). It is also important to remember to check whether the patient whose nocturnal asthma is difficult to control has a history of snoring or apneas.

☞ Key points box 21.4

Treatment steps

1. Optimize baseline asthma control—usually achieved by increasing preventive therapy, such as inhaled corticosteroids

2. If step I fails to achieve adequate symptom control or peak flow, add a long acting bronchodilator:

   Beta-agonists (salmeterol, formoterol)
   Theophylline

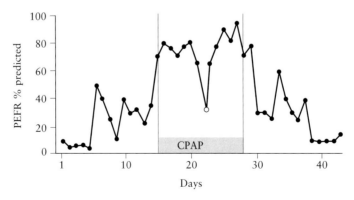

Fig 21.6 Peak expiratory flow rate (PEFR), as percentage predicted, at 3 A.M. in a snoring asthmatic person measured during a control period, during a period of nocturnal continuous positive airway pressure (CPAP) therapy, and during a subsequent period after CPAP withdrawal. The open circle during the CPAP period represents a single night when CPAP period was withdrawn. (Redrawn from Chan CS, Woolcock AJ, Sullivan CE: Nocturnal asthma: role of snoring and obstructive sleep apnea. Am Rev Respir Dis 1988; 137:1502–1504.)

CONCLUSIONS

Nocturnal asthma causes significant inconvenience to large numbers of people. The development of inhaled long-acting bronchodilators has made management significantly easier.

REFERENCES

1. Kerr HD. Diurnal variation of respiratory function independent of air quality. Arch Environ Health 1973; 26:144–53.

2. Hetzel MR, Clark TJH. Comparison of normal and asthmatic circadian rhythms in peak expiratory flow rate. Thorax 1980; 35:732–738.

3. Hetzel MR, Clark TJH. Does sleep cause nocturnal asthma? Thorax 1979; 34:749–754.

4. Connolly CK. The effect of bronchodilators on diurnal rhythms in airway obstruction. Br J Dis Chest 1981; 75:197–203.

5. Catterall JR, Rhind GB, Stewart IC, et al. Effect of sleep deprivation on overnight bronchoconstriction in nocturnal asthma. Thorax 1986; 41:676–680.

6. Whyte KF, Douglas NJ. Posture and nocturnal asthma. Thorax 1989; 44:579–581.

7. Connolly CK. Diurnal rhythms in airway obstruction. Br J Dis Chest 1979; 73:357–366.

8. Davies RJ, Green M, Schofield NM. Recurrent nocturnal asthma after exposure to grain dust. Am Rev Respir Dis 1976; 114: 1011–1019.

9. Ryan G, Latimer KM, Dolovich J, et al. Bronchial responsiveness to histamine: relationship to diurnal variation of peak flow rate, improvement after bronchodilator and airway calibre. Thorax 1982; 37:423–429.

10. Platts-Mills TAE, Mitchell EB, Nock P, et al. Reduction of bronchial hyper-reactivity during prolonged allergen avoidance. Lancet 1982; 2:675–677.

11. Perpina M, Pellicer C, Marco V, et al. The significance of the reflex bronchoconstriction provoked by gastroesophageal reflux in bronchial asthma. Eur J Respir Dis 1985; 66:91–97.

12. Chan CS, Woolcock AJ, Sullivan CE. Nocturnal asthma: role of snoring and obstructive sleep apnea. Am Rev Respir Dis 1988; 137:1502–1504.

13. Baust W, Bohnert B. The regulation of heart rate during sleep. Exp Brain Res 1969; 7:169–180.

14. Morrison JF, Pearson SB, Dean HG. Parasympathetic nervous system in nocturnal asthma. Br Med J 1988; 296:1427–1429.

15. Catterall JR, Rhind GB, Whyte KF, et al. Is nocturnal asthma caused by changes in airway cholinergic activity? Thorax 1988; 43:720–724.

16. Mackay TW, Fitzpatrick MF, Douglas NJ. Non-adrenergic, non-cholinergic nervous system and overnight airway calibre in asthmatic and normal subjects. Lancet 1991; 338:1289–1292.

17. Clark TJH, Hetzel MR. Diurnal variation of asthma. Br J Dis Chest 1977; 71:87–92.

18. Morrison JFJ, Teale C, Pearson SB, et al. Adrenaline and nocturnal asthma. Br Med J 1990; 301:473–476.

19. Mackay TW, Wallace WAH, Howie SEM, et al. Role of inflammation in nocturnal asthma. Thorax 1994; 49:257–262.

20. Oosterhoff Y, Kauffman HF, Rutgers B, et al. Inflammatory cell number and mediators in bronchoalveolar lavage fluid and peripheral blood in subjects with asthma with increased nocturnal airways narrowing. J Allergy Clin Immunol 1995; 2:219–229.

21. Catterall JR, Douglas NJ, Calverley PM, et al. Irregular breathing and hypoxaemia during sleep in chronic stable asthma. Lancet 1982; 1:301–304.

22. Montplaisir J, Walsh J, Malo JL. Nocturnal asthma features of attacks, sleep and breathing patterns. Am Rev Respir Dis 1982; 125:18–22.

23. Fitzpatrick MF, Engleman H, Whyte KF, et al. Morbidity in nocturnal asthma: sleep quality and daytime cognitive performance. Thorax 1991; 46:569–573.

24. White DP, Doughlas NJ, Pickett CK, et al. Sleep deprivation and the control of ventilation. Am Rev Respir Dis 1983; 128:984–986.

25. Deegan PC, McNicholas WT. Continous non-invasive monitoring of evolving acute severe asthma during sleep. Thorax 1994; 6:613–614.

26. Issa FG, Sullivan CE. Respiratory muscle activity in thoracoabdominal movement during acute episodes of asthma during sleep. Am Rev Respir Dis 1985; 132:999–1004.

27. Horn CR, Clark TJH, Cochrane GM. Is there a circadian variation in respiratory morbidity? Br J Dis Chest 1987; 81:248–251.

28. British Thoracic Association. Death from asthma in two regions of England. Br Med J 1982; 285:1251–1255.

29. Hetzel MR, Clark TJH, Branthwaite MA. Asthma: analysis of sudden deaths and ventilatory arrests in hospital. Br Med J 1977; 1:808–811.

30. Horn CR, Clark TJH, Cochrane GM. Inhaled therapy reduces morning dips in asthma. Lancet 1984; 1:1143–1145.

31. Fitzpatrick MF, Mackay T, Driver H, et al. Salmeterol in nocturnal asthma: a double blind, placebo controlled trial of a long acting inhaled β_2 agonist. Br Med J 1990; 301: 1365–1368.

32. Maesen FPV, Smeets JJ, Gubbelmans HLL, et al. Formoterol in the treatment of nocturnal asthma. Chest 1990; 98: 866–870.

33. Lockey RF, DuBuske LM, Friedman B, et al. Nocturnal asthma: effect of salmeterol on quality of life and clinical outcomes. Chest 1999; 3:666–673.

34. Barnes PJ, Greening AP, Neville L, et al. Single-dose slow-release aminophylline at night prevents nocturnal asthma. Lancet 1982; 1:299–301.

35. Milledge JS, Morris J. A comparison of slow-release salbutamol with slow-release aminophylline in nocturnal asthma. J Int Med Res 1979; 7:106–110.

36. Crompton GK, Ayres JG, Basran G, et al. Comparison of oral bambuterol and inhaled salmeterol in patients with symptomatic asthma and using inhaled corticosteroids. Am J Respir Crit Care Med 1999; 3:824–828.

37. Scott PH, Tabachnik E, MacLeod S, et al. Sustained-release theophylline for childhood asthma: evidence for circadian variation of theophylline pharmacokinetics. J Pediatr 1981; 99:476–479.

38. Rhind GB, Connaughton JJ, McFie J, et al. Sustained release choline theophyllinate in nocturnal asthma. Br Med J 1985; 291:1605–1607.

39. Fitzpatrick MF, Engleman HM, Boellert F, et al. Effect of therapeutic theophylline levels on the sleep quality and daytime cognitive performance of normal subjects. Am Rev Respir Dis 1992; 145:1355–1358.

40. Selby C, Engleman HM, Fitzpatrick MF, et al. Inhaled salmeterol or oral theophylline in nocturnal asthma? Am J Resp Crit Care Med 1997; 155:104–108.

41. Brambilla C, Chastang C, George D, et al. Salmeterol compared with slow release terbutaline in nocturnal asthma. A multi-centre randomised double-blind double dummy sequential clinical trial. Allergy 1994; 49:421–426.

42. Weersink EJ, Douma RR, Postma DS, et al. Fluticasone propionate, salmeterol xinafoate and their combination in the treatment of nocturnal asthma. Am J Respir Crit Care Med 1997; 155:1241–1246.

43. Mullarkey MF, Lammert JK, Blumenstein BA. Long term methotrexate treatment in corticosteroid dependent asthma. Ann Intern Med 1990; 112:577–581.

22 SLEEP IN CHRONIC OBSTRUCTIVE PULMONARY DISEASE

Walter T McNicholas

INTRODUCTION

Sleep has well-recognized effects on breathing which in normal persons have no adverse impact. These effects include a mild degree of hypoventilation with consequent hypercapnia and a diminished responsiveness to respiratory stimuli. However, in patients with chronic lung disease such as chronic obstructive pulmonary disease (COPD), these physiological changes during sleep may have a profound effect on gas exchange, and episodes of profound hypoxemia may develop, particularly during rapid eye movement (REM) sleep (1), which may predispose to death at night (2). Furthermore, COPD has an adverse impact on sleep quality itself (3), which may contribute to the complaints of fatigue and lethargy that are well-recognized features of the condition (4).

⊶ Key points box 22.1

Impact of sleep in COPD

1. Impaired gas exchange
   Hypoxemia—may be severe in REM sleep
   Hypercapnia—usually mild

2. Disturbed sleep quality
   Diminished slow wave and REM sleep
   Frequent arousals

EFFECTS OF SLEEP ON RESPIRATION

The control of breathing during sleep is covered extensively in Chapter 1, but it is summarized in this chapter to highlight the interaction of the physiological changes in respiration during sleep with the abnormalities in lung mechanics and respiratory control associated with COPD.

The respiratory center is influenced by chemical inputs from chemoreceptors responding to changes in PaO_2, $PaCO_2$, and pH, by mechanoreceptors in the airway, lungs, and chest wall, and by behavioral inputs from higher cortical centers, transmitted via the reticular activating system (5). Removal of these inputs can markedly reduce ventilation, and in some experimental settings may produce complete cessation of spontaneous breathing (6). Sleep is associated with a number of effects on respiration, including changes in central respiratory control, airways resistance, and muscular contractility.

CENTRAL RESPIRATORY EFFECTS

The onset of sleep is associated with a diminished responsiveness of the respiratory center to chemical and mechanical inputs and to a major reduction in the stimulant effects of cortical inputs (5). These effects are more pronounced as sleep deepens, particularly during (REM) sleep. Ventilatory responsiveness to both hypoxia and hypercapnia are diminished. Furthermore the respiratory muscles' responsiveness to respiratory center outputs are also diminished during sleep, particularly REM sleep, although the diaphragm is less affected than the accessory muscles in this regard. There is a decrease in minute ventilation (V_E) during non-REM (NREM) sleep (7), predominantly due to a reduction in tidal volume, which is associated with a rise in end-tidal PCO_2. However, part of this hypoventilation during sleep is likely a response to the lower metabolic rate during sleep, since O_2 consumption and CO_2 production diminish during sleep compared to wakefulness (8). During REM sleep, both tidal volume and respiratory frequency are much more variable than in NREM sleep (7), particularly during phasic REM, when there are bursts of REM, as opposed to tonic REM during which eye movements tend to be absent. Minute ventilation is lower during phasic REM than during tonic REM sleep.

These physiological changes are not associated with any clinically significant deterioration in gas exchange among normal subjects, but they may produce profound hypoxemia in patients with respiratory insufficiency such as COPD (1, 3). This finding is principally due to the fact that normal subjects have PaO_2 levels on the flat portion of the oxyhemoglobin dissociation curve, and thus modest falls in PaO_2 as a consequence of hypoventilation during sleep are not associated with significant falls in oxygen saturation (SaO_2) (7). However, COPD patients tend to have PaO_2 levels at or near the steep portion of the oxyhemoglobin dissociation curve, and thus equivalent modest falls in PaO_2 during sleep may result in clinically significant falls in SaO_2 (1). The drop in SaO_2 during sleep in COPD is further compounded by the increased work of breathing associated with chronic airflow limitation, which likely also aggravates the effects of the reduction in respiratory drive during sleep.

AIRWAY RESISTANCE

Upper airway resistance increases during sleep compared to wakefulness (9), which predisposes to upper airway occlusion and obstructive sleep apnea syndrome (OSAS) in susceptible persons. In addition, lower airway patency may also be compromised during sleep. The majority of normal subjects have circadian changes in airway caliber

with mild nocturnal bronchoconstriction. Such bronchoconstriction may be exaggerated in patients with asthma, who can demonstrate falls in peak flow rate to 50% or more, compared to an average of 8% in normal subjects (10).

RIB CAGE AND ABDOMINAL CONTRIBUTION TO BREATHING

In the supine resting state, breathing is predominantly a function of diaphragmatic contraction (11). During NREM sleep there is an increased ribcage contribution to breathing and an associated increase in the respiratory electromyographic (EMG) activity of intercostal muscles (12), with respiratory activity of the diaphragm being little increased or unchanged. The resulting expansion of the rib cage may improve mechanical efficiency of diaphragmatic contraction by optimizing the length or radius of curvature of the diaphragm (13). This increased efficiency of the diaphragm is reflected in an increase in the transdiaphragmatic pressure developed for a given level of diaphragmatic EMG activity.

In contrast, a reduction in rib cage contribution to breathing has been reported during REM sleep compared to wakefulness, due to a marked reduction in intercostal muscle activity (14). Diaphragmatic EMG activity is substantially increased, whereas transdiaphragmatic pressure falls significantly, which implies a decrease in diaphragmatic efficiency, a pattern opposite to that seen during NREM sleep.

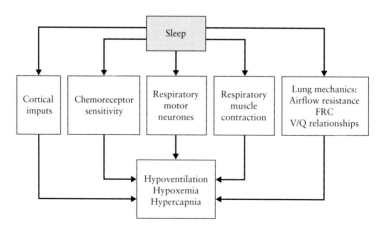

Fig 22.1 *Schematic diagram of the effects of sleep on respiration. In each case, sleep has a negative influence, which has the overall impact of producing hypoventilation with or without hypoxemia and hypercapnia. FRC, Functional residual capacity; V/Q = ventilation-perfusion.*

NEUROMUSCULAR CHANGES DURING SLEEP

The loss of stimulant input from the cerebral cortex is an important contributor to the hypoventilation of sleep described above, but in addition, during REM sleep, a marked loss of tonic activity occurs in the tongue and in the pharyngeal, laryngeal, and intercostal muscles. There appears to be supraspinal inhibition of gamma motoneurons (and to a lesser extent alpha motoneurons), in addition to presynaptic inhibition of afferent terminals from muscle spindles. The diaphragm, being driven almost entirely by alpha motoneurons and, with far fewer spindles than intercostal muscles, has little tonic (postural) activity; therefore, it escapes reduction of this particular drive during REM sleep (5). This helps to explain the increase in abdominal contribution to breathing in REM sleep.

The fall in intercostal muscle activity assumes particular clinical significance in patients who are particularly dependant on accessory muscle activity to maintain ventilation, such as those with COPD (15), since hyperinflation of the lungs results in flattening of the diaphragm and an associated reduction in the efficiency of diaphragmatic contraction. Diaphragmatic efficiency is further compromised by the supine posture since the pressure of abdominal contents against the diaphragm by gravitational forces contrasts with the effect of gravity in the erect posture, which tends to move abdominal contents away from the diaphragm. This pressure impairs diaphragmatic contraction as this moves the diaphragm in a caudal direction to produce lung expansion.

FUNCTIONAL RESIDUAL CAPACITY

A modest, but statistically significant, fall in functional residual capacity (FRC) has been noted in healthy sleeping adults in both NREM and REM sleep (16). This fall is not considered to be sufficient to cause significant ventilation-to-perfusion mismatching in healthy subjects, but it could do so, with resulting hypoxemia, in patients with chronic lung disease (17). Possible mechanisms responsible for this reduction in FRC include respiratory muscle hypotonia, cephalad displacement of the diaphragm, and a decrease in lung compliance (15).

OVERALL EFFECTS DURING SLEEP

The above account illustrates the complex effect of sleep on respiratory function, with the overall trend being a reduction in ventilation compared to wakefulness. In nor-

mal persons, arterial blood gases change little from wakefulness to sleep (7). However, when subjects with daytime hypoxemia due to underlying respiratory disease develop abnormal breathing patterns during sleep, life-threatening hypoxemia may occur (1). This partly results from the fact that a similar drop in PaO_2 will be associated with a much greater drop in SaO_2 when the subject is already hypoxemic and on the steep part of the oxyhemoglobin dissociation curve. Furthermore, the changes in rib cage and abdominal contribution to breathing and the changes in FRC may result in worsening ventilation-perfusion relationships, which will also aggravate any tendency to hypoxemia. In addition, the reduction in ventilatory drive and the changes in breathing pattern during sleep attenuate the compensatory hyperventilation seen during wakefulness in these patients. This effect on ventilation is particularly seen during periods of REM sleep. A schematic outline of the effects of sleep on respiration is given in Figure 22.1.

SLEEP IN COPD

Patients with COPD are adversely affected by sleep in different ways. First, as indicated above, the physiological

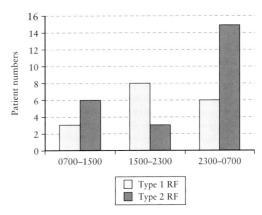

Nocturnal Deaths in COPD

Fig 22.2 Time of death among patients with COPD comparing those with type 1 and type 2 respiratory failure (RF) and demonstrating a significant excess of death at night among those with type 2 failure. (Adapted from McNicholas WT, FitzGerald MX. Nocturnal death among patients with chronic bronchitis and emphysema. B M J 1984; 289:878).

changes that occur during sleep predispose to abnormalities in ventilation and gas exchange. Second, sleep quality is impaired in patients with COPD, which likely represents a significant factor in the complaints of fatigue and lethargy frequently exhibited by these patients.

Sleep-related hypoxemia and hypercapnia are well recognised in COPD, particularly during REM sleep, and may contribute to the development of cor pulmonale (18) and nocturnal death (2). These abnormalities are most common in 'blue-bloater' type patients, who also have a greater degree of awake hypoxemia and hypercapnia than 'pink-puffer' type patients (18). A previous report from this department has demonstrated that patients who die in hospital with an exacerbation of COPD are significantly more likely to die at night, in contrast to patients who die from stroke or neoplasm (2). The excess nocturnal mortality is particularly seen in patients with severe hypoxemia and hypercapnia (Type 2 respiratory failure) (Fig. 22.2). Many patients with awake PaO_2 levels in the mildly hypoxemic range can also develop substantial nocturnal oxygen desaturation, which appears to predispose to the development of pulmonary hypertension (19).

MECHANISMS OF NOCTURNAL OXYGEN DESATURATION IN COPD
Hypoventilation

Studies using noninvasive methods of quantifying respiration have shown clear evidence of hypoventilation, particularly during REM sleep, associated with periods of hypoxemia in patients with COPD (20, 21), but the semi-quantitative nature of these measurements makes it difficult to determine if this is the sole mechanism of oxygen desaturation, or whether other factors are involved. A recent report (22), in which ventilation, SaO_2 and transcutaneous PCO_2 ($PtcCO_2$) were continuously recorded during sleep in a group of patients with severe but stable COPD, demonstrated that falls in SaO_2 were accompanied by a rise in $PtcCO_2$, and REM sleep, in particular, was frequently characterized by irregular, low tidal volume respiration and a high $PtcCO_2$. These observations support hypoventilation as the major cause of nocturnal desaturation in COPD, particularly during REM sleep.

Impact of the Oxyhemoglobin Dissociation Curve

Numerous reports have demonstrated a close relationship between awake PaO_2 and nocturnal SaO_2 levels (21–23),

and it has been proposed that nocturnal oxygen desaturation in patients with COPD is largely the consequence of the combined effects of physiological hypoventilation during sleep and the fact that hypoxemic patients show a proportionately greater fall in SaO_2 with hypoventilation than normoxemic persons, because of the effects of the oxyhemoglobin dissociation curve. However, it has been shown (22) that PaO_2 falls to a greater degree during sleep among patients who show a major degree of nocturnal oxygen desaturation compared to the fall in PaO_2 during sleep among those with minor desaturations, which indicates that the greater fall in SaO_2 during sleep among more severely hypoxemic COPD patients is not simply a consequence of their being on the steep portion of the oxyhemoglobin dissociation curve, and that other factors must also play a part in the blood gas changes observed in these patients during sleep.

Altered Ventilation-Perfusion Relationships

The changes in respiratory muscle function during sleep, particularly the loss of accessory muscle contribution to breathing, also result in a decreased FRC and contribute to worsening ventilation-perfusion relationships during sleep, which also aggravate hypoxemia in COPD (15, 21–23).

Support for a role for ventilation-perfusion disturbances in the pathophysiology of nocturnal oxygen desaturation in COPD comes from the observation that PCO_2 levels rise to a similar extent in those patients who developed major nocturnal oxygen desaturation as in those who developed only a minor degree of desaturation (22), which suggests a similar degree of hypoventilation in both groups, despite the different degrees of nocturnal oxygen desaturation. The much larger fall in PaO_2 among the patients with major desaturation as compared to those with minor desaturation, in conjunction with the similar rise in $PtcCO_2$ in both patient groups, suggests that in addition to a degree of hypoventilation operating in all patients, other factors such as ventilation-perfusion mismatching must also play a part in the excess desaturation of some COPD patients. Nonetheless, awake PaO_2 remains the factor that best predicts a likelihood of nocturnal oxygen desaturation.

Co-existing Sleep Apnea (Overlap Syndrome)

An early study on the mechanisms of nocturnal oxygen desaturation in COPD proposed that nocturnal oxygen desaturation was due to the presence of coexisting OSAS (24). However, this report was flawed by the fact that patients included in that study had been referred because of a clinical suspicion of sleep apnea, and later reports have found sleep apnea in only a minority of patients with COPD who show evidence of nocturnal oxygen desaturation (25). Various reports suggest a prevalence of sleep apnea in patients with COPD of about 10–15% percent (26, 27), which is higher than would be expected in a normal population of similar age. Factors that may predispose to sleep apnea in patients with COPD include impaired respiratory drive, particularly in 'blue-bloater' type COPD patients. Patients with coexisting COPD and sleep apnea are prone to develop episodic profound hypoxemia during sleep because such patients may be hypoxemic at the commencement of each apnea, whereas in patients with isolated sleep apnea resaturation to normal SaO_2 levels tends to occur in between apneas. Therefore, these are patients particularly prone to the complications of chronic hypoxemia, such as corpulmonale and polycythemia (26).

O— **Key points box 22.2**

Mechanisms of nocturnal oxygen desaturation
1. Hypoventilation: most important factor
2. Ventilation-perfusion mismatching
3. Coexisting sleep apnea: in about 12–15% of cases
4. Impact of oxyhemoglobin dissociation curve

CONTRASTS WITH EXERCISE

The mechanisms of hypoxemia during sleep contrast with those during exercise, during which the normal physiological increase in ventilation and in lung volumes during exercise are limited in COPD because of the effects of increased airflow resistance, inadequate ventilatory response, and lack of reduction in dead space. These factors combine to cause relative hypoventilation and ventilation-perfusion disturbances, leading to hypoxemia in some patients (28).

In patients with COPD, desaturation is more than twice as much during sleep than during maximal exercise (22), which contrasts with the findings in patients with interstitial lung disease, who develop greater desaturation during exercise than sleep (29). This greater O_2 desaturation dur-

ing sleep supports the finding (30) that in patients with COPD, the demand for coronary blood flow during episodes of nocturnal hypoxemia can be transiently as great as during maximal exercise. This increased myocardial oxygen demand may be a factor in the nocturnal arrhythmias (31) and in the higher nocturnal death rate among patients with COPD (2), particularly since the level of exercise achieved during these studies was much greater than patients would normally reach during daily activities. Nocturnal oxygen desaturation also appears to be important in the development of pulmonary hypertension, even in the absence of significant awake hypoxemia (32).

SLEEP QUALITY IN COPD

Sleep quality is impaired in patients with COPD (3), which is likely an important factor in the chronic fatigue, lethargy, and overall impairment in quality of life described by these patients (4). Sleep tends to be fragmented, with frequent arousals and diminished amounts of slow wave sleep (SWS) and REM sleep. Unfortunately, sleep impairment is an aspect of COPD that is frequently ignored by many physicians, even in research protocols designed to assess the impact of COPD on quality of life (33–36). This aspect assumes particular importance in the context of assessing the impact of pharmacological therapy on quality of life in patients with COPD (37), since pharmacological agents that improve sleep quality in COPD (38) are likely to have a beneficial clinical impact over and above that simply associated with improvements in lung mechanics and gas exchange, particularly in terms of fatigue and overall energy levels.

O— **Key points box 22.3**

Consequences of nocturnal hypoxemia
1. Cor pulmonale
2. Nocturnal arrhythmias
3. Nocturnal death

INVESTIGATION OF SLEEP-RELATED BREATHING DISTURBANCES IN COPD

The serious and potentially life-threatening disturbances in ventilation and gas exchange that may develop during sleep in patients with COPD raise the question of appropriate investigation of these patients. However, it is widely accepted that sleep studies are not routinely indicated in patients with COPD associated with respiratory insufficiency, particularly since the awake PaO_2 level provides a good indicator of the likelihood of nocturnal oxygen desaturation (17). Sleep studies are only indicated when there is a clinical suspicion of an associated sleep apnea syndrome or manifestations of hypoxemia not explained by the awake PaO_2 level, such as corpulmonale or polycythemia. In most situations in which sleep studies are indicated, a limited study focusing on respiration and gas exchange should be sufficient.

MANAGEMENT OF RESPIRATORY ABNORMALITIES DURING SLEEP IN COPD

A summary of management options for patients with sleep-related breathing problems in COPD is given in Table 22.1. These options can be viewed as a stepwise approach, and in many instances, careful attention to detail with the earlier options such as optimizing the patient's general condition in addition to appropriate use of supplemental oxygen and pharmacological therapy, can obviate more aggressive interventions such as assisted ventilation.

Table 22.1. Management options for COPD patients in respiratory failure

General Measures
- Optimize therapy of underlying condition
- Physiotherapy
- Prompt therapy of infective exacerbations

Supplemental Oxygen
- Low flow to minimize risk of CO_2 retention

Pharmacological therapy
- Theophyllines
- Anticholinergic agents
- Almitrine
- Protriptyline

Assisted ventilation
- Noninvasive by nasal mask

GENERAL PRINCIPLES

The first principle of management should be to optimize the underlying condition, since this will almost invariably have beneficial effects on breathing during sleep. In the case of obstructive airway diseases such as COPD and asthma, optimizing bronchodilator therapy has been shown to improve gas exchange during sleep (38–40). Prompt therapy of infective exacerbations is also important, since these will almost inevitably be associated with worsening of nocturnal oxygen desaturation.

OXYGEN THERAPY

The most serious consequence of hypoventilation, particularly during sleep, is hypoxemia, and appropriate oxygen therapy plays an important part in the management of any disorder associated with respiratory insufficiency during sleep. Care must be taken that correction of hypoxemia is not complicated by hypercapnia in patients with COPD, since respiratory drive in such patients is partly dependent on the stimulant effect of hypoxemia. Therefore, the concentration of added oxygen should be carefully titrated to bring the PaO_2 up into the mildly hypoxemic range to minimize the tendency to CO_2 retention, particularly during sleep.

However, the risk of CO_2 retention with supplemental oxygen therapy in such patients may have been overstated in the past, and there is evidence that CO_2 retention with oxygen supplementation is often modest and usually is nonprogressive (41).

The need for monitoring oxygen levels during sleep in patients with respiratory insufficiency is debatable. Although SaO_2 almost invariably falls during sleep in patients with respiratory insufficiency, the degree of fall is most closely related to the awake SaO_2 levels (21, 17, 41), which indicates that a knowledge of the awake PaO_2 is the most important variable needed to predict the likelihood of nocturnal oxygen desaturation, and it is usually not necessary to record SaO_2 during sleep unless there is a perceived requirement for nocturnal ventilatory support. However, the relationship of awake to sleep SaO_2 is variable, and previous reports have described nocturnal oxygen desaturation in patients without significant awake hypoxemia (18). Therefore, it would be appropriate to monitor nocturnal SaO_2 in patients without significant awake hypoxemia who have complications suggestive of chronic hypoxemia, such as cor pulmonale or polycythemia, since unrecognized nocturnal hypoxemia may be an important factor in the pathogenesis of these complications (18).

The most common methods of low flow oxygen therapy are nasal cannulae and Venturi face masks. Patients requiring long-term oxygen therapy are usually given oxygen via nasal cannulae, but in patients with acute respiratory failure, face masks are often preferred because of the ability to deliver higher concentrations of oxygen and to give better control of the inspired oxygen concentration (FiO_2). However, face masks are less comfortable and are much more likely to become dislodged during sleep than nasal cannulae (42). These factors should be considered when choosing the method of oxygen delivery, and the relative importance of accurate control of FiO_2 and compliance must be determined when selecting the route of oxygen delivery for each patient. Patients with hypercapnic respiratory failure benefit from the more accurate control of FiO_2 provided by face masks, but care must be taken to ensure adequate compliance, since the abrupt withdrawl of oxygen supplementation may result in more severe hypoxemia than prior to supplementation (43). Therefore, patients in this category who tolerate face masks poorly may be better managed by nasal cannulae.

PHARMACOLOGICAL THERAPY
Theophylline

In addition to being a bronchodilator, theophylline has important effects on respiration, which may be beneficial in patients with COPD, including central respiratory stimulation (44) and improved diaphragmatic contractility (45). This agent has been demonstrated to have beneficial effects on nocturnal oxygen saturation and CO_2 levels in COPD (39). The beneficial effect in COPD appears to be mainly due to a reduction in trapped gas volume rather than bronchodilatation. However, the principal limiting effects of theophyllines in this context are adverse effect on sleep quality (39) (which appears to differ from the effects on sleep quality of normal subjects (46)), and the relatively high prevalence of gastrointestinal intolerance.

Anticholinergic agents

Cholinergic tone is increased at night and it has been proposed that this contributes to airflow obstruction and deterioration in gas exchange during sleep in patients with obstructive airways disease. A recent report has demonstrated improvements in both sleep quality and gas exchange in patients with COPD treated with ipratropium (38). The improved sleep quality in this report provides a distinct advantage for anticholinergic agents over theophyllines.

Beta agonists

Only limited data exist on the efficacy of beta agonists in the management of sleep-related breathing abnormalities in COPD. One report found a long-acting theophylline superior to salbutamol in terms of nocturnal gas exchange and overnight fall in spirometry with no difference in effects on sleep quality (47). However, there are no studies of the impact of long-acting beta agonists on sleep and breathing in COPD.

Almitrine

Almitrine is a powerful carotid body agonist, which stimulates ventilation (48). Almitrine also improves ventilation-perfusion relationships within the lung (49, 50), probably by an enhancement of hypoxic pulmonary vasoconstriction. The overall effect is to lessen hypoxemia (51), and the agent is a useful addition in the management of conditions associated with hypoxemia, particularly in COPD patients with type 2 respiratory failure. Important side effects include pulmonary hypertension, dyspnea (presumably due to the respiratory stimulant effect in patients with chronic airflow limitation), and peripheral neuropathy (52). The last-mentioned complication can be minimized by giving the drug on an intermittent basis with a 1 month holiday after each 2 months of active therapy.

Protriptyline

Protriptyline is a tricyclic antidepressant with a number of other effects that may be beneficial in some patients with sleep-related respiratory insufficiency. The most important of these effects is a fragmentation of REM sleep, since sleep-related breathing abnormalities tend to be most severe in this sleep stage, particularly in COPD. Short-term studies have shown a benefit in both awake and sleep blood gas levels in patients with COPD (53), although this benefit may not persist with long-term use of the drug (54). Furthermore, long-term use is significantly limited by side effects, particularly anticholinergic effects. Therefore, despite its theoretical role, this agent is rarely used in the management of sleep-related breathing disturbance in COPD.

NONINVASIVE VENTILATION

Patients with COPD associated with respiratory insufficiency who fail to respond to the above measures should be considered for some form of assisted ventilation. In an acute setting, this may require intubation and ventilation, but over the past decade increasing attention has been directed towards noninvasive methods of ventilatory support, particularly during sleep (55, 56). Long-term noninvasive ventilation can also be considered in COPD patients with chronic respiratory failure. Assisted ventilation is usually confined to sleep if possible, for obvious practical reasons, but beneficial effects on gas exchange during wakefulness have been reported in patients treated with nocturnal ventilatory support (57), in addition to improvements in respiratory muscle strength and endurance (58). An example of the beneficial effect of noninvasive ventilation by nasal intermittent positive pressure ventilation (NIPPV) on oxygenation during sleep in a patient with chronic respiratory failure due to an old thoracoplasty and COPD is given in Figure 22.3.

The past decade has seen the widespread introduction of NIPPV by nasal mask, and this technique has now largely replaced other forms of noninvasive ventilation during sleep, such as negative pressure ventilation (59, 60). NIPPV is dependent on the patient's maintaining exclusive nasal breathing for efficacy, but it is helped by the fact that humans are semi-obligate nose-breathers, particularly during sleep. Some patients do breathe through the mouth while on NIPPV, but this problem can usually be overcome by wearing a chin strap.

Many studies have reported an improvement in daytime blood gas levels respiratory muscle strength with NIPPV (58, 61–63). The mechanism by which NIPPV produces improvements in daytime blood gas values likely involves a number of factors, which include resting of the respiratory muscles (61–63). This resting does not appear to occur with nocturnal negative pressure ventilation in COPD (64). Respiratory muscle fatigue seems to be an important factor in the development of hypercapnia among patients with COPD (65). Other factors that may be important include resetting of respiratory drive, particularly at the chemoreceptor level; in addition improved ventilatory responsiveness to hypercapnia has been demonstrated in COPD after NIPPV (57). A reduc-

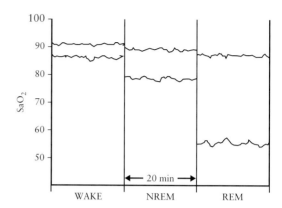

Fig 22.3 *Oxygen saturation levels (SaO$_2$) during sleep before and after nasal intermittent positive pressure ventilation (NIPPV) in a 65 year old man with chronic respiratory failure due to COPD and an old thoracoplasty for tuberculosis. Each section represents 20 min continuous record of SaO$_2$ in each of wakefulness, NREM, and REM sleep. The lower tracings in each panel represent SaO$_2$ levels before NIPPV while the patient was receiving 28% supplemental oxygen by Ventimask. The upper tracings represent the values while on NIPPV in addition to 4 L/min supplemental oxygen through the nasal mask.*

tion in residual volume and in the degree of gas trapping has also been demonstrated with NIPPV, implying a reduction in respiratory load (57). In some cases in which the PaCO$_2$ fails to fall during NIPPV, this failure is due to CO$_2$ rebreathing through the standard exhalation device, and use of an appropriate alternative exhalation device can eliminate the problem (66). Short-term withdrawal of NIPPV for periods of up to 2 weeks may be associated with persistence of the improvement in daytime blood gas levels, but not in night-time gas exchange (67).

Recently, NIPPV has been used successfully in the management of acute exacerbations of COPD associated with respiratory failure and has been shown to reduce the need for intubation and mechanical ventilation in such patients (68). There is also considerable evidence that NIPPV may help patients with COPD who are in chronic respiratory failure (59, 61, 69). Sleep quality and diurnal PaO$_2$ and PaCO$_2$ levels are better with NIPPV plus supplemental oxygen than with supplemental oxygen alone (61). Early studies of NIPPV in patients with stable COPD (69) indicated that the treatment was poorly tolerated, but a more recent report in patients with more severe awake blood gas derangement found that NIPPV was well tolerated by the vast majority of patients (61). One factor that may influence patient acceptance of NIPPV is the length of time spent initiating therapy; compliance may be improved if therapy is commenced as an inpatient.

The reported benefits of NIPPV in severe COPD contrast with the findings from several studies of negative pressure ventilation (70, 71) in COPD, which have failed to show improvements in daytime blood gas values, exercise performance, or quality of life, although other studies have shown benefit (72).

The findings from studies of NIPPV in COPD offer exciting new prospects for the treatment of patients with advanced disease who are in chronic respiratory failure, particularly because of the associated improvements in quality of life and possible improved survival. However, the health care resource implications of this therapy are potentially enormous, particularly because of the common nature of the condition. Although it is clear from the literature that NIPPV will play an increasing role in the management of patients with advanced COPD over the coming years, it is likely that only a subset of patients with advanced COPD will benefit from this therapy. In view of the evolving experience with NIPPV in different patient populations, it is not possible at this time to provide precise patient selection criteria. However, the objective documentation of nocturnal respiratory failure by overnight respiratory monitoring should represent a minimum inclusion criterion, and it is most unlikely that this form of therapy would benefit patients with severe dyspnea without associated hypoxemia. These considerations emphasize the importance of outcome studies that evaluate the efficacy of this therapy in patients with COPD.

REFERENCES

1. Douglas NJ, Calverley PMA, Leggett RJE, et al. Transient hypoxaemia during sleep in chronic bronchitis and emphysema. Lancet 1979; 1:1–4.

2. McNicholas WT, FitzGerald MX. Nocturnal death among patients with chronic bronchitis and emphysema. Br Med J 1984; 289:878.

3. Cormick W, Olson LG, Hensley MJ, et al. Nocturnal hypoxaemia and quality of sleep in patients with chronic obstructive lung disease. Thorax 1986; 41:846–854.

4. Breslin E, Van der Schans C, Breubink S, et al. Perception of fatigue and quality of life in patients with COPD. Chest 1998; 114:958–964.

5. Phillipson EA. Control of breathing during sleep. Am Rev Respir Dis 1978; 118:909–939.

6. Phillipson EA, Duffin J, Cooper JD. Critical dependence of respiratory rhythmicity on metabolic CO_2 load. J Appl Physiol 1981; 50:45–54.

7. Stradling JR, Chadwick GA, Frew AJ. Changes in ventilation and its components in normal subjects during sleep. Thorax 1985; 40:364–370.

8. White DP, Weil JV, Zwillich CW. Metabolic rate and breathing during sleep. J Appl Physiol 1985; 59:384–391.

9. Hudgel DW, Martin RJ, Johnson BJ, et al. Mechanics of the respiratory system and breathing pattern during sleep in normal humans. J Appl Physiol 1984; 56:133–137.

10. Hetzel MR, Clark TJH. Comparison of normal and asthmatic circadian rhythms in peak expiratory flow rate. Thorax 1980; 35:732–738.

11. Sharp JT, Goldberg NB, Druz WS, et al. Relative contributions of rib cage and abdomen to breathing in normal subjects. J Appl Physiol 1975; 39:608–618.

12. Tabachnik E, Muller NL, Bryan AC, et al. Changes in ventilation and chest wall mechanics during sleep in normal adolescents. J Appl Physiol 1981; 51:557–564.

13. Pengelly LD, Alderson AM, Milic-Emili J. Mechanics of the diaphragm. J Appl Physiol 1971; 30:797–805.

14. Tusiewicz K, Moldofsky H, Bryan AC, et al. Mechanics of the ribcage and diaphragm during sleep. J Appl Physiol 1977; 43:600–602.

15. Johnson MW, Remmers JE. Accessory muscle activity during sleep in chronic obstructive pulmonary disease. J Appl Physiol 1984; 57:1011–1017.

16. Hudgel DW, Devadetta P. Decrease in functional residual capacity during sleep in normal humans. J Appl Physiol 1984; 57:1319–1322.

17. Connaughton JJ, Caterall JR, Elton RA, et al. Do sleep studies contribute to the management of patients with severe chronic obstructive pulmonary disease? Am Rev Resp Dis 1988; 138:341–344.

18. DeMarco FJ Jr, Wynne JW, Block AJ, et al. Oxygen desaturation during sleep as a determinant of the "blue and bloated" syndrome. Chest 1981; 79:621–625.

19. Fletcher EC, Luckett RA, Miller T, et al. Pulmonary vascular hemodynamics in chronic lung disease patients with and without oxyhemoglobin desaturation during sleep. Chest 1989; 95:757–766.

20. Martin RJ. The sleep-related worsening of lower airways obstruction: understanding and intervention. Med Clin North Am 1990; 74:701–714.

21. Caterall JR, Calverley PMA, McNee W, et al. Mechanism of transient nocturnal hypoxemia in hypoxic chronic

bronchitis and emphysema. J Appl Physiol 1985; 59: 1698–1703.

22. Mulloy E, McNicholas WT. Ventilation and gas exchange during sleep and exercise in patients with severe COPD. Chest 1996; 109:387–394.

23. Stradling JR, Lane DJ. Nocturnal hypoxaemia in chronic obstructive pulmonary disease. Clin Sci 1983; 64:213–222.

24. Guilleminault C, Cummiskey J, Motta J. Chronic obstructive airflow disease and sleep studies. A Rev Respir Dis 1980; 122:397–406.

25. Catterall JR, Douglas NJ, Calverley PMA, et al. Transient hypoxemia during sleep in chronic obstructive pulmonary disease is not a sleep apnea syndrome. Am Rev Respir Dis 1983; 128:25–29.

26. Chaouat A, Weitzenbum E, Krieger J, et al. Association of chronic obstructive pulmonary disease and sleep apnea syndrome. Am J Respir Crit Care Med 1995; 151:82–86.

27. Bradley TD, Rutherford R, Lue F, et al. Role of diffuse airway obstruction in the hypercapnia of obstructive apnea. Am Rev Respir Dis 1986; 134:920–924.

28. Gallagher CG. Exercise and chronic obstructive pulmonary disease. Med Clin North Am 1990; 74:619–641.

29. Midgren B, Hansson L, Erikkson L, et al. Oxygen desaturation during sleep and exercise in patients with interstitial lung disease. Thorax 1987; 42:353–356.

30. Shepard JW, Schweitzer PK, Kellar CA, et al. Myocardial stress. Exercise versus sleep in patients with COPD. Chest 1984; 86:366–374.

31. Flick MR, Block AJ. Nocturnal vs. diurnal arrhythmias in patients with chronic obstructive pulmonary disease. Chest 1979; 75:8–11.

32. Fletcher EC, Luckett RA, Miller T, et al. Pulmonary vascular hemodynamics in chronic lung disease patients with and without oxyhemoglobin desaturation during sleep. Chest 1989; 95:757–766.

33. Ping-Shin T, McDonnell M, Spertus JA, et al. A new self-administered questionnaire to monitor health-related quality of life in patients with COPD. Chest 1997; 112:614–622.

34. Jones PW, Quirk FH, Baveystock CM, et al. A self-complete measure of health status for chronic airflow limitation. Am Rev Respir Dis 1992; 145:1321–1327.

35. Tsukino M, Nishimura K, Ikeda A, et al. Physiological factors that determine the health-related quality of life in patients with COPD. Chest 1996; 110:896–903.

36. Ketelaars CAJ, Schlosser MAG, Mostert R, et al. Determinants of health-related quality of life in patients with chronic obstructive pulmonary disease, Thorax 1996; 51:29–43.

37. Jones PW, Bosh TK. Quality of life changes in COPD patients treated with salmeterol. Am J Respir Crit Care Med 1997; 155:1283–1289.

38. Martin RJ, Bucher BL, Smith P, et al. Effect of ipratropium bromide treatment on oxygen saturation and sleep quality in COPD. Chest 1999; 115:1338–1345.

39. Mulloy E, McNicholas WT. Theophylline improves gas exchange during rest, exercise and sleep in severe chronic obstructive pulmonary disease. A Rev Respir Dis 1993; 148:1030–1036.

40. Fitzpatrick MF, Mackay T, Driver H, Salmeterol in nocturnal asthma: a double blind placebo controlled trial of a long acting β_2 agonist. Br Med J 1990; 301:1365–1368.

41. Goldstein RS, Ramcharan V, Bowes G, et al. Effects of supplemental oxygen on gas exchange during sleep in patients with severe obstructive lung disease. N Engl J Med 1984; 310:425–429.

42. Costello R, Liston R, McNicholas WT. Compliance at night with low-flow oxygen therapy: a comparison of nasal cannulae and Venturi face masks. Thorax 1995; 50:405–406.

43. West JB. Oxygen therapy. In: Pulmonary pathophysiology Baltimore: Williams & Wilkins; 1977; 169–183.

44. Eldrige FL, Millhorn DE, Waldrop TG, et al. Mechanism of respiratory effects of methylxanthines. Respir Physiol 1983; 53:239–261.

45. Murciano D, Aubier M, Lecocguic Y, et al. Effects of theophylline on diaphragmatic strength and fatigue in patients with chronic obstructive pulmonary disease. N Engl J Med 1984; 311: 349–353.

46. Fitzpatrick MF, Engleman HM, Boellert F, et al., Effect of therapeutic theophylline levels on the sleep quality and daytime cognitive performance of normal subjects. Am Rev Respir Dis 1992; 145:1355–1358.

47. Man GC, Chapman KR, Ali SH, et al. Sleep quality and nocturnal respiratory function with once-daily theophylline (Uniphil) and inhaled salbutamol in patients with COPD. Chest 1996; 110:648–653.

48. Laubie M, Schmitt H. Long-lasting hyperventilation induced by almitrine: evidence for a specific effect on carotid and thoracic chemoreceptors. Eur J Pharmacol 1980; 61:125–136.

49. Simonneau G, Meignan M, Denjean A, et al. Cardiopulmonary effects of a single oral dose of almitrine at rest and on exercise in patients with hypoxic chronic airflow obstruction. Chest 1986; 89:174–179.

50. Reyes A, Roca J, Rodriguez-Roisin R, et al. Effect of almitrine on ventilation-perfusion distribution in adult respiratory distress syndrome. Am Rev Respir Dis 1988; 137:1062–1067.

51. Bell RC, Mullins RC, West LG, et al. The effect of almitrine bismesylate on hypoxaemia in chronic obstructive pulmonary disease. Ann Intern Med 1986; 105:342–346.

52. Howard P. Hypoxia, almitrine, and peripheral neuropathy. Thorax 1989; 44:247–250.

53. Carroll N, Parker RA, Branthwaite MA. The use of protriptyline for respiratory failure in patients with chronic airflow limitation. Eur Respir J 1990; 3:746–751.

54. Series F, Cormier M, LaForge J. Long-term effects of pro-triptyline in patients with chronic obstructive pulmonary disease. Am Rev Respir Dis 1993; 147:1487–1490.

55. Branthwaite MA. Assisted ventilation 6. Non-invasive and domiciliary ventilation: positive pressure techniques. Thorax 1991; 46:208–212.

56. Fauroux B, Howard P, Muir JF. Home treatment for chronic respiratory insufficiency: the situation in Europe in 1992. The European Working Group on Home Treatment for Chronic Respiratory Insufficiency. Eur Respir J 1994; 7:1721–1726.

57. Elliott MW, Mulvey DA, Moxham J, et al. Domiciliary nocturnal nasal intermittent positive pressure ventilation in COPD: mechanisms underlying changes in arterial blood gas tensions. Eur Resp J 1991; 4:1044–1052.

58. Goldstein RS, De Rosie JA, Avendano MA, et al. Influence of noninvasive positive pressure ventilation on inspiratory muscles. Chest 1991; 99:408–415.

59. Waldhorn RE. Nocturnal nasal intermittent positive pressure ventilation with bi-level positive airway pressure (BiPAP) in respiratory failure. Chest 1992; 101:516–521.

60. Elliott MW, Simonds AK, Carroll MP, et al. Domiciliary nocturnal nasal intermittent positive pressure ventilation in hypercapnic respiratory failure due to chronic obstructive lung disease: effects on sleep and quality of life. Thorax 1992; 47:342–348.

61. Meecham Jones DJ, Paul EA, Jones PW, et al. Nasal pressure support ventilation plus oxygen compared with oxygen therapy alone in hypercapnic COPD. Am J Respir Crit Care Med 1995; 152:538–544.

62. Ambrosino N, Nava S, Bertone P, et al. Physiologic evaluation of pressure support ventilation by nasal mask in patients with stable COPD. Chest 1992; 101:385–391.

63. Renston JP, DiMarco AF, Supinski GS. Respiratory muscle rest using nasal BiPAP ventilation in patients with stable severe COPD. Chest 1994; 105:1053–1060.

64. Belman MJ, Soo Hoo GW, Kuei JH, et al. Efficacy of positive vs. negative pressure ventilation in unloading the respiratory muscles. Chest 1990; 98:850–856.

65. Oliven A, Kelsen SG, Deal EC, et al. Mechanisms underlying CO_2 retention during flow-resistive loading in patients with COPD. J Clin Invest 1983; 71:1442–1449.

66. Ferguson GT, Gilmartin M. CO_2 re-breathing during BiPAP ventilatory assistance. Am J Respir Crit Care Med 1995; 151:1126–1135.

67. Masa Jimenez JF, Sanchez de Cos Escuin J, Disdier V C, et al. Nasal intermittent positive pressure ventilation. Analysis of its withdrawal. Chest 1995; 107:382–388.

68. Brochard L, Mancebo J, Wysocki M, et al. Noninvasive ventilation for acute exacerbations of chronic obstructive pulmonary disease. N Engl J Med 1995; 333:817–822.

69. Strumpf DA, Millman RP, Carlisle CC, et al. Nocturnal positive pressure ventilation by nasal mask in patients with severe chronic obstructive pulmonary disease. Am Rev Respir Dis 1991; 144:1234–1239.

70. Celli B, Lee H, Criner G, et al. Controlled trial of external negative pressure ventilation in patients with severe airflow limitation. Am Rev Respir Dis 1989; 140:1251–1256.

71. Shapiro SH, Ernst P, Gray-Donald JG, et al. Effect of negative pressure ventilation in severe chronic obstructive pulmonary disease. Lancet 1992; 340:1425–1429.

72. Cropp A, DiMarco AF. Effects of intermittent negative pressure ventilation on respiratory muscle function in patients with severe chronic obstructive pulmonary disease. Am Rev Respir Dis 1987; 135:1056–1061.

23

SLEEP IN PATIENTS WITH NEUROMUSCULAR AND CHEST WALL DISORDERS

Roger S Goldstein, Dina Brooks, and Lori Davis

INTRODUCTION

For persons with neuromuscular disease (NMD) or thoracic restrictive disease (TRD), sleep far from being a period of tranquillity and recuperation, represents an important physiological challenge that may actually influence the clinical course, stability, and long-term outcome of their conditions. Such patients may be especially vulnerable at night, when the changes in respiratory mechanics and control of breathing observed during sleep among healthy individuals are imposed on a ventilatory system that already has altered respiratory mechanics and control of breathing, either as a primary or as a secondary consequence of underlying disease. The recognition of respiratory changes during sleep is important as it may result in an approach that could reduce morbidity and even mortality for those with nonobstructive respiratory conditions. Management of sleep disorders may result in an improved health-related quality of life and a better functional exercise capacity. Therefore, an assessment of respiratory function during sleep should form part of the clinical evaluation of patients with nonparenchymal restrictive disorders. In this chapter, we describe typical clinical presentations, review the factors underlying the sleep disturbances, and discuss current management strategies.

CLINICAL PRESENTATION

PULMONARY FUNCTION TESTS

The reduced lung volumes associated with NMD and TRD are compounded by the hypoventilation and reduced lung volumes that occur during sleep. In addition, both NMD and TRD result in reductions in respiratory muscle strength and endurance. In patients aged 13 to 62 years with kyphoscoliosis, cardiorespiratory symptoms

occurred when the deformity was greater than 100 degrees by radiological measurement (1). The vital capacity fell to 35% of predicted values, even when such values were predicted on the basis of height (which underestimates the impairment). In our own experience (2) in the vital capacity of 30 patients with kyphoscoliosis and respiratory failure was 27 ± 9% predicted. Our patients also had severe weakness of their respiratory muscles. Their maximum inspiratory pressure was 35 ± 14% predicted and their maximum expiratory pressure was 73 ± 50% predicted. In patients with neuromuscular diseases and reduced respiratory muscle strength, vital capacity was not only reduced but fell further when they changed from the seated to the supine position (3–7).

The relationship between altered pulmonary function and disordered sleep is not a precise one. In patients with amyotrophic lateral sclerosis (ALS), neither forced vital capacity nor negative inspiratory pressure could reliably predict changes in sleep-disordered breathing (8). However, in patients with myasthenia gravis, pulmonary function tests represented an associated risk factor for abnormal breathing during sleep (9).

ARTERIAL BLOOD GASES

As the condition progresses, impaired mechanics are accompanied by altered resting awake arterial gas tensions, with $PaCO_2$ levels of 56–61 mm Hg and PaO_2 levels of 37–70 mm Hg in representative studies (10–13). Not surprisingly, the relationship between altered arterial blood gasvalues and pulmonary function was not precise. A study designed to determine at what level of mechanical impairment respiratory failure was likely to occur evaluated 53 patients with proximal myopathies. The authors reported that hypercapnia occurred when respiratory muscle strength fell below 30% predicted in uncomplicated myopathy and when the vital capacity fell below 55% predicted in those with or without parenchymal involvement (14). Reports that have included measurements of gas exchange during sleep have identified nocturnal falls in SaO_2 and elevations in $PaCO_2$ (2–5). When measurements for non–rapid eye movement sleep (NREM) and REM sleep have been reported separately, $PaCO_2$ has generally been higher throughout REM sleep and SaO_2 has generally been lower. Furthermore, the highest individual $PaCO_2$ and

the lowest SaO_2 values have invariably occurred during REM sleep (Fig. 23.1).

POLYSOMNOGRAPHY

In reports that include full respiratory polysomnographic measurements (2–4, 10), rapid shallow breathing during quiet wakefulness and NREM sleep is a consistent observation in patients with NMD and chest wall disorders (Fig. 23.2). The pattern of breathing in NREM sleep

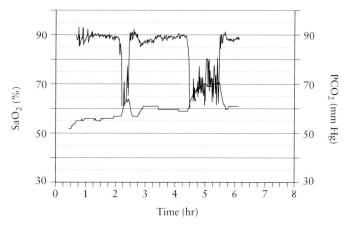

Fig 23.1 *Two channel recording in a patient with muscular dystrophy. Oximetry (upper channel) reflects a stable baseline (88%). During REM sleep, saturation falls and has an oscillating profile. Transcutaneous PCO_2 (lower channel) rises slowly, with the highest values corresponding to REM sleep.*

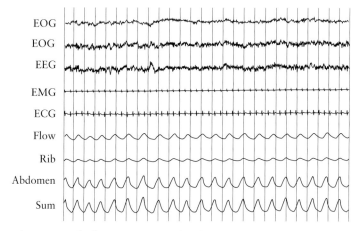

Fig 23.2 *Polysomnograph (60 s epoch) from a patient with ankylosing spondylitis during stage 2 (NREM) sleep shows rapid, shallow breathing (respiratory rate of 24 breaths/min). Channels from top to bottom: Electro-oculogram (EOG); electroencephalogram (EEG); submental electromyogram (EMG); electrocardiogram (ECG); oronasal airflow (flow); excursion of the rib cage (rib), abdomen (abdomen); and their sum (sum).*

becomes more pronounced in REM sleep with a further decrease in rib cage and abdominal excursion, which may result in a fall in saturation. Hypoventilation is sometimes associated with apneic episodes. Although central apneas predominate (Fig. 23.3), both obstructive and mixed apneas have been reported (10, 15). In 10 patients with postpoliomyelitis syndrome, sleep architecture was disrupted by frequent arousals associated with apneas (16). Patients with bulbar involvement had more frequent apneic events than those without bulbar involvement. Irrespective of whether the events were central, obstructive, or mixed, the longest apneas occurred during REM sleep (4, 9).

Sleep disruption may translate into clinical symptoms during the daytime. In a recent review of 17 polysomnograms from patients with ALS, sleep disruption correlated with complaints of orthopnea and daytime sleepiness (8). Similarly, all patients with myasthenia gravis and REM-related respiratory events complained of disturbed sleep as well as breathlessness (9). The natural progression of TRD and NMD to chronic pulmonary hypertension, cor pulmonale, right heart failure, and death may depend at least in part on the severity of the desaturation during sleep. Many reports have documented the development of jugular venous distention, cardiomegaly, leg edema, polycythemia, and pulmonary hypertension during sleep, in addition to symptoms such as morning headaches, hypersomnolence, intellectual dysfunction, and generalized fatigue (6, 8, 12).

⊶ Key points box 23.1

In patients with neuromuscular and chest wall disorders:

- sleep, particularly REM sleep, may be accompanied by marked falls in arterial O_2 saturation and increases in $PaCO_2$.
- apneas, particularly central apneas, are common during sleep and may result in considerable sleep disruption, daytime sleepiness and fatigue.

FACTORS UNDERLYING SLEEP DISTURBANCES IN PATIENTS WITH NEUROMUSCULAR AND CHEST WALL DISORDERS

The factors responsible for sleep-related respiratory dysfunction in patients with NMD and TRD reflect both reductions in alveolar ventilation ($\dot{V}_A$) and regional mismatching of ventilation and perfusion ($\dot{V}/\dot{Q}$). Attempts have been made to correlate the extent of the disturbance in gas exchange during sleep with several indices of respiratory function (4, 8, 9, 17). Broadly, those with the most severe mechanical derangement are likely to have the most disturbed gas exchange. There appears to be lit-

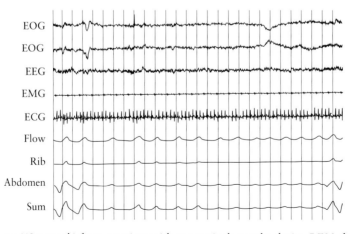

Fig 23.3 *Polysomnogram (60 s epoch) from a patient with myotonic dystrophy during REM sleep shows central hypoventilation. Channels as in Figure 23.2.*

tle predictive value between the degree of thoracic deformity, muscle weakness, results of simple pulmonary function tests, measurements of chemoresponsiveness, and extent to which gas exchange deteriorates during sleep. It is likely that the relationship between daytime respiratory function and nocturnal changes in blood gas tensions will vary, depending at least in part on the cause of the respiratory condition (e.g., generalized NMD, isolated muscle weakness, idiopathic scoliosis) and the extent to which primary or secondary changes in respiratory control have occurred.

TRD and NMD both result in altered ventilatory mechanics and respiratory control. The extent to which such changes occur varies among diagnostic groups, among patients within a particular group, and within a single patient at different times. Gilmartin et al. (6) compared breathing and oxygenation during sleep in patients with myotonic dystrophy and in patients without myotonic dystrophy but with a comparable respiratory muscle weakness. There was a higher frequency of apneas and hypopneas in the myotonic dystrophy group than in the other group, especially in NREM sleep.

Reduced lung volumes is a frequent observation, which if associated with a high closing volume will predispose to peripheral atelectasis and $\dot{V}/\dot{Q}$ mismatching. Decreased compliance of the respiratory system in TRD will increase the work of breathing required of muscles that may themselves be less able to endure the necessary contractile activity because of their architectural distortion and altered length-tension relationships. In NMD, even though the work of breathing may remain normal, the primary involvement of respiratory muscles will reduce their endurance. Reduced expiratory muscle function will impair cough effectiveness and promote secretion retention, further aggravating $\dot{V}/\dot{Q}$ mismatching.

Respiratory control may be affected by the underlying disease, as in bulbar poliomyelitis, or be involved as a consequence of the ongoing sleep disruption or secondary to chronic hypoxemia and hypercapnea. In addition, when the physiological changes of sleep are imposed on the abnormalities of control and ventilatory mechanics that characterize NMD and TRD, changes in $\dot{V}_A$ and in $\dot{V}/\dot{Q}$ ratios will aggravate the blood gas disturbances described above.

Accordingly, a qualitative 'equation' can be written in schematic terms that describes the interaction between the pathophysiological elements of restrictive ventilatory disease and the physiological elements of REM sleep. Although the relative importance of each of these interactions will vary, Figure 23.4 summarizes some of the important changes that occur. On the left panel are changes in respiratory drive and mechanics that are a consequence of diseases that result in restrictive ventilatory failure, and on the right panel are changes in respiratory drive and mechanics that have been described in healthy persons during REM sleep. The summation of these two panels results in physiological consequences shown to the right. It is by means of these physiological consequences that arterial blood gases deteriorate further.

RESPIRATORY DRIVE

During REM sleep there is a reduction in overall central neural output, resulting in hypopneas and occasionally in central apneas (18). In the healthy person, these transient reductions in ventilation are of little clinical importance. In contrast, for patients with restrictive ventilatory failure, in whom alveolar ventilation may be compromised, a further reduction in breathing will produce a marked decrement in alveolar ventilation. Moreover, because of the inverse hyperbolic relationship between $\dot{V}_A$ and $PaCO_2$ (19), a small decrease in $\dot{V}_A$ in patients who are already hypercapnic while awake may result in a greater change in CO_2 tension than would a comparable decrease in $\dot{V}_A$ in healthy subjects. For the same decrement in arterial oxygen tension, patients who already have a reduced PaO_2 will experience more profound desaturation because they are operating on the steeper part of the oxyhemoglobin dissociation curve. Another characteristic feature of REM sleep is that of rapid, shallow, and irregular respiration when compared with NREM sleep or quiet wakefulness. As these effects are imposed on the rapid, shallow pattern of breathing associated with ventilatory restriction, the resulting increase in dead space ventilation is likely to further reduce effective alveolar ventilation. Finally, because ventilatory responses to hypoxia, hypercapnia, and elastic loads may be blunted in patients with restrictive disease, the superimposed decrement in chemoresponsiveness and load compensation that may occur in REM sleep may leave the patient with little ability to respond to the additional asphyxic stimuli that accumulate during periods of reduced alveolar ventilation, thereby prolonging the duration of such events.

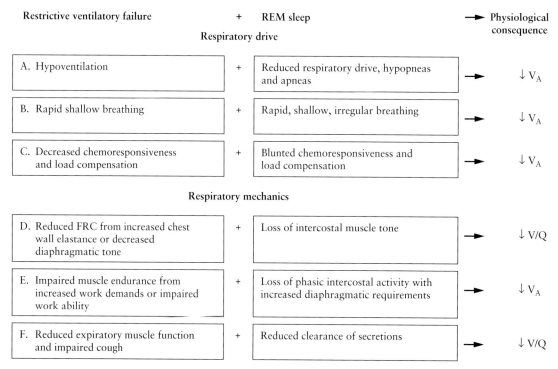

Fig 23.4 *Schematic equation that describes changes in respiratory drive and mechanics that occur when restrictive ventilatory failure and REM sleep are combined. The physiological consequences that result are shown on the right side of the figure.*

VENTILATORY MECHANICS

In healthy persons there is a decrease in the contribution of the rib cage excursion to breathing during REM sleep, reflecting the decreased contribution of the intercostal muscles. Tidal volume is maintained by a compensatory increase in diaphragm activity (20, 21). In subjects with restrictive ventilatory failure, the diaphragm may be distorted consequent on changes in thoracic architecture, or it may be involved primarily in the underlying neuromuscular process. Therefore, the diaphragm may be unable to increase its contribution to respiration in response to the inhibition of phasic intercostal and accessory muscle function that occurs during REM sleep. Any attempt to increase diaphragmatic activity may aggravate a situation of 'chronic dysfunction,' which has been hypothesized to occur as a consequence of increased work of breathing or of decreased muscular ability. Thus, there is a further reduction in tidal volume and a further reduction of $\dot{V}_A$. Of additional importance is that the decrease in the rest-ing tone of the intercostal and accessory muscles during REM sleep may reduce the functional residual capacity (FRC). In such patients, the FRC is already below the closing volume. Therefore, the mismatching between ventilation and perfusion is further increased. Although the muscle hypotonia of REM may also increase upper airway resistance, respiratory load compensation is impaired during REM and therefore ventilation may be reduced. If (as is often the case) the work of breathing is already increased, the imposition of increased upper airway resistance will result in a marked reduction in alveolar ventilation.

The cough reflex is normally depressed during REM sleep, and mucous clearance is impaired. As a result of this impairment there may be an excessive accumulation of airway secretions in subjects in whom the cough reflex has already been impaired by dysfunction of expiratory muscles. The resultant regional V/Q mismatching will further influence gas exchange.

Respiratory changes in TRD, NMD and REM sleep
- Sleep-related respiratory dysfunction in patients with neuromuscular and chest wall disorders is related to the interaction between the underlying pathophysiological features of the disease and the physiological events of sleep, particularly REM sleep.
- These events include reductions in central respiratory drive, a rapid and shallow pattern of breathing, decreased ventilatory chemoresponses, reduced intercostal muscle activation, and a depressed cough reflex.

MANAGEMENT OF SLEEP DISORDERS

Patients who develop sleep-related disturbance may have a variety of signs and symptoms, such as nocturnal restlessness, frequent awakening, snoring, daytime sleepiness, fatigue, or headaches. Polysomnography is helpful in distinguishing among the different types of sleep disturbances and in assessing their severity.

The management of hypoventilation is based on the premise that preventing further reductions in alveolar ventilation during sleep will result in an improvement in nighttime and subsequently daytime arterial blood gases, a reduction in pulmonary hypertension and cor pulmonale, and the prevention of premature death. It is important to note that to date there have been no prospective randomized controlled trials regarding the management of respiratory failure in such patients. Nevertheless, compelling clinical evidence suggests that elective mechanical ventilatory support, preferably with a noninvasive technique, is effective in achieving the above goals.

Oxygen alone, although preventing the nocturnal desaturation, often results in unacceptably high levels of $PaCO_2$ (Fig. 23.5 A, B). Diuretics and tracheostomy alone (1), although providing a temporary improvement, will at best delay the need for mechanical ventilatory support (Fig. 23.6 A, B).

EFFECTIVENESS OF MECHANICAL VENTILATION

The idea that ongoing ventilatory support can improve the status of patients with respiratory failure is not new. Weirs et al. (22) tailored cuirass shells to fit four patients with TRD who subsequently returned home, having recovered from acute respiratory failure. Garray et al. (23) described eight patients in whom noninvasive ventilation was maintained at home for 11 ± 3.5 years, and in whom sustained improvements in arterial blood gases were associated with a return to a productive lifestyle. Curran (24) reported the effectiveness of nighttime support in improving gas exchange and allowing for a higher level of independence among patients with late stage Duchenne muscular dystrophy.

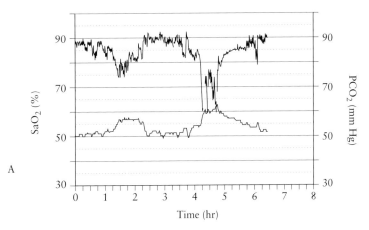

A

Fig 23.5A

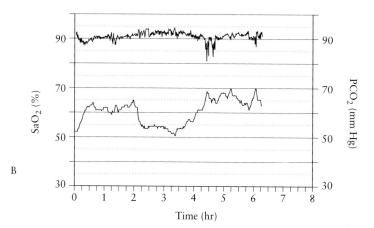

Fig 23.5 *Two channel recording in a patient with kyphoscoliosis (vital capacity 35% predicted, total lung capacity 52% predicted). Channels as in Figure 23.1. A, Patient is breathing room air. Note desaturation (mean SaO$_2$ 83%, range 48–94%) and elevated transcutaneous PCO$_2$ (mean PCO$_2$ 54 mm Hg, range 49–63 mm Hg). B, Patient is receiving supplemental oxygen at 1 L/min via nasal prongs. Note saturation has improved (mean SaO$_2$ 91%, range 79–95%), but transcutaneous PCO$_2$ is substantially higher (mean PCO$_2$ 60 mm Hg, range 50–70 mm Hg).*

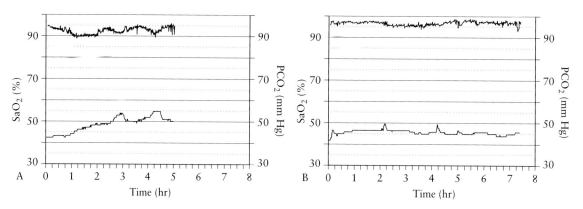

Fig 23.6 *Two channel recording in a patient with olivoponto cerebellar degeneration breathing room air. Channels as in Figure 23.1. A, Saturation is adequate but the PCO$_2$ increases gradually through the night. B, After a tracheostomy for vocal cord dysfunction, patient is breathing spontaneously through an uncuffed, nonfenestrated tracheostomy tube. Note good saturation and reduced stable PCO$_2$.*

Home mechanical ventilation has been defined as 'the longer term application of ventilatory support to patients who are no longer in acute respiratory failure and do not need the sophistication of an intensive care setting' (25). A task force of the American College of Chest Physicians identified the goals of long-term mechanical ventilation as increasing longevity, decreasing morbidity, enhancing quality of life, and maximizing the cost effectiveness of medical care (26).

Patients do succumb to the chronic respiratory insufficiency associated with advanced NMD or TRD (27, 28). Mechanical ventilation can improve their survival. In

1983, Splaingard et al. (29) reviewed 26 adults and 21 children discharged from hospital with tracheostomies and positive pressure ventilators. The patients had either severe restrictive NMD, had thoracic deformity, or reduced ventilatory drive during sleep. The 3 year survival was 74% for patients without spinal cord injury and 63% for those with spinal cord injury. The same authors reported their experience with negative pressure ventilation in the home (30). The survival of 40 adults with NMD who received nighttime ventilatory support with tank respirators was 76% and 61% at 5 and 10 years, respectively. Complications were minor and occurred at a rate of less than one per year per patient. A shorter term study in 51 patients with respiratory failure secondary to TRD or NMD revealed a two year survival of 90% (31). All but 10 patients were treated with negative pressure ventilation. In general, these patients demonstrated a sustained improvement in symptoms, arterial blood gases, breathlessness, and exercise tolerance as well as a low rate of hospital admission. Their outcomes were independent of the severity or the duration of their respiratory failure.

Leger et al. (32) reported on 276 patients with multiple causations of NMD who received nasal intermittent positive pressure ventilation (NIPPV) for up to 5 years. Improvements in gas exchange and in the number of days in hospital were observed, especially among patients with

kyphoscoliosis and those with posttuberculosis sequelae. Bach and Tilton (33) reported that patients with ALS survived a mean of 4.4 years using noninvasive IPPV. Thirty-seven of 89 patients were still alive at the completion of the study. Simonds and Elliott (34) examined the 5 year survival of 180 patients who received (NIPPV). Their hypercapneic respiratory failure was attributed to chest wall restriction, NMD, or chronic obstructive pulmonary disease. Their 5 year survival was 70% for early-onset scoliosis, 100% for previous poliomyelitis, and 82% for NMD.

CHOICE OF MECHANICAL SUPPORT

If a patient has previously required prolonged ventilation and has a tracheostomy in place, IPPV using a portable volume-cycled pressure-limited ventilator may be the most immediately effective treatment (Fig. 23.7). However, the management of a tracheostomy at home presents psychological and medical problems in addition to the patient and caregiver being taught tracheostomy care. Therefore, decannulation is always considered before a tracheostomy is regarded as permanent. If ventilation is initiated electively, more options are available. Patients may try various mechanical ventilatory support systems and choose the one that is most comfortable as well as appropriate to their home environment.

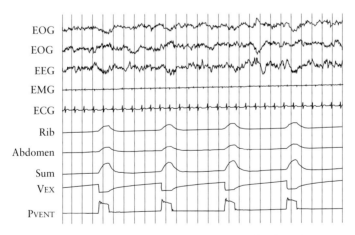

Fig 23.7 Polysomnogram (30 s epoch) from a patient with kyphoscoliosis and asthma during stage 3 (NREM) sleep. Patient is being ventilated through a Bivona 6.5 cm cuffed tracheostomy tube attached to a volume cycled ventilator with a tidal volume of 450 ml and a respiratory rate of 12 breaths/min. Mean SaO$_2$ is 98%, mean PCO$_2$ is 48 mm Hg. Channels as in Figure 23.2 plus the addition of the measured exhaled volume (V$_{EX}$) and the ventilating pressure (P$_{vent}$).

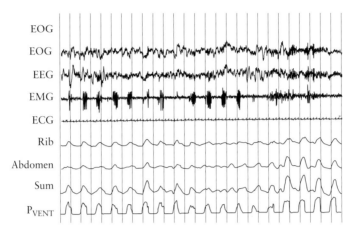

Fig 23.8 *Polysomnogram (60 s epoch) from a patient with kyphoscoliosis. The patient is ventilated noninvasively using a volume cycled ventilator with a nasal mask. The tidal volume is 620 ml and the respiratory rate is 20 breaths/min.*

Negative pressure ventilation can be very effective, although the large size, the weight, and the lack of maneuverability of the tank may be a deterrent for some patients. The poncho and cuirass both require considerable adjustment and depend for their effectiveness on a reasonable chest configuration. The complication of upper airway obstruction can be managed successfully with a tricyclic medication or with nasal continuous positive airway pressure (CPAP) (35, 36).

NIPPV has enabled many patients to return to the community (5, 11, 13, 35–38). A close-fitting face mask will reduce leakage (Fig. 23.8). However, some air does leak through the mouth during sleep when nasal pressure-limited systems are used (39). This air leakage occurs more frequently in slow-wave sleep and results in sleep fragmentation (37, 39). The improvements in nighttime saturation, and daytime arterial blood gases and the decreased risk of pulmonary complications still occur despite varying degrees of insufflation leakage (37).

EFFECT OF MECHANICAL VENTILATION ON PHYSIOLOGICAL VARIABLES

A number of reports (5, 10–13, 35–38) have documented the reversal of sleep-induced hypoventilation and chronic respiratory failure among patients with restrictive ventilatory impairments by the use of elective nocturnal mechanical ventilatory support. Studies that have included detailed measurements of saturation and CO_2 tension during sleep have shown such values to be markedly improved during mechanical ventilation compared with a control (unassisted) night.

The mechanisms by which patients improve are likely to include resting the respiratory muscles, decreasing their metabolic demand, resetting chemoreceptors, expanding areas of atelectasis, improving the ventilation-perfusion ratio, assisting inspiratory muscle function, and increasing lung compliance (37).

A reduction in diaphragmatic and accessory muscle electromyographic (EMG) activity during assisted ventilation has been demonstrated in healthy volunteers (15, 40), negative pressure ventilation (11, 15), and positive pressure ventilation (40). It has been postulated that the beneficial effects of ventilatory support may be mediated by a reduction in inspiratory muscle work. Conceivably, inspiratory muscles are in a state of 'chronic dysfunction' as a result of either increased work or decreased endurance consequent on their primary or secondary involvement with the disease process. Inspiratory muscle endurance is reduced by hypoxia (41), and therefore improved muscle endurance is to be expected consequent upon an improvement in nocturnal SaO_2. One study (36) observed an improvement in measured inspiratory muscle endurance from 7.1 ± 3.4 min at baseline to 14.8 ± 7.6 min at 3 months after nightly assisted ventilation.

The influence of mechanical ventilation on respiratory muscle strength and lung volumes is less clear, with slight increases being reported by some authors (10, 42) and no improvement by others (11, 36).

Nocturnal ventilation should prevent the decreased compliance associated with hypoventilation (1), thereby decreasing the daytime work of breathing and reducing the demands made on the inspiratory muscles. Alternatively, improved nocturnal blood gases could result in a resetting of respiratory control with an increase in chemosensitivity and a reduction in the body bicarbonate pool. Any nocturnal increase in $PaCO_2$ would then be accompanied by a more appropriate response in minute ventilation. Although a decrease in ventilatory response to CO_2 has been documented in patients with alveolar hypoventilation, there is limited information regarding chemoresponsiveness in such circumstances (35).

Clinical Sequelae of Mechanical Ventilation

Although the precise mechanisms by which patients improve remain to be defined, clinical reports have consistently observed that nocturnal ventilatory support improved nocturnal gas exchange (5, 11, 35–37). Subsequently daytime arterial blood gas tensions returned toward normal values within 4–6 weeks. These changes are associated with a reduction in hemoglobin (12), a reduction in pulmonary hypertension (23), an improvement in daytime exercise tolerance (11, 36), and level of functioning. Patients who had been previously disabled by profound dyspnea, sleep fragmentation, cor pulmonale, and unstable respiratory failure have in many instances returned to full-time activities (11, 12, 36). In a longer term study, eight patients with NMD received 18 months of NIPPV. They maintained normal daytime arterial blood gases and had improved nocturnal respiratory events and better sleep quality (43).

Although an extensive literature now exists demonstrating the improvement in daytime function after long-term nocturnal ventilation, there is less information on the influence of subsequently withdrawing the ventilator on unassisted breathing during sleep. If the ventilator is withdrawn, nocturnal gas exchange deteriorates even after a prolonged period of stability. Garray et al., (23) withdrew ventilatory support for 2 weeks in eight patients after a 1 year period of nightly use. Within 2 weeks, nighttime gas exchange had deteriorated, as had daytime arterial blood gas values. Symptoms

such as morning headaches, daytime drowsiness, and generalized fatigue returned. These changes were reversed by the resumption of nocturnal ventilatory assistance. Piper and Sullivan (44) noted improved respiratory muscle function, respiratory drive during sleep, and wakefulness and arousal responses in 14 patients after 6 months of nasal ventilatory support. In the absence of support, blood gases during sleep remained abnormal.

Mechanical ventilation may also have a positive effect on health-related quality of life. This term refers to a patient's perception of performance in at least one of four important domains: somatic sensation, physical function, emotional state, and social interaction (45, 46). Such measures provide evidence of the effects of ventilatory support other than physiological measures of impairment and disability.

In the absence of specific measures designed for patients who are mechanically ventilated, life satisfaction scales as well as general instruments such as the Sickness Impact Profile have been used (33, 47–51).

In addition, the user perspectives among the diverse group of patients who receive home mechanical ventilation have been assessed (52). This information can be derived from open-ended interviewer administered questionnaires. Responses have shown that ventilator users adapt well to ongoing ventilatory support and recognize the positive impact of such support on their lives.

⚷ Key points box 23.3

Managing respiratory failure in TRD and NMD

- Patients with neuromuscular or chest wall disorders, nocturnal restlessness, daytime fatigue and sleepiness, or morning headache should undergo overnight polysomnography.

- The management of such patients is aimed at preventing further reductions in alveolar ventilation during sleep, which can be best achieved by mechanical ventilatory assistance.

- Mechanical ventilatory support at night usually results in improved daytime blood gas values, exercise tolerance, and quality of life.

CONCLUSIONS

In patients with restrictive ventilatory failure, the worst arterial blood gases are to be found during sleep, especially during REM sleep. Although supplemental oxygen will temporarily improve oxygen saturation, mechanical ventilatory support is a more effective treatment. It is preferable to introduce it electively and to use a noninvasive system when possible. Nocturnal ventilatory support reduces respiratory events during sleep, improves daytime arterial blood gas values, and increases functional exercise capacity. Since well-ventilated patients spend less time in hospital, this treatment approach is also cost effective. If the ventilator is withdrawn, even after a prolonged period of stabilization, the arterial blood gases deteriorate. Therefore, assisted ventilation should be maintained on an ongoing basis.

REFERENCES

1. Bergofsky EH. Respiratory failure in disorders of the thoracic cage. Am Rev Resp Dis 1979; 119:643–669.

2. Goldstein RS, Molotiu N, Skrastins R, et al. Reversal of sleep induced hypoventilation and chronic respiratory failure by nocturnal negative pressure ventilation in patients with restrictive ventilatory impairment. Am Rev Respir Dis 1987; 135:1049–1055.

3. Ellis ER, Bye PTP, Bruderer JW, et al. Treatment of respiratory failure during sleep in patients with neuromuscular disease. Am Rev Respir Dis 1987; 135: 148–152.

4. Mezon BL, West P, Israels J, et al. Sleep breathing abnormalities in kyphoscoliosis. Am Rev Respir Dis 1980; 122–617–621.

5. Bach JR, Alber AS. Management of chronic alveolar hypoventilation by nasal ventilation. Chest 1990; 97: 52–57.

6. Gilmartin JJ, Cooper BG, Griffiths CJ, et al. Breathing during sleep in patients with myotonic dystrohy and nonmyotonic respiratory muscle weakness. Q J Med 1991; 78: 21–31.

7. Finnimore AJ, Jackson RV, Morton A, et al. Sleep hypoxia in myotonic dystrophy and its correlation with awake and respiratory function. Thorax 1994; 49:66–70.

8. David WS, Bundlie SR, Madhavi Z. Polysomnographic studies in amyotrophic lateral sclerosis. J Neurol Sci 1997; 152:S29–S35.

9. Quera-Salva MA, Guilleminault C, Chevret S, et al. Breathing disorders during sleep in myasthenia gravis. Ann Neurol 1992; 31:86–92.

10. Ellis ER, Grunstein RR, Chan S, et al. Non invasive ventilatory support during sleep improves respiratory failure in kyphoscoliosis. Chest 1988; 984: 811–815.

11. Goldstein RS, Avendano MA, De Rosie JA, et al. Influence of non-invasive positive pressure ventilation on inspiratory muscles. Chest 1991; 99:408–415.

12. Hoeppner VH, Cockroft DW, Dosman JA, et al. Nighttime ventilation improves respiratory failure in secondary kyphoscoliosis. Am Rev Respir Dis 1984; 129: 240–243.

13. Kirby GR, Mayer LS, Pingleton SK. Nocturnal positive pressure ventilation via nasal mask. Am Rev Respir Dis 1987; 135:738–740.

14. Braun NMT, Aurora NS, Rochester DF. Respiratory muscle and pulmonary function in polymyositis and other proximal myopathies. Thorax 1983; 38:316–323.

15. Guilleminault C, Kurlund G, Winkle R, et al. Severe kyphoscoliosis—breathing and sleep. Chest 1981; 79:626–630.

16. Dean AC, Graham BA, Dalakas M. Sleep apnea in patients with postpolio syndrome. Ann Neurol 1998; 43: 661–664.

17. Newsom Davis J, Goldman M, Loh L, et al. Diaphragm function and alveolar hypoventilation. Q J Med 1976; 177: 87–100.

18. Phillipson EA. Control of breathing during sleep. Am Rev Respir Dis 1978; 118:909–939.

19. Otis AB. Quantitative relationships in steady-state gas exchange. In: Fenn WO Rahn, eds. Handbook of physiology (section 3). Respiration (vol. 1). Washington, DC.: American Physiological Society; 1964, 681–698.

20. Stradling JR, Chadwick GA, Frew AJ. Changes in ventilation and its components in normal subjects during sleep. Thorax 1985; 40:364–370.

21. Tabachnik E, Muller NL, Brian AC, et al. Changes in ventilation in chest wall mechanics during sleep in normal adolescents. J Appl Physiol 1981; 51:557–564.

22. Weirs PWJ, Le Coultre R, Dallinga OT, et al. Cuirass respirator treatment of chronic respiratory failure in scoliotic patients. Thorax 1977; 32:221–228.

23. Garray SM, Turino GM, Goldring RM. Sustained reversal of chronic hypercapnia in patients with alveolar hypoventilation syndromes. Long-term maintenance with non-invasive nocturnal mechanical ventilation. Am J Med 1981; 70:269–274.

24. Curran FJ. Night ventilation by body respirators for patients in chronic respiratory failure due to late stage Duchenne muscular dystrophy. Arch Phys Med Rehabil 1981; 270–274.

25. Muir J-F. Home mechanical ventilation. In: Simond AK, Muir J-F, Person DJ, eds. Pulmonary rehabilitation, London: BMJ Publishing Group; 1996.

26. O'Donahue WJ, Giovannoni RM, Goldberg AI, et al. Long-term mechanical ventilation. Guidelines for management in the home and at alternate community sites. Report of the Ad Hoc Committee, Respiratory Care Section, ACCP. Chest 1986; 90(Suppl):1–37.

27. Vianelloe A, Bevilacqua M, Salvador V, et al. Long-term nasal intermittent positive pressure ventilation in advanced Duchenne's muscular dystrophy. Chest 1994; 105:445–448.

28. Pehrsson K, Larsson S, Oden A, et al. Long-term follow-up of patients with untreated scoliosis. A study of mortality, causes of death, and symptoms. Spine 1992; 17:1091–1096.

29. Splaingard ML, Frates RC, Harrison GM, et al. Home positive pressure ventilation—20 years experience. Chest 1983; 84:276–282.

30. Splaingard ML, Frates RC, Jefferson LS, et al. Home negative pressure ventilation: Report of 20 Years of experience in patients with neuromuscular disease. Arch Phys Med Rehabil 1985; 66:239–242.

31. Sawicka EH, Loh L, Branthwaite. Domiciliary ventilatory support: an analysis of outcome. Thorax 1988; 43: 31–35.

32. Leger P, Jennequin J, Gerard M, et al. Home ventilation via nasal mask for patients with neuromuscular weakness or restrictive lung or chest-wall disease. Respir Care 1989; 34:73–77.

33. Bach JR, Tilton MC. Life satisfaction and well-being measures in ventilator assisted individuals with traumatic tetraplegia. Arch Phys Med Rehabil 1994; 75: 626–632.

34. Simonds AK, Elliott MW. Outcome of domiciliary nasal intermittent positive pressure ventilation in restrictive and obstructive disorders. Thorax 1995; 50:604–609.

35. Ellis ER, McCauley VB, Mellis C, et al. The treatment of alveolar hypoventilation in a 6 year-old girl with intermittent positive pressure ventilation through a nose mask. Am Rev Respir Dis 1987; 136:188–191.

36. Goldstein RS, Molotiu N, Skrastins R, et al. Assisting ventilation in respiratory failure by negative pressure ventilation and by rocking bed. Chest 1987; 92:470–474.

37. Bach JR, Robert D, Leger P, et al. Sleep fragmentation in kyphoscoliotic individuals with alveolar hypoventilation treated by NIPPV. Chest 1995; 107: 1552–1558.

38. Carroll N, Branthwaite MA. Intermittent positive pressure ventilation by nasal mask: technique and applications. Intens Care Med 1988; 14:115–117.

39. Meyer TJ, Pressman MR, Benditt J, et al. Air leaking through the mouth during nocturnal nasal ventilation: effect on sleep quality. Sleep 1997; 20:561–569.

40. Carrey Z, Gottfried S, Levy R. Ventilatory muscle support in respiratory failure with nasal positive pressure ventilation. Chest 1990; 97:15–58.

41. Jardim J, Farkas G, Prefaut C, et al. The failing inspiratory muscles under normoxic and hypoxic conditions. Am Rev Respir Dis 1981; 124:274–279.

42. Marino W, Braun NMT. Reversal of the clinical sequelae of respiratory muscle fatigue by intermittent mechanical ventilation. Am Rev Respir Dis 1982; 125:85.

43. Barbe F, Quera-Salva MA, de Lattre J, et al. Long-term effects of nasal intermittent positive-pressure ventilation on pulmonary function and sleep architecture in patients with neuromuscular diseases. Chest 1996; 110:1179–1183.

44. Piper AJ, Sulivan CE. Effects of long-term nocturnal nasal ventilation on spontaneous breathing during sleep in neuromuscular and chest wall disorders. Eur Respir J 1996; 9:1515–1522.

45. Guyatt GH, Feeny DH, Patrick DL. Measuring health-related quality of life. Ann intern Med 1993; 118: 622–629.

46. Lacasse Y, Wong E, Guyatt G, et al. Health status measurement instruments in chronic obstructive pulmonary disease. Can Respir J 1997; 4:152–164.

47. Bach JR, Campagnolo DI, Hoeman S. Life satisfaction of individuals with Duchenne muscular dystrophy using long-term mechanical ventilatory support. Am J Phys Med Rehabil 1991; 70:129–135.

48. Bach JR, Campagnolo DI. Psychosocial adjustment of post-poliomyelitis ventilator assisted individuals. Arch Phys Med Rehabil 1992; 73:934–939.

49. Gelinas DF, O'Connor P, Miller RG. Quality of life for ventilator-dependent ALS patients and their caregivers. J Neurol Sci 1998; 160(Suppl 1): S134–S136.

50. Janssens J-P, Penalosa B, Degive C, et al. Quality of life of patients under home mechanical ventilation for restrictive lung diseases: a comparative evaluation with COPD patients. Monaldi Arch Chest Dis 1996; 51:178–184.

51. Pehrsson K, Olofson J, Larsson S, et al. Quality of life of patients treated by home mechanical ventilation due to restrictive ventilatory disorders. Respir Med 1994; 88:21–26.

52. Goldstein RS, Psek JA, Gort EH. Home mechanical ventilation: demographics and users perspectives. Chest 1995; 108:1581–1586.

24

SLEEP IN CYSTIC FIBROSIS, INTERSTITIAL LUNG DISEASE, AND OTHER RESPIRATORY DISORDERS

Peter M A Calverley

INTRODUCTION

As has already been detailed in other chapters of this book, the onset of sleep poses specific problems for the maintenance of normal gas exchange and alveolar ventilation. Additionally, sleep modifies the physiological response to stimuli such as increased arterial CO_2 tensions and increased respiratory impedance, which usually provoke compensatory consciousness-related modifications in respiratory center output and timing. Secondarily, many respiratory diseases can themselves disrupt the subject's ability to initiate sleep or maintain it, especially when further alterations in lung mechanics occur during established sleep. It is not surprising that sleep disruption and daytime fatigue are concomitant nonspecific complaints in many respiratory illnesses.

SLEEP AND RESPIRATORY DISORDERS

Despite the range of different pathologies producing impairments in the respiratory system, their effects on sleep are relatively stereotyped and largely reflect the altered respiratory physiology produced by day rather than any specific sleep-modifying effect of the individual disease. Among these are impairments of upper airway function secondary to specific pathology, which can be as varied as laryngeal tumors and amyloid deposition in the pharynx related to pulmonary sepsis. The pathophysiology of these processes together with the much commoner causes of upper airway dysfunction have been discussed in other chapters. Disordered or inappropriate respiratory control can induce significant problems as a consequence of sleep-related events. Thus, patients with central alveolar hypoventilation can have features of daytime central cyanosis and peripheral edema, which can be corrected by nocturnal positive pressure ventilation.

Conversely, an intact chemoreceptor response to persistent hypoxia can produce sustained hypocapnia at altitude, sleep disruption, headaches, and acute mountain sickness. Both aspects of this form of respiratory dysfunction have been reviewed in other chapters of this book.

LOWER RESPIRATORY TRACT DISORDERS

Most respiratory diseases affect the lower respiratory tract and, surprisingly, systematic studies of sleep disturbance are lacking even in a number of common conditions, usually because sleep-related symptoms are attributed to secondary changes associated with the primary illness. Thus, bronchial tumors can develop in large or small airways, presenting in a variety of ways. These include hemoptysis, lung collapse, or distant spread but are not associated with specific sleep complaints until the terminal stage of the illness, when the effects of cachexia and opiate-related drug treatment disrupt normal sleep rhythms. The same appears to be true for processes such as pleural effusions of whatever cause and for many immunologically mediated lung disease with limited physiological impact. Some illnesses, such as acute pneumonia and especially pulmonary tuberculosis and lung abscesses, are associated with persistent febrile responses, which promote sleep inappropriately. These are briefly considered below.

The most important physiological responses to chronic lung damage are the development of airflow limitation, so-called obstructive lung disorders, and the development of reduced pulmonary or chest wall compliance, characterized by a restrictive physiological defect. Chronic obstructive pulmonary disease and bronchial asthma have been reviewed elsewhere in this book, but the problems of patients with cystic fibrosis are considered here as a number of features of this illness have been examined specifically in sleep-related investigations. Likewise, a limited amount of data are available about the effects of interstitial lung disease that produces restrictive physiological problems due to pulmonary fibrosis reducing lung compliance.

SLEEP AND FEVER

Febrile responses are characteristic of patients with bacterial lobar pneumonia, atypical pneumonic illnesses secondary to agents such as Mycoplasma and Chlamydia pneumoniae and viral illnesses such as influenza. The body temperature usually fluctuates significantly and has peaks ranging from 39–40° C with periods of normal body temperature between times. Consciousness is often impaired, with relatively brief periods of unrefreshing sleep being characteristic. In contrast, infections with pulmonary tuberculosis are associated with a persistent lower grade pyrexia often accompanied by nighttime sweating attacks (1). No objective measurements of sleep quality or daytime sleepiness have been made in these illnesses.

The biochemical basis underlying febrile responses is now better characterized. A number of specific cytokines including interleukin-1 (IL-1) and tumor necrosis factor (TNF) interact with their receptors in the third ventricle and adjacent structures to release prostaglandin E2 (PGE2), which modifies the activity of the thermoregulatory centre and changes the body temperature set point (2). Studies of the effect of these cytokines in rabbits have shown that exogenous TNF-alpha promotes non–rapid eye movement (REM) sleep in a dose dependent fashion (3), and this is seen with a number of synthetic TNF fragments. However, it was possible to dissociate the sleep-promoting and febrile responses of this molecule. IL-1 is thought to be important in regulating the amount of NREM sleep; and its effects have been blocked in rabbits when synthetic IL-1 receptor fragments (amino acids 86–95) are injected intracysternally (4). Muramyl peptides are derived from bacterial cell walls and have a specific sleep-promoting properties when administered to animals. Injection of the IL-1 receptor blocks the effects of these agents on sleep (4), suggesting that they also regulate endogenous IL-1 activity. Muramyl peptides can be taken up by primary microglial cells in culture, and these elaborate cytokines and other products, which promote NREM sleep when injected into rabbits (5).

As yet these intriguing observations have not been translated to human disease but are providing a theoretical basis for the sleep-promoting effects of febrile illness, such as occur in respiratory disease in humans.

CYSTIC FIBROSIS

Cystic fibrosis (CF) is an autosomal recessive disorder and is the most common single gene mutation in the Western world (6). A substantial number of individual genetic abnormalities have now been described within the CF gene, the most important being characterized by a failure of the cystic fibrosis transmembrane conductance regulator (CFTR) protein to successfully transport chloride across the apical cell membrane. As a result of this, secondary changes occur in mucus production primarily affecting the respiratory tract and the pancreas and, in the former case, leading to the development of chronic respiratory infection and bronchiectasis. The illness has its onset in childhood. Twenty years ago survivors beyond adolescence were almost unknown. Improved clinical care, early treatment with antibiotics, and pancreatic enzyme supplements now permit a majority of patients to reach early adulthood. Nonetheless, those with fully developed disease will pursue an inexorable downhill course with the development of airflow limitation, persistent bronchial sepsis, and, ultimately, respiratory failure often associated with persistent hypoxemia and cor pulmonale. Concern about the factors that might promote pulmonary hypertension and cor pulmonale led to the earliest observations about the role of sleep-disordered breathing in this disease. It was recognized that pulmonary function testing and the arterial oxygen tension during the day appeared to be poor predictors of the onset of pulmonary hypertension. Moreover, observations that nocturnal desaturation was frequently seen in hypoxemic chronic obstructive pulmonary disease (COPD) and was associated with elevations of pulmonary artery pressure during sleep (7) stimulated investigations of oxygen desaturation in these younger patients. The resulting literature has been focused on observations about this aspect of sleep-related breathing disorders and about the relationship of treatment to nighttime oxygenation.

HYPOXEMIA DURING SLEEP IN CF

The mechanisms producing hypoxemic episodes in CF are not substantially different from those investigated in patients with COPD (see Chapter 22). Episodes of sleep-related oxygen desaturation were identified in some, but not all, patients with CF (8–14) and were more likely in persons with severe disease (8). Despite differences in the end point chosen—minimum nighttime oxygen saturation, time spent below 94% saturated—it is clear that clinical indices of disease severity, symptom scores, and resting pulmonary function are poor predictors of the risk that desaturation will occur. In contrast, resting arterial oxygen tensions were more predictive. Thus, in a study of 14 patients monitored at home, those with a $PaO_2 < 60$ mm Hg were likely to spend greater than 80% of the night's sleep with an SaO_2 of $< 90\%$, whereas this was unlikely if the resting PaO_2 was > 70 mm Hg (12). Studies of transcutaneous CO_2 monitoring ($PtcCO_2$) proved more acceptable than arterial blood gas measurements in these younger frail patients, but their interpretation is limited by the recurrent problems of instrumental drift (11). Nonetheless, small rises in $PtcCO_2$ appear to accompany falls in oxygen saturation at night. These studies are less specific about whether global mean oxygen saturation (SaO_2) during sleep is the most important variable determining pathophysiological change or whether equivalent information is obtained from assessing the lowest SaO_2 reached. Certainly, CF patients with persistent low SaO_2 values were the ones who showed indirect evidence of pulmonary hypertension in one early study (8).

When compared to age-matched controls, CF patients show greater desaturation during REM and NREM sleep (8). Several mechanisms are likely to explain this. First, desaturation is more likely during sleep in those who already show a degree of resting hypoxemia. The physiological fall in minute ventilation that occurs in all adults during the transition from wakefulness to NREM sleep will produce a greater change in SaO_2 in persons close to the steep part of the oxygen dissociation curve (15). This process is well recognized in COPD patients (16) and helps explain the relationship with waking PaO_2 already noted. Second, there is evidence that patients with CF do show relatively greater degrees of nocturnal hypoventilation than normal control subjects. The extent of this is shown in Figure 24.1 Tepper et al. (17) used a calibrated respiratory inductance plethysmograph that has technical limitations but seemed to be associated with more normal sleep and some stage REM, unlike the more direct measurements of Ballard et al. (18) (Fig. 24.1). These changes in breathing pattern were accompanied, by evidence of gas trapping as assessed from helium dilution lung volume

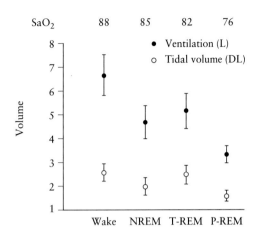

Fig 24.1 *Breathing pattern in six patients with stable CF recorded by calibrated Respitrace during different stages of sleep. T-REM and P-REM refer to tonic and phasic REM sleep identified from the density of the REM on the electro-oculogram (EOG) channel of the polysomnogram. Data are derived from Tepper et al. (17). These data indicate a lower resting and sleeping ventilation than those of Ballard et al. (18), in which no stage REM was recorded and the patients slept in an adapted horizontal body plethysmograph. Changes in breathing pattern from wake to NREM sleep were much smaller in this study, and no changes in directly measured upper or lower airways resistance were seen.*

measurements, reflecting closure of the smaller airways. This reduction in lung volume available for gas exchange is also supported by noninvasive measurements of rib cage and abdominal movement in CF patients when magnetometers have been used, to suggest that functional residual capacity (FRC) falls below the closing capacity of the small airways (14, 19). As a result, there is further ventilation-perfusion mismatching, which will exaggerate the degree of hypoxemia. The effect of sleep on mucociliary clearance in CF has not been studied, but this is likely to be impaired. Localized mucus plugging provides a further factor that will impair ventilation-perfusion matching in this illness and may go some way to explain the poor relationship between daytime pulmonary function testing and nighttime measurements in these patients.

Sleep apnea does not appear to contribute to oxygen desaturations in CF, as a mean of only eight apneic episodes per night were seen in 12 children (7–17 years old) with mild to severe CF who underwent detailed polysomnography (20).

Other attempts at estimating the severity of nocturnal desaturations have proven disappointing. Thus, in a study of 13 hypoxemic and 8 normoxemic patients a relationship was found between the waking oxygen saturation and that during sleep, but oxygen desaturation during exercise was unrelated to the maximum falls in oxygen saturation seen during sleep (10). This is likely to reflect the absence of airway closure during exercise and the relatively greater effects of increased cardiac output in waking exercise compared with the hypoventilation that predominates during sleep-related desaturations. In contrast, other workers studying younger subjects found that the mean lowest nocturnal SaO_2 was correlated with the minimal SaO_2 on exercise, although this relationship was still weaker than that with the waking SaO_2 (13).

THERAPY

To date, there is no conclusive evidence that isolated desaturation during sleep in CF is an independent predictor of survival. Data from patients with Duchenne muscular dystrophy in whom oxygen desaturation also occurs episodically during sleep in advanced disease, have failed to show an independent effect of desaturations on future mortality (21). However, concerns about the clinical significance of these findings have not prevented investigations of a number of possible treatments relevant to the CF patients, principally those designed to reduce nocturnal hypoxemia.

Theophylline

The methylxanthine group of drugs have complex effects in respiratory disease, some of which may be helpful in reducing nocturnal oxygen desaturation. They are weak bronchodilators, may reduce the degree of air trapping associated with severe airflow obstruction (a particular problem in CF—see above), and have desirable effects on respiratory muscle function (22). They are also nonspecific neuroleptics and appear to increase respiratory drive in waking subjects and, hence, minute ventilation. Whether this effect is achieved by enhancing cerebral hypoxia (23) is debatable, but it is clear that sleep quality is impaired in normal persons and in those with asthma when the therapeutic doses of theophylline are maintained (24). Children may be more sensitive to sleep disruption from these drugs, which is seen in a small study of 12 CF

children (age mean 11.8 years), in whom only five achieved therapeutic levels of > 10 mmol/L (20). These children had fewer oxygen desaturations during sleep but poorer sleep quality, tempting the observation that not sleeping is an effective way of preventing sleep-related events. Therapeutically, these drugs have little to offer to the CF patient.

Oxygen Therapy

Increasing the inspired oxygen concentrations is a relatively simple way of improving daytime and nocturnal oxygenation and is effective in increasing survival in hypoxemic COPD (25, 26). In a crossover study 10 adolescent CF patients were given air or 2 L of O_2/min to breathe overnight in a single blind trial (27). Nocturnal hypoxemia was abolished by the O_2, but the usual increase of 5.6 mm Hg in the transcutaneous CO_2 tension during air-breathing sleep rose by a further 5.1 mmHg on the oxygen night. Similar changes in $PtcCO_2$ were seen in chronically hypercapnic CF patients given increasing O_2 flow rates during sleep, although the authors of this study concluded that CO_2 retention with supplementary oxygen during sleep is not a clinically important problem at customary O_2 flow rates (28).

In a carefully conducted randomized control trial of 28 patients with hypoxemic CF studied with a mean follow-up time of 26 months, no difference was found between patients recently O_2 treatment and control subjects (29). Particular care was taken to examine important secondary end points, such as left ventricular function, neuropsychological state, and pulmonary hypertension, none of which showed any differences between the two limbs of the trial. The authors noted that the onset of clinical cor pulmonale cannot be related to any baseline measurement, including the severity of the O_2 desaturation during sleep, and they questioned the role of regular O_2 treatment before an episode of significant fluid retention occurs. Compliance was similar in air and O_2 treated groups, 5.3 and 7.0 hours/night, respectively. The limitations of this study are the relatively small trial size, suggesting the possibility of a type II error, and the restriction of active treatment to the nighttime, at least 15 hours of supplementary oxygen per day being needed to show an effect in the studies of cor pulmonale in COPD. However, if any effect is present from nocturnal O_2 therapy, it is unlikely to be a large one.

Noninvasive Positive Pressure Ventilation (NIPPV)

Nocturnal hypoventilation plays an important part in the genesis of nocturnal oxygen desaturation in CF as impaired lung mechanics secondary to both airflow limitation and localized mucus plugging are significant contributors to patient morbidity. The development of simple pressure-cycled, patient-triggered ventilation using the bilevel technique and administered predominantly overnight has had a significant impact on many illnesses in which nocturnal hypoventilation is a major problem (30). Modification of nasal continuous positive airway pressure (CPAP) equipment has proven suitable for patients to use overnight and has been applied to persons with CF. Low-flow O_2 and NIPPV have been compared in six patients (31). Both produced comparable improvements in overnight O_2 saturation, but NIPPV prevented the hypercapnia seen with O_2 therapy. In an open study of four hypercapnic CF patients unresponsive to other treatments, NIPPV reduced waking CO_2 tensions, increased respiratory muscle strength, and improved sleep quality (32). These hospitalized patients were discharged home on the treatment and remained well 18 months later.

No randomized clinical trial of this approach has yet been conducted, and there is uncertainty over its practicality.

Key points box 24.1

Cystic fibrosis (CF)

- CF is the most common single gene mutation in the Western world.
- Improved patient care has resulted in survival into adulthood.
- Nocturnal hypoxemia is common and due to similar mechanisms as in COPD.
- Awake PaO_2 is superior to other indices of disease severity in predicting a likelihood of nocturnal oxygen desaturation.
- There is no convincing evidence that isolated nocturnal oxygen desaturation affects survival.
- Oxygen therapy corrects nocturnal hypoxaemia, and noninvasive positive pressure ventilation has also been used successfully in severely affected patients.

Nonetheless, the ability to sustain ventilation at night even in an illness like CF, in which bronchiectasis and sputum production might impede its use, has led to the widespread use of nasal ventilation in CF centers. This is confined to those patients reaching the end stage of their illness who are having problems maintaining nocturnal oxygenation or who need additional support while waiting for a suitable transplant donor organ to become available.

INTERSTITIAL LUNG DISEASE

Interstitial lung disease (ILD) is a term given to a number of pulmonary disorders associated with alveolar inflammation or fibrosis (or both) that diffusely affects the lung parenchyma and can progress to involve the peribronchiolar and peribronchial tissues (33). Such diffuse lung injury can be produced by a wide range of causes and although some (such as abnormal reactions to drugs or pulmonary vasculitis) are well recognized, others (such as cryptogenic fibrosing alveolitis) have still to be explained. There is increasing recognition that diffuse lung disease occurs in collagen vascular disorders such as progressive systemic sclerosis and rheumatoid arthritis as well as in response to inorganic dusts such as asbestos. Physiologically, the elastic recoil of the lung is reduced, producing falls in the vital capacity and residual volume and an increase in the FEV_1/VC ratio. However, some persons who smoke and develop these problems have a mixed mechanical and gas exchange defect (34). Normally, resting gas exchange is preserved until the disease becomes advanced, but patients typically show profound falls in arterial oxygenation during exercise, reflecting their inability to maintain alveolar ventilation in these circumstances. The significant increase in elastic inspiratory loading leads to a rapid, shallow breathing pattern, as predicted from acute elastic loading studies in healthy persons.

As noted previously, sleep symptoms are not prominent in these illnesses, although cough during the day and at night is a troublesome symptom. A small number of studies have examined sleep structure oxygenation and breathing pattern in interstitial lung disease, although only one small study has been reported in the last decade (35).

GENERAL CONSIDERATIONS

Sleep quality in patients with ILD is poor compared with controls, with patients spending 34% of total sleep time in stage 1 and only 12% in stage REM, compared to 13.5% and 20%, respectively, in similar age-matched control subjects (36). Similar data have been reported by other investigators (37), although all these studies lack acclimatization days and so it is difficult to know how much effect instrumentation has had upon these results.

Several authors have studied breathing patterns in ILD, which provides a useful model of persistent elastic loading and differs from the complex mixed load seen in chronic obstructive pulmonary disease, in which hypoxemia is more frequent. Early studies by Perez-Padilla et al. (36) found in 11 subjects (9 snorers) that waking respiratory frequency, inspiratory time, and expiratory time were shortened in ILD compared to control subjects while cycle was the same (36). These author found no consistent effect of sleep, unlike Shea et al. (38) (Fig. 24.2). These latter workers studied similar patients with ILD and control subjects and confirmed the differences in waking

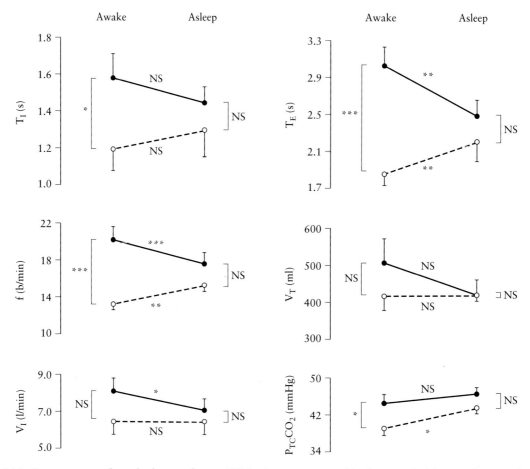

Fig 24.2 *Group means and standard error of mean (SEM) of respiratory variables during wakefulness and stage 4 sleep in normal subjects (open circles) and in patients with ILD (closed circles); 8 subjects per group. T_I = inspiratory time; T_E = expiratory time, f = respiratory frequency; V_T = tidal volume; V_I = ventilation; $P_{tc}CO_2$ = transcutaneous Pco_2. Significant differences in group means, derived from t-tests, between groups within each state and between states within each group are indicated: * = p < 0.05, ** = p < 0.01, *** = p < 0.001, NS = no significant difference (i.e., p > 0.1, except for the fall in V_T from wakefulness to sleep in the normal group were p = 0.09). (From Perez-Padilla R, West P, Lertzman M, et al. Breathing during sleep in patients with interstitial lung disease. Am Rev Respir Dis 1985; 132:224–229.)*

breathing pattern. During sleep, both groups of subjects where given supplementary O_2 to breathe so as to minimize any effect of hypoxic ventilatory stimulation. The authors compared wakefulness to stage 4 sleep, when behavioral influences are believed to be least important. The patients with ILD showed significant falls in ventilation and respiratory frequency (f) in deep NREM sleep compared with wakefulness. This latter change was due to an increased expiratory time (Te), unlike the situation in healthy controls, in whom f increased and ventilation was unchanged. These findings differed from reports on more hypoxemic patients, in whom f was unaffected by sleep (36), whereas these data are similar to the report in another clinical study (37). Although the results of the Shea et al. (38) study might have been due to differences in blood gas tensions or system dead space, the most likely explanation is the reduction in cortical perception of respiratory effort evident in stage IV sleep.

Several studies have looked at the frequency of nocturnal O_2 desaturation in ILD. The first of these was that of Bye et al. (39), who studied 13 ILD patients (mean FVC 66% predicted), all of whom had episodes of oxygen desaturation when asleep. This was marked in two persons, but four of this population snored. Similar falls in SaO_2 during REM sleep were seen by Perez-Padilla et al. (36), who noted that the severity of the desaturation was related to the waking SaO_2. ILD patients spent 44 (15%) of total sleep time with SaO_2 less than 90%. These data suggest that O_2 desaturation might be a frequent finding in ILD, but as with patients with COPD, the severity of REM related desaturation was dictated by waking levels of oxygenation rather than any specific sleep pathology.

McNicholas et al. (37) confirmed the presence of O_2 desaturation in seven ILD patients, but these were noted to be brief, the SaO_2 changes from wake to sleep being from 93% to 91%. This change was highly correlated with waking SaO_2. Unlike other workers, they specifically avoided including anyone with symptoms of sleep apnea. Their findings were supplemented by a series of studies by Midgren et al. (40), who found similar wake-to-sleep changes in mean SaO_2 in 16 ILD patients. They noted brief falls in SaO_2 with the minimum value ranging from 70–92% but considered that these were likely to be clinically unimportant. In a further series of studies, ILD patients were compared with COPD and kyphoscoliotic patients to assess the relative magnitude of the changes in gas exchange during sleep. The ILD and COPD subjects showed similar falls in SaO_2 and elevations in transcutaneous CO_2 while the maximum changes in both variables were seen in those persons with kyphoscoliosis.

Several attempts have been made to relate falls in SaO_2 during sleep in ILD patients to the transient reductions in oxygenation seen during exercise. The latter are likely to be influenced by the type of patients selected, the exercise protocol used, and whether or not treadmill or cycle exercises were employed to test the subject. This is likely to explain the contradictory results reported so far. In the study of Bye et al. (39), oxygen desaturation at night was more dramatic than that seen at the end of exercise. However, Midgren et al. (40) found much larger falls in SaO_2 during exercise in ILD than during sleep (mean exercise desaturation 4.5% versus 0.5% during sleep). Only one study has looked at chemical control of breathing in ILD patients (41); the authors of this study performed polysomnography in 14 patients with ILD and measured their hypercapnic ventilatory responses when awake. They confirmed the dependence of the minimal nocturnal SaO_2 during REM sleep on the waking value, but unlike reports in other illnesses, found an inverse relationship between the minimum SaO_2 and the hypercapnic ventilatory response. These data may reflect the impact of abnormal lung mechanics on ventilatory response to CO_2 rather than any true central failure of respiratory control of function in this disease. As such, persons in whom the ventilatory response to CO_2 did not increase are likely to have the highest respiratory system impedance and will experience most difficulty maintaining ventilation during stage REM, when it is particularly dependent on

---

⌕ Key points box 24.2

Interstitial Lung Disease (ILD)

- Sleep quality is impaired in patients with ILD.
- Ventilation falls in sleep, predominantly due to a reduction in breathing frequency.
- Nocturnal oxygen desaturation is common and of similar magnitude to that seen in patients with COPD.
- Studies that have compared nocturnal oxygen desaturation between sleep and exercise have produced differing results.

diaphragm function. A similar relationship was reported for the occlusion pressure response to CO_2, but this may be due to the correlation between this response and the waking SaO_2 and is likely not to be causally related (Fig. 24.3).

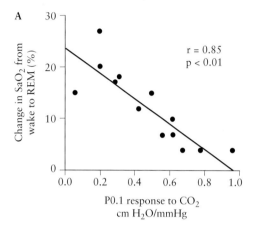

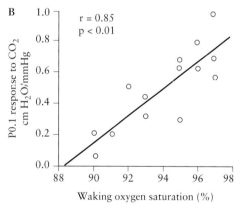

*Fig 24.3 Relationship between mouth occlusion response to CO_2 and the change in O_2 saturation from wakefulness to the minimum in stage REM sleep in patients with interstitial lung disease (redrawn from data in Tatsumi et al. [41]). A indicates that persons with the lowest ventilatory response show the greatest falls in SaO_2 during REM sleep. However, the fall during REM sleep is also related to the waking SaO_2, and when this is plotted against the occlusion pressure response **B** a strong correlation is again seen. Thus, the association between respiratory drive when awake and desaturation during sleep may be an epiphenomenon rather than a causal one.*

CONCLUSIONS

Systematic studies of sleep dysfunction have not been undertaken in many areas of respiratory medicine. It is likely that as simpler tests become available—which will more accurately reflect sleep disruption—the impact of respiratory disease on sleep quality will be shown to be significant. Likewise, febrile illnesses produce transient and reversible modifications of sleep behavior, which are likely to be mediated by cytokines or other chemical messengers. For most patients with lower respiratory tract problems, the altered lung mechanics that characterize their daytime symptoms also dictate their tendency to nocturnal hypoventilation and may well contribute to impaired sleep quality. The correction of hypoxemia alone does not appear to be particularly beneficial in CF before the onset of fluid retention. In ILD nocturnal hypoxemia appears less frequent than might be anticipated from lung mechanical abnormalities measured by day, at least until late in the illness. Much is still to be learned about the importance of sleep in modulating respiratory compensatory responses that function during the day as well as how it contributes to the symptoms of patients with many respiratory illnesses.

REFERENCES

1. Ormerod LP. Respiratory tuberculosis. In: Davies PDO, ed. Clinical tuberculosis. London: Chapman and Hall; 1998:155–174.

2. Dinarello CA, Wolff SM. Pathogenesis of fever and the acute phase responses. In: Maidell GL, Bennett JC, Dolin R, eds. Principles and practise of infectious diseases. New York: Churchill Livingstone; 1995:530–536.

3. Kapas L, Hong L, Cady AB, et al. Somnogenic, pyrogenic and anorectic activities of tumor necrosis factor-alpha and TNF-alpha fragm. Am J Physiol 1992; 263: R708–R715.

4. Takahashi S, Kapas L, Fang J, et al. An interleukin-1 receptor fragment inhibits spontaneous sleep and muramyl dipeptide-induced sleep. Am J Physiol 1996; 271: R101–108.

5. Fincher EF, Johannsen L, Kapas L, et al. Microglia digest *Staphylococcus aureus* into low molecular weight biologically active compounds. Am J Physiol 1996; 271: R149–R156.

6. Rosenstein BJ, Zeitlin PL. Cystic fibrosis. Lancet 1998; 351:277–282.

7. Douglas NJ, Calverley PM, Leggett RJ, et al. Transient hypoxaemia during sleep in chronic bronchitis and emphysema. Lancet 1979; 1:1–4.

8. Francis PW, Muller NL, Gurwitz D, et al. Hemoglobin desaturation: its occurrence during sleep in patients with cystic fibrosis. American Journal of Diseases of Children 1980; 134:734–740.

9. Braggion C, Pradal U, Mastella G. Hemoglobin desaturation during sleep and daytime in patients with cystic fibrosis and severe airway obstruction. Acta Paediatr 1992; 81:1002–1006.

10. Coffey MJ, Fitzgerald MX, McNicholas WT. Comparison of oxygen desaturation during sleep and exercise in patients with cystic fibrosis. Chest 1991; 100:659–662.

11. Pradal U, Braggion C, Mastella G. Transcutaneous blood gas analysis during sleep and exercise in cystic fibrosis. Pediatr Pulmonol 1990; 8:162–167.

12. Montgomery M, Wiebicke W, Bibi H, et al. Home measurement of oxygen saturation during sleep in patients with cystic fibrosis. Pediatr Pulmonol 1989; 7:29–34.

13. Versteegh FG, Bogaard JM, Raatgever JW, et al. Relationship between airway obstruction, desaturation during exercise and nocturnal hypoxaemia in cystic fibrosis patients. Eur Respir J 1990; 3:68–73.

14. Stokes DC, McBride JT, Wall MA, et al. Sleep hypoxemia in young adults with cystic fibrosis. Am J Dis Child 1980; 134:741–743.

15. Connaughton JJ, Catterall JR, Elton RA, et al. Do sleep studies contribute to the management of patients with severe chronic obstructive pulmonary disease? Ame Rev Respir Dis 1988; 138:341–344.

16. Douglas NJ. Sleep in patients with chronic obstructive pulmonary disease. Clin Chest Med 1998; 19:115–125.

17. Tepper RS, Skatrud JB, Dempsey JA. Ventilation and oxygenation changes during sleep in cystic fibrosis. Chest 1983; 84:388–393.

18. Ballard RD, Sutarik JM, Clover CW, et al. Effects of non-REM sleep on ventilation and respiratory mechanics in adults with cystic fibrosis. Am J Respir Crit Care Med 1996; 153:266–271.

19. Muller NL, Francis PW, Gurwitz D, et al. Mechanism of hemoglobin desaturation during rapid-eye-movement sleep in normal subjects and in patients with cystic fibrosis. Am Rev Respir Dis 1980; 121:463–469.

20. Avital A, Sanchez I, Holbrow J, et al. Effect of theophylline on lung function tests, sleep quality, and nighttime SaO$_2$ in children with cystic fibrosis. Am Rev Respir Dis 1991; 144:1245–1249.

21. Phillips MF, Smith PE, Carroll N, et al. Nocturnal oxygenation and prognosis in Duchenne muscular dystrophy. Am J Respir Crit Care Med 1999; 160:198–202.

22. Moxham J. Aminophylline and the respiratory muscles. Clin Chest Med 1988; 9:325–336.

23. Nishimura M, Suzuki A, Yoshioka A, et al. Effect of aminophylline on brain tissue oxygenation in patients with chronic obstructive lung disease. Thorax 1992; 47: 1025–1029.

24. Rhind G, Connaughton JJ, McFie J, et al. Sustained release choline theophyllinate in nocturnal asthma. Br Med J 1985; 1605–1607.

25. Continuous or nocturnal oxygen therapy in hypoxemic chronic obstructive lung disease: a clinical trial. Nocturnal Oxygen Therapy Trial Group. Ann Intern Med 1980; 93:391–398.

26. Long-term domiciliary oxygen therapy in chronic hypoxic cor pulmonale complicating chronic bronchitis and emphysema. Report of the Medical Research Council Working Party. Lancet 1981; 1:681–686.

27. Spier S, Rivlin J, Hughes D, et al. The effect of oxygen on sleep, blood gases, and ventilation in cystic fibrosis. Am Rev Respir Dis 1984; 129:712–718.

28. Hazinski TA, Hansen TN, Simon JA, et al. Effect of oxygen administration during sleep on skin surface oxygen and carbon dioxide tensions in patients with chronic lung disease. Pediatrics 1981; 67:626–630.

29. Zinman R, Corey M, Coates AL, et al. Nocturnal home oxygen in the treatment of hypoxemic cystic fibrosis patients. J Pediatr 1989; 114:368–377.

30. Ellis ER, Bye PTP, Bruderer JW, et al. Treatment of respiratory failure during sleep in patients with neuromuscular disease: positive pressure ventilation through a nose mask. Am Rev Respir Dis 1987; 135:148–152.

31. Gozal D. Nocturnal ventilatory support in patients with cystic fibrosis: comparison with supplemental oxygen. Eur Respir J 1997; 10:1999–2003.

32. Piper AJ, Parker S, Torzillo PJ, et al. Nocturnal nasal IPPV stabilizes patients with cystic fibrosis and hypercapnic respiratory failure. Chest 1992; 102:846–850.

33. British Thoracic Society. The diagnosis, assessment and treatment of diffuse parenchymal lung disease in adults. Thorax 1999; 54 (Suppl 1):S1–S30.

34. Doherty MJ, Pearson MG, O'Grady EA, et al. Cryptogenic fibrosing alveolitis with preserved lung volumes. Thorax 1997; 52:998–1002.

35. Hira HS, Sharma RK. Study of oxygen saturation, breathing pattern and arrythmias in patients of interstitial lung disease during sleep. Indian J Chest Dis 1997; 39:157–162.

36. Perez-Padilla R, West P, Lertzman M, et al. Breathing during sleep in patients with interstitial lung disease. Am Rev Respir Dis 1985; 132:224–229.

37. McNicholas WT, Coffey M, Fitzgerald MX. Ventilation and gas exchange during sleep in patients with interstitial lung disease. Thorax 1986; 41:777–782.

38. Shea SA, Winning AJ, McKenzie E, et al. Does the abnormal pattern of breathing in patients with interstitial lung disease persist in deep, non-rapid eye movement sleep? Am Rev Respir Dis 1989; 139:653–658.

39. Bye PTP, Issa F, Berthon-Jones M, et al. Studies of oxygenation during sleep in patients with interstitial lung disease. Am Rev Respir Dis 1984; 129:27–32.

40. Midgren B, Hansson L, Eriksson L, et al. Oxygen desaturation during sleep and exercise in patients with interstitial lung disease. Thorax 1987; 42:353–356.

41. Tatsumi K, Kimura H, Kunitomo F, et al. Arterial oxygen desaturation during sleep in interstitial pulmonary disease. Correlation with chemical control of breathing during wakefulness. Chest 1989; 95:962–967.

INDEX

Note: Page references in *italics* refer to Figures; those in **bold** refer to Tables